A Clinician's Pearls and Myths in Rheumatology

A Clinician's Pearls and Myths in Rheumatology

John H. Stone

Editor

A Clinician's Pearls and Myths in Rheumatology

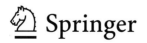 Springer

John H. Stone, M.D., M.P.H.
Director, Clinical Rheumatology
Massachusetts General Hospital
55 Fruit Street / Yawkey 2
Boston, MA. 02114

ISBN: 978-1-84800-933-2   e-ISBN: 978-1-84800-934-9
DOI: 10.1007/978-1-84800-934-9
Springer Dordrecht Heidelberg London New York

Library of Congress Control Number: 2009933269

Springer is part of Springer Science+Business Media (www.springer.com)

Once when I was an intern, an attending rheumatologist bemoaned the number of decisions he had to make when caring for a single complex patient. *Which dose of prednisone? When to taper? Which steroid-sparing agent to add, or whether to add one at all? Was an ACE inhibitor a good idea in a patient with a serum creatinine of 3.5 mg/dL? When to employ Pneumocystis prophylaxis, and when to stop it?* These struck me as highly interesting questions, but as an intern more concerned that my beeper might sound again any moment to signal my next "hit," I took only passing note of the remark and evinced little sympathy for the beleaguered attending. At least he was going to get some sleep that night!

Some years later, having differentiated into a rheumatologist myself, I pursued training in clinical investigation, wrote papers, conducted randomized clinical trials, and developed a stable of complex patients of my own. Only then did I recall the attending's remark with empathy and observe just how few of the clinical decisions I made were based upon rigorous evidence. Indeed, even if the budget at the National Institutes of Health were once again to double within a short period of time and then to double again, the highly nuanced nature of rheumatic disease would yield to "Grade A evidence" on only a minority of important clinical decision points. In our discipline, there will always remain ample room for the keen clinical "*Gestalt*."

This inevitably brings chagrin to advocates of comparative effectiveness studies, among whom I count myself a member. The application of clinical evidence (when available) to major treatment decisions is critical to conscientious and effective patient care. But the dozens of smaller decisions that comprise the craft of medicine are still rooted in a clinician's direct experience; in clinical intuition; in nuggets of wisdom handed down from mentors; and in tips imparted to practitioners by patients themselves. Rheumatology training and practice rely, in short, on the understanding and application of clinical Pearls. Further, becoming a good clinician and an effective teacher also involves the ability to recognize and debunk Myths: those specious concepts and harebrained ideas that cling to the body of medical knowledge like gum to a shoe, despite being fundamentally wrong.

Pearls and Myths are a substantial, ancient, and ever-renewed portion of the medical canon. When Hippocrates sat beneath the shade of his plane tree on the island of Kos and formulated aphorisms, he generated Pearls that continue to influence the fabric of medical practice down to the present day. Rheumatology fellows on the wards today will do well to recall Hippocrates' Pearl that "A woman does not take the gout, unless her menses be stopped". And even great clinicians are not immune to the unwitting propagation of Myths from time to time. No less an authority than Sir William Osler advocated the use of arsenic for the treatment of pernicious anemia.

The discipline of rheumatology is more conducive than most to teaching and learning by Pearls and Myths. Rheumatologists pride themselves on the idea that no subspecialty relies so heavily upon the history and physical examination – the laying on of hands – for rendering diagnoses. Astute rheumatologists can leap broadly to speculations on prognosis after an examination of only a patient's fingers and hands. At the same time, rheumatology rivals any subspecialty for its array of diagnostic tests that appear arcane to outsiders: *What are the clinical implications of a high-titer ANA with a speckled pattern? And the oligodot pattern?*

Pearls and Myths in Rheumatology is a compilation of the wisdom of some of the most experienced clinicians and insightful clinician-scientists whose work touches upon rheumatic disease. No fewer than 126 contributors, experts all, have written the Pearls and Myths for this book:

73 rheumatologists for adults
19 pediatric rheumatologists
2 dermatologists
1 dermatologist/rheumatologist
3 otolaryngologists
4 orthopedists
2 internists
3 pathologists
1 dentist
3 neurologists
1 endocrinologist
2 neuroophthalmologists
1 ophthalmologist
1 ocular immunologist
1 pediatric infectious disease specialist
1 nephrologist
4 pulmonologists
1 clinical immunologist
2 clinical geneticists
1 undifferentiated stem cell (medical student), but an expert nonetheless

Of course, nearly all of these contributors wear more than one hat. They are clinical investigators, educators, epidemiologists, basic scientists, or accomplished practitioners of other disciplines in which they engage when not doing clinical work. They hail from 13 countries: Austria, Belgium, Canada, Denmark, Germany, Great Britain, Greece, Italy, Japan, the Netherlands, Spain, Turkey, and the United States. Together, they have written 48 chapters of Rheumatology Pearls and Myths. Their chapters comprise a total of more than 1,400 such packets of knowledge (836 Pearls and 610 Myths, actually). Their points are driven home by 400 illustrative elements, including 300 clinical photographs.

Finally, a word about the book's dedication. *Pearls & Myths in Rheumatology* is dedicated to my father, Dr. John Stone III (1936–2008). My father served as the Director of Admissions at the Emory University School of Medicine for more than 20 years. He was a cardiologist, poet, teacher – and an extraordinary clinician. Much of what I know about taking a history I learned from hearing him recount the details of patients he had cared for. As a child, I was thrilled by opportunities to accompany him to the hospital or on the occasional home visit. From time to time as a young boy, some of my playmates were his pediatric patients from the institution that Atlanta once called the "Crippled Children's Clinic": children with congenital or acquired heart disease. As an undergraduate pursuing pre-medical studies, I occasionally tagged along on Cardiology Consult Rounds, where I strained my ears to discern the pericardial friction rub of a 22-year-old woman with end-stage renal disease caused by lupus. And as a medical student performing a visiting clerkship at Grady Memorial Hospital and examining a man alleged to have syphilitic aortitis, I endeavored unsuccessfully to distinguish the potential Austin Flint murmur of aortic regurgitation from the rumble of mitral stenosis caused by rheumatic heart disease. *(I still wonder if the underlying cause of the patient's aortic regurgitation was not giant cell arteritis....)*

I regret that my father's superb cardiac auscultation skills, acquired by dint of many years of hard practice, were not bestowed upon me by right of primogeniture, but it is only fitting that *Pearls and Myths in Rheumatology* is devoted to him: in memory of my finest role model and in celebration of the many cases we enjoyed discussing together. How I wish that those discussions could continue, and go on and on.

I hope you will enjoy, learn from, and pass along the Pearls you deem worthy, all in the spirit of "See one, do one, teach one." Moreover, I hope you will see fit to debunk loudly any Myths described herein (some of which have been passed off as "fact" for generations). Remember only that clinical medicine, described by Lewis Thomas as "The Youngest Science," is ever changing. This will bring, in short order, not only a whole new generation of Pearls and Myths, but also the realization that some of today's Pearls are to become tomorrow's Myths. The converse is also true. These are the principal purposes, perhaps, of second editions.

John H. Stone, MD, MPH
Massachusetts General Hospital
Boston, Massachusetts
jhstone@partners.org

References:

Hippocrates. The genuine works of Hippocrates, volumes 1 and 2. Translated and edited by Adams F. New York: Wood; 1886.
Osler W, McCrae T. The Principles and Practice of Medicine. 8th Edition. D. Appleton and Company; 1912.
Thomas L. The Youngest Science: Notes of a medicine-watcher. Viking; 1983.

Contents

Contributors

Rachel Abuav Johns Hopkins University, Department of Dermatology, 600 N. Caroline Street, Baltimore, MD 21287, USA

Yuri Agrawal Johns Hopkins University, Department of Otolaryngology, 600 N. Caroline Street, Baltimore, MD. 21287, USA

Daniel Aletaha Medical University of Vienna, Department of Rheumatology, Waehringer Guertel 18-20, A-1090, Vienna, Austria

Roy D. Altman University of California, Los Angeles, Internal Medicine/Rheumatology, 9854 W. Bald Mountain Court, Agua Dulce, California 91390

Grant J. Anhalt Johns Hopkins University, Department of Dermatology, 600 N. Caroline Street, Baltimore, MD 21287, USA

Pamela Aubert National Institute of Arthritis & Musculoskeletal Disease, National Institutes of Health, 10 Center Drive, Bethesda, Maryland 20892-1828 USA

Ingeborg M. Bajema Department of Pathology, Leiden University Medical Center, Leiden, The Netherlands

Robert P. Baughman University of Cincinnati, Internal Medicine, 1001 Homles, Eden Avenue, Cincinnati, OH 45267, USA

Joseph J. Biundo Tulane University Health Science Center, 4315 Houma Blvd., Ste 303, Metairie, LA 70006, USA

Dimitrios Boumpas University of Crete. Department of Medicine, Greece

Jürgen Braun Ruhr University Bochum, Rheumazentrum Ruhrgebiet, Landgrafenstrasse 15, Herne NRW 44652, Germany

David A. Cabral British Columbia Children's Hospital, Pediatrics, 4480 Oak Street, V6H 3V4 Canada

Leonard H. Calabrese Cleveland Clinic Foundation, Department of Rheumatology & Immunology, 9500 Euclid Avenue, Cleveland, OH 44195 USA

David A. Chad Neurology Department, Massachusetts General Hospital, 165 Cambridge Street, Suite 820, Boston, MA 02114, USA

Hyon K. Choi Department of Medicine, Boston University School of Medicine, 650 Albany Street, Suite 200, Boston, MA 02118, USA

Andrew Churg Department of Pathology, University of British Columbia, 2211 Wesbrook Mall Vancouver, BC, Canada V6T 2B5

William E. St. Clair Medicine Department, Duke University Medical Center, Box 3874 DUMC, Durham, NC 27710, USA

Daniel Clauw Medicine and Psychiatry, Chronic Pain and Fatique Research Center, University of Michigan, 24 Frank Lloyd Wright Dr., Domino Farms, Lobby M. Ann Arbor, MI 48105, USA

Philip J. Clements UCLA Medical School, Box 951670, 1000 Veterans Avenue Rehab Center, Los Angeles, California 90095-1670 USA

Megan E.B. Clowse Medicine, Division of Rheumatology and Immunology, Duke University, Box 3535 Trent Dr., Durham, NC 27710, USA

Shawn E. Cowper Yale Nephrogenic Systemic Fibrosis Registry, Yale University School of Medicine, Yale Dermatopathology Service, 15 York Street, LMP 5031, New Haven, CT 06520-8059, USA

Bruce N. Cronstein NYU Langone Medical Center, Clinical Pharmacology/Rheumatology/ Medicine, 550 First Avenue, NBV16NI, New York, NY 10016, USA

Troy E. Daniels University of California at San Franscisco School of Medicine and Dentistry, Orofacial Sciences Box 0422, 521 Parnassus Avenue, San Francisco, CA. 94143-2206

David P. D'Cruz St. Thomas Hospital, Lupus Research Unit, Rayne Institute, Lambath Palace Road, London SE1 7EH England

Atul Deodhar Oregon Health Sciences University, Division of Rheumatology, Portland, Oregon 97021

Rajiv K. Dixit Medicine Department, University of California, San Francisco, 120 La Casa Via, Suite 204, Walnut Creek, CA 94598, USA

Anne De Paepe Medical Genetics Department, Ghent University Hospital, De Pintelaan 185, 9000Gent, Belgium

N. Lawrence Edwards University of Florida, Division of Rheumatology 100-277, Gainesville, Florida 32610 USA

Brian M. Feldman University of Toronto/SickKids, Rheumatology, 555 University Avenue,Room 8253 Elm Wing, Toronto, Ontario M5G 1X8, Canada

Polly J. Ferguson Department of Pediatrics / Rheumatology, Children's Hospital of Iowa, 200 Hawkins Drive 2534JCP, Iowa City, Iowa 52242

Robert I. Fox Rheumatology Clinic, Scripps Memorial Hospital, 9850 Genesee Avenue, Suite 910, La Jolla, CA 92037, USA
6565 Caminito Sinnecock, La Jolla, CA 92037, USA

George E. Fragoulis National University of Athens Medical School Department of Pathophysiology 75 Mikras Asias Str Athens 115 27 Greece

Howard W. Francis Johns Hopkins University School of Medicine, Otolaryngology – Head and Neck Surgery, 601 N. Caroline Street, JHOC 6251, Baltimore, MD 21287, USA
6008 Lakehurst Dr., Baltimore, MD 21210, USA

Daniel E. Furst UCLA Medical School, Box 951670, 1000 Veterans Avenue Rehab Center, Los Angeles, California 90095-1670 USA

Marco Gattorno University of Genova, Pediatria H, Instituto G. Gaslini, Genova 16147, Italy

Terence Gibson Medicine Department, Guy's and St. Thomas' Hospitals,
60B Copers Cope Road, Beckenham, Kent BR31RJ, UK
Department of Rheumatology, Guy's Hospital, London SE1 9RT, UK

Dafna D. Gladman Toronto Western Hospital 399 Bathurst St. RM1E-4OB Toronto,
Ontario M5T 2S8 Canada

Fiona Goldblatt Royal Adelaide Hospital North Terrace, Adelaide SA 5000, AUSTRALIA

Raphaela Goldback-Mansky National Institute of Arthritis & Musculoskeletal Disease,
National Institutes of Health, 10 Center Drive, Bethesda, Maryland 20892-1828 USA

Don L. Goldenberg Newton-Wellesley Hospital Newton, Massachusetts 02462 USA

Mark Gourley National Institute of Arthritis and Musculoskeletal Diseases,
National Institutes of Health, 10 Center Drive MSC 1616 Bethesda, Maryland 20892-1616

Robert W. Hoffman Chief Division of Rheumatology and Immunology,
University of Miami Miller School of Medicine, Medicine, 1120 N.W. 14th Street,
Suite 968, Miami, FL 33101, USA

Laura K. Hummers Johns Hopkins Scleroderma Center, Johns Hopkins University,
5501 Hopkins Bayview Circle, Baltimore, MD 21224, USA

Robert D. Inman Rheumatology, University of Toronto and Toronto Western Hospital,
399 Bathurst Street, Toronto, Ontario M5T 2S8, Canada

David Isenberg University College of London Center for Rheumatology Research Windeyer
Building Room 331 London W1T 4JF England

Cees G.M. Kallenberg University Medical Groningen Clinical Immunology/Rheumatology
T3 242 Hanzeplein 1 Groningen 9713 GZ The Netherlands

Andrew Keat Northwick Park Hospital, Watford Rd., Harrow HA1 3UJ, England

Karina Keogh Division of Pulmonary and Critical Care Medicine, May Clinic,200 First
Street, SW, Rochester, MN 55905, USA

Munther Khamashta The Lupus Research Unit, The Rayne Institute,
Kings College School of Medicine, Street Thomas' Hospital, London SE1 7EH, UK

Dinesh Khanna UCLA Medical School, Box 951670, 1000 Veterans Avenue Rehab Center,
Los Angeles, California 90095-1670 USA

Nancy E. Lane Medicine, University of California at Davis Medical School,
4800 Second Avenue, Suite 2600, Sacramento, CA 95817, USA

Carol A. Langford Cleveland Clinic Foundation, Department of Rheumatology &
Immunology, 9500 Euclid Avenue, Cleveland, OH 44195 USA

Simmons Lessell Massachusetts Eye & Ear Infirmary, Boston, Massachusetts, USA

Carol B. Lindsley Chief Pediatric Rheumatology, University of Kansas Medical Center,
Pediatrics, 3901 Rainbow, Kansas City, KS 66160, USA

John R. Looney University of Rochester Division of Rheumatology 601 Elmwood Avenue
Rochester, New York 14642 USA

Elyse E. Lower University of Cincinnati, Internal Medicine, 1001 Holmes, Eden Avenue,
Cincinnati, OH 45267, USA

Harvinder S. Luthra Rheumatology Department, Mayo Medical School,
200 First Street SW, Rochester, MN 55905, USA

Mike S. McGrath Sinai Hospital of Baltimore, Center for Join Preservation and
Reconstruction, Rubin for Advanced Orthopedics, 2401 W. Belvedere Avenue, Baltimore,
MD 21215, USA

Alberto Martini University of Genova, Pediatria H, Instituto G. Gaslini, Genova 16147,
Italy

Eric L. Matteson Mayo Clinic, Division of Rheumatology, 200 First Street SW,
Rochester, MN 55095, USA

Maureen D. Mayes University of Texas-Houston Health Science Center/Rheumatology
6431 Fannin MSB 5.270 Houston, Texas 77030, USA

Philip Mease Seattle Rheumatology Associates 1101 Madison Street, Suite 1000 Seattle,
Washington 98104

Thomas Medsger University of Pittsburgh Medicine/Rheumatology 3500 Terrace Street 7S
BST Pittsburgh, Pennsylvania 15261

Fransiska Malfait Medical Genetics Department, Ghent University Hospital,
De Pintelaan 185, 9000Gent, Belgium

Frederick W. Environmental Autoimmunity Group National Institutes of Health / NIEHS
Building 10-2330 9000 Rockville Pike MSC 1301Bethesda, Maryland 20892-1301

Elinor Mody Brigham & Women's Hospital Division of Rheumatology Boston,
Massachusetts 02115

Eamonn S. Molloy Cleveland Clinic, Rheumatic and Immunologic Diseases,
Desk A50, 9500 Euclid Avenue, Cleveland, OH 44195, USA

Michael A. Mont Sinai Hospital of Baltimore, Center for Join Preservation and
Reconstruction, Rubin for Advanced Orthopedics, 2401 W. Belvedere Avenue,
Baltimore, MD 21215, USA

Sarah L. Morgan Division of Clinical Nutrition Department of Nutrition Sciences1714 9th
Ave S # Lrc354 Birmingham, AL 35205-3606

Haralampos M. Moutsopoulos National University of Athens Medical School Department
of Pathophysiology 75 Mikras Asias Str Athens 115 27 Greece

Chester V. Oddis University of Pittsburgh Medicine/Rheumatology 3500 Terrace Street 7S
BST Pittsburgh, Pennsylvania 15261

James R. University of Nebraska Medical Center Department of Internal Medicine Omaha,
Nebraska 68198-3025 USA

Shoichi Ozaki St. Marianna University School of Medicine Department of Internal
Medicine 2-16-1 Sugao Miyamae-ku Kawasaki 216-8511 Japan

Seza Ozen Department of Pediatric Nephrology and Rheumatology, Hacettepe University
Faculty of Medicine, Sihhiye 06100 Ankara, Turkey

Lauren M. Pachman Department of Pediatrics, Division of Rheumatology,
Children's Memorial Research Center, Children's Memorial Hospital, Northwestern
University, Feinberg School of Medicine, 2340 N. Halsted Street, Box 212, Chicago,
IL 60614-4314, USA

George N. Papaliodis Massachusetts Eye & Ear Infirmary Ocular Immunology Clinic
Boston, Massachusetts 02114

Mark A. Perazella Yale University Medical Center Division of Nephrology New Haven, Connecticut USA

Michelle Petri Medicine, Johns Hopkins University School of Medicine, 1830 East Monument Street, Suite 7500, Baltimore, MD 21205, USA

Clarissa A. Pilkington Great Ormond Street Rheumatology Department University College London London England

Michael H. Pillinger NYU Medical Center, Rheumatology/Medicine, 550 First Avenue, New York, NY 10016, USA

Nicolo Pipitone Arcispedale S Maria Nuova Viale Risorgimento 80 42100 Reggio Emilia Italy

Misha Pless Massachusetts General Hospital Department of Neurology55 Fruit StreetBoston, Massachusetts 02114

Paul H. Plotz Arthritis and Rheumatism Branch, National Institute of Arthritis and Musculoskeletal and Skin Diseases, National Institutes of Health, 9000 Rockville Pike, Bethesda, MD 20892, USA

Janet E. Pope St. Joseph Health Care London 268 Grosvenor St. London, Ontario N6A 4V2 Canada

Manuel Ramos-Casals Servei de Malalties Autoimmunes, Hospital Clínic, C/Villarroel, 170, 08036-Barcelona, Spain

Rosalind Ramsey-Goldman Northwestern University Division of Rheumatology FSM-300 240 E. Huron Street Chicago, Illinois 60611 USA

Niels Rasmussen Rigshospitalet, Otolaryngology – Head and Neck Surgery, Blegdamsvej 9, Copenhagen 2100, Denmark

Ann M. Reed Mayo Clinic 200 First Street SW Rochester, Minnesota 55905 USA

Lisa G. Rider Environmental Autoimmunity Group National Institutes of Health / NIEHS Building 10-2352 9000 Rockville Pike MSC 1301 Bethesda, Maryland 20892-1301

Christopher Ritchlin Rheumatology Department, University of Rochester, 601 Elmwood Avenue, Box 695, Rochester, NY 14642, USA 4459 Middle Cheshire Road, Canandaigua, NY 14424, USA

Neal W. Roberts Medical College of Virginia Department of Internal Medicine 11th & Marshall - Box 9890647 Richmond, VA. 23298-0001

James T. Rosenbaum Department of Ophthalmology, Division of Arthritis and Rheumatic Diseases, Oregon Health and Science University, Casey Eye Institute, 2275 SW Terwilliger Blvd, Portland, OR 97239, USA

Ann K. Rosenthal Medical College of Wisconsin Division of Rheumatology 9200 W. Wisconsin Avenue Milwaukee, Wisconsin 53226

Anne H. Rowley Department of Microbiology/Immunology Ward 12-140, Pediatrics W-140, Northwestern University Medical School, Chicago, IL 60611-3008, USA

Kenneth G. Saag Department of Medicine, Division of Clinical Immunology and Rheumatology, University of Alabama at Birmingham, 510 Twentieth Street, South, Suite 820, Birmingham, AL 35233, USA FOT 820, 1530 Third Avenue, South Birmingham, AL 35294-3408, USA

George H. Sack Johns Hopkins University School of Medicine, Medicine and Biological Chemistry, 725 N. Wolfe Street, Physiology G15, Baltimore, MD 21205, USA

Carlo Salvarani Arcispedale S Maria NuovaViale Risorgimento 80 42100 Reggio Emilia Italy

Frank T. Saulsbury University of Virginia Medical Center Department of Pediatrics P.O. Box 800386 Charlottesville, Virginia 22908 USA

Joseph H. Schwab Massachusetts General Hospital Department of Orthopedics 55 Fruit Street Boston, Massachusetts 02114

James Seibold University of Michigan Medical Center Division of Rheumatology Ann Arbor, Michigan USA

Margaret Seton Rheumatology, Allergy and Immunology, Harvard Medical School, Massachusetts General Hospital, 55 Fruit Street, Boston, MA 02114, USA

Peter Siao Neurology Department, Massachusetts General Hospital,165 Cambridge Street, Suite 820, Boston, MA 02114, USA

Earl D. Silverman Pediatrics, Division of Rheumatology, Hospital for Sick Children, University of Toronto, 555 University Avenue, Toronto, Ontario M5G 1X8, Canada

Aneesh B. Singhal Neurology, MGH Stroke Research Center, Harvard Medical School, Massachusetts General Hospital, 175 Cambridge Street, Suite 300, Boston, MA 02114, USA

Fotini N. Skopouli National University of Athens Medical School Department of Pathophysiology 75 Mikras Asias Str Athens 115 27 Greece

Josef S. Smolen Medical University of Vienna, Department of Rheumatology, Waehringer Guertel 18-20, A-1090, Vienna, Austria

Ulrich Specks Division of Pulmonary and Critical Care Medicine, May Clinic, 200 First Street, SW, Rochester, MN 55905, USA

Virginia Steen Georgetown University Medical Center Department of Rheumatology 3800 Reservoir Road Washington, D.C. 20007 USA

John H. Stone Massachusetts General Hospital, 55 Fruit Street / Yawkey 2, Rheumatology Clinic, Boston, Massachusetts, 02114

James R. Stone Massachusetts General Hospital Department of Pathology 55 Fruit Street Boston, Massachusetts 02114

Robert P. Sundel Children's Hospital, Harvard Medical School, 300 Longwood Avenue, Boston, MA 02115, USA

Ira N. Targoff Oklahoma Medical Research Foundation Arthritis & Immunology 825 NE 13th Street Oklahoma City, Oklahoma 73104 USA

Robert A. Terkeltaub VA Division of Rheumatology, VA Healthcare San Diego, University of California, San Diego, 3350 La Jolla Village Drive 111k, San Diego, CA 92161, USA

Shirley M.L. Tse University of Toronto/SickKids, Rheumatology, 555 University Avenue, Room 8253 Elm Wing, Toronto, Ontario M5G 1X8, Canada

Dimitrios Vassilopoulos Athens University School of Medicine, Hippokration General Hospital, 2nd Department of Medicine, 114 Vass. Sophias Avenue, 115 27 Athens, Greece

Amy H. Warriner Division of Endocrinology & Metabolism 2000 6th Ave S # 4Birmingham, AL 35233-2110

Michael H. Weisman Division of Rheumatology, Cedars Sinai Medical Center, 8700 Beverly Blvd., Room B131, Los Angeles, CA 90201, USA

Victoria P. Werth University of Pennsylvania Dermatology 3600 Spruce Street / Rhoads Pavilion Philadelphia, Pennsylvania 19104 USA

John P. Whitcher University of Californa-San Francisco Department of Ophthalmology San Francisco, California

Patience H. White Arthritis Foundation Department of Public Health 2011 Pennsylvania Avenue, Suite 610 Washington, D.C. 20006 USA

Patricia Woo Centre for Paediatric and Adolescent Rheumatology, University College London, London England

Yusuf Yazici New York University Hospital for Joint Diseases Division of Rheumatology 246 East 20th Street New York, New York 10003 USA

Hasan Yazici University of Istanbul/Cerrahpasa Medical Faculty, Division of Rheumatology, Department of Medicine, Askaray, Istanbul 34098, Turkey Safa sok. 17/7, Kadikoy, Istanbul 34170, Turkey

David Tak Yan Yu UCLA Medical School, Box 951670, 1000 Veterans Avenue Rehab Center, Los Angeles, California 90095-1670 USA

Michael G. Zywiel Sinai Hospital of Baltimore, Center for Join Preservation and Reconstruction, Rubin for Advanced Orthopedics, 2401 W. Belvedere Avenue, Baltimore, MD 21215, USA

Rheumatoid Arthritis

1

James R. O'Dell, Josef S. Smolen, Daniel Aletaha, Dwight R. Robinson, and E. William St. Clair

1.1 Overview of Rheumatoid Arthritis

> Rheumatoid arthritis (RA) affects all ethnic groups. Women are nearly three times more likely than men to develop the disease.

> The pattern of arthritis typically favors distal and symmetrical involvement.

> The most commonly involved joints are the wrists, metacarpophalangeal, proximal interphalangeal, and metatarsophalangeal joints. However, many other joints can also be involved. Shoulder, elbow, hip, knee, or neck disease (particularly at the atlanto-axial joint, C1–C2) are frequently observed.

> Most presentations are subacute in nature, with the insidious onset of fatigue, morning stiffness, and arthritis. More explosive onsets of disease are also described.

> If untreated, RA is a chronic, progressive disorder that leads to joint damage, disability, and early mortality.

> A variety of extraarticular features are typical of "seropositive" RA (RA associated with the presence of rheumatoid factor in the serum). These include rheumatoid nodules, secondary Sjögren's syndrome, interstitial lung disease, scleritis, and rheumatoid vasculitis.

> Approximately 70% of patients with RA are rheumatoid factor positive. An approximately equal percentage has antibodies directed against cyclic citrullinated peptides (i.e., anti-CCP antibodies). There is substantial but not complete overlap between groups of patients who are rheumatoid factor positive and those who have anti-CCP antibodies.

> Some patients have RA that appears in every way to be typical disease yet do not have either rheumatoid factor or anti-CCP antibodies. These patients are said to have "seronegative RA."

> Radiographic studies in RA reveal joint space narrowing, erosions, deformities, and periarticular osteopenia.

> Treatment approaches now emphasize early interventions designed to suppress joint inflammation entirely as soon as possible after the onset of clinical disease.

1.1.1 Diagnosis

Myth: A patient must fulfill at least four of the seven American Rheumatism Association (now called the American College of Rheumatology; ACR) classification criteria to be diagnosed as having rheumatoid arthritis (RA).

Reality: Diagnostic criteria do not exist for RA. The ACR classification criteria developed in 1987 were not intended for the purpose of diagnosing individual patients, but rather for defining patient populations that are comparable across different clinical studies (Table 1.1) (Arnett 1988).

In addition, the RA classification criteria were developed in patients with *established* RA, not in patients with early inflammatory arthritis. Thus, they have limited applicability for classifying patients with early disease, who may lack several of the relevant criteria (e.g., erosions or rheumatoid nodules) (Aletaha et al. 2005b). Among patients with early RA, many do not fulfill at least four of the seven ACR criteria. Conversely, many patients with early arthritis have diagnoses other than RA yet do fulfill the criteria, at least temporarily (Harrison et al. 1998; Machold 2006). The gold standard for the diagnosis of RA continues to be the clinical pronouncement by a rheumatologist.

1.1.2 Clinical Features

Myth: Rheumatoid arthritis patients rarely get gout.

Reality: Adequate data on this association are lacking, but this myth is almost certainly an artifact of mid-twentieth century RA treatment regimens. High-dose aspirin, a uricosuric agent, was used in majority of RA patients in that era. With the development of more effective treatment regimens for RA that do not involve high-dose aspirin, it is not rare to see the two diseases in the same patient.

Myth: RA burns out with time in many patients.

Reality: Some clinicians refer to "burned out" RA. Patients to whom this monicker is applied generally have long-standing

Table 1.1 1987 Revised ARA criteria for the classification of rheumatoid arthritis

For classification purposes, a patient is said to have RA if he or she has satisfied at least four of the following seven criteria. Criteria 1–4 must have been present for at least 6 weeks. Patients with two clinical diagnoses are not excluded. Designation as classic, definite, or probable RA is not to be made

1. Morning stiffness

   Morning stiffness in and around the joints, lasting at least 1 h before maximal improvement

2. Arthritis of three or more joint areas

   At least 3 joint areas simultaneously have had soft tissue swelling or fluid (not bony overgrowth alone) observed by a physician; the 14 possible joint areas are right or left proximal interphalangeal (PIP) joints, metacarpophalangeal (MCP) joints, wrist, elbow, knee, ankle, and metatarsophalangeal (MPT) joints

3. Arthritis of hand joints

   At least 1 area swollen (as defined above) in a wrist, MCP or PIP joint

4. Symmetric arthritis

   Simultaneous involvement of the same joint areas (see 2 above) on both sides of the body (bilateral involvement of PIPs, MCPs, or MTPs is acceptable without absolute symmetry)

5. Rheumatoid nodules

   Subcutaneous nodules, over bony prominences, or extensor surfaces, or in juxta-articular regions, observed by a physician

6. Serum rheumatoid factor

   Demonstration of abnormal amounts of serum rheumatoid factor by any method for which the result has been positive in <5% of normal control subjects

7. Radiographic changes

   Radiographic changes typical of RA on posteroanterior hand and wrist radiographs, which must include erosions or unequivocal bony decalcification localized to or most marked adjacent to the involved joints (osteoarthritis changes alone do not qualify)

disease, severe joint damage, and little evidence of synovitis. Most are on minimal therapy for RA, albeit some have tried multiple agents in the past.

Most patients with "burned out" RA have at least moderately elevated acute phase reactants. More importantly, they often continue to deteriorate radiographically, despite having symptoms that are minimal when compared with patients with early disease. If patients with "burned out" RA are treated, their symptoms improve. Thus, the label of "burned out" applies only on rare occasions. Strong consideration should be given to treating patients who fit the operative definition of this condition with DMARDs.

Myth: Clinically detectable synovitis and radiographic progression in RA are linked tightly, such that the control of one leads to control of the other.

Reality: This impression is a classic example of dogma that was believed widely for decades, but which is now recognized as false. Several trials have shown that excellent control of clinical features of disease activity may be achieved in the face of continued radiographic deterioration. The converse is also true;

i.e., patients who show no radiologic evidence of damage can have flagrant clinical signs of ongoing synovitis. As an example, clinical trials of denosumab (an antiRANK-ligand monoclonal antibody) have demonstrated that this medication halts radiographic progression but exerts comparatively little effect on clinical measures of disease activity (Cohen et al. 2008).

Myth: Rheumatoid nodules are an important finding in early RA.

Reality: Rheumatoid nodules are one of the seven ACR criteria for established RA. However, rheumatoid nodules are usually not present within the first few months of the onset of synovitis. Thus, their absence at presentation does not reliably exclude the diagnosis of RA.

Pearl: Troublesome rheumatoid nodules can be injected with glucocorticocoids.

Comment: Nodules that are painful or interfere with function require an intervention. Direct injection of the nodule with a mixture of local anesthetic and glucocorticoids may be beneficial. Surgical excision is necessary for some nodules.

Glucocorticoid injections of nodules are often effective in decreasing the size of these lesions. This Pearl was illustrated in a study of 24 nodules in 11 patients with RA (Ching 1992). Each injection was assigned randomly to be performed with glucocorticoids or with placebo. Among the nodules injected with glucocorticoids, 9 of 12 shrank by more than 50%, compared with only 1 of 12 injected with placebo.

The procedure for injecting rheumatoid nodules is as follows. Up to 0.3 mL of methylprednisolone or triamcinolone hexacetonide 40 mg/mL is mixed in 1:1 ratio with 1% lidocaine. Following local anesthesia of the overlying skin, the needle is inserted directly into the center of the nodule. The medication is injected slowly as the needle is withdrawn. Considerable force on the plunger of the syringe is needed in some cases to express the mixture into the nodule.

Myth: Rheumatoid nodules occur in the heart and cause conduction defects.

Reality: Although mentioned in most textbooks as an extra-articular complication of RA, there is only one case reported in the world's literature (Thery 1974). Don't expect to see this vanishingly rare complication in a clinic near you any time soon.

Pearl: Rheumatoid pleural effusions can mimic empyemas.

Comment: RA is one of the few causes of a low pH in pleural effusions. Two other major ones are empyema and esophageal rupture. Pleural effusions in RA are exudates, characterized by high protein and lactate dehydrogenase levels and very low glucose. White blood cell counts are frequently elevated in RA effusions. In contrast to empyemas, lymphocytes tend to predominate over neutrophils unless the fluid collection is tapped early (Avnon et al. 2007).

Pearl: Amyloidosis and possibly rheumatoid vasculitis pose less of a threat than they did before the availability of effective therapy.

Comment: Two potentially lethal complications of RA are the development of secondary amyloidosis and the occurrence of rheumatoid vasculitis. Secondary amyloidosis caused by uncontrolled RA is now rarely seen in countries where modern therapies are available. Even before the age of biologic therapies for RA, the adoption of methotrexate as the standard of care in the 1980s had led to improvements in disease control and patient survival (Choi 2002).

Most RA experts believe that cases of rheumatoid vasculitis are also now less common than in the past. However, as described in the chapter on rheumatoid vasculitis, the epidemiologic data on this issue are mixed (see Chapter 2, Rheumatoid Vasculitis).

1.1.3 Rheumatoid Arthritis Mimickers

Myth: Gout and RA are always easily differentiated from each other.

Reality: Acute gout usually involves the joints of the lower extremities and is episodic. In addition, it tends to involve one joint or only a few (i.e., it is oligoarticular). These features contrast clearly with typical RA. However, chronic tophaceous gout can cause persistent inflammatory disease of multiple joints of both upper and lower extremities, a condition that mimics RA more closely. Tophi, which occur typically over bony prominences, can be mistaken for rheumatoid nodules. More than one seasoned clinician has been fooled by gout and mistaken this disorder for RA (Doherty and Dieppe 1986; De Souza 2005).

Myth: Symmetrical polyarthritis at presentation is the rule for RA.

Reality: Classic RA involves the joints in a symmetrical manner, affecting the joint areas on both sides of the body in a relatively equal manner. However, in early disease, symmetry is often not apparent (Rantapaa-Dahlqvist 2005; Masi 1983). Approximately one-third of patients with RA have single joint disease as the initial manifestation.

Conversely, symmetrical swelling and deformity of peripheral joints including the metacarpophalangeal joints are not always due to RA. As an example, Jaccoud's arthropathy is seen in patients with rheumatic fever and SLE. Jaccoud's arthropathy is characterized by swelling, ulnar deviation, and volar subluxation of the MCP joints. Such changes may mimic RA closely. The deformity in SLE results from ligamentous laxity rather than the destructive synovial pannus of RA.

Jaccoud's arthropathy can be differentiated from RA radiographically. Bone erosions are absent in Jaccoud's, even in patients with longstanding disease and severe joint deformities (Fernandez et al. 2006). In one study, MRI revealed images described as bony erosions, but these lesions were not shown to progress to bone loss (Ostendorf et al. 2003). When patients with SLE do develop bony erosions, their disorder is often termed "rhupus" (Van Vugt et al. 1998). Such patients have serological features of both RA and SLE (Chan 2008).

Pearl: Calcium pyrophosphate dihydrate (CPPD) arthropathy can mimic rheumatoid arthritis.

Comment: CPPD arthropathy often presents as pseudogout, usually in a monoarticular pattern and most commonly in the knee. However, chronic polyarticular disease can also occur, with variable degrees of synovitis. The radiographic and clinical examination may be similar to osteoarthritis, but polyarticular CPPD disease involves joints that are not typically affected in osteoarthritis, such as the wrist, shoulder, and metacarpophalangeal joints (Fig. 1.1). Involvement of these joints is much more typical of RA.

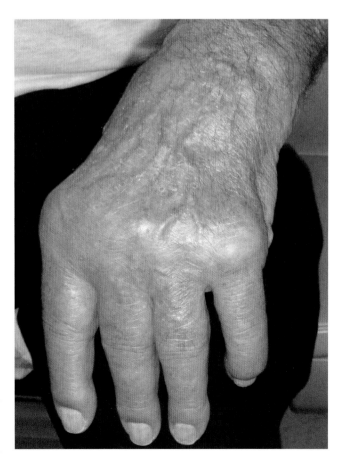

Fig. 1.1 Involvement of the wrist and metacarpophalangeal joints in a patient with calcium pyrophosphate dehydrate (CPPD) deposition disease

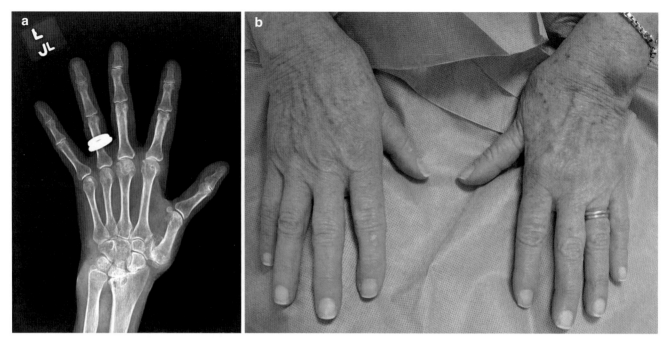

Fig. 1.2 (**a**) Articular cartilage loss and subchondral cysts are common in CPPD deposition disease. (**b**) This patient also had pronounced swelling the ulnar styloid region, a finding common to rheumatoid arthritis. Knee radiographs showed CPPD deposition within cartilage (Courtesy of Dr Greg Emkey)

Articular cartilage loss and subchondral cysts are common in CPPD deposition disease (Fig. 1.2), but the marginal erosions of RA are not found. The finding of CPPD deposition disease in a young patient raises the spectre of hemochromatosis (Axford 1991).

Pearl: Parvovirus infection can mimic RA precisely, even down to the presence of autoantibodies.

Comment: Before starting methotrexate for an acute, symmetrical polyarthritis affecting small joints of the hands, wrists, and feet, one is strongly advised to check serologies for parvovirus B. Parvovirus B infection has the uncanny ability to pose as RA. Acute infections with this virus tend to cause the classic "slapped cheek" skin rash ("fifth disease" Young and Brown 2004) in children. Fifth disease is not associated with significant joint manifestations in the majority of pediatric patients. However, the opposite is true in adults, in whom cutaneous features are unusual but the arthropathy is paramount (Young and Brown 2004).

Parvovirus infection not only causes an arthropathy compatible with RA in adults, it can also be associated with a host of autoantibodies (e.g., rheumatoid factor) that provide further misleading evidence of RA or another connective tissue disease such as lupus (Lunardi et al. 2008). In this setting, however, a positive IgM assay for antibodies to parvovirus leads to the correct diagnosis. Fortunately, the great majority of symptomatic parvovirus infections subside within 2 months. Virtually, all patients' joint symptoms have subsided by 6–12 months.

Pearl: Not all destructive polyarthritis is rheumatoid or psoriatic arthritis.

Comment: Erosive osteoarthritis is a subset of osteoarthritis characterized by destructive disease of the proximal and distal interphalangeal joints. The joints develop osteophytes, often accompanied by inflammatory pain and swelling. There are histologic changes of inflammation in the synovium (Bellhorn and Hess 1993).

The distal interphalangeal joint involvement characteristic of erosive osteoarthritis can cause particular confusion with psoriatic arthritis. Bony erosions are evident characteristically in the center of the joints on plain radiographs (Fig. 1.3). This is accompanied by sclerosis of the remaining subchondral bone, giving a gull-winged appearance typical of osteoarthritis. This appearance differs from the marginal erosions that occur in rheumatoid arthritis (Fig. 1.4). Loss of motion and fusion of interphalangeal joints can occur in erosive osteoarthritis, but metacarpophalangeal joint involvement is uncommon.

Acute phase reactants, rheumatoid factor, and anti-CCP antibody assays are typically normal in erosive osteoarthritis, further helping to differentiate this entity from RA and psoriatic arthritis (Morozzi et al. 2005). Finally, the symptoms of EO fail to respond to immunomodulatory agents such as methotrexate.

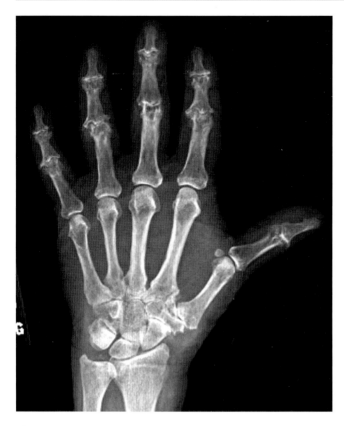

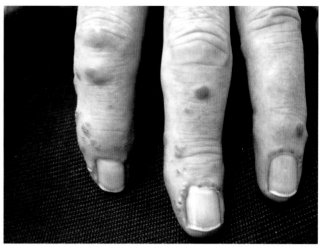

Fig. 1.5 Multicentric reticulohistiocytosis is usually accompanied by erythematous, nodular swelling of the skin that has been referred to as a "coral beads" (Courtesy of Dr Jeffrey Callen)

There appears to be a strong heritable component to erosive osteoarthritis, with expression of the trait particularly common in women in successive generations within families. The same is true for "conventional" osteoarthritis of the hands.

Pearl: For a real zebra, consider the possibility of multicentric reticulohistiocytosis in a case of aggressive, polyarticular joint disease.

Comment: Reticulohistiocytosis causes a symmetrical polyarthritis that focuses on the small joints of the hands and therefore often resembles aggressive RA (Kalajian and Callen 2008). A distinctive histiocytic infiltration of the synovium that is associated with multinucleated giant cells leads to destruction of the joints and juxta-articular bone. Multicentric reticulohistiocytosis is usually accompanied by erythematous, nodular swelling of the skin that has been referred to as a "coral beads" (Fig. 1.5).

Multicentric reticulohistiocytosis is often accompanied by an underlying malignancy. The disease is usually refractory to conventional anti-inflammatory medications, but sporadic reports describe responses to antiTNF agents.

Fig. 1.3 Erosive osteoarthritis. Bony erosions are evident characteristically in the center of the joints, rather than at the margins. Note the sparing of the MCP joints, typical of osteoarthritis, but the involvement of the distal and proximal interphalangeal joints and the degenerative changes at the base of the thumb

1.1.4 Serological Features and Radiology

Pearl: High titers of rheumatoid factor (RF) are of diagnostic and prognostic value.

Comment: RA is characterized by the presence of autoantibodies, among which RF was the first described. The finding of a serum RF is relatively non-specific in the sense that it may be associated with a variety of other conditions that can cause an

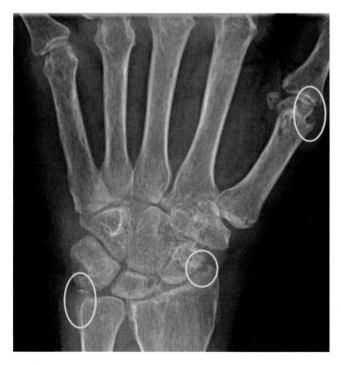

Fig. 1.4 Marginal joint erosions characteristic of rheumatoid arthritis

inflammatory arthritis, particularly connective tissue diseases and chronic hepatitis. In addition, up to 15% of the healthy elderly population have RF, albeit usually in low titers.

Several studies have shown that a high cut-off point for a positive assay (e.g., 50 IU/mL) enhances the positive predictive value of RF for RA (Nell et al. 2005; Sinclair and Hull 2003). One meta-analysis of 50 studies that evaluated the operating characteristics of RF pegged the sensitivity of this test at 69% and its specificity at 85% (Nishimura et al. 2007). High titers of RF are a marker for patients at risk for aggressive, destructive joint disease and extra-articular complications of RA, such as interstitial lung disease and rheumatoid vasculitis.

Assays for anti-CCP antibodies have a sensitivity that rivals that of RF, but a higher specificity (Schellekens et al. 2000; Nell et al. 2005). The sensitivity and specificity of anti-CCP antibodies in the meta-analysis mentioned above were 67% and 95%, respectively (Nishimura et al. 2007). Moreover, anti-CCP antibodies also have prognostic value. They identify a subset of patients more likely to suffer erosive disease and also indicate a greater likelihood of a treatment response to methotrexate or tumor necrosis factor inhibitors (Kroot et al. 2000). Some data indicate that anti-CCP antibodies predict erosive disease even more accurately than do high titers of RF. However, most patients with anti-CCP antibodies are also RF positive, and vice versa. Only a small percentage of patients have one of these antibodies but not the other.

Pearl: In patients with early polyarthritis, anti-CCP antibody positivity is an excellent predictor of an RA diagnosis.

Comment: A study from the Netherlands demonstrated convincingly that in patients with early undifferentiated arthritis who are anti-CCP antibody positive, at least 93% have definite diagnoses of RA 3 years later (or earlier). Among the patients who were anti-CCP antibody negative, only 25% had developed RA by 3 years (van Gaalen et al. 2004).

1.1.5 Risk Factors

Pearl: Cigarette smoking is bad if one is otherwise genetically predisposed to the development of RA.

Comment: This warning is in addition, of course, to the other reasons that cigarette smoking is bad Several studies show a significant and independent association between cigarette smoking and increased susceptibility to RA (Silman et al. 1996). This environmental exposure interacts in RA with the HLA-DRB1 shared epitope to increase susceptibility to RA (Padyukov et al. 2004). Smoking is also associated with the presence of extraarticular manifestations and serum rheumatoid factor (Turesson et al. 2003; Saag et al. 1997; Mattey

et al. 2002). Whether smoking independently worsens established disease remains controversial, as retrospective case-control studies have shown divergent results on radiographic progression (Finckh et al. 2007).

Cigarette smoking also has been associated with an increased risk of anti-CCP antibody-positive RA among individuals who have the HLA-DRB1 shared epitope alleles (Klareskog et al. 2006). These results suggest a model in which smoking triggers anti-CCP antibodies in patients with RA and the shared epitope. However, other studies have failed to confirm the links among smoking, the shared epitope, and anti-CCP antibodies (Lee et al. 2007; Mikuls et al. 2008).

1.1.6 Disease Assessment

Pearl: A simple clinical index that does not depend on laboratory data allows outcome measures to be employed prospectively in the clinic.

Comment: Prospective data indicate that the adjustment of RA therapies every 8–12 weeks with the goal of controlling specific indices of disease activity leads to improved patient outcomes (Grigor et al. 2004; Verstappen et al. 2007; Goekoop-Ruiterman et al. 2005; Smolen et al. 2003a). Thus, the assessment of disease activity is important in both clinical trials and clinical practice.

Composite disease activity indices are superior to individual variables in the assessment of disease activity. Two major factors pose potential barriers to the routine use of validated disease activity indices in clinical practice. First, many validated scores are so complex that they require a calculator for computation. Second, some composite indices require the results of laboratory tests (e.g., an ESR or C-reactive protein level) before they can be completed. Both of these issues dramatically reduce the utility of such scores.

The Clinical Disease Activity Index (CDAI) is a simple numerical index that is calculated by summing the number of tender and swollen joints using the 28-joint count and the patient and physician global assessments on a 10-cm visual analog scale (Fig. 1.6). The CDAI has proven to be a valid, reliable, and sensitive measure to change as reflected by ACR responses, the DAS28, and the Simplified Disease Activity Index, all of which rely on laboratory tests (Smolen et al. 2003b).

The CDAI ranges from 0 to 76. The cutpoints for remission and various degrees of activity are as follows:

- Remission ≤ 2.8
- Low disease activity ≤ 10
- Moderate disease activity ≤ 22
- High disease activity > 22

The CDAI provides the most stringent remission criteria available and correlates with outcomes such as the Health

Complete Disease Activity Index (CDAI)

Swollen joint count

+

Tender joint count

CDAI = +

Patient global assessment

+

Evaluator global assessment

Fig. 1.6 The Complete Disease Activity Index (CDAI). The CDAI is composed of the count of swollen joints (SJC), the number of tender joints (TJC), the patient global assessment (PGA), and the evaluator global assessment (EGA)

Assessment Questionnaire (HAQ) and radiographic progression (Aletaha et al. 2005b; Mierau et al. 2007; Smolen et al. 2003b, 2009a). Treatment modifications should be considered every 3 months if patients do not reach a CDAI ≤ 10 (Aletaha et al. 2007).

Myth: Assessing joint counts and composite indices is too time-consuming to be practical in routine clinical care.

Reality: The 28-joint count is valid, reliable, and correlates well with the total joint count. More importantly, the 28-joint count requires only a minute or two for a trained person to calculate. The clinician's 28-joint count is combined with the physician's disease assessment and the patient global assessment to form the CDAI.

1.1.7 Treatment

The Treatment section is divided into three subsections:

- Treatment strategy
- Glucocorticoids, Methotrexate, and conventional DMARDs
- Biologic agents

1.1.7.1 Treatment Strategy

Myth: RA is a benign disease for which therapy can be delayed safely for a while.

Reality: A cardinal feature of RA is its propensity to destroy joints. Joint destruction can lead to irreversible physical disability, additional comorbidities (e.g., complications of joint surgery), economic losses, and a reduction in life expectancy (Yelin et al. 2002; Kobelt and Jönsson 2008; Michaud and

Wolfe 2007). Radiographic evidence of joint disease is detected in a large percentage of seropositive RA patients within 2 years of diagnosis, and within several months in some patients (Plant et al. 1998). Both joint damage and subsequent disability are related directly to the activity of inflammation in many patients (Drossaers-Bakker et al. 1999). These facts underscore the importance of treating RA early, aggressively, and effectively.

Pearl: Remission is the aim of therapy.

Comment: Only the complete and sustained clinical control of RA activity is associated with the cessation of joint damage (Smolen et al. 2008a). Even states of low disease activity are associated with the progression of joint damage (Smolen et al. 2008a). Functional impairment is higher in states of low disease activity than in remission. Attaining remission is the ultimate therapeutic goal. The achievement of low disease activity constitutes an appropriate intermediate aim.

Pearl: Effective treatment in RA involves prompt changes of therapy if clinical responses are not observed within several months.

Comment: The long-term clinical outcome can be predicted reliably in the majority of RA patients within 3–6 months of starting therapy (Aletaha et al. 2007). The maximal efficacy of RA treatment is observed within the first few months. Patients who have not responded with significant improvement by 6 months are unlikely to do so if the same medications are continued. These patients should be switched to other treatment approaches (Aletaha et al. 2007; Goekoop-Ruiterman et al. 2005; Smolen et al. 2003a).

Myth: Evidence-based data from randomized controlled trials confirm that a variety of conventional and biologic DMARDs are highly effective for the treatment of an RA patient who has five tender joints and five swollen joints.

Reality: Most major clinical trial has been performed to address this patient population. Most major randomized controlled trials published in the last 15 years have required at least six tender joints and six swollen joints. All 3 of the phase III golimumab trials required 4 tender and 4 swollen joints, so "all" is no longer formally correct. Other studies have shown that the vast majority of patients in rheumatologists' clinics do not have disease that is sufficiently active to qualify for clinical trials. There is, therefore, a gap in our knowledge regarding these patients. Rightly or wrongly, the results from the published clinical trials are extrapolated to this patient population.

1.1.7.2 Glucocorticoids, Methotrexate, and Conventional DMARDs

Myth: Once an RA patient is started on glucocorticoids, he or she will never be able to discontinue the medication.

Reality: Clinical trials in the era of biologic agents have shown that this oft-heard refrain is a Myth. With use of effective DMARD therapy – conventional, biological, or both – RA patients can be tapered to low doses of glucocorticoids and many discontinue them entirely.

Glucocorticoids are an effective therapy for RA, but 60 years after their introduction we still struggle to understand the optimal way to use them. As discussed below, some patients should be maintained on a low dose of prednisone (e.g., 5 mg/day).

Pearl: Glucocorticoids are an important part of early RA therapy.

Comment: Glucocorticoids provide important benefits in the treatment of early RA, whether they are administered in moderately high doses or low doses (Boers et al. 1997; Mottonen et al. 1999; Wassenberg et al. 2005; Svensson et al. 2005). The COBRA study employed an aggressive glucocorticoid regimen that began patients with early RA on 60 mg of prednisone/day (Boers et al. 1997). Other trials have employed substantially lower starting doses (Mottonen et al. 1999; Wassenberg et al. 2005; Svensson et al. 2005). Regardless of the starting dose used, the addition of glucocorticoids provides significant advantages when compared with treatment approaches that employ methotrexate alone or combinations of synthetic DMARDs.

The upshot of these data is that the optimal therapeutic approach for RA is a blend of the old and the new. Methotrexate is the cornerstone of initial RA treatment and should be used in combination with glucocorticoids at the start of therapy. Most clinicians also employ low-dose glucocorticoids. If methotrexate is insufficiently effective in this scheme, a biologic agent should be added within 3–6 months, possibly with another glucocorticoid boost at the initiation of this new treatment.

Pearl: Glucocorticoids act as DMARDs in RA.

Comment: The Empire rheumatism studies of the 1950s demonstrated that glucocortiosteroid therapy significantly slowed radiographic progression of disease. Many clinicians did not believe these data and avoided prescribing glucocorticoids because of their well-known adverse effects. Well-designed randomized, controlled clinical trials have subsequently confirmed the findings from the Empire rheumatism studies (Kirwan 1995).

Adjunct medications such as bisphosphonates and statins now attenuate many of the potential drawbacks to glucocorticoids. Many clinicians should probably be more liberal in the use of these medications, which are remarkably cheap and effective therapy.

Myth: When using methotrexate, start low and go slow.

Reality: Methotrexate has been the cornerstone of treatment for RA since the mid-1980s. In the early years of methotrexate

use, the prevailing maxim was to "start low and go slow." Most clinicians began methotrexate at 7.5 mg/week and advanced the dose slowly over many months, never exceeding 15 mg/week for many patients.

In an ironic twist, clinical trials of the biologic agents changed the way methotrexate is used in practice. A comparatively aggressive methotrexate regimen was used in the comparison arm of a randomized, double-blind clinical trial that compared etanercept to methotrexate over a 6-month period (Bathon 2000). Patients in the methotrexate arm began treatment with 15 mg/week and quickly escalated their dose to a mean of approximately 20 mg/week. The results were dramatic: although the etanercept group had a superior "area under the curve" disease activity analysis at 6 months, patients in the methotrexate group had a similar ACR20 response rate at 12 months as the etanercept group.

Methotrexate therapy in most patients should begin at 10–15 mg/week, and then be escalated to 20 mg/week over the next 4 weeks, as tolerated. The dose can be increased to 25 mg/week or even higher in some cases.

Myth: When administered weekly in low doses (10–25 mg/week), methotrexate often accumulates to dangerous levels in physiologic third spaces, such as peritoneal effusions, pleural effusions, and pericardial effusions.

Reality: Methotrexate has been reported to accumulate in physiologic third spaces, such as pleural and peritoneal fluid during high-dose MTX therapy for cancer (Li and Gwilt 2002). In these cases, the presence of a physiologic third space may prolong the half-life of MTX and cause unanticipated toxicity. Such toxicity has not been reported in patients with RA who are receiving standard weekly arthritis doses. The issue of methotrexate "third-spacing" probably would not be a significant concern in RA unless the patient has significant renal insufficiency.

Pearl: Leflunomide remains in the body for years after administration.

Comment: Because of its extensive enterohepatic re-circulation, leflunomide persists in the body for years after the medication has been discontinued. This is an important fact when toxicities occur or if pregnancy is considered, because leflunomide has significant teratogenic potential. In these situations, a washout with cholestyramine may be desired. If the persistence of leflunomide is a potential concern, blood levels may be checked.

Myth: Antibiotics are not effective in the treatment of RA.

Reality: There is little to no evidence that the antibacterial effects of some DMARDs are important in the treatment of RA. However, sulfasalazine and minocycline, both of which have significant antibacterial effects, also have some efficacy in RA. Whether the antibacterial effects of these drugs are important with regard to their activity against RA is unclear.

In the case of minocycline, a number of other mechanisms of action may be important (O'Dell 1999). Minocycline has substantial immunomodulatory actions, some of which contribute to its well-known ability to induce lupus. Minocycline is unique among antibiotics in terms of its ability to inhibit metalloproteinases and among DMARDs because of its ability to inhibit peptidyl arginine deiminase.

Myth: Hydroxychloroquine is not an effective DMARD.

Reality: There is a paucity of direct evidence that hydroxychloroquine slows radiographic progression in RA. However, multiple studies have shown that if hydroxychloroquine is started early in the course of disease, patients experience better outcomes, including less radiographic progression. The combination of methotrexate and hydroxychloroquine is the most common tandem DMARD regimen used for the treatment of RA. In addition, some data suggest that the use of hydroxychloroquine markedly reduces the incidence of diabetes among patients with RA (Wasko et al. 2007).

The potency of the MTX-HCQ combination may be explained at least in part by a patient's increased exposure to MTX (e.g., increased area under the curve) when MTX is administered together with HCQ (Carmichael et al. 2002).

Myth: Combination therapy with conventional (i.e., non-biologic) DMARDs is uniformly effective when compared with MTX alone.

Reality: Combination therapies of traditional DMARDs were advocated strongly for the treatment of RA until well into the 1990s. One major trial that preceded the era of biologic treatments indicated that the combination of methotrexate, sulfasalazine, and hydroxychloroquine was superior to methotrexate alone (O'Dell 1996). However, most clinical trials comparing combination therapy to monotherapy have not shown superiority of the combination therapy arms (summarized in Smolen et al. 2005).

Pearl: Gold shots are dramatically efficacious for the treatment of RA in one of every five patients.

Comment: No one knows for certain whether or not this statement is a Pearl or a Myth, but it is echoed widely by practitioners who treated RA in the heyday of chrysotherapy. Because of unequivocal advances in RA treatment since the 1980s, the truth or falseness of this statement is likely to remain uncertain. However, when injections of gold sodium thiomalate were compared with weekly MTX therapy in a double-blind, randomized trial, gold produced twice as many clinical remissions as the latter (24.1% vs. 11.5%) (Rau et al. 1997). Gold was also associated with more side effects and withdrawals due to toxicity.

Table 1.2 Treatment arms in the BeSt study

- Group 1 (sequential monotherapy) – Sequential monotherapy began with methotrexate. The following agents were added in succession if the disease remained poorly controlled:
  - Sulfasalazine (methotrexate discontinued)
  - Leflunomide (sulfasalazine discontinued)
  - Methotrexate plus an anticytokine agent (leflunomide discontinued)
- Group 2 (step-up) – Step-up therapy began with methotrexate. The following agents were added together (one at a time) if the disease remained poorly controlled:
  - Sulfasalazine
  - Hydroxychloroquine
  - Prednisolone
  - An anticytokine agent (with discontinuation of sulfasalazine and hydroxychloroquine)
- Group 3 (initial combination DMARD plus prednisolone) – Initial combination treatment consisted of the combination of methotrexate, sulfasalazine, and prednisolone. Persistent disease led to the addition of:
  - Cyclosporine (sulfasalazine discontinued)
  - Methotrexate (prednisolone discontinued)
- Group 4 (combination methotrexate and infliximab) – Initial combination treatment consisted of methotrexate and infliximab. Persistent disease led to the addition (one at a time) of:
  - Sulfasalazine
  - Leflunomide
  - Methotrexate, cyclosporine, and prednisolone

1.1.7.3 Biologic Agents

Myth: Nearly all patients with RA respond to tumor necrosis factor inhibitors.

Reality: The BeSt study randomly assigned 508 DMARD-naive patients with RA of less than 2 years duration to one of four different treatment strategies. The four treatment groups included in this study are shown in Table 1.2. Approximately 22% of patients randomized to the TNF inhibitor arm, a combination of infliximab and methotrexate, failed treatment (Goekoop-Ruiterman et al. 2005).

Myth: When a TNF inhibitor fails, other TNF inhibitors are unlikely to work.

Reality: Several open-label studies or analyses from registries have suggested that a second TNF inhibitor can be efficacious following the failure of a first TNF inhibitor (Gomez-Reino and Carmona 2006; van Vollenhoven 2004; Hyrich et al. 2007). This appears to be true even if the first and second TNF inhibitors are pharmacologically similar; for example, the case of adalimumab following infliximab (both medications are monoclonal antibodies).

These data from uncontrolled investigations have now been expanded in a double-blind, controlled clinical trial of golimumab (Smolen et al. 2008b). These data reveal that a third TNF inhibitor can be effective even after two have failed. However, if all three other TNF inhibitors (etanercept, infliximab, and adalimumab) have failed before golimumab, then golimumab is unlikely to be effective.

Pearl: TNF inhibitors work better in combination with methotrexate than alone.

Comment: All clinic trials that have addressed this question have found that the combination of methotrexate plus infliximab, etanercept, or adalimumab is more effective than methotrexate alone or any of the TNF inhibitors by themselves. This is true for both clinical response (ACR20 or DAS) and radiographic outcomes. In addition, observational studies have strongly suggested that protection against cardiovascular morbidity and mortality by the TNF inhibitors is dependent on the concomitant use of methotrexate.

The synergistic effects of methotrexate extend beyond TNF inhibitors. Abatacept and rituximab also work better when prescribed in combination with methotrexate.

Pearl: Neutralizing antibodies (human antichimeric antibodies [HACA]) may decrease the efficacy of infliximab over time.

Comment: Secondary failure, i.e., the loss of a response after an initial improvement, may be due in part to the development of neutralizing antibodies. Strategies for managing this potential complication of infliximab include concomitant use of an immunosuppressive agent such as MTX and avoidance of intermittent therapy with infliximab. Prolonged intervals between stopping and re-starting infliximab are associated with a greater risk of HACA development.

Myth: B cells are depleted for life after therapy with rituximab.

Reality: B cells eventually return. This return often begins as early as 4–6 months after completion of the rituximab infusions but is not complete for years. B cell numbers do correlate with response to rituximab in groups of patients, implying that more investigation is required to understand why rituximab works (when it works) for autoimmune conditions (Breedveld et al. 2007).

1.1.8 Co-Morbidities and Adverse Effects

Myth/Pearl: RA is associated with an increased incidence of cancer.

Comment: This statement may be regarded as either a Myth or a Pearl, depending on the type of malignancy to which one refers. The incidence of lymphoma is increased in RA; most studies suggest at least a twofold increase compared with the general population. Lung cancers are also overrepresented in patients with RA, perhaps because smoking is a potent risk factor for

RA. Gastrointestinal cancers, however, appear to be decreased among patients with RA, probably by a factor of 3 or 4.

The decrease in colon cancers among patients with RA led investigators to hypothesize that NSAIDs slow polyp formation. This led, in turn, to randomized trials of COX-2 inhibitors designed to prove this hypothesis – and to the unexpected finding that certain COX-2 inhibitors are associated with an increased risk of myocardial infarction.

Pearl: Severe COPD and exposure to cyclophosphamide may be risk factors for malignancy in patients treated with TNF inhibition.

Comment: Most long-term observational data on TNF inhibition are reassuring with regard to the risk of malignancy. The overall incidence of cancer does not appear to be elevated dramatically. However, it may be wise to avoid TNF inhibition in some patient subsets.

A randomized clinical trial in Wegener's granulomatosis found an increased risk of solid tumors in patients who were exposed to etanercept (Stone et al. 2006). All patients who developed solid malignancies also had histories of exposure to cyclophosphamide. These data suggest that it is wise to avoid TNF inhibitors in patients who are on cyclophosphamide at the same time or who have significant histories of cyclophosphamide use.

A trial of infliximab therapy for severe COPD suggested an increase in early lung cancers in the patients treated with infliximab (Rennard et al. 2007).

Pearl: All TNF inhibitors are not alike when it comes to toxicity.

Comment: Infliximab is associated much more often with the reactivation of tuberculosis than is etanercept (Wallis et al. 2004). Data from Europe suggest that the risk of tuberculosis with adalimumab is similar to that of infliximab and higher than etanercept. Infliximab is also more likely to be associated with histoplasmosis, coccidioidomycosis, and listeriosis (Wallis et al. 2004). Conversely, etanercept has been linked more commonly to demyelinating diseases.

Pearl: The effects of TNF inhibition in patients with viral hepatitis diverge widely depending on the specific form of hepatitis.

Comment: Well-documented, life-threatening, or fatal flares of hepatitis B virus infection have occurred in patients treated with TNF inhibitors or rituximab (Calabrese et al. 2006). Thus, both medications are relatively contraindicated in patients with a history of hepatitis B, but TNF inhibitors have been used in patients with hepatitis B virus infection kept on antiviral agents. In contrast, hepatitis C virus infection does not appear to be a contraindication for therapy with TNF inhibition. Limited data suggest a possible beneficial effect of TNF inhibition on the liver disease during treatment for hepatitis C.

Myth: Biologic agents can be used safely in combination to treat RA.

Reality: All available data suggest that when two biologic agents are used in tandem, toxicity (particularly from infections) rises significantly. Studies of biologic combinations of etanercept and anakinra and etanercept and abatacept have shown only marginal, if any, improvements in efficacy, but significantly increased rates of infections in the combination group when compared with either biologic alone (Furst in press). Clinicians should avoid using two of the currently available biologic agents at the same time.

Myth: AntiTNF agents are safe in pregnancy.

Reality: Only anecdotal data about the impact of TNF inhibition on pregnancy are available. These seemingly reassuring outcomes have led some clinicians to believe "so far, so good" and allow pregnant women to use TNF inhibitors. It is too early to judge whether TNF inhibitors are safe in pregnancy. Two reports raise at least some concern. One abstract has reported a possible increase in a distinctive pattern of birth defects called VACTERL (or Vater syndrome) where V = verterbral anomalies, A = anal atresia, C = cardivascular anomalies, T = tracheoesophageal fistula, E = esoghageal atresia, R = renal and/or radial abnormalities, and L = limb anomalies (Carter et al., 2009). A second report suggested an increased risk of miscarriage among women exposed to TNF agents early in pregnancy.

A prudent approach is to discontinue TNF inhibitors when conception is confirmed or, even better, before conception (to the extent that pregnancy can be planned). Patients and clinicians alike hope for the temporary remission of RA that frequently accompanies pregnancy once TNF inhibitor use has been suspended (see Chap 17).

Pearl: RA is an independent risk factor for cardiovascular disease.

Comment: Several studies show that cardiovascular disease is the leading cause of death in patients with RA. In a recent meta-analysis, the risk of cardiovascular death was 50% higher in patients with RA when compared with the general population (Aviña-Zubieta et al. 2008).

Pearl or Myth: DMARD and/or biologic therapy reduce the occurrence of adverse cardiovascular events in RA.

Comment: Retrospective case-control studies suggest that MTX and TNF inhibitors decrease cardiovascular morbidity and mortality in RA, but these positive outcomes have not been substantiated by evidence from prospective studies or randomized, controlled clinical trials. A verdict on this will require additional prospective work.

Myth: Cardiovascular risk factors confer the same risk for cardiovascular outcomes in patients with RA as they do in the general population.

Reality: One retrospective study has shown that male gender, smoking, and personal cardiac history had weaker associations with cardiovascular events among patients with RA than they do among individuals who do not have RA (Gonzalez et al. 2006). In contrast, the risks imparted by other risk factors – hypertension, dyslipidemia, body mass index, diabetes mellitus, and family history – were no different between the two groups.

1.2 Immunizations in RA

Myth: Methotrexate monotherapy has been generally associated with a profoundly reduced response to the influenza vaccine.

Reality: Therapy with methotrexate has been associated with little (if any) reduction in the response to the influenza vaccine.

Myth: Influenza vaccination is NOT recommended for patients receiving a TNF inhibitor.

Reality: Although the serological responses are less robust in patients with RA receiving a TNF inhibitor when compared with that of healthy individuals, their use does not raise any safety concerns and the titers are sufficiently high to warrant influenza vaccination in all RA patients. However, a large proportion of patients with RA may not respond to pneumococcal vaccination while they are taking MTX and a TNF inhibitor. The optimal approach to vaccination in these patients, therefore, is to administer the pneumococcal vaccination before starting treatment with these agents.

References

Aletaha D, Nell VPK, Stamm T, ct al Acute phase reactants add little to composite disease activity indices for rheumatoid arthritis: Validation of a clinical activity score. Arthritis Res 2005a; 7:R796–R806

Aletaha D, Ward MM, Machold KP, et al Remission and active disease in rheumatoid arthritis: Defining criteria for disease activity states. Arthritis Rheum 2005b; 52:2625–2636

Aletaha D, Breedveld FC, Smolen JS. The need for new classification criteria for rheumatoid arthritis. Arthritis Rheum 2005c; 52: 3333–3336

Aletaha D, Funovits J, Keystone EC, Smolen JS. Disease activity early in the course of treatment predicts response to therapy after one year in rheumatoid arthritis patients. Arthritis Rheum 2007; 56(10): 3226–3235

Arnett FC, Edworthy SM, Block DA, et al The American Rheumatism Association 1987 revised criteria for the classification of rheumatoid arthritis. Arthritis Rheum 1988; 31:315–324

Aviña-Zubieta JA, Choi HK, Sadatsafavi M, et al Risk of cardiovascular mortality in patients with rheumatoid arthritis: A meta-analysis of observational studies. Arthritis Rheum 2008; 59:1690–1697

Avnon LS, Abu-Shakra M, Flusser D, et al Pleural effusion associated with RA Rheum International 2007; 27:919–925

Axford JS. Rheumatic manifestations of haemochromatosis. Baillieres Clin Rheumatol 1991; 5:351–365

Bathon JM, Martin RW, Fleischmann RM, et al A comparison of etanercept and methotrexate in early rheumatoid arthritis. N Engl J Med 2000;343:1586–93

Bellhorn LR, Hess EV. Erosive osteoarthritis. Semin Arthritis Rheum 1993; 22:298–306

Boers M, Verhoeven AC, Markusse HM, et al Randomised comparison of combined step-down prednisolone, methotrexate and sulphasalazine with sulphasalazine alone in early rheumatoid arthritis: A randomised trial. Lancet 1997; 350:309–318

Breedveld F, Agarwal S, Yin M, et al Rituximab pharmacokinetics in patients with rheumatoid arthritis: B-cell levels do not correlate with clinical response. J Clin Pharmacol 2007; 47:1119–1128

Calabrese LH, Zein NN, Vassilopoulos D. Hepatitis B virus (HBV) reactivation with immunosuppressive therapy in rheumatic diseases: assessment and preventive strategies. Ann Rheum Dis 2006; 65: 983–989

Carmichael SJ, Beal J, Day RO, Tett SE. Combination therapy with methotrexate and hydroxychloroquine for rheumatoid arthritis increases exposure to methotrexate. J Rheumatol 2002; 29: 2031–2033

Carter JD, Ladhani A, Ricca LR, et al A safety assessment of tumor necrosis factor antagonists during pregnancy: A review of the Food and Drug Administration database. J Rheumatol 2009; 36:3

Chan MT. Owen P. Dunphy J, et al Associations of erosive arthritis with anti-cyclic citrullinated peptide antibodies and MHC Class II alleles in systemic lupus erythematosus. J Rheumatol 2008; 35 (1):77–83

Ching DW, Petrie JP, Klemp P, et al Injection therapy of superficial rheumatoid nodules. Br J Rheumatol 1992; 31:775

Choi HK, Hernan MA, Seeger JD, et al Methotrexate and mortality in patients with rheumatoid arthritis: A prospective study. Lancet 2002; 359(9313):1173–1177

Cohen SB, Dore RK, Lane NE, et al Denosumab treatment effects on structural damage, bone mineral density, and bone turnover in rheumatoid arthritis: A twelve-month, multicenter, randomized, double-blind, placebo-controlled, phase II clinical trial. Arthritis Rheum 2008; 58(5):1299–1309

De Souza AW, Fernendes V, Ferrari AJ. Female gout: Clinical and laboratory features. J Rheumatol 2005; 32:2186–2188

Doherty M, Dieppe PA. Crystal deposition disease in the elderly. Clin Rheum Dis 1986; 12:97–116

Drossaers-Bakker KW, de Buck M, van Zeben D, et al Long-term course and outcome of functional capacity in rheumatoid arthritis: The effect of disease activity and radiologic damage over time. Arthritis Rheum 1999; 42:1854–1860

Fernandez A, Quintana G, Rondon F, et al Lupus arthropathy: A case series of patients with rhupus. Clin Rheumatol 2006; 25:164–167

Finckh A, Dehler S, Costenbader KH, et al Cigarette smoking and radiographic progression in rheumatoid arthritis. Ann Rheum Dis 2007; 66:1066–1071

Furst DE. The risk of infections with biologic therapies for rheumatoid arthritis. Semin Arthritis Rheum 2009 (in press)

Genovese MC, Becker JC, Schiff M, et al Abatacept for rheumatoid arthritis refractory to tumor necrosis factor alpha inhibition. N Engl J Med 2005; 353(11):1114–1123

Goekoop-Ruiterman YP, De Vries-Bouwstra JK, Allaart CF, et al Clinical and radiographic outcomes of four different treatment strategies in patients with early rheumatoid arthritis (the BeSt study): A randomized, controlled trial. Arthritis Rheum 2005; 52: 3381–3390

Gomez-Reino JJ, Carmona L. Switching TNF antagonists in patients with chronic arthritis: An observational study of 488 patients over a four-year period. Arthritis Res Ther 2006; 8(1):R29

Gonzalez A, Kremers HM, Crowson CS, et al Do cardiovascular risk factors confer the same risk for cardiovascular outcomes in rheumatoid arthritis as in non-rheumatoid arthritis patients? Ann Rheum Dis 2006; 67:64–69

Grigor C, Capell H, Stirling A, et al Effect of a treatment strategy of tight control for rheumatoid arthritis (the TICORA study): A single-blind randomised controlled trial. Lancet 2004; 364:263–269

Harrison BJ, Symmons DP, Barret EM, Silman AS. The performance of the 1987 ARA classification criteria for rheumatoid arthritis in a population based cohort of patients with early inflammatory polyarthritis. J Rheumatol 1998; 25(2324):2330.

Hyrich KL, Lunt M, Watson KD, et al Outcomes after switching from one anti-tumor necrosis factor alpha agent to a second anti-tumor necrosis factor alpha agent in patients with rheumatoid arthritis: Results from a large UK national cohort study. Arthritis Rheum 2007; 56(1):13–20

Kalajian A, Callen J. Multicentric reticulohistiocytosis successfully treated with infliximab: An illustrative case and evaluation of cytokine expression supporting anti-tumor necrosis factor therapy. Arch Dermatol 2008; 144:1360–1366

Kirwan JR, The Arthritis and Rheumatism Council Low-Dose Glucocorticoid Study Group. The effect of glucocorticoids on joint destruction in rheumatoid arthritis. N Engl J Med 1995; 333: 142–146

Klareskog L, Stolt P, Lundberg K, et al A new model for an etiology of rheumatoid arthritis: Smoking may trigger HLA-DR (shared epitope)-restricted immune reactions to autoantigens modified by citrullination. Arthritis Rheum 2006; 54:38–46

Kobelt G, Jönsson B. The burden of rheumatoid arthritis and access to treatment: Outcome and cost-utility of treatments. Eur J Health Econ 2008; 8 (Suppl 2):S95–S106

Kroot EJ, de Jong BA, van Leeuwen MA, Swinkels H, et al The prognostic value of anti-cyclic citrullinated peptide antibody in patients with recent-onset rheumatoid arthritis. Arthritis Rheum 2000; 43(8):1831–1835

Lee H, Irigoyen P, Kern M, et al Interaction between smoking, the shared eiptope, and anti-cyclic citrullinated peptide: A mixed picture in three large North American rheumatoid arthritis cohorts. Arthritis Rheum 2007; 56:1745–1753

Li J, Gwilt P. The effect of malignant effusions on methotrexate disposition. Cancer Chemother Pharmacol 2002; 50:373–382

Lunardi C, Tinazzi E, Bason C, et al Human parvovirus B19 infection and autoimmunity. Autoimmun Rev 2008; 8:116–120

Machold KP, Stamm TA, Nell VP, et al Very recent onset rheumatoid arthritis: Clinical and serological patient characteristics associated with radiographic progression over the first years of disease. Rheumatology (Oxford) 2006 [Epub 2006 Aug 9 ahead of print]

Masi, AT. Articular patterns in the early course of rheumatoid arthritis. Am J Med 1983; 75:16

Mattey DL, Dawes PT, Clarke S, et al Relationship among the HLA-DRB1 shared epitope, smoking, and rheumatoid factor production in rheumatoid arthritis. Arthritis Care Res 2002; 47:403–407

Michaud K, Wolfe F. Comorbidities in rheumatoid arthritis. Best Pract Res Clin Rheumatol 2007; 21(5):885–906

Mierau M, Schoels M, Gonda G, et al Assessing remission in clinical practice. Rheumatology 2007; 46:975–979 [Epub 2007 Mar 6]

Mikuls TR, Huges LB, Westfall AO, et al Cigarette smoking, disease severity, and autoantibody expression in African Americans with recent-onset rheumatoid arthritis. Ann Rheum Dis 2008; 67: 1529–1534

Morozzi G, Bellisai F, Fioravanti A, Galeazzi M. Absence of anti-cyclic citrullinated peptide antibodies in erosive osteoarthritis: Further serological evidence of the disease as a subset of osteoarthritis. Ann Rheum Dis 2005; 64:1095–1096

Mottonen T, Hannonen P, Leirisalo-Repo M, et al Comparison of combination therapy with single-drug therapy in early rheumatoid arthritis: A randomised trial. FIN-RACo trial group. Lancet 1999; 353(9164):1568–1573

Nell V, Machold KP, Stamm TA, et al Autoantibody profiling as early diagnostic and prognostic tool for rheumatoid arthritis. Ann Rheum Dis 2005; 64:1731–1736 [Epub 2005 May 5]

Nishimura K, Sugiyama D, Kogata Y, et al Meta-analysis: Diagnostic accuracy of anti-cyclic citrullinated peptide antibody and rheumatoid factor for rheumatoid arthritis. Ann Intern Med 2007; 146:797–808

O'Dell J. Treatment of rheumatoid arthritis with methotrexate alone, sulfasalazine and hydroxychloroquine, or a combination of all three medications. N Engl J Med 1996; 334:1287–1291

O'Dell R. Is there a role for antibiotics in the treatment of patients with rheumatoid arthritis? Drugs 1999; 57:279–282

Ostendorf B, Scherer A, Specker C, et al Jaccoud's arthropathy in systemic lupus erythematosus: Differentiation of deforming and erosive patterns by magnetic resonance imaging. Arthritis Rheum 2003; 48:157–165

Padyukov L, Silva C, Stolt P, et al A gene-environment interaction between smoking and shared epitope genes in HLA-DR provides a high risk of seropositive rheumatoid arthritis. Arthritis Rheum 2004; 50:3085–3092

Plant MJ, Jones PW, Saklatvala J, et al Patterns of radiological progression in rheumatoid arthritis: Results of an 8 year prospective study. J Rheumatol 1998; 25:417–426

Rantapaa-Dahlqvist S. Diagnostic and prognostic significance of autoantibodies in early rheumatoid arthritis. Scand J Rheumatol 2005;34:83

Rau R, Herborn G, Menninger H, Blechschmidt J. Comparison of intramuscular methotrexate and gold sodium thiomalate in the treatment of early erosive rheumatoid arthritis: 12 month data of a double-blind parallel study of 174 patients. Br J Rheumatol 1997; 36:345–352

Rennard SI, Fogarty C, Kelsen S, et al The safety and efficacy of infliximab in moderate to severe chronic obstructive pulmonary disease. Am J Respir Crit Care Med 2007; 175:926–934

Saag KG, Cerhan JR, Kolluri S, et al Cigarette smoking and rheumatoid arthritis severity. Ann Rheum Dis 1997; 56:463–469

Schellekens GA, Visser H, de Jong BA, et al The diagnostic properties of rheumatoid arthritis antibodies recognizing a cyclic citrullinated peptide. Arthritis Rheum 2000; 43:155–163.

Silman AJ, Newman J, MacGregor AJ. Cigarette smoking increases the risk of rheumatoid arthritis. Arthritis Rheum 1996; 39:732–735

Sinclair D, Hull RG. Why do general practitioners request rheumatoid factor? A study of symptoms, requesting patterns and patient outcome. Ann Clin Biochem 2003; 40(Pt 2):131–137

Smolen JS, Sokka T, Pincus T, Breedveld FC. A proposed treatment algorithm for rheumatoid arthritis: Aggressive therapy, methotrexate, and quantitative measures. Clin Exp Rheumatol 2003a; 21(5 Suppl 31):S209–S210

Smolen JS, Breedveld FC, Schiff MH, et al A simplified disease activity index for rheumatoid arthritis for use in clinical practice. Rheumatology 2003b; 42:244–257

Smolen JS, Aletaha D, Keystone E. Superior efficacy of combination therapy for rheumatoid arthritis. Fact or Fiction? Arthritis Rheum 2005; 52:2975–2983

Smolen JS, Han C, Van der Heijde DM, et al Radiographic changes in rheumatoid arthritis patients attaining different disease activity states with methotrexate monotherapy and infliximab plus methotrexate: The impacts of remission and TNF blockade. Ann Rheum Dis 2009; (6):823–7

Smolen J, Kay J, Doyle MK, et al Golimumab, a new human anti-TNF alpha monoclonal antibody, subcutaneously administered every 4 weeks in patients with active rheumatoid arthritis who were previously treated with anti-TNF-alpha agent(s): Results of the randomized, double-blind, placebo-controlled trial. Ann Rheum Dis 2008b; 67(Suppl II):50

Stone JH, Holbrook JT, Marriott MA, et al, for the Wegener's Granulomatosis Etanercept Trial Research Group. Solid malignancies among patients in the Wegener's Granulomatosis Etanercept Trial. Arthritis Rheum 2006; 54:1608–1618

Svensson B, Boonen A, Albertsson K, et al Low-dose prednisolone in addition to the initial disease-modifying antirheumatic drug in patients with early active rheumatoid arthritis reduces joint destruction and increases the remission rate: A two-year randomized trial. Arthritis Rheum 2005; 52:3360–3370

Thery C, Lekieffre J, Gosselin B, et al Atrio-ventricular block in rheumatoid polyarthritis. Arch Mal Coeur Vaiss 1974; 67:1181–1191

Turesson C, O'Fallon WM, Crowson CS, et al Extra-articular disease manifestation in rheumatoid arthritis: Incidence, trends, and risk factors over 46 years. Ann Rheum Dis 2003; 62:722–727

van der Heijde DM, van Riel PL, van Leeuwen MA, et al Prognostic factors for radiographic damage and physical disability in early rheumatoid arthritis. A prospective follow-up study of 147 patients. Br J Rheumatol 1992; 31(8):519–525

van der Helm-van Mil AH, le Cessie S, van Dongen H, et al A prediction rule for disease outcome in patients with recent-onset undifferentiated arthritis: How to guide individual treatment decisions. Arthritis Rheum 2007; 56:433

van Gaalen FA, Linn-Rasker SP, van Venrooij WJ, de Jong BA, Breedveld FC, Verweij CL, Toes RE, Huizinga TW. Autoantibodies to cyclic citrullinated peptides predict progression to rheumatoid arthritis in patients with undifferentiated arthritis: A prospective cohort study. Arthritis Rheum 2004; 50:709–715

van Vollenhoven R. Switching between biological agents. Clin Exp Rheumatol 2004; 22(Suppl 5):S115–S121

van Vugt RM, Derksen RH, Kater L, Bijlsma JW. Deforming arthropathy or lupus and rhupus hands in systemic lupus erythematosus. Ann Rheum Dis 1998; 57: 540–544

Verstappen SM, Jacobs JW, Heurkens AH, et al Intensive treatment with methotrexate in early rheumatoid arthritis: Aiming for remission. Computer Assisted Management in Early Rheumatoid Arthritis (CAMERA, an open-label strategy trial). Ann Rheum Dis 2007; 66(11):1443–1449

Wallis RS, Broder MS, Wong JY, Hanson ME, Beenhouwer DO. Granulomatous infectious diseases associated with tumor necrosis factor antagonists. Clin Infect Dis 2004; 38(9):1261–1265

Wasko MC, Hubert HB, Lingala VB, Elliott JR, Luggen ME, Fries JF, Ward NM. Hydroxychloroquine and risk of diabetes in patients with rheumatoid arthritis. JAMA 2007; 298:187–193

Wassenberg S, Rau R, Steinfeld P, Zeidler H. Very low-dose prednisolone in early rheumatoid arthritis retards radiographic progression over two years: A multicenter, double-blind, placebo-controlled trial. Arthritis Rheum 2005; 52:3371–3380

Yelin E, Trupin L, Wong B, Rush S. The impact of functional status and change in functional status on mortality over 18 years among persons with rheumatoid arthritis. J Rheumatol 2002; 29(9):1851–1857

Young NS, Brown KE. Parvovirus B19. N Engl J Med 2004; 350: 586–597

Rheumatoid Vasculitis

John H. Stone and Eric L. Matteson

2

2.1 Overview of Rheumatoid Vasculitis

> Rheumatoid arthritis (RA) is associated with vasculitis in approximately 1% of patients.
> Rheumatoid vasculitis (RV) refers specifically to a destructive inflammatory process with protean clinical features that center on the blood vessel wall. The disease strongly resembles polyarteritis nodosa in its predilection for particular organs: the skin, peripheral nerves, gastrointestinal tract, and heart.
> RV can affect a wide range of blood vessel types, from medium-sized muscular arteries to smaller arterioles even post-capillary venules (the size of blood vessels involved in many forms of small-vessel vasculitis).
> RV usually occurs in patients with severe, longstanding, nodular, destructive RA.
> Palpable purpura, cutaneous ulcers (particularly in the malleolar region), digital infarctions, and peripheral sensory neuropathy are common manifestations.
> Tissue biopsy establishes the diagnosis of RV. Deep skin biopsies from the border of ulcers may capture medium-sized vessels that are involved. Nerve conduction studies help identify involved nerves for biopsy. Muscle biopsies should be performed simultaneously with nerve biopsies to increase the diagnostic yield of the procedure.

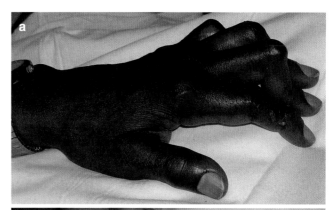
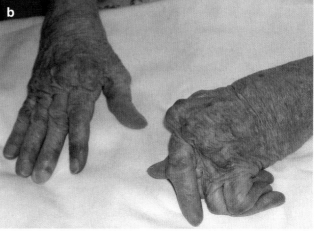

Figs. 2.1 (a, b) RV tends to occur in patients with burnt-out joint disease (Figures courtesy of Dr. John Stone)

Pearl: RV tends to occur in patients with "burnt-out" RA.

Comment: This very good rule of thumb, seldom violated, remains one of the many mysteries surrounding rheumatoid disease. RV singles out patients who have had severe, destructive RA whose joint disease is no longer active (Figs. 2.1a and b). Thus, the classic patient with this complication is one with a longstanding history of nodular, seropositive, destructive RA who, after years of ineffectual disease-modifying antirheumatic drugs (DMARDs) and too much prednisone, has minimal synovitis. The life-threatening nature of RV

unfortunately means that the patient now needs intensive therapy – glucocorticoids and possibly cyclophosphamide – more than ever.

In addition to RA duration, other risk factors for RV include the presence of other extraarticular manifestations of RA, especially rheumatoid nodulosis, scleritis, amyloidosis, and the presence of rheumatoid factor and antiCCP antibody (Turesson et al. 2003; Turesson and Matteson 2008; Van Gaalen et al. 2004). There appears to be a genetic predisposition toward developing RV, as HLA-DRB1 shared epitope

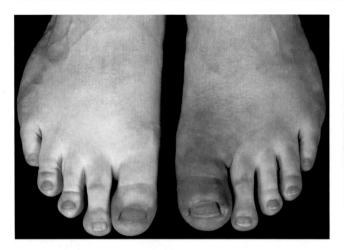

Fig. 2.2 Vasculitis of the left great toe in a patient with RA of 5 months duration treated with methotrexate and hydroxychloroquine. Minimal synovitis is present. Biopsy of the skin was consistent with a leukocyto-clastic vasculitis. The patient developed a foot drop from mononeuritis, which responded to oral prednisone, at an initial dose of 1 mg/kg/daily (Figure courtesy of Dr. Eric Matteson)

phenotypes are strongly associated with extraarticular disease manifestations including RV (Turesson et al. 2005).

Although the occurrence of RV in patients with longstanding disease is the rule, cases developing early in the course of RA have been reported (Fig. 2.2) (Voskuyl et al. 1996).

Myth: Nailfold infarcts in RA are a harbinger of serious vasculitis and should trigger an intensification of treatment.

Reality: Bywaters' lesions are cutaneous infarctions that occur around the nailbeds in patients with RA (Bywaters 1949, 1957) (Fig. 2.3a and b). These lesions do not imply the need for intensive immunosuppression. Although such lesions do tend to occur in patients with seropositive RA, they do not correlate with systemic vasculitis in other organs (Watts et al. 1995; Price-Forbes et al. 2002).

Pearl: The development of pericarditis in a patient with RA should not be considered an "intercurrent event".

Comment: Pericarditis is the cardiac manifestation most likely to present early in the setting of RV. Its development should trigger an evaluation for other hallmarks of vasculitis: subtle neurological symptoms of peripheral nerve disease, skin lesions, higher than baseline elevations of acute phase reactants, or hypocomplementemia. One series of 50 patients documented cardiac manifestations in approximately one-third of patients (Scott et al. 1981). These complications included pericarditis, arrhythmia, and aortic incompetence, and myocardial infarction.

Myth: RV is high on the differential diagnosis when a patient with RA has a myocardial infarction.

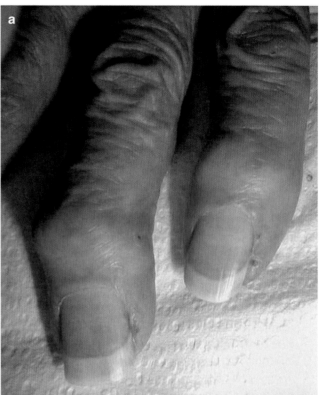

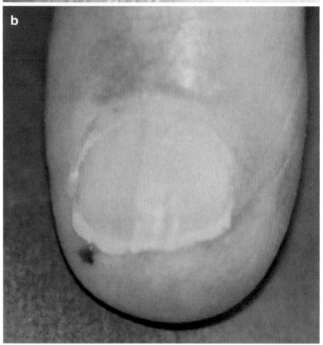

Figs. 2.3 Bywaters' Lesions. (**a**) Seventy-four-year-old woman with osteoarthritis and RA for 15 years treated with methotrexate and prednisone (5 mg daily). The patient developed recurrent periungual and terminal digit infarctions over an 8-month period. These healed without intervention. No active synovitis was present at the time the infarctions developed (Figures courtesy of Dr. Eric Matteson). (**b**) Bywaters' lesions in another patient with RA (Figure courtesy of Dr. John Stone)

Reality: Cases of coronary vasculitis are well-documented in the medical literature (Sokoloff 1953; Cruikschank 1954; Johnson et al. 1969). However, myocardial infarction as a direct result of coronary arteritis in RV is unusual (Van Albada-Kuipers et al. 1986). Clinically manifest coronary vasculitis is likely to occur only in RA patients with clearcut evidence of vasculitis in other organ systems.

Despite the rarity of true coronary vasculitis in RV, one of the most important determinants of the increased mortality in RA patients is an elevated risk of cardiovascular disease. This appears to represent a significant acceleration of common atherosclerosis (Wallberg-Jonsson et al. 2002; Park et al. 2002; Kumeda et al. 2002; Hurlimann et al. 2002).

Myth: Leg ulcers in RA are almost certainly due to vasculitis.

Reality: Other clinical entities often cause leg ulcers in RV. Pyoderma gangrenosum occurs occasionally in RA, but is significantly less common than ulcers due to RV. Indeed, because of the absence of a diagnostic histopathology of pyoderma gangrenosum and the frequency with which biopsies in RV are non-diagnostic, many cases of "pyoderma gangrenosum" associated with RA in the past were probably in fact actually a manifestation of RV.

Another factor that may contribute to the development of leg ulcers in RA is the combination of venous stasis disease and chronic glucocorticoid use, the latter of which leads to increased skin fragility and a tendency to ulcerations with minor trauma. Thus, not all skin ulcerations in RA represent RV.

Leg ulcers in patients with RA often occur due to minor trauma. There may be an underlying vasculitis that promotes the lesion. However, ulcer expansion and chronicity are influenced much more by other factors, including concomitant immunodeficiency, arterial insufficiency, trauma, and dependent edema (Turesson 2004; Puechal et al. 2008). Chronic glucocorticoid use and smoking also promote development of these chronic ulcers. Approximately 30% of patients with Felty's syndrome (neutropenia, splenomegaly, and RA) develop skin ulcers.

The development of leg ulcers should trigger a thorough evaluation for the possibility of RV including, if appropriate, a skin biopsy. Patients with leg ulcers must be monitored closely, particularly those who have high titers of rheumatoid factor, low complement, and cryoglobulins, as more ominous manifestations of RV including digital infarcts and sensory motor neuropathy can occur in these patients (Fig. 2.4).

Appropriate treatment of leg ulcers in patients with RA includes aggressive wound management. This may include skin grafting. Aggressive immunosuppressive therapy and aggressive antiTNF therapy, including the use of biologics, is usually not warranted (Turesson 2004). High-dose glucocorticoids are not warranted; the chronic use of glucocorticoids

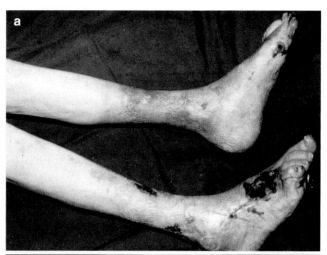

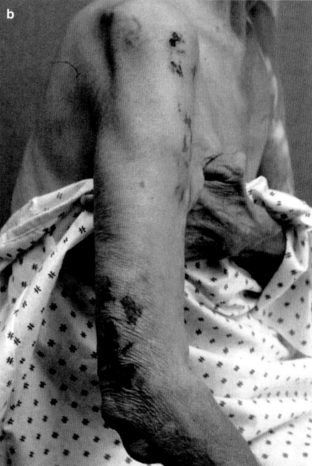

Figs. 2.4 Mononeuritis multiplex with bilateral foot drop on the right and extensive foot ulcerations in a 69 year-old man with a 20-year history of RA. There had been multiple previous episodes of vasculitis; extensive tissue atrophic changes especially of the over the soft tissues of the calf are evident (**a**) The patient also suffered upper extremity ulcerations (**b**) Note, in these figures, the rheumatoid deformities of the feet, the olecranon nodules, left thumb deformity and left-hand muscle atrophy (Figures courtesy of Kenneth Calamia, MD, Mayo Clinic Jacksonville)

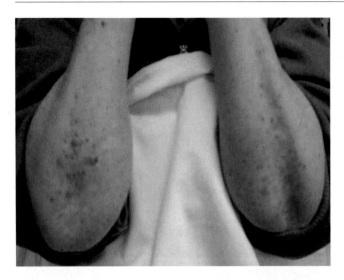

Fig. 2.5 Palpable purpura occurring 4 months after the initiation of etanercept therapy for rheumatoid arthritis in a 61-year-old woman. Biopsy of a lesion revealed leukocytoclastic vasculitis. The lesions resolved with discontinuation of etanercept. Oral prednisone was initiated at 20 mg daily and tapered over 6 weeks (Figure courtesy of Dr. Eric Matteson)

promotes arterial sclerosis and may promote occlusive vasculopathy in patients with vasculitis.

Pearl: TNF inhibitors can cause a drug-induced vasculitis, but this is not "RV".

Comment: Figure 2.5 illustrates a case of small-vessel, leukocytoclastic vasculitis induced by etanercept. The form of vasculitis, limited to the skin and involving small blood vessels only, is a different entity from RV. TNF inhibitor-induced vasculitis is usually self-limited, resolves with discontinuation of the agent, and is unlikely to develop if other TNF inhibitors are used.

Pearl: RV overlaps substantially with polyarteritis nodosa and tends to affect the same types of organs.

Comment: Parallels between RV and polyarteritis nodosa have been recognized for more than half a century (Ball 1954). Both disorders tend to involve medium-sized arteries and to affect the skin, peripheral nerves, gastrointestinal tract, heart, and other organs. RV is somewhat less likely to cause microaneurysms than is polyarteritis nodosa, but microaneurysms complicating the vasculitis of rheumatoid disease have certainly been described (Achkar 1995; Pagnoux et al. 2005).

Pearl: RV is associated with other extraarticular disease, including scleromalacia perforans.

Comment: Vasculitis of RA almost always occurs in patients with other extraarticular features, including nodulosis and inflammatory eye disease. The vasculitis may involve systemic organs including the viscera and the cranial arteries. The involvement of parenchymal organs is often catastrophic

and requires aggressive management (Turesson 2004; Puechal et al. 2008).

Effective control of RA is important in RV. However, once RV is established, the role for antiTNF therapy for management of the vasculitis of RA is uncertain. Some reports claim benefits of this approach, others suggest no benefit or disease worsening while patients are on TNF inhibitors (Puechal et al. 2008).

Decisions about the treatment of RV must be made on a case-by-case basis. However, high-dose glucocorticoids and cyclophosphamide are the standard of care for disseminated disease involving multiple organs.

Pearl: A rise in the white blood cell count, thrombocytosis, and acute phase reactants may precede or accompany RV.

Comment: A marked increase in acute phase reactants may reflect active joint disease as well as extraarticular manifestations. There is no single test that predicts the development of RV, but patients with RV often have high titers of rheumatoid factor and/or antiCCP antibodies, anemia, elevated acute phase reactants, thrombocytosis, and leukocytosis (Turesson and Matteson 2008). Patients with antinuclear antibodies and antineutrophil cytoplasmic antibodies that cause perinuclear (P-ANCA) staining by immunofluorescence have higher frequencies of extraarticular manifestations of RA, including vasculitis.

Myth: Distal, symmetric polyneuropathy occurring in a patient who has longstanding RA is likely to be a vasculitic neuropathy.

Reality: The inclination is to lump most patients who have symmetrical sensory symptoms into the category of distal peripheral neuropathy, along with the 400 or so other causes of this disorder (including diabetic neuropathy and alcoholic neuropathy). In patients who have RA who are the typical substrate for RV, however, the cause of such symptoms is often vasculitic neuropathy (Puechal et al. 1995). Careful evaluations of these patients and an increase in their RA therapy may be required, even if no specific therapy for vasculitis is initiated.

In contrast to the myriad other causes of peripheral neuropathy (e.g., diabetes-associated and alcohol-related peripheral nerve dysfunction), the onset of vasculitic neuropathy in rheumatoid vasculopathy can be quite rapid. An unusually swift tempo may be the telltale piece of information indicating that further evaluation is required.

Myth: The first symptom of mononeuritis multiplex is pain or weakness.

Reality: As a rule, pain is not striking at the onset of vasculitic neuropathy; rather, the predominant symptom is anesthesia. Within days or weeks of the start of sensory symptoms, muscle weakness caused by motor nerve infarction may ensue (Said and Lacroix 2005). Patients often experience their first symptoms – numbness, tingling, or other sensory symptoms – after a period of sleep (Schmid et al. 1961).

Myth: Mononeuritis multiplex is always asymmetric.

Reality: Mononeuritis multiplex has three clinical hallmarks: asymmetry, asynchrony, and a predilection for distal nerves. Early in the process, nerve involvement is likely to affect one side more than the other (e.g., the left peroneal nerve, leading to a unilateral foot drop). Within days to weeks, however, the process can develop a more symmetrical appearance, as distal peripheral nerves are affected in an additive fashion.

The full development of motor dysfunction within a given nerve often occurs within the day of onset. There is maximal damage at the time the condition is recognized, followed by deficits that persist for weeks, months, and sometimes forever.

Myth: Diagnosing vasculitic neuropathy in RA often means recognizing fire through a lot of smoke. This is true even in the interpretation of histopathology.

Reality: Sural nerve biopsies sometimes show active arteritis, particularly if the patient has been treated intensively before the procedure. However, the finding of a proliferative endarteritis of the epineurium reflects the healed stage of a previous acute arteritis (Conn et al. 1972). Clinicopathologic correlation is essential in such cases. In the optimal situation, this means sitting down at the microscope with the neuropathologist and correlating the histopathologic findings with the patient's clinical presentation, serologic features, and electrodiagnostic study results.

Pearl: Vasculitis is a crucial feature in the formation of rheumatoid nodules.

Comment: Vascular inflammation has long been considered a primary event in the formation of rheumatoid nodules (Sokoloff 1953). A small-vessel vasculitis that leads to fibrinoid necrosis forms the core of the lesion in rheumatoid nodules. This core is surrounded by a proliferation of fibroblasts.

Although RV is strongly associated with rheumatoid nodules, only a minority of patients with nodules develop RV. The nodules of one patient who did are shown in Fig. 2.6.

Myth: The incidence of RV is diminishing.

Reality: Although the assumption that more effective therapy will lead to the observation of less RV in the future, there remain few data on the impact of biologic agents on the incidence of RV. Data from the era just preceding the common availability of biologics are contradictory on the changing incidence of RV (Watts et al. 2004; Turesson 2004).

In a population-based study from Norfolkshire in the United Kingdom that covered the years from 1988 to 2002, a decrease in the annual incidence of RV from about 12 per

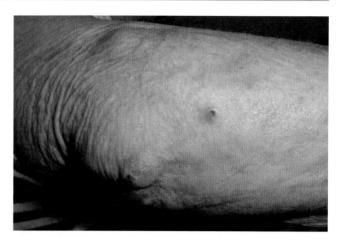

Fig. 2.6 Healing, superficial infarctions of rheumatoid nodules. The patient developed several ulcers and mononeuritis multiplex of the lower extremities approximately 4 months after the onset of these elbow and finger infarctions (Figure courtesy of Dr. Eric Matteson)

million individuals to less than 4 per million was reported (Watts et al. 2004). In contrast, in a population-based study from Olmsted County, Minnesota that examined data covering a period of 40 years observed no decrease in either the incidence of RV or other extra-articular manifestations of RA (Turesson 2004). Data on the impact of biologic agents on RV is awaited eagerly.

Pearl: The development of scleritis in a patient with RA is often the first indication of RV.

Comment: In a patient with longstanding, seropositive RA, scleritis equals vasculitis, even if histopathological proof is difficult to obtain. In one series of nine patients with RA and necrotizing scleritis, scleral biopsies confirmed vasculitis in each case (Fong 1991).

Scleritis can occur in either anterior or posterior locations (Okhravi et al. 2005). Bilateral disease is quite common, though one eye can be affected more severely than the other. Anterior forms of scleritis are evident from the appearance of the eye. In contrast to episcleritis (which may occur in the absence of an underlying condition), scleritis is usually highly symptomatic and cannot be ignored by the patient.

Anterior scleritis is subdivided further into three clinical variants:

1. Diffuse (least severe) (Fig. 2.7a)
2. Nodular (intermediate in severity) (Fig. 2.7b)
3. Necrotizing (most severe) (Fig. 2.7c)

These variants are largely non-overlapping. Progression from one variant to another is unusual. The necrotizing form of scleritis may lead to scleromalacia perforans.

In contrast to anterior scleritis, obvious on clinical examination, posterior scleritis must be diagnosed by inference from the patient's symptoms – primarily a deep-seated pain

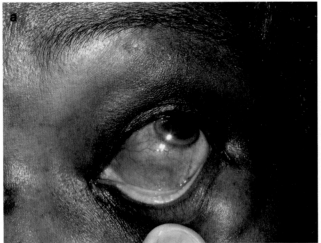

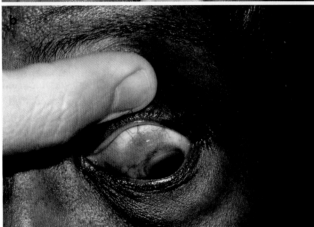

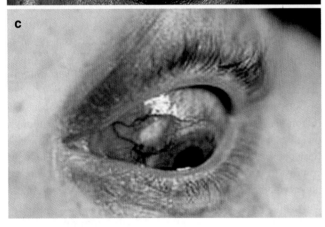

Fig. 2.7 (a–c) Diffuse, nodular, and necrotizing scleritis in patients with rheumatoid arthritis (Figures courtesy of Dr. John Stone)

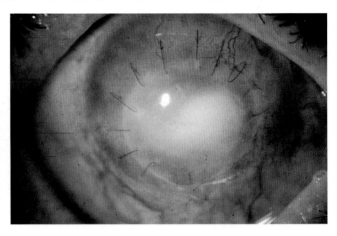

Fig. 2.8 Patch sewn over a perforated cornea that resulted from rheumatoid vasculitis and the corneal melt syndrome. The patient is blind in this eye, but may benefit in the future from a corneal transplant. (Figure courtesy of Dr. John Stone)

and ocular tenderness, but also visual blurring. The posterior coat of the eye is observed to be thickened on orbital ultrasonography or magnetic resonance imaging (McCluskey et al. 1999). Posterior scleritis should be considered in patients with RA who present with severe headaches.

Pearl: Beware the "corneal melt" syndrome in the RA patient with a painful red eye.

Comment: Two terms rheumatologists must know in order to converse with their ophthalmology colleagues and avoid ocular disasters are PUK (an acronym for peripheral ulcerative keratitis, generally spelled out: "P – U – K"), and its potential consequence, corneal melt. A corneal transplant in the eye of a patient with PUK and corneal melt is shown in Fig. 2.8.

PUK can be thought of as necrotizing scleritis that is situated in a highly unfortunate portion of the eye: the outer rim of the cornea or the kerato-scleral junction. PUK and necrotizing scleritis often occur together. In PUK, inflammatory cells infiltrate the peripheral area of the cornea, leading to a crescent-shaped ulceration near the corneoscleral junction. The principal complication of PUK is a "corneal melt" syndrome, in which corneal keratolysis, perforation of the globe, and visual failure can result within days (Squirrell et al. 1999). Following the occurrence of a corneal melt, patients often lose all useful vision in the eye. Both necrotizing scleritis and PUK require urgent therapy with high doses of immunosuppressive medications, generally both high-dose glucocorticoids and cyclophosphamide.

Myth: The finding of rheumatoid nodules in the lungs usually coincides with RV.

Reality: Although rheumatoid nodules occur in the lungs and pathologic evidence of vasculitis is an inherent feature of rheumatoid nodules wherever they are found, most patients with rheumatoid nodules in the lungs do not have evidence of systemic vasculitis (Sokoloff et al. 1953; Yousem et al. 1985). The biggest problem that pulmonary rheumatoid nodules cause is the concern that they may actually represent a malignancy.

Pearl: Two types of renal disease occur in RV: a PAN-like medium-vessel renal arteritis, and a pauci-immune glomerulonephritis. Both of these complications are rare.

Comment: Both renal artery involvement similar to that which occurs in polyarteritis nodosa and glomerulonephritis that is reminiscent of microscopic polyangiitis, or Wegener's granulomatosis are well described (Ball 1954; Johnson 1959; Harper et al. 1997; Boers et al. 1987). Medium-vessel arteritis involving the renal vessels rarely leads to microaneurysms, in contrast to PAN. The glomerular pathology caused by vasculitis in RA is a pauci-immune glomerulonephritis, sometimes associated with crescent formation.

This type of glomerular disease contrasts with common beliefs about the pathophysiology of RV in other organs, which is generally considered to result from an immune complex-mediated process characterized by the organ deposition of rheumatoid factor, complement components, and other immunoreactants (Epstein and Engleman 1959). Antineutrophil cytoplasmic antibodies (ANCA) do not play a role in the glomerulonephritis that occasionally complicates rheumatoid disease. If a patient has ANCA directed against either proteinase-3 or myeloperoxidase, then a second process is present.

Pearl: The strongest risk factor for the development of RV is a high serum titer of rheumatoid factor.

Comment: Vasculitis in seronegative RA is rare (Mongan et al. 1969; Geirsson et al. 1987). High titers of rheumatoid factor are reported consistently to be the strongest predictor of the development of RV (Vollertsen et al. 1986 (Medicine); Geirsson et al. 1987). Few data exist to date on the correlation between antiCCP antibodies, but this correlation is undoubtedly high. Serum levels of IgM rheumatoid factor – the serotype usually measured – are poor markers of disease activity (Scott et al. 1981; 38).

Myth: Cyclophosphamide should not be used if the only manifestation of RV is skin ulceration.

Reality: Some baseball managers err by "going to the bullpen" – i.e., bringing on a relief pitcher – too late. Some clinicians make the same mistake by leaving cyclophosphamide on the bench for too long.

Clinicians rightly resent having to contemplate cyclophosphamide for "skin-only" disease. However, in some patients, cyclophosphamide is an essential drug, without which, healing will not occur. The baleful direct effects (pain, reduced mobility, increasing incapacitation), and the substantial complications of leg ulcers (infection, sepsis), underscore the need to suppress and heal these lesions as quickly as possible.

High doses of prednisone, conventional DMARDs, and biologic agents should be considered before cyclophosphamide. However, for disease that is severe at the time of diagnosis and for vasculitis that does not continue to improve as glucocorticoids are tapered, the use of cyclophosphamide earlier rather than later may be the correct choice.

Myth: RV can cause an immune complex-mediated glomerulonephritis.

Reality: The histological findings in RV may include: (1) leukocytoclastic vasculitis associated with immune complex deposition in venules, capillaries, and arterioles; and (2) pauci-immune lesions (i.e., inflammation associated with sparse deposition of immunoreactants) in medium-sized arteries and renal glomeruli. One paradoxical finding in RV is that although glomeruli are considered small blood vessels – the renal equivalent of capillaries – the well-documented cases of renal involvement in RV are generally associated with pauci-immune glomerulonephritis.

References

Achkar AA, Stanson AW, Johnson CM et al Rheumatoid vasculitis manifesting as intra-abdominal hemorrhage. Mayo Clin Proc 1995; 70(6):565–9

Ball J. Rheumatoid arthritis and polyarteritis nodosa. Ann Rheum Dis 1954; 13:277–290

Boers M, Croonen AM, Dijkmans BAC, et al Renal findings in rheumatoid arthritis: Clinical aspects of 132 necropsies. Ann Rheum Dis 1987; 46:658–663

Bywaters EGL. A variant of rheumatoid arthritis characterized by recurrent digital pad nodules and palmar fasciitis, closely resembling palindromic rheumatism. Ann Rheum Dis 1949; 8:1–30

Bywaters EGL. Peripheral vascular obstruction in rheumatoid arthritis and its relationship to other vascular lesions. Ann Rheum Dis 1957; 16:84–103

Conn DL, Schroeter AL, McDuffie FC. Immunopathologic study of sural nerves in rheumatoid arthritis. Arthritis Rheum 1972; 15:135

Cruikschank B. The arteritis of rheumatoid arthritis. Ann Rheum Dis 1954; 13:136–145

Epstein WV, Engleman EP. The relation of the rheumatoid factor content of serum to clinical neurovascular manifestations of rheumatoid arthritis. Arthritis Rheum 1959; 2:250–258

Fong LP, Sainz de la Maza M, Rice BA et al Immunopathology of scleritis. Ophthalmology 1991; 98(4):472–9

Geirsson AJ, Sturfelt G, Truedsson L, et al Clinical and serological features of severe vasculitis in rheumatoid arthritis: Prognostic implications. Ann Rheum Dis 1987; 46:727–733

Harper L, Cockwell P, Howie AJ, et al Focal segmental necrotizing glomerulonephritis in rheumatoid arthritis. QJM 1997; 90:125

Hazes JM. Management of Extraarticular Disease and Complications. In: Hochberg MC, Silman AJ, Smolen JS, Weinblatt ME, Weisman MH (eds) Extraarticular Features of Rheumatoid Arthritis and Systemic Involvement. Rheumatology (4th edn). Philadelphia, PA, Mosby, 2008, pp. 897–914

Hurlimann D, Forster A, Noll, G et al Anti-tumor necrosis factor-alpha treatment improves endothelial function in patients with rheumatoid arthritis. Circulation 2002; 106:2184

Johnson RL, Smyth CJ, Holt GW, et al Steroid therapy and vascular lesions in rheumatoid arthritis. Arthritis Rheum 1959; 2:224–249

Kumeda, Y, Inaba, M, Goto, H, et al Increased thickness of the arterial intima-media detected by ultrasonography in patients with rheumatoid arthritis. Arthritis Rheum 2002; 46:1489

McCluskey PJ, Watson PG, Lightman S, et al Posterior scleritis: Clinical features, systemic associations, and outcome in a large series of patients. Ophthalmology 1999; 106:2380–2386

Mongan ES, Cass RM, Jacox RF, et al A study of the relation of seronegative and seropositive rheumatoid arthritis to each other and to necrotizing vasculitis. Am J Med 1969; 47:23–35

Okhravi N, Odufuwa B, McCluskey P, et al Scleritis. Surv Ophthalm 2005; 50(4):351–363

Pagnoux, C, Mahr, A, Cohen, P, Guillevin, L. Presentation and outcome of gastrointestinal involvement in systemic necrotizing vasculitides: Analysis of 62 patients with polyarteritis nodosa, microscopic polyangiitis, Wegener granulomatosis, Churg-Strauss syndrome, or rheumatoid arthritis-associated vasculitis. Medicine (Baltimore) 2005; 84:115

Park YB, Ahn CW, Choi HK, et al Atherosclerosis in rheumatoid arthritis: Morphologic evidence obtained by carotid ultrasound. Arthritis Rheum 2002; 46:1714

Price-Forbes AN, Watts RA, Lane SE, et al Do we need to treat isolated nailfold vasculitis (NFV) in rheumatoid arthritis (RA) more aggressively? Abstract 848, American College of Rheumatology annual scientific meeting, October 2002

Puechal X, Said G, Hilliquin P, et al Peripheral neuropathy with necrotizing vasculitis in rheumatoid arthritis. A clinicopathologic and prognostic study of thirty-two patients. Arthritis Rheum 1995; 38:1618–1629

Puechal X, Miceli-Richard C, Mejjad O, et al Anti-tumour necrosis factor treatment in patients with refractory systemic vasculitis associated with rheumatoid arthritis. Ann Rheum Dis 2008; 67:880–884

Said G, Lacroix C. Primary and secondary vasculitis neuropathy. J Neurol 2005; 252:633–641

Schmid FR, Cooper NS, Ziff M, et al Arteritis in rheumatoid arthritis. Am J Med 1961; 30:56–83

Scott DG, Bacon PA, Tribe CR. Systemic rheumatoid vasculitis: A clinical and laboratory study of 50 cases. Medicine (Baltimore) 1981; 60:288

Sokoloff L. The heart in rheumatoid arthritis. Am Heart J 1953; 45:635

Sokoloff L, McCluskey RT, Bunim JJ. Vascularity of the early subcutaneous nodule in rheumatoid arthritis. Arch Pathol 1953; 55: 475–479

Squirrell DM, Winfield J, Amos RS. Peripheral ulcerative keratitis "corneal melt" and rheumatoid arthritis: A case series. Rheumatology 1999; 1245–1248

Turesson C, Matteson EL. Management of extraarticular disease manifestations in rheumatoid arthritis. Curr Opin Rheum 2004;16:206–211

Turesson C, Matteson EL. Extraarticular features of rheumatoid arthritis and systemic involvement. In: Hochberg MC, Silman AJ, Smolen JS, Weinblatt ME, Weisman MH (eds) Rheumatology (4th edn). Philadelphia, PA, Mosby, 2008, pp. 773–783

Turesson C, O'Fallon WM, Crowson C, et al Extraarticular disease manifestations in rheumatoid arthritis: Incidence, trends, and risk factors over 46 years. Annals of Rheumatic Disease 2003; 62:722–727

Turesson, C, McClelland, R, Christianson, TJ, Matteson, EL. No decrease over time in the incidence of vasculitis or other extra-artic-ular manifestations in rheumatoid arthritis (abstract). Arthritis Rheum 2004; 50:S380

Turesson C, Schaid DJ, Weyand CM, et al The impact of HLA-DRB1 genes on extraarticular disease manifestations in rheumatoid arthritis. Arthritis Res Ther 2005; 7:R1386–R1393

Van Albada-Kuipers GA, Bruijn JA, Westedt ML, et al Coronary arteritis complicating rheumatoid arthritis. Ann Rheum Dis 1986; 45:963

Van Gaalen FA, Linn-Rasker SP, van Venrooij WJ, et al Autoantibodies to cyclic citrullinated pepties predict progression to rheumatoid arthritis in patients with undifferentiated arthritis. Arthritis Rheum 2004; 50(3):709–715

Vollertsen RS, Conn DL, Ballard DJ, et al Rheumatoid vasculitis: Survival and associated risk factors. Medicine 1986; 65(6):365–375

Voskuyl AE, Zwinderman AH, Wested ML, et al The mortality of rheumatoid vasculitis compared with rheumatoid arthritis. Arthritis Rheum 1996; 39:266–271

Wallberg-Jonsson, S, Cvetkovic, JT, Sundqvist, KG, et al Activation of the immune system and inflammatory activity in relation to markers of atherothrombotic disease and atherosclerosis in rheumatoid arthritis. J Rheumatol 2002; 29:875

Watts RA, Carruthers DM, Scott DG. Isolated nail fold vasculitis in rheumatoid arthritis. Ann Rheum Dis 1995; 54:927

Watts RA, Mooney J, Lane SE, Scott DG. Rheumatoid vasculitis: Becoming extinct?. Rheumatology (Oxford) 2004; 43:920

Yousem SA, Colby TV, Carrington CB. Lung biopsy in rheumatoid arthritis. Am Rev Respir Dis 1985; 131:770

Adult-Onset Still's Disease

3

Michael H. Weisman

3.1 Overview of Adult-Onset Still's Disease

> Adult-onset Still's disease (AOSD) was described originally by Eric Bywaters in 1971.
> AOSD closely resembles systemic-onset juvenile idiopathic arthritis, a pediatric disorder known originally as Still's disease.
> An intensely inflammatory, multiorgan system disorder characterized by a polyarthritis, high spiking fevers, and an evanescent, salmon-colored rash (Figs. 3.1a–c).
> The rash is described as small macules that disappear during the night but reappear the next day, usually coincident with a fever spike.
> Peripheral joint involvement can be fleeting but also may settle into a refractory, destructive arthritis marked by a tendency in some joints for fusion.
> AOSD is typically seronegative. Patients do not have rheumatoid factor or antibodies to cyclic citrullinated peptides.
> Other common features are leukocytosis, thrombocytosis, elevations of the serum hepatic aminotransferase concentrations, splenomegaly, and serositis.
> Pharyngitis is often the initial symptom.

Pearl: Still's disease should not be regarded as a category of "juvenile rheumatoid arthritis".

Comment: AOSD strongly resembles the pediatric condition known as "Still's disease". Bywaters wrote that Still's disease was often referred to as "juvenile rheumatoid arthritis" (JRA), a name that (he believed) prejudged the issue of the disorder's appropriate classification (Bywaters 1971). Bywaters questioned whether Still's disease was really related directly to the JRA/RA disease spectrum, or whether it comprised an entirely separate condition. Bywaters strongly favored the hypothesis that AOSD and Still's disease formed a spectrum of disease that is separate from that of RA and JRA (JRA is now termed juvenile idiopathic arthritis (Chap. 4).

Pearl: Bywaters anticipated the relationship between AOSD and the group of conditions now termed "autoinflammatory syndromes" (Chapter 5).

Comment: Bywaters commented on the similarities between AOSD, familial Mediterranean fever, and an entity now known as the Muckle–Wells syndrome (Chapter 5). These other disorders, now grouped as autoinflammatory syndrome, are characterized by an urticarial rash, "aguey bouts" (malarial fever), and amyloidosis, all features typical of AOSD.

In truth, Bywaters' original paper is almost all one needs to know about AOSD. Little of any major significance has been written since those papers, with the important exception being the identification of AOSD in many patients as an IL-1 mediated disease (see below).

Pearl: The fever curve is the most important diagnostic criterion for AOSD.

Comment: Very few conditions mimic the fevers of AOSD, with their tendency to decline to normal temperatures at least once every 24-h period. Most other rheumatic conditions associated with fever (and most infectious or malignant causes) tend to be associated with more continuous patterns of fever if left untreated, with temperature elevations sustained over days.

Bywaters described the fever of AOSD as dramatic and remittent, often mistaken for sepsis and treated energetically but in vain with a succession of antibiotics. Patients' temperatures should be measured every 4h to demonstrate the characteristic quotidian (or "double-quotidian") pattern, because fever spikes can occur at any time in the 24h period.

Myth: AOSD is a benign, self-limited condition that does not produce joint damage or disability.

Reality: This statement is a total myth. The original papers by Bywaters and Aptekar in the early 1970s emphasized the benign nature of AOSD (Bywaters 1971; Aptekar et al. 1973), but almost every large series since then has indicated that the disease becomes chronic, if intermittent, in the majority of

J. H. Stone (ed.), *A Clinician's Pearls and Myths in Rheumatology,*
DOI:10.1007/978-1-84800-934-9_3, © Springer Science + Business Media B.V. 2009

Fig. 3.1 The evancescent, salmon-colored rash of adult-onset Still's disease (Figures courtesy of Dr. John Stone)

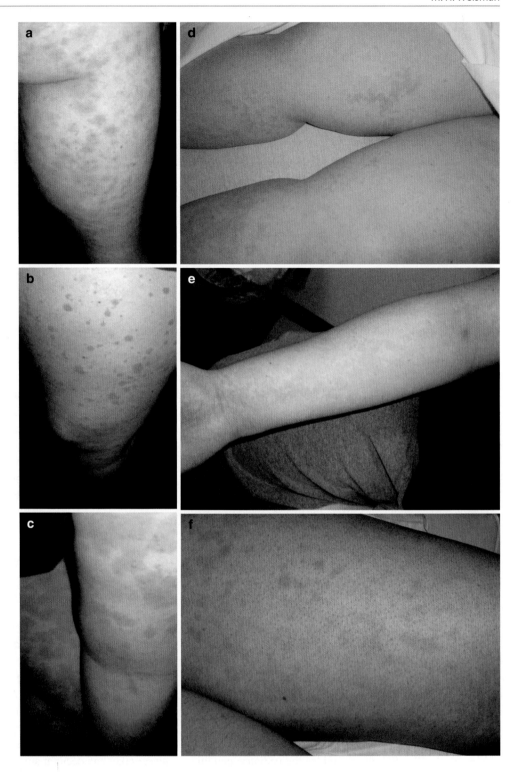

patients. In addition, it can be notoriously difficult to treat. The joint manifestations and the systemic features may be out of sync with each other: one can dominate the clinical picture while the other remains quiet. This creates challenges in selecting how aggressive to be with therapy.

Joint destruction can occur in AOSD patients. Hip or knee replacements are not uncommon sequellae of this disease. The wrists are particularly prone to damage in AOSD and often develop joint fusion. Joint damage can occur in AOSD

in multiple joints in a symmetric fashion, with a distribution similar to that of seropositive RA.

The state of the literature on AOSD is that it is difficult to make anything other than general conclusions about its natural history, because of the many different definitions used to characterize the disease course, the varying length of follow-up of different studies, and the selection bias inherent in many of the cohorts reported (Esdaile 2008). One reasonable statement about AOSD is that 30–50% of patients will display a chronic course, and the remainder are divided equally between those who have self-limited disease and those who experience intermittent disease exacerbations. The initial enthusiasm that AOSD is a benign, self-limited condition is clearly not the case most of the time.

Pearl: Arthritis may be absent in the initial stages of AOSD.

Comment: Joint pain is common in the early stages, but frank arthritis may not be evident. Many patients with AOSD present as fevers of unknown origin. In this setting, joint involvement can be masked or ignored by the overwhelming nature of the systemic disease features such as fever, rash, anemia, leukocytosis, and thrombocytosis. The absence of arthritis as a dominant symptom makes the diagnosis difficult in the early stages and probably accounts for the oft-quoted diagnostic delays, which frequently approach 6 months.

In some patients, mild joint involvement is not accompanied by obvious swelling or synovitis. However, if joint symptoms have not become more obvious within 6 months of the patient's presentation, then the diagnosis of AOSD should be held in some doubt.

Pearl: The rash of AOSD does not itch, burn, or sting, and may therefore be missed by patient and clinician alike.

Comment: Aside from its salmon-colored appearance and characteristically evanescent nature, there are few other rules about the AOSD rash except that is it generally asymptomatic. The rash has a tendency to affect the trunk but certainly occurs on the extremities, as well.

It has been written that the rash of AOSD accompanies the fever spike in the afternoon when the rounding physicians are not in attendance, and that clinicians who see the patient only in the early morning or late in the day will miss the rash entirely. This statement flies in the face of the fact that the fevers of AOSD can occur at any time. The more important point is that repeated examinations and vigilance for observation of the rash may be required to detect the AOSD exanthema. The poor lighting of most hospital rooms and failure to examine the patient's skin thoroughly probably both contribute to the elusiveness of the rash. Dermatographism, a common feature of AOSD, is non-specific.

Myth: AOSD disease management is fairly straightforward and tends to follow the approach once used in RA. Nonsteroidal anti-inflammatory drugs (NSAIDs) should be attempted first, followed by disease-modifying antirheumatic drugs (DMARDs), and then anti-TNF agents. There is no role for systemic glucocorticoids.

Reality: Unfortunately, these statements contain not one but several myths. First, the management of AOSD patients is anything but straightforward. Patients seldom have a complete, sustained response to NSAIDs alone. The author sometimes uses a high dose up to 200 mg/day of indomethacin to get the biggest bang for the buck, yet additional therapies are required in most cases. No clinical trial data are available to support the efficacy of traditional DMARDs in this disease, e.g., methotrexate, sulfasalazine, and hydroxychloroquine. Finally, much against expectations, anti-TNF therapies for AOSD have demonstrated only marginal (read largely disappointing) results (Husni et al. 2002; Fautrel et al. 2005).

The second major myth uttered above pertains to glucocorticoids. In fact, high doses of systemic glucocorticoids are often required to gain control of the acute disease manifestations. If a relapse of symptoms occurs during the glucocorticoid taper, then methotrexate should be started with a rapid titration of the dose toward 25 mg/week. Clinical experience suggests that the combination of glucocorticoids and methotrexate suffices to control AOSD in a sizeable proportion of patients, but not all.

The extrapolation of IL-1 inhibition strategies to AOSD made perfect sense in view of the similarities between AOSD and the autoinflammatory syndromes, most of which are mediated by abnormalities in the IL-1 pathway. Multiple reports indicate a rapid and sustained reduction in signs and symptoms along with parallel improvement of inflammatory markers (Fitzgerald et al. 2005; Bresnihan 2008). Some patients with treatment-resistant AOSD have experienced striking responses to IL-1 inhibition. This author has even used responsiveness to anakinra as a diagnostic test for AOSD in some patients.

However, anakinra is a difficult drug to use, not only because of the requirement for daily parenteral injections but also the frequent and sometimes dramatic skin rashes associated with this agent. Such reactions tend to resolve within a few weeks of continued administration, but newer IL-1 blocking agents with greater ease of administration are welcome.

Myth: The presence of hepatic, pulmonary, and cardiac involvement decreases the likelihood of AOSD and adds new urgency to the search for vasculitis or an infectious etiology of the patient's problems.

Reality: Disease manifestations in the liver, lungs, and heart were present but not emphasized clearly in the initial reports of Bywaters, Aptekar, and colleagues (Bywaters 1971; Aptekar et al. 1973). In the decades since those original descriptions, a fuller picture of the disease has emerged.

AOSD patients can present with dramatic liver function abnormalities. As a result, various forms of hepatitis must be considered and excluded. A reactive hemophagocytic syndrome must also be considered. Pleural effusions and even interstitial lung disease have been observed, as well. Pericarditis is evident in some patients.

In a disease for which there exists no single diagnostic test, one must always keep an open mind about other etiologies. However, the presence of liver, lung, or cardiac disease does not necessarily exclude AOSD.

Pearl: Primary renal involvement does not occur in AOSD.

Comment: Despite the protean nature of AOSD, this Pearl holds up. Primary renal disease is not characteristic of this disorder. Of course, one must account for the possibility that renal dysfunction might result from intercurrent problems, e.g., acute tubular necrosis caused by NSAIDs. But the guiding principle that primary renal involvement does not occur in AOSD can be very useful in differentiating AOSD from various forms of vasculitis, lupus, or malignancies.

Pearl: The diagnosis of AOSD can be made without actually seeing the patient and with the aid of a cell-phone camera.

Comment: This outrageous Pearl is actually true in some cases. Few disease entities reproduce the fever curve of AOSD and if a reliable nursing record of temperature recordings can be obtained, the consultant can make the diagnosis from the nurses' station. Photodocumentation of the rash before meeting the patient in person can add further certainty to the diagnosis.

Pearl: Severe sore throat can be both a misleading clue as well as a helpful adjunct to the diagnosis of AOSD.

Comment: Some patients with AOSD present with severe sore throats, even to the point of having difficulty swallowing. Despite the severity of this symptom, patients with this complaint generally manifest no physical evidence of tonsillar, laryngeal, or tracheal inflammation. These patients usually undergo courses of antibiotics, often have multiple visits to otolaryngologists, and even sometimes undergo endoscopic procedures in efforts to understand the source of this complaint.

Sore throat is as common as rash and arthritis as the presenting complaint of AOSD (Nguyen and Weisman 1997). Thus, to the knowledgeable clinician, a severe sore throat that defies the conventional explanation can be a clue to the diagnosis of AOSD.

Myth: An elevated ferritin level is diagnostic for AOSD.

Reality: There are no diagnostic tests for AOSD. The serum ferritin is nearly always elevated in AOSD, but because of the low specificity of this test its positive predictive value is poor. Other acute phase reactants are also elevated, and often strikingly so. As examples, an increased ESR is nearly universal; the platelet count can exceed one million per cubic millimeter. A significant leukocytosis is also very common.

The negative predictive value of a serum ferritin level normal or only moderately elevated is probably quite high, but this has not been tested in a prospective study. Moreover, the incremental improvement in terms of diagnosis offered by an elevated serum ferritin level compared with measurements of other acute phase reactants is not clear.

Pearl: Advances in our understanding of innate immunity mediated diseases and certain auto-inflammatory conditions (especially in children) have enabled us to diagnose and treat AOSD more effectively.

Comment: The observations that certain "autoinflammatory syndromes" are under genetic control and that many of those conditions can be traced to mutations which cause increased IL-1 production have opened our eyes to new therapeutic targets for AOSD (Allantaz et al. 2007). The discovery of the importance of the IL-1 pathway in the pathogenesis of AOSD and related conditions has increased our understanding of the inflammasome and opened the door for the successful treatment of many AOSD patients with IL-1 antagonists.

References

Allantaz F, Chaussabel D, Banchereau J, Pascual V. Microarray-based identification of novel biomarkers in IL-1-medicated diseases. Curr Opin Immunol 2007; 19:623–632

Aptekar RG, Decker JL, Bujak JS, Wolff SM. Adult onset juvenile rheumatoid arthritis. Arthritis Rheum 1973; 16:715–718

Bresnihan B. Cytokine neutralizers: IL-1 inhibitors. In: Hochberg MC, Silman AJ, Smolen JS, Weinblatt ME, Weisman MH (eds) Rheumatology (4th edn). Edinburgh, UK, Mosby, 2008, pp. 495–500

Bywaters, EGL. Still's disease in the adult. Ann Rheum Dis 1971; 30:121–132

Esdaile J. Adult Still's disease. In: Hochberg MC, Silman AJ, Smolen JS, Weinblatt ME, Weisman MH (eds) Rheumatology (4th edn). Edinburgh, UK, Mosby, 2008, pp. 785–792

Fautrel B, Sibilia J, Mariettte X, et al Tumor necrosis factor alpha blocking agents in refractory adult Still's disease: An observational study of 20 cases. Ann Rheum Dis 2005; 64:262–266

Fitzgerald AA, LeClercq SA, Yan A, et al Rapid responses to anakinra in patients with refractory adult-onset Still's disease. Arthritis Rheum 2005; 52:1794–1803

Husni ME, Maier AL, Mease PJ, et al Etanercept in the treatment of adult patients with Still's disease. Arthritis Rheum 2002; 46:1171–1176

Nguyen KH, Weisman MH. Severe sore throat as a presenting symptom of adult-onset still's disease: A case series and review of the literature. J Rheumatol 1997; 24:592–597

Juvenile Idiopathic Arthritis

4

Patience H. White, Patricia Woo, and Carol B. Lindsley

4.1 Overview of Juvenile Idiopathic Arthritis

> Juvenile idiopathic arthritis (JIA) is an umbrella term for a group of persistent arthritides of unknown etiology that affect children under the age of 16, and last for more than 6 weeks (Petty et al. 2004). The clinically defined categories are shown in Table 4.1.

> The pathogenesis of these diseases involves both autoimmune and genetic factors. Dysregulation of the immune and inflammatory systems are observed. In addition, hormonal, infectious, and other environmental agents yet to be identified probably participate in the disease-diagnosing process.

> The diagnosis of JIA is rendered from the combination of data derived from the history, physical examination, and laboratory testing.

> The prevalence of JIA varies depending on subtypes. As a group, the prevalence is generally agreed to be 1:1,000 children.

> For the vast majority of patients with JIA, the immunogenetic associations, clinical course and functional outcome are quite different from adult-onset rheumatoid arthritis. In addition, certain specific disease subsets are not observed at all or are seen very rarely in adults. These subsets include the oligoarticular pattern of arthritis associated with uveitis and antinuclear antibodies, and sJIA (sJIA).

> Most patients with JIA do not achieve a remission and require long-term treatment. However, the use of new therapies such as methotrexate and the biologic agents has improved the outcome of JIA.

Myth: Systemic-onset juvenile idiopathic arthritis (sJIA) represents a homogeneous disease subset.

Reality: The classic clinical signs of quotidian fevers, macular rashes, and arthritis separate patients with sJIA (sometimes termed "Still's disease") from the oligoarticular and polyarticular JIA subtypes. However, clinicians have long recognized that sJIA has a broad clinical spectrum that includes patients with mild to severe arthritis, transient to persistent systemic features, variable disease duration, differing propensities to relapse, and disparate responses to standard therapies.

Patients with sJIA tend to respond to methotrexate less well than do those with other forms of JIA (Woo 2006). Fewer than 50% of patients with sJIA achieve good clinical responses on methotrexate and even these are often not sustained (Lovell 2006). Some patients show dramatic improvement with IL-1 receptor antagonist therapy, but overall the percentage of patients who respond to this intervention is less than 50% (Lequerre and Quartier 2008). Finally, a substantial proportion of patients with sJIA appear to respond to IL-6 blockade (Yokota et al. 2008). These results suggest strongly that subtypes of sJIA exist.

Other systemic inflammatory disorders that mimic the clinical features of sJIA (e.g., the autoinflammatory/periodic fever syndromes) have specific single-gene mutations that lead to an imbalance toward a proinflammatory state. These conditions include the chronic infantile neurological cutaneous arthropathy (CINCA) syndrome, the Muckle–Wells syndrome, the hyper-IgD syndrome, and the tumor-necrosis receptor associated periodic syndromes (TRAPSs). All of these conditions are associated with urticarial or macular rashes, periodic fevers, constitutional disturbances, and arthralgia or arthritis – disease features that mimic those of sJIA closely. Gene association studies have revealed many cytokine genes that alter the homeostasis of the sJIA inflammatory response (Woo 2000). Thus, although sJIA and the autoinflammatory syndromes can bear striking resemblance to each other clinically, the genetic background of sJIA appears to be far more complex.

J. H. Stone (ed.), *A Clinician's Pearls and Myths in Rheumatology,*
DOI:10.1007/978-1-84800-934-9_4, © Springer Science + Business Media B.V. 2009

Table 4.1 International league against rheumatism classification of JIA (Petty 2004)

• Oligorticular – persistent or extended
• Polyarticular – rheumatoid factor negative
• Polyarticular – rheumatolod factor positive
• Systemic
• Psoariatic
• Enthesitis related
• Unclassified

Note 1: Arthritis related to inflammatory bowel disease is excluded
Note 2: sJIA is often now classified as an autoinflammatory disease

Table 4.2 Blood abnormalities in patients with sJIA

• Elevated erythrocyte sedimentation rate
• Leukocytosis
• Thrombocytosis
• Anemia
• Hypoalbuminemia
• Mild increases in the hepatic transaminases
• Elevated D-dimer levels
• Dramatic increases in serum ferritin levels

Pearl: Patients with sJIA are at risk for the macrophage activation syndrome.

Comment: More recently, the development of macrophage activation (or secondary hemophagocytic histiocytosis, HLH) has been recognized to be more prevalent in sJIA patients. Genetic studies indicate that patients with the macrophage activation syndrome are a disease subset in which the individuals share genetic risk factors with patients who have familial HLH (Zhang et al. 2008).

Pearl: Certain clinical features may indicate the emergence of the macrophage activation syndrome in a patient with sJIA.

Comment: Children with systemic JRA have a host of abnormal findings in the blood (Table 4.2). All of these abnormalities return to normal when the disease becomes less active. The macrophage activation syndrome (MAS) can occur in sJIA and shares many features of that disorder, but also occurs in patients with intracellular viral infections and in patients who have no known risk factors. The following features are typical of MAS:

- Fever
- Hepatosplenomegaly
- Encephalopathy, manifested by dizziness, lethargy, and disorientation
- An extraordinarily high serum ferritin level
- Elevated serum triglyceride levels
- Coagulopathy (increasing D-dimer levels and abnormal PT and PTT) and bruising
- Decreasing ESR (as opposed to the elevation typical of sJIA)

- Cytopenias (leucopenia, thrombocytopenia, and anemia, in contrast to the leucocytosis and thrombocytosis of sJIA)
- Extremely elevated serum hepatic transaminase levels
- The bone marrow aspirate characteristically shows hemophagocytosis

Paradoxically, the arthritis of sJIA may improve as MAS develops. Thus, an improvement in the patient's arthritis, a decline in the ESR, and decreases in the white blood cell and platelet counts can all signal improvement in sJIA, and may also herald the complication of MAS, a life-threatening condition (Stephen et al. 1993).

Myth: JIA will "burn out" when the child grows up.

Reality: Many children with JIA who have a persistent oligoarthritis, particularly those with a monoarthritis, eventually experience disease remission. However, some patients experience the recurrence of arthritis in the same joints involved earlier by JIA, or the extension of inflammatory arthritis to other joints much later in life (unpublished clinical observation).

Recent presentations of gene expression profiles in polyarticular JIA patients who are in remission showed abnormal expression patterns compared to controls, strengthening the impression that the immune system is balanced in remission but not in the same way as those without JIA (Jarvis et al. 2006). This preliminary finding is consistent with the fact that there are genes associated with JIA that alter the innate and adaptive immune responses in these patients (Prahalad and Glass 2008). Thus, triggers such as serious viral infections can alter the balance to a persistent inflammatory state again, leading in theory to the recurrence of arthritis. Therefore, the term "burnt out" should be avoided.

Myth: IgM rheumatoid factor is usually positive in patients with polyarticular JIA. This assay is therefore helpful in distinguishing inflammatory disease from other forms of arthropathy in children.

Reality: The polyarticular subset comprises about 40% of the children with JIA. However, only about 5% of JIA patients test positively for rheumatoid factor. JIA patients who are seropositive tend to be adolescents with aggressive disease and significant involvement of the small joints of the hands. Thus, a negative rheumatoid factor assay in a child or adolescent with arthritis does not exclude the diagnosis of JIA.

Rheumatoid nodules are also unusual in JIA, but when present tend to occur in patients who have rheumatoid factor.

Myth: Anti-CCP antibodies are helpful in identifying disease subtypes.

Reality: Anti-CCP antibodies have a low prevalence in JIA but are increased in HLA-DR4 positive patients with polyarticular disease. They are associated with erosive disease and rheumatoid factor positivity, and therefore have little relevance beyond this small JIA subtype.

Pearl: In oligoarticular JIA, the activity of the eye disease is independent of the activity of the joint disease.

Comment: The activity of the uveitis that occurs in JIA is independent of the disease activity in the joints. Uveitis precedes the onset of arthritis in about 10% of patients with olgioarticular JIA. Uveitis occurs simultaneously with arthritis in 30%, and develops after arthritis in 60% (Rosenberg and Oen 1986). Even when both arthritis and uveitis are present in the same patient, the activity of these disease manifestations may be incongruent. Thus, children with oligoarticular JIA must be screened regularly according to recommended guidelines (an example of USA guidelines can be found in Table 4.3) (Cassidy et al. 2006), even if the arthritis appears well controlled. Uveitis can proceed insidiously and lead to significant ocular damage in the absence of eye symptoms (Figs. 4.1 and 4.2).

Pearl: Single-digit arthritis is often an early sign of psoriatic arthritis.

Comment: Psoriatic arthritis in children often begins with diffuse, sausage-like swelling in one or more digits. Over the

Table 4.3 Screening guidelines for uveitis in patients with pauciarticular JIA in the USA (adapted from Cassidy et al. 2006)

Type	ANA	Onset (years)	Duration (years)	Risk	Examination
Oligo/	+	≤6	≤4	High	q 3 m
Poly	+	≤6	>4	Moderate	q 6 m
	+	≤6	>7	Low	q 12 m
	+	>6	≤4	Moderate	q 6 m
	+	>6	>4	Low	q 12 m
	–	≤6	≤4	Moderate	q 6 m
	–	< or >6	>4	Low	q 12 m
Systemic	NA	NA	NA	Low	q 12 m

q: every; m: months

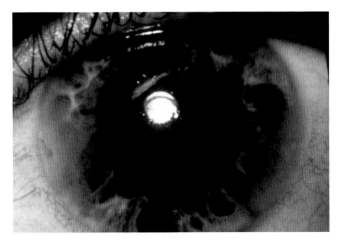

Fig. 4.1 Uveitis – band keratopathy

long term, psoriatic arthritis in children demonstrates a pattern of joint involvement that is asymmetric. The onset of cutaneous psoriasis may follow the presentation of arthritis by several years. Therefore, queries about the patient's family history with regard to psoriasis and inspection of the nails for the characteristic pitting are important aspects of assembling the entire picture and recognizing psoriatic arthritis early (Fig. 4.3).

Pearl: Bone and muscle growth abnormalities are affected substantially by joint inflammation and use (or disuse) of the extremities.

Comment: Overgrowth, undergrowth, and maturation of the bone growth plates are affected by variations in blood flow that occur during the course of JIA. The presence of inflammation

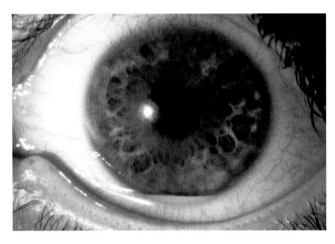

Fig. 4.2 Uveitis – irregular pupil with synechiae

Nail Pits

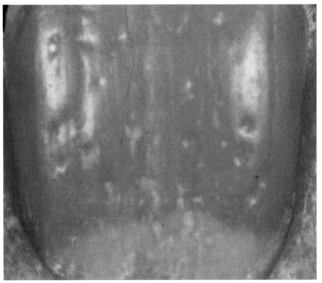

Fig. 4.3 Pitting of the nails in a pediatric patient with psoriatic arthritis

can accelerate bone age and lead to increased bone length. Alternatively, inflammation can lead to early closure of the epiphysis, resulting in a shorter bone. If an extremity is underutilized, stunting of the extremity's growth may occur. A typical example in JIA is shortening of the forefoot resulting from poorly-controlled ankle arthritis. Physical therapy and control of the inflammation are essential to ensuring growth patterns that are as normal as possible.

Another functional complication of oligoarthritis is muscle atrophy on both sides of the affected joint. This can often be observed strikingly in the quadriceps muscle. Muscle atrophy occurs quickly and patients require lengthy periods of time to recover muscle mass, even if remission is achieved and physical therapy efforts are active.

Pearl: Enthesitis can occur in sJIA.

Comment: Gross swelling of tendon insertions can occur in sJIA in certain individuals. These swelling are sometimes mistaken for arthritis or for muscle abscesses. Ultrasound and MRI studies show amorphous material in the tendon near the enthesis (Fig. 4.4) and aspiration is often difficult. The common sites of enthesitis in sJIA are the bicipital tendons near the shoulder and the gastrocnemius tendons behind the knee.

Myth: In a girl who has antinuclear antibodies and a knee monoarthritis that has persisted for 6 months, polyarticular disease will not occur.

Reality: Chronic arthritis in one to four joints over the initial 6 months of disease meets the criteria for oligoarthritis. However, 20–30% of children with oligoarthritis evolve to a polyarticular pattern of disease (extended oligoarthritis) over the ensuing few years.

Myth: Back pain is uncommon in children and most always means pathology.

Reality: Back pain is common in the general pediatric population in developed countries and occurs in 11–36% of school age children. Among pediatric patients referred to orthopedists for back pain, 50% have no explanation for their pain. Scheuermann's disease, spondylolysis, disc prolapse, infection, and tumor are other causes of back pain in children (Tumer 1989, Feldman 2000).

Myth: The onset of sacroiliitis does not occur before the teen years.

Reality: Epidemiologic studies from areas in which pediatric spondylitis is prevalent indicate that inflammation of the sacroiliac joints can occur in the pre-teen years (Huerta-Sil et al. 2006). The use of contrast-enhanced MRI studies in appropriate clinical settings has facilitated the diagnosis in these cases (Fig. 4.5).

Myth: Children with the psoriatic arthritis subset of JIA are likely to develop axial arthritis.

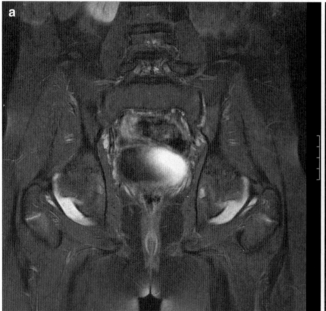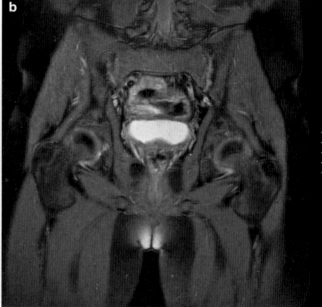

Fig. 4.4 (**a**) An 11-year-old boy with symptoms of left buttock pain and bilateral hip (groin) pains. This sagittal view of an MRI study shows enhancement of the left sacroiliac and hip joints on this T1-weighted sequence. (**b**) Repeat MRI after 1 year while on methotrexate treatment. There is bilateral involvement of the sacroiliac joints

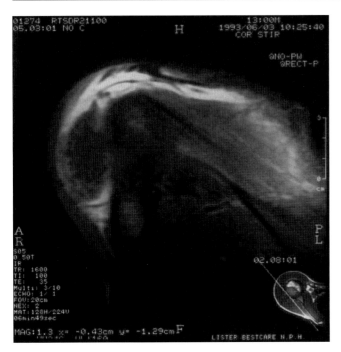

Fig. 4.5 Enthesitis of the bicipital tendon and inflammation of the deltoid muscle in a patient with systemic-onset JIA

Reality: In adults, sacroiliitis or spondylitis occurs in less than 40% of patients with psoriatic arthritis (Lambert and Wright 1977). For children with psoriatic arthritis identified using the so-called "Vancouver criteria", less than 5% develop sacroiliac disease (Robertson et al. 1989; Stoll et al. 2006). Children identified by the JIA subcategory of psoriatic arthritis are even less likely to develop sacroiliitis and spondylitis, because of the associated exclusion criteria.

Pearl: Pediatric psoriatic arthritis patients should be screened for uveitis, just as patients with pauciarticular JIA are screened for this complication.

Comment: Many pediatric rheumatologists consider psoriatic arthritis to be an entity separate from the spondyloarthropathies. This view is bolstered by the fact that children with psoriatic arthritis rarely develop painful iritis but are at moderate risk of the development of asymptomatic eye inflammation. Pediatric patients with psoriatic arthritis should be screened routinely for uveitis in the same manner in which patients with oligoarticular JIA are screened.

Myth: Leukemia is easily distinguished from JIA.

Reality: Distinguishing leukemia from JIA and in particular from sJIA can be a challenge. About 20–40% of children with leukemia have arthritis at the presentation of their disease. The hematologic findings can be normal in leukemia for weeks or months after onset of musculoskeletal symptoms, so repeated evaluations are needed and a bone marrow examination is usually required.

In about half of all patients with leukemic arthritis, a single joint – most often the knee – is involved. The finding of an oligoarthritis is also common. The pain of leukemic arthritis is more severe than JIA and tends to be focused over the metaphysis rather than the joint itself. The ESR in leukemia is normally elevated out of proportion to the small number of effected joints. In contrast, oligoarticular JIA is usually associated with a low or normal ESR.

In leukemia, low white blood cell and platelet counts are the norm, in contrast to the leukocytosis and thrombocytosis that are characteristic of JIA. A striking elevation of the serum lactic dehydrogenase level should also make the clinician suspect leukemia. A bone scan can distinguish between malignancy and JIA when the musculoskeletal complaints are generalized (Cabral and Tucker 1999).

References

Cabral DA, Tucker LB. Malignancies in children who initially present with rheumatic complaints. J Pediatr 1999; 1345:53–57

Cassidy J, Kivlin J, Lindsley C, Nocton J. Opthalmologic examinations in children with juvenile rheumatoid arthritis. Pediatrics 2006; 117:1843–1845

Ferucci ED, Majka DS, Parrish LA, Moroldo MB, Ryan M, Passo M, Thompson SD, Deane KD, Rewers M, Arend WP, Glass DN, Norris JM, Holers VM. Arthritis Rheum. 2005 Jan;52(1):239–46

Huerta-Sil G, Casasola-Vargas JC, Londoño JD, et al Low grade radiographic sacroiliitis as prognostic factor in patients with undifferentiated spondyloarthritis fulfilling diagnostic criteria for ankylosing spondylitis throughout follow up. Ann Rheum Dis 2006; 65(5):642–646

Jarvis JN, Petty HR, Tang Y, et al Evidence for chronic peripheral activation of neutrophils in polyarticular juvenile rheumatoid arthritis. Arthritis Res Ther 2006; 8:R154

Lambert JR, Wright V. Psoriatic spondylitis: a clinical and radiological description of the spine in psoriatic arthritis. QJ Med 1977; 46(184): 411–425

Lequerre T, Quartier P, et al Interleukin-1 receptor antagonist treatment in patients with systemic-onset juvenile idiopathicarthritis or adult onset Still dieases: Preliminary experience in France. Ann Rheum Dis 2008; 67:281–282

Lovell DJ. Update on treatment of arthriits in children: New treatment, new goals. Bull NYU Hosp Jt Dis 2006; 64 (1–2):72–76

Petty RE, Southwood TR, Manners P, Baum J, Glass DN, Goldenberg J, IIe X, Maldonado-Cocco J, Orozco-Alcala J, Prieur AM, Suarez-Almazor ME, Woo P. International League of Associations for Rheumatology. J Rheumatol 2004 Feb; 31(2):390–392

Prahalad S, Glass DN. A comprehensive review of the genetics of juvenile idiopathic arthritis. Paedr Rheumatol Online J 2008; 6:11

Robertson DM, Cabral DA, Malleson PN, Petty RE. Juvenile psoriatic arthritis: Follow-up and evaluation of diagnostic criteria. J Rheumatol 1989; 32:1007–1013

Rosenberg A, Oen K. The relationship between ocular and articular disease activity in children with JRA and associated uveitis.Arthritis Rheum 1986; 29:797

Stephen JL, Zeller J, Hubert PH, et al Macrophage Activation syndrome and rheumatic disease in childhood: A report of four cases. Clin Exp Rheumatol 1993; 11:451–456

Stoll ML, Zurakowski D, Nibrovic LE, et al Patients with juvenile psoriatic arthritis comprise two distinct populations. Arthritis Rheum 2006; 54:3564–3572

Woo, P. Systemic juvenile idiopathic arthritis. Nat Clin Pract Rheumatology 2006; 2:28–34

Yokota S, Imagawa T, Mori M, et al Efficacy and safety of tocilizumab in patients with systemic onset juvenile idiopathic arthritis: A randomised double-blind, placebo-controlled, withdrawal phase III trial. Lancet 2008 Mar 22; 371(9617):998–1006

Zhang K, Biroschak J, Glass DN, Thompson SD, Finkel T, Passo MH, Binstadt BA, Filipovich A, Grom AA. Macrophage activation syndrome in patients with systemic juvenile idiopathic arthritis is associated with MUNC13-4 polymorphisms. Arthritis Rheum 2008; 58:2892–2896.

Monogenic Autoinflammatory Syndromes

5

Marco Gattorno, Alberto Martini, Raphaela Goldbach-Mansky, Pamela Aubert, and Polly J. Ferguson

5.1 Overview of the Monogenic Autoinflammatory Syndromes

> "Autoinflammatory syndromes" is the broad name given to a group of heritable conditions that initially consisted of a group of diseases termed *hereditary periodic fever syndromes*. Autoinflammatory syndrome is the preferred name for these conditions, because not all of the disorders that have been added to this class of inflammatory disorde rs present with periodic febrile episodes.

> In contrast to autoimmune diseases such as systemic lupus erythematosus and rheumatoid arthritis, autoantibodies and antigen-specific T cells do not play a role in the pathogenesis of the autoinflammatory syndromes.

> Although the term *autoinflammatory syndrome* is now commonly used to include polygenic diseases such as Behcet's syndrome, Still's disease, and even Type 2 diabetes, this chapter addresses the monogenic autoinflammatory syndromes.

> These syndromes demonstrate a Mendelian inheritance pattern, and their genetic causes have been identified. The disorders typically present in childhood.

> The disorders are divided into different clinical syndromes that include mixtures of clinical manifestations in the joints, the bones, the skin, the abdomen, and the lymph nodes. The seven currently identified monogenic autoinflammatory syndromes are shown in Table 5.1.

> Intermittent febrile episodes of noninfectious origin can occur throughout life in patients with some autoinflammatory syndromes. Febrile episodes, which last for variable periods according to the specific autoinflammatory syndrome, are accompanied by an intense acute phase response.

> Most autoinflammatory syndromes are caused by mutations that lead to a gain-of-function of the affected innate immune pathway; for example, the genetic mutations lead to inappropriately elevated levels of inflammatory cytokines, such as interleukin-1.

> Most autoinflammatory syndromes can be differentiated on the basis of their clinical features (Table 5.2).

5.1.1 Familial Mediterranean Fever

- Familial Mediterranean fever (FMF) is an autosomal recessive disease.
- Mutations in the MEFV gene, located on the short arm of chromosome 16, cause FMF.
- MEFV gene encodes a protein named pyrin, which is expressed in neutrophils, macrophages, and eosinophils but not lymphocytes.
- More than 70 mutations in the MEFV gene have been described, but the six most prevalent mutations account for 80% of all FMF cases.
- Painful serositis accompanied by fever is a hallmark of the disease.
- The synovitis of FMF is intense but nondestructive, and tends to involve only one joint.
- Skin lesions mimic erysipelas or acute infectious cellulitis and usually affect the lower extremities (Fig. 5.1).
- Secondary amyloidosis is a major long-term complication of FMF that affects patients' longevity. Colchicine use is essential to prevent this complication.
- Proteinuria (>0.5 g/24 h) suggests amyloidosis.

Myth: FMF is a disease of the Mediterranean people.

Reality: The term *Mediterranean* is somewhat misleading. Ethnic groups with the highest disease prevalence are of Mediterranean ancestry, e.g., Armenians, Turks, Arabs, and Jews (Sephardic > Ashkenazi). However, the disease is uncommon in Mediterranean populations such as Greeks, Italians, and Spanish. In fact, the clinical symptoms have been well documented to occur in a variety of ethnicities that lack any Mediterranean background (Samuels et al. 1998).

Table 5.1 Epidemiology and genetic inheritance

	Ethnic group predilection	Mutation	Protein	Mode of inheritance
FMF	Jewish, Armenian, Arab, Turkish, Italian	*MEFV* (16p13)	Pyrin/marenostrin	Autosomal recessive
TRAPS	Any ethnic group	*TNFRS1A* (12p13)	Tumor necrosis factor receptor 1	Autosomal dominant
HIDS	European (originally described among Dutch children)	*MVK* (12q24)	Mevalonate kinase	Autosomal recessive
CAPS				
FCAS	Mostly European	*CIAS1/NLRP3/NALP3/ PYPAF-1* (1q44) Exon 3	Cryopyrin	Autosomal dominant
MWS	Northern European	*CIAS1/NLRP3/NALP3/ PYPAF-1* (1q44) Exon 3	Cryopyrin	Autosomal dominant
NOMID	Any ethnic group	*CIAS1/NLRP3/NALP3/ PYPAF-1* (1q44) Exon 3	Cryopyrin	Autosomal dominant/de novo
CRMO	Any ethnic group	(murine) *PSTPIP2* 18p	(murine) PSTPIP2	Sporadic
Majeed's syndrome	Any ethnic group	*LPIN2* (18p11)	Lpin2	Autosomal recessive
PAPA	Caucasian American	*CD2BP1* (15q24)	Pstpip1/CD2-binding protein 1	Autosomal dominant
Cherubism				

Pearl: FMF patients may have persistently elevated acute phase reactants between attacks.

Comment: Febrile attacks are associated invariably with marked elevations of acute phase proteins. Even during periods of clinical quiescence, however, many FMF patients have persistent elevations of the erythrocyte sedimentation rate (ESR) and C-reactive protein (CRP) and serum amyloid A (SAA) levels (Lachmann et al. 2006).

Myth: A negative family history of FMF excludes the diagnosis.

Reality: In countries with large families and high carrier rates, it is common to elicit a family history of FMF. However, only 50% presents a positive family history (Kastner 2008).

Pearl: The arthritis of FMF can mimic a septic joint.

Comment: The arthritis of FMF often presents as an acute, exquisitely painful, monoarticular arthritis associated with fever, acute phase reactant elevations, and a neutrophil-rich joint effusion (Kastner 2008). A sterile synovial fluid culture and the absence of crystals should lead one to consider FMF as a diagnostic possibility in this setting.

Myth: Pericarditis is common form of serositis in FMF.

Reality: Although recurrent serositis is one of the hallmarks of FMF, symptomatic pericarditis is relatively rare in FMF. However, asymptomatic pericardial effusions are relatively common (Kastner 2008). A sterile peritonitis is the most common form of serositis in FMF.

Myth: A diagnosis of FMF requires the detection of two mutations in the MEFV gene.

Reality: Despite the elucidation of the genetic basis for FMF, the diagnosis of FMF remains predicated upon clinical grounds (The International FMF Consortium 1997; The French FMF Consortium 1997). This does not minimize the importance of genetic testing but rather reflects the fact that current mutation detection methods do not identify 100% of the mutant alleles. The most striking example of this is in the Arabic population, in which as many as half of the mutant alleles are not identifiable in a cohort of well-characterized FMF patients (El-Shanti et al. 2006).

Pearl: FMF may present as functional abdominal pain in childhood.

Comment: In the high risk ethnic populations, FMF should be on the differential diagnosis of functional abdominal pain; as many as twenty percent of Arabic and Jewish children with functional abdominal pain are homozygous for MEFV mutations (Brik et al. 2001; El-Shanti et al. 2006).

Myth: Among Jewish people, FMF affects primarily non-Ashkenazi Jews.

Reality: FMF is an autosomal recessive disease with variable penetrance. The three major mutations in MEFV are M694V,

Table 5.2 Cardinal clinical findings

	Age at presentation	Flare/fever pattern	Skin	Ocular	Musculo-skeletal	Distinguishing features	Treatment
FMF	Eighty percent of the cases occur before the age of 20	1–3 days	Erysipeloid erythema of lower extremity	Rare	Arthralgia, oligoarthritis, myalgia	Serosal inflammation, amyloidosis	Colchicine, thalidomide, etanercept, anakinra
TRAPS	Median age of onset 3 years	1–4 weeks	Migratory rash	Conjunctivitis	Arthralgia, arthritis	Serosal inflammation, amyloidosis	Corticosteroids, anakinra, etanercept
HIDS	Median age of onset 6 months	3–7 days	Rare	Conjunctivitis, episcleritis	Arthralgia	Some with elevated IgD, diarrhea, lymphadeno-pathy	NSAIDs, anakinra, etanercept, simvastatin
CAPS							Interleukin-1 inhibition
FCAS	First 6 months of life	<24 h	Cold-induced urticaria-like rash	Conjunctivitis	Arthralgia	Cold-induced symptoms	Cold avoidance, NSAIDs, anakinra, rilonacept
MWS	Infancy to adolescence	24–48 h	Urticaria-like rash	Conjunctivitis, episcleritis	Arthralgia	Sensorineural hearing loss; amyloidosis (30%)	anakinra, NSAIDs, rilonacept
NOMID	Neonatum or Early infancy	Continuous with flares	Urticarial rash	Conjunctivitis, episcleritis, uveitis, papilledema	Arthralgia, arthropathy secondary to osseous overgrowth	Chronic aseptic meningitis, sensorineural hearing loss, characteristic facies, amyloidosis (rare)	Anakinra, Corticosteroids for severe CNS manifestations and acute hearing loss
CRMO	Childhood (as early as <2 years as late as 55years)	Uncommon	Palmoplantar pustulosis, psoriasis	None	Recurrent, multifocal osteolytic sterile bone lesions	Association with IBD	NSAIDs, corticosteroids, bisphosphonates, interferon α and γ, azithromycin, etanercept
Majeed's syndrome	Early infancy (1–19 months)	Common	Sweet's syndrome, psoriasis in carriers	None	Bone pain, osteitis, early onset CRMO	Cultures negative, organomegaly, microcytic dyserythropoietic anemia	NSAIDs or corticosteroids. Other possible treatments include bisphosphonates, interferon α and γ, sulfasalazine, azithromycin, etanercept
PAPA	Early childhood	Weeks-months	Cystic acne, pyoderma gangrenosum	None	Sterile pyogenic arthritis	Skin findings begin at puberty	Intra-articular and oral glucocorticoids, etanercept, anakinra
Cherubism	Early childhood	Not applicable	None	Up turned eyes	Marked expansion of the jaw bones	Typical facies with marked enlargement of the jaw and upturned eyes	No effective treatment is known. Based on murine model and role of osteoclasts, TNF inhibitors and bisphosphonates may prove useful

Figs. 5.1 (a, b) The skin lesions in familial Mediterranean fever (FMF) can mimic erysipelas or acute infectious cellulitis and usually affect the lower extremities

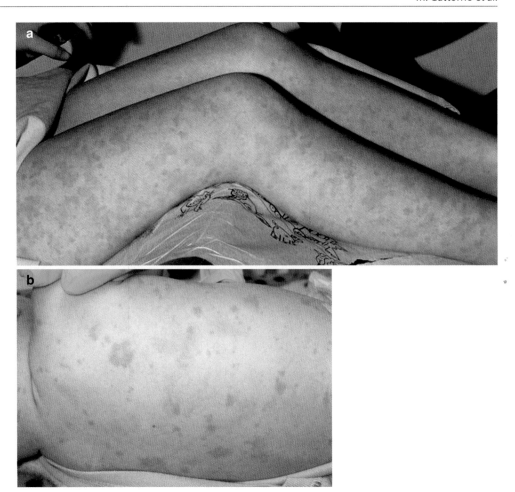

V726A, and E148Q. The M694V mutation, which is observed across a number of ethnic groups, is by far the predominant mutation in North African (Sephardic) Jews. M694V homozygosity increases an individual's risk for early age of onset, more frequent attacks, and systemic amyloidosis.

The carrier frequency of FMF in non-Ashkenazi (mostly Sephardic) Jews is estimated to be between 1:5 and 1:16. Several studies have found that approximately 1 in 5 Ashkenazi Jews also carries mutations that can cause FMF, the most common being E148Q and P369S (Aksentijevich et al. 1999; Stoffman et al. 2000). The higher than expected carrier frequency among the Ashkenazi Jewish population suggests that some mutations, particularly E148Q, are not fully penetrant. Indeed, milder mutations with lower penetrance such as E148Q and V726A are more common than M694V in Ashkenazi Jews compared with Sephardic Jews.

Pearl: Renal amyloidosis may be the first manifestation of FMF.

Comment: Amyloid A (AA) type amyloidosis is the most severe long-term complication of FMF. This protein is a cleavage product of SAA, an acute phase reactant produced by the liver. The most common clinical manifestation of

amyloidosis is proteinuria. A specific genotype, homozygosity for the M694V mutation of the MEFV gene, is the most relevant risk factor for the development of amyloidosis. This genotype is found most commonly in Armenia, Israel, and Arab countries (Touitou et al. 2007).

Renal involvement is usually observed after a variable time from the onset of the disease (phenotype I). However, in some patients, renal amyloidosis is the first manifestation of FMF (phenotype II). In an international, multicenter study of FMF, amyloidosis was diagnosed in 73 of the 371 patients, and was the presenting clinical manifestation in seven patients (Mimouni et al. 2000).

Myth: Long-term colchicine treatment affects fertility and has mutagenic and teratogenic effects during pregnancy.

Reality: Colchicine is believed to affect fertility because of its potential to inhibit cell division. However, no clear relationship exists between female infertility and colchicine therapy. Several reports have described women with FMF who were receiving colchicine but who were fertile (Kallinich et al. 2007). With regard to males, although adverse effects of colchicine on male fertility are alleged, sperm analyses in volunteers and patients with FMF who received therapeutic doses of colchicine were normal.

Spontaneous abortions occurred in 12% of pregnant women with FMF who were treated with colchicine, compared with 20% of women in the same cohort who were not treated (Kallinich et al. 2007). In theory, mutagenic and teratogenic effects of colchicine are possible because the drug crosses the placenta. However, there is no clear evidence for human teratogenicity or increased rate of aneuploidy. In some reports, colchicine therapy during conception and the first trimester of pregnancy had no adverse effects on the offspring (Kallinich et al. 2007). The current approach for most female patients with FMF is to continue colchicine before conception and during pregnancy (Ben-Chetrit et al. 2003).

Pearl: FMF patients who are lactose intolerant may develop dose-limiting side effects of colchicine.

Comment: Some FMF patients experience abdominal pain and diarrhea as a side effect of chronic colchicine therapy. In such patients, it is worth considering the possibility that the symptoms are due to acquired lactose deficiency. A case–control study in FMF patients receiving colchicine confirmed the experimental animal data that had suggested the gastrointestinal side effects of colchicine therapy to be often caused by lactose intolerance induced by the medication (Fradkin et al. 1995). These patients should be managed with lactose avoidance or Lactaid in order to permit the continuation of colchicine therapy.

Pearl: Patients undergoing renal transplant who receive cyclosporine and colchicine can develop colchicine toxicity.

Comment: FMF patients who receive renal allografts because of amyloidosis-associated end-stage renal disease can develop serious colchicine toxicity if immunosuppressive therapy with cyclosporine is coadministered with colchicine. The side effects are mild to moderate in many cases, consisting of diarrhea and muscle weakness, but can result in multiple organ failure (Cohen et al. 1989; Minetti et al. 2003; Eleftheriou et al. 2008).

Colchicine is secreted into the bile as a major pathway of elimination (Speeg et al. 1992). Renal excretion accounts for 10–20% of drug elimination. Colchicine toxicity is induced by cyclosporine by several mechanisms, the most important of which is the modulation of the P-glycoprotein (also known as P-gp or gp-170), a 170-kDa cell surface glycoprotein encoded by the MDR-1 (multidrug resistance) gene. P-glycoprotein is expressed in enterocytes, renal tubular cells, hepatocytes, and some endothelial cells. Cyclosporine inhibits P-glycoprotein expression, leading to increased intracellular drug concentrations.

Both hepatic and renal colchicine secretion probably depend on the MDR-1 transport system. Thus, both the elimination pathways are potentially inhibited by cyclosporine. Other factors include reduced renal elimination of colchicine caused by cyclosporine-induced reductions in the glomerular filtration rate, but this appears to be of lesser importance when compared towith the effects of cyclosporine on the MDR-1 transport system. The net effect is an increase in the plasma concentration of colchicine and a higher likelihood of toxic drug effects (Minetti et al. 2003).

Most cases of gastrointestinal side effects and muscle weakness caused by colchicine administration in the setting of cyclosporine use disappear within a few days of stopping cyclosporine (Cohen et al. 1989). However, the coadministration of cyclosporine and colchicine should be avoided. This poses substantial challenges in the management of FMF patients who undergo renal transplantation.

Pearl: FMF-associated amyloidosis rarely affects the heart, the tongue, or the peripheral nerves.

Comment: Systemic AA amyloidosis is the most devastating long-term complication of FMF. This complication results from the organ deposition of AA protein, a cleavage product of SAA that is produced by the liver. In systemic AA amyloidosis, the kidneys, adrenal glands, intestine, and the spleen are most often involved. The AA protein is deposited only rarely in the heart, the musculoskeletal system, and the nervous system (Altiparmak et al. 2002; Yildiz et al. 2001; Kavukçu et al. 1997).

The most common outcomes of systemic amyloidosis are nephrotic syndrome and chronic renal failure. Most FMF patients who develop amyloidosis present such complications by the age of 40 years (Samuels et al. 1998). The prevalence of amyloidosis differs among various ethnic groups. Country of residence (foremost Armenia and Turkey), homozygosity of the M694V mutation in MEFV, male gender, and the a/a genotype of serum amyloid A1 (SAA1) gene are the risk factors for the development of amyloidosis (Touitou et al. 2007).

Amyloidosis and chronic renal disease are less common in Arabs with FMF than in other ethnic groups often affected by the disease. The frequency of amyloidosis ranges from 0.4% in Jordanian patients to 2% in a mixed Arab population residing in Kuwait. In contrast, the frequency of amyloidosis in Sephardic Jews, Armenians, and Turks has been estimated to range from 24 to 60%. The low rate of occurrence of FMF-related amyloidosis reported in Arabs is probably a result of the fact that these figures were obtained after the establishment of colchicine as the standard of care (El-Shanti et al. 2006).

Colchicine remains the mainstay of treatment for FMF. At low doses, colchicine is effective in controlling acute febrile flares, while high doses are required for the prevention of amyloidosis (Samuels et al. 1998).

5.1.2 Tumor Necrosis Factor Receptor-Associated Periodic Syndrome (TRAPS)

- TRAPS is inherited in an autosomal dominant fashion.
- The median age of onset is 3.
- TRAPS is caused by mutations in TNFRFSF1A, located on chromosome 12p13. This gene encodes the main surface receptor for TNF.
- More than 50 mutations in this gene have been associated with TRAPS. The precise mechanism through which these mutations lead to the clinical TRAPS syndrome is not known precisely. However, two hypotheses relate to defective shedding of TNF receptors (TNFR) from the cell membrane and misfolding of the TNFR.
- Febrile episodes in TRAPS are often of longer duration (up to several weeks) than those of other periodic fever syndromes.
- Localized myalgia usually afflicts the limbs during periods of fever. This symptom, probably caused by a monocytic fasciitis, can be severe.
- Erythematous macules and patches are also found on the limbs during febrile episodes.
- Abdominal pain, usually less severe than that of FMF but sometimes accompanied by vomiting, constipation, or even bowel obstruction, occurs in almost all patients.
- Eye manifestations of TRAPS are diverse, and include: conjunctivitis, uveitis, iritis, and periorbital edema.

Myth: TRAPS is a disorder of individuals of northern European stock.

Reality: TRAPS, formerly known as familial Hibernian fever, was described in 1982 in a kindred of Irish-Scottish descent (Williamson et al. 1982). TRAPS is caused by mutations in the p55 TNF Receptor (TNFR1) and inherited in an autosomal dominant fashion. TNFR1 is encoded by the TNF Super Family Receptor 1A gene (TNFRSF1A) (McDermott et al. 1999). Fewer than 200 families have been reported worldwide, but this is likely an underestimate of the true number.

Till date, TRAPS has been reported mainly in the people of northern European ancestry. However, the disease has been described in almost every ethnic group, including patients from Mediterranean countries (Italy, Spain), Africa (Mauritius), Central America (Puerto Rico, Mexico), and Asia (India and Japan) (Aksentijevich et al. 2001; Aganna et al. 2003). The prevalence of TNFRSF1A mutations in non-Ashkenazi Jews, Arabs, Turks and Armenian populations is yet to be tested.

Pearl: The absence of a clear history of recurrent fever attacks does not exclude the diagnosis of TRAPS.

Comment: TRAPS-associated mutations usually lead to severe inflammatory episodes. Most patients present in the pediatric age group. Attacks of intermittent fever with body temperatures above 38–39°C last from 1 to 3 weeks and are interspersed by intervals of variable duration during which the patient feels completely well. Febrile episodes are associated with acute phase reactant elevations, leukocytosis, and anemia.

In adulthood, febrile episodes generally become less frequent and patients experience milder disease courses, characterized by intermittent abdominal pain, arthralgias, myalgias, ocular findings (e.g., conjunctivitis, uveitis), and slight but persistent acute phase reactant elevations. SAA levels are usually elevated in TRAPS.

Some patients carrying mutations in the TNFRSF1A gene have been reported, who present with the typical clinical manifestations of TRAPS but without fever. These patients have had mutations that do not affect cysteine residues (Y20H and T50M). One patient with the T50M mutation developed severe renal AA amyloidosis in her second decade without any preceding febrile episodes or other TRAPS-associated clinical manifestations earlier in life (Kallinich et al. 2006).

Myth: Low serum levels of the p55 TNFR1 during febrile attacks should be used as a screening test before proceeding with a molecular analysis of TNFRSF1A gene.

Reality: Following cell activation, the extracellular portion of the p55 and p75 TNFR undergo metalloprotease-dependent cleavage (shedding) from the cell membrane. Shedding of free TNFRs from the membrane produces a pool of soluble receptors that may scavenge the circulating TNF by competing with membrane-bound receptors. It has been suggested that some TNFRSF1A mutations may interfere with this process of TNFR shedding.

Consistent with this hypothesis, is the finding that leukocytes from TRAPS patients display a reduced cleavage rate of the p55 TNFR but not the p75 isoform following cell stimulation (Aksentijevich et al. 2001; D'Osualdo et al. 2006). Impaired elevation of the soluble p55 TNFR during fever episodes has been adopted as a screening test in patients suspected of having TRAPS. Unfortunately, the potential utility of this assay is impaired substantially by the large variability in serum p55 TNFR levels during systemic inflammation, both in healthy individuals and in other inflammatory conditions. Moreover, recent observations have shown that some TNFRSF1A mutations are not associated with a defect in TNFR shedding (Huggins et al. 2004).

Pearl: Anti-IL-1 treatment controls fevers in TRAPS.

Comment: Fever episodes usually respond to glucocorticoids. However, due to the possible long duration of fever attacks and the tendency to a chronic course, patients may become steroid-dependent.

Many other immunosuppressive medications appear to be ineffective in reducing the frequency and the intensity of the inflammatory episodes and in preventing amyloidosis (Hull et al. 2002). The observation of a defect in TNFRI shedding led to the proposal of TNF inhibition as a potential treatment strategy (Aksentijevich et al. 2001; Hull et al. 2002; Galon et al. 2000). However, incomplete treatment responses have been reported (Arostegui et al. 2005; Jacobelli et al. 2007).

An excellent short-term response to the treatment with the recombinant receptor antagonist for IL-1 (IL-1Ra, Anakinra) was observed in one TRAPS patient (Simon et al. 2004a) and supported by the findings, in a long-term, of the efficacy and safety of this approach in five patients with TRAPS (Gattorno et al. 2008a). As described below, IL-1 blockade is also efficacious in some other monogenic autoinflammatory diseases.

Pearl: Low-penetrant TNFRFS1A mutations are usually associated with mild disease courses.

Comment: Mutations that result in cysteine substitutions demonstrate a higher penetrance of the clinical phenotype. Patients with these mutations have severe disease courses and an increased probability of developing renal amyloidosis. In contrast, low-penetrance mutations such as the R92Q and P46L mutations are usually associated with a more heterogeneous clinical presentation, a milder disease course, and a lower incidence of amyloidosis (Aksentijevich et al. 2001).

In a recent study of a pediatric population, TRAPS patients with missense substitutions of cysteine residues had more aggressive disease, compared with that of patients with other mutations (D'Osualdo et al. 2006). Cysteine residue mutations were associated with febrile episodes of longer duration (mean: 23 days), higher glucocorticoids requirement, and a higher incidence of amyloidosis. Conversely, children carrying a R92Q substitution had febrile episodes that lasted for a mean of only 4.1 days and responded more quickly to glucocorticoids.

5.1.3 Hyper Immunoglobulin D and Periodic Fever Syndrome

- Hyper IgD syndrome (HIDS) is caused by mutations in the mevalonate kinase gene (MVK), which is located on the long arm of chromosome 12 (12q24).
- The mechanism by which reduced activity of MVK leads to an autoinflammatory condition is not understood completely.
- Patients with HIDS have recurrent fever attacks that last approximately 4 to 6 days. Attacks begin early in childhood and often recur every 4 to 6 weeks.
- Febrile attacks in HIDS generally begin with chills, followed by a swift and steep temperature elevation.
- Cervical adenopathy and abdominal pain, with vomiting and diarrhea, occur during periods of HIDS activity.

- Cutaneous findings in HIDS are common. These include erythematous maculopapular lesions, urticarial, and a variety of other rashes. Genital and oral ulcers occur in some patients.
- Patients with HIDS have normal life expectancies, and both the frequency and the severity of the episodes tend to decrease after childhood.
- Serum levels of immunoglobulin D are persistently elevated in most patients with HIDS. However, levels of IgD do not correlate with disease activity.

Pearl: HIDS is not limited to the people of Dutch ancestry.

Comment: Periodic fever associated with mevalonate kinase deficiency (MKD) was originally identified in 1984, in six patients of Dutch ancestry who had long histories of recurrent attacks of fever of unknown cause and high serum IgD levels (van der Meer et al. 1984). For this reason, this disorder has also been named HIDS or Dutch fever.

After the identification of the molecular defect, it became clear that the distribution of MKD is not limited to Dutch or other northern European populations. Patients have been observed also among populations living around the Mediterranean basin (Italy) (D'Osualdo et al. 2001) and Asia (Japan) (Drenth et al. 1994), and even in ethnic groups, in which there is a high prevalence of FMF (e.g., Turks and Arabs) (Gattorno et al. 2008b; Demirkaya et al. 2007).

Myth: HIDS and mevalonic aciduria have two completely distinctive phenotypes.

Reality: HIDS is caused by mutations in the MVK gene, encoded on chromosome 12q24. MVK is an essential enzyme in the isoprenoid biosynthesis pathway. The complete deficiency of this enzyme causes a distinct syndrome called mevalonic aciduria, which is characterized clinically by severe mental retardation, ataxia, failure to thrive, myopathy, cataracts, and recurrent fever attacks (Hoffman et al. 1993). The most common mutation in MVK gene is the V377I variant, which is associated exclusively with the mild phenotype of HIDS and some residual MVK activity (Houten et al. 1999). It is therefore clear that mevalonic aciduria and HIDS associated with MKD represent the two extremities of a broad clinical spectrum. Intermediate clinical scenarios are sometimes observed (Simon et al. 2004b).

Pearl: Splenomegaly and gastrointestinal manifestations during fever attacks are suggestive of HIDS.

Comment: In a recent study, 228 consecutive children with a clinical history of periodic fever were screened for mutations of the MVK, TNFRSF1A, and MEFV genes (Gattorno et al. 2008b). Clinical variables such as a positive family history, early age of onset, presence of abdominal and chest pain, diarrhea, and the absence of aphthosis correlated highly with the probability of relevant mutations in genes known to be associated with periodic fever.

Fever durations of less than 2 days were associated with FMF. In contrast, febrile periods longer than 7 days were characteristic of TRAPS. Among patients who presented with fevers between 3 and 6 days duration, the differential diagnosis usually focused on two entities: FMF and MKD.

Splenomegaly and vomiting strongly suggest HIDS, even though these symptoms can be present in patients with FMF, as well. Figure 5.2 shows a flow chart to guide the genetic testing for children with recurrent fever of unknown origin (Gattorno et al. 2008b). Additional information is available at http://www.printo.it/periodicfever.

Myth: HIDS is a self-limited, benign disorder that has a good long-term prognosis.

Reality: HIDS is essentially a pediatric disease. The onset of symptoms in HIDS occurs very early in life – usually in infancy. Almost all the patients become symptomatic during the first decade of life. Fever attacks have an abrupt onset and last for 4–6 days. The symptoms of HIDS persist for years but may become less prominent over time. Nevertheless, a study from the international HIDS study group indicated that more than 12 attacks per year still occurred in 18% of the patients who were older than 20 years, compared with 24% of those between the ages of 10 and 20 (van der Hilst et al. 2008). Amyloidosis has been reported in a small number of patients with MKD (D'Osualdo et al. 2005; Siewert et al. 2006).

Myth: High serum levels of IgD are the hallmark of HIDS.

Reality: High IgD plasma levels (>100 UI/mL) during fever episodes and in basal conditions were used as a diagnostic hallmark until mutations in the MVK gene were identified in 1999. However, the sensitivity and the specificity of these findings are debated (D'Osualdo et al. 2005; Demirkaya et al. 2007). In a recent series of 50 patients, the sensitivity of a high IgD value for the diagnosis of HIDS was 79% (Ammouri et al. 2007). In five patients with MVK mutations, IgD levels were found to be in the normal range. Elevated levels of IgD are also found in other inflammatory conditions, including FMF.

An increased urine excretion of mevalonic acid is observed during fever spikes, and decreased MVK activity may also suggest the diagnosis. However, these determinations require highly specialized laboratories, and their utility as screening tests is therefore limited. Thus, the decision to undergo the molecular analysis of MVK gene in a child with periodic fever is usually taken on clinical grounds.

5.1.4 Cryopyrin-Associated Periodic Syndromes

- The cryopyrin-associated periodic syndromes (CAPS) include three overlapping conditions.

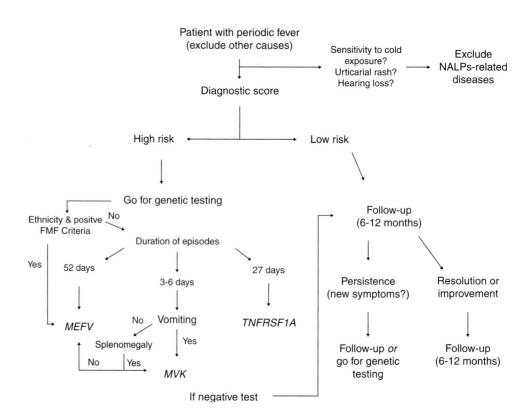

Fig. 5.2 Flow chart for the genetic testing of children with recurrent fevers of unknown origin

- The familial cold autoinflammatory syndrome (FCAS).
- The Muckle-Wells syndrome (MWS).
- The neonatal onset multisystem inflammatory disorder, which is also known as the chronic infantile neurologic, cutaneous, and articular syndrome (NOMID/CINCA).
- These three disorders represent a spectrum of disease severity with overlapping clinical features. The clinical features found in each of these entities are fever, an urticaria-like skin rash, and varying degrees of arthralgia and arthritis.
- The CAPS disorders also have similar laboratory profiles, characterized by neutrophil-mediated inflammation and elevated acute-phase reactants (Stojanov et al. 2005; Aksentijevich et al. 2007).
- All patients present in childhood, usually in the perinatal period.

Pearl: The determination of the precise clinical phenotype has important prognostic implications in this spectrum of disease.

Comment: The FCAS has the mildest phenotype and the best prognosis; MWS has an intermediate phenotype and prognosis; and NOMID has the worst of both. In addition to the symptoms that are commonly shared by them, these three disorders have distinguishing characteristics:

- As its name implies, the FCAS is characterized by attacks that are precipitated by exposure to cold and or drafts of air. Hearing loss and amyloidosis are rare but are reported complications of FCAS (Thornton et al. 2007).
- Symptoms of the MWS seldom have any clear association with cold temperatures, but most develop sensorineural hearing loss during their teens or twenties. Deafness is a common complication of MWS, and the prevalence of secondary AA amyloidosis reaches 30% among untreated patients.
- In the NOMID/CINCA syndrome, inflammation-induced organ damage occurs early in life. Central nervous system inflammation with aseptic meningitis and cognitive impairment are common in NOMID/CINCA. Increased intracranial pressure leads to frequent headaches and papilledema. Progressive optic nerve atrophy and sensorineural hearing loss usually occurs in the first decade of life. Joint and bone abnormalities include patellar bony enlargement, joint deformity, and severe contractures (Hill et al. 2007).

Pearl: FCAS, MWS, and NOMID/CINCA are all caused by mutations in CIAS1, which encodes the protein cryopyrin.

Comment: These mutations are autosomal dominant. Mutations in CIAS1 lead to the oversecretion of interleukin-1 (IL-1) in vitro (Agostini et al. 2004). The FCAS and MWS occur mostly as familial diseases with the presence of founder mutations in FCAS (Hoffman et al. 2003). Sporadic cases

also occur (Aksentijevich et al. 2007; Goldbach-Mansky et al. 2008). The NOMID/CINCA syndrome occurs almost exclusively as a sporadic mutation, because most untreated patients with NOMID/CINCA are not able to reproduce.

Pearl: Never stop treatment with anakinra in patients with CAPS, even during infections or surgery.

Comment: The pivotal role of IL-1 oversecretion in CAPS is confirmed by the marked response to interleukin-1 (IL-1) blockade in patients with CAPS. Treatment with daily injections of anakinra, a recombinant antagonist of the human IL-1 receptor, results in markedly improved clinical and laboratory manifestations in patients with FCAS, MWS, and NOMID/CINCA. Withdrawal leads to recurrence of symptoms (Hawkins et al. 2004; Hoffman et al. 2004; Goldbach-Mansky et al. 2006). In a prospective withdrawal trial of anakinra in 18 patients with NOMID, the discontinuation of anakinra uniformly resulted in disease relapses, sometimes within hours of stopping the medication (Goldbach-Mansky et al. 2006). Therefore, anakinra should not be discontinued, even during an infection.

Controlled data on the development of infections on IL-1 blockade are derived from a recent placebo-controlled trial in patients with FCAS and MWS using the long acting IL-1 inhibitor called rilonacept. Rilonocept is an IL-1 trap, a soluble receptor molecule that binds IL-1 and prevents its interaction with the cell surface IL-1 receptor. In this study, 18% of patients on IL-1 inhibition had infections, compared with 22% in the placebo group (Hoffman et al. 2008). Unpublished data suggest that infections heal as expected in patients on continuous IL-1 inhibition, and that the risk of infection during IL-1 blockade does not appear to be increased significantly over the risk before treatment.

Myth: The rash in CAPS is urticarial.

Reality: The rash in CAPS is often mistaken for "classic urticaria." In FCAS, the rash is induced by cold, usually within the first 6 months of life. In the MWS and NOMID/CINCA syndromes, the rash is typically present at birth and does not require cold for induction. The rash of CAPS is difficult to distinguish clinically from an urticarial, allergic rash.

The histopathological features of CAPS are consistent with a neutrophilic dermatosis (Fig. 5.3), in contrast to the typical lymphocytic or eosinophilic infiltrate of classic urticaria (Leslie et al. 2006). The epidermis is normal in CAPS, but there is a superficial and a deep perivascular and interstitial cellular infiltrate predominantly composed of neutrophils, some lymphocytes, and rare eosinophils (Prieur 2001; Hoffman et al. 2001b; Shinkai et al. 2008; Kilcline et al. 2005).

Confusion frequently exists in distinguishing the skin rash of FCAS from that of cold urticaria, a common form of physical urticaria that can be primary (idiopathic) or secondary (acquired). True cold urticaria is nonfamilial and is not caused by mutations in CIAS1. The diagnosis can be established

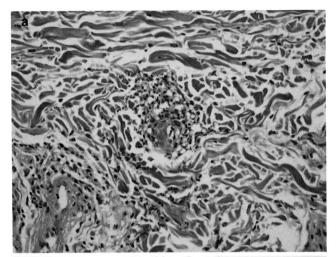

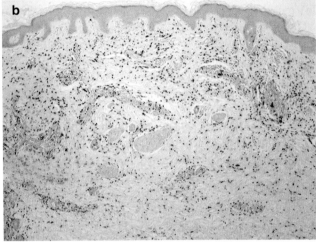

Fig. 5.3 (**a, b**) Neutrophilic dermatosis in a patient with a cryopyrin-associated periodic syndrome (CAPS)

with the use of an ice cube test or an ice water immersion test, in which a wheal reaction appears on the exposed skin 10–20 min after exposure (Neittaanmäki et al. 1985). The ice cube test is negative in patients with FCAS, MWS or NOMID/CINCA (Delorme et al. 2002; Hoffman et al. 2001a).

Pearl: There is a subset of patients with classical CAPS who are negative for mutations in CIAS1 but respond similarly to IL-1 blockade as patients who are CIAS1 mutation positive.

Comment: All the three CAPS syndromes are caused by autosomal dominant mutations in exon 3 of the CIAS1 gene on chromosome 1q44 (Cuisset et al. 1999; Hoffman et al. 2001a, b; Feldman 2002; Aksentijevich et al. 2002). Although there is some genotype/phenotype correlation observed within the spectrum of these diseases, there also appears to be the role of background genes and environmental factors in controlling disease expression (Hawkins et al. 2004). In addition, not all patients with unequivocal CAPS have detectable mutations in CIAS1 (Neven et al. 2004; Aksentijevich et al. 2007). This is especially true for NOMID, in which up

to 40% of the patients are negative for CIAS1 mutations (Aksentijevich et al. 2002).

Patients without CIAS1 mutations detectable by routine analysis may have somatic mutations (Saito et al. 2008). Regardless of their mutation status, patients of the entire CAPS spectrum respond equally well to IL-1 blocking therapy (Hawkins et al. 2004; Hoffman et al. 2004; Goldbach-Mansky et al. 2006; Gattorno et al. 2007).

Pearl: Bony deformities, which result from derangements of the growth plate, are unique to the NOMID/CINCA syndrome.

Comment: Joint pain and swelling occur occasionally during febrile exacerbations of all three CAPS syndromes, but is particularly characteristic of the NOMID/CINCA syndrome. In CAPS, synovitis can present with warm, swollen, stiff joints and increased synovial fluid production, reminiscent of juvenile idiopathic arthritis (Prieur et al. 1987; Kilcline et al. 2005). However, the joint manifestations of the FCAS and MWS are usually limited to arthralgias and limb pain and synovitis, if present, is mild. In contrast, joint involvement in NOMID can be much more severe and is among the diagnostic criteria for the disease.

The onset of arthropathy in NOMID/CINCA is usually within the first year of life. The knees are the most commonly affected joints. Other sites of involvement, by order of decreasing frequency, include the ankles, the elbows, the wrists, the hips, and the small joints. The axial joints are not affected in NOMID/CINCA (Yarom et al. 1985; Prieur 2001; Stankovic et al. 2007).

The musculoskeletal changes in NOMID/CINCA are characterized by endochondral bony overgrowth and premature ossification that originate in the growth plate. These lesions lead to deformities in the adjacent metaphysis and epiphysis (Hill et al. 2007). Premature patellar and epiphyseal long bone ossification and resultant osseous overgrowth often develop early in life and lead to severe contractures, deforming arthropathy, and long-term disability (Fig. 5.4) (Prieur et al. 1987; Yarom et al. 1985; Kilcline et al. 2005).

Pearl: Hearing loss in CAPS, caused by cochlear inflammation, responds to IL-1 inhibition.

Comment: Central nervous system manifestations are among the most devastating sequelae of CAPS. They tend to occur in the more severe phenotypes. Sensorineural hearing loss develops in patients with MWS in the second to fourth decade of life. NOMID patients show signs of hearing loss in the first decade of life. The sensorineural hearing loss is progressive and can lead to complete hearing loss.

The presence of cochlear enhancement on FLAIR sequences of magnetic resonance imaging in almost all NOMID patients suggests that hearing loss is caused by cochlear inflammation. Treatment with anakinra for 6 months led to a decrease and even elimination of the cochlear enhancement within 3 months

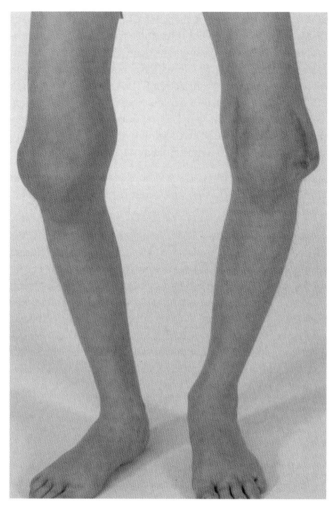

Fig. 5.4 The arthropathy of NOMID/CINCA

of treatment (Goldbach-Mansky et al. 2006). One third of the patients showed improved hearing on audiometry and the remainder showed stability in their hearing deficits. Additional case reports in NOMID and MWS patients confirmed improved hearing by audiometry after treatment with anakinra (Yamazaki et al. 2008; Rynne et al. 2006).

5.1.5 Chronic Recurrent Multifocal Osteomyelitis

• Chronic recurrent multifocal osteomyelitis (CRMO) is characterized by chronic recurrent multifocal sterile osteomyelitis that commonly affects the metaphysis of long bones, but that can be found in many other sites including the clavicle, spine, and the pelvic bones.
• Patients with CRMO can have both symptomatic and asymptomatic bone lesions.
• An association exists between inflammatory skin conditions, inflammatory bowel disease, and CRMO.

• Majeed's syndrome is a syndromic form of CRMO caused by an autosomal recessive alteration in the LPIN2 gene on the short arm of chromosome 18.
• Majeed's syndrome is characterized by an early onset of CRMO, congenital dyserythropoietic anemia (CDA), and inflammatory neutrophilic dermatosis.
• Although mutations in the PSTPIP2 gene mapped to chromosome 18 cause chronic multifocal osteomyelitis in a murine model, the genetic cause for the more common presentations of CRMO in humans has not yet been discovered.

Myth: CRMO is a benign, self-limited disorder with little long-term morbidity.

Reality: CRMO has been described as a benign, self-limited disorder, yet this conclusion is based upon data from short-term follow-up. Estimates of the likelihood of active disease at long-term follow-up have varied widely. The incidence of permanent bone deformity leading to leg length discrepancies is high (Duffy et al. 2002). CRMO has also been reported to evolve into spondyloarthropathy. The outcome for children with an early onset of CRMO (onset <2 years of age) is more guarded; they tend to have severe disease often associated with failure to thrive, secondary joint contractures, and the need for long-term immune suppression.

Pearl: CDA that accompanies the Majeed syndrome is typically microcytic and may be mild.

Comment: The Majeed syndrome is an autosomal recessive disorder caused by mutations in LPIN2. Classic cases of the Majeed syndrome present with the triad of early-onset CRMO, CDA, and a neutrophilic dermatosis (Majeed et al. 1989, 2000, 2001; Al-Mosawi et al. 2007; Ferguson et al. 2005). However, skin involvement may be absent and the anemia is mild, posing substantial challenges in the diagnosis of the Majeed syndrome. One helpful clue is that the anemia of the Majeed syndrome is microcytic. This feature contrasts sharply with other well-described CDA, which are either macrocytic or normocytic (Majeed et al. 1989, 2000, 2001; Al-Mosawi et al. 2007).

Bone marrow aspiration should be included in the work-up of all children who present with CRMO before the age of two. The Majeed syndrome should be suspected if CDA is present. This in turn, leads to the evaluation of mutations in LPIN2.

Pearl: Inflammatory disorders of the skin and the gut are frequently present in individuals with CRMO.

Comment: In the late 1970s, several reports noted the frequent cooccurrence of CRMO and pustulosis palmoplantaris. The link between psoriasis and CRMO was recognized in the late 1980s. Since then, multiple inflammatory skin disorders have been associated with CRMO including generalized pustulosis, pyoderma gangrenosum, severe acne, Sweet's syndrome, and Crohn's disease.

Myth: In CRMO, tubular long bone involvement is confined to the metaphysis.

Reality: Involvement of the metaphyses of the long bones is the most common site for CRMO lesions. Diaphyseal involvement is typically in the area immediately adjacent to active metaphyseal lesions. The presence of isolated diaphyseal lesions should prompt a second look for an alternative diagnosis. In addition, a substantial number of children with CRMO never have long bone involvement but have lesions in other sites including the clavicles, vertebral bodies, pelvis, ribs, feet, sternum, jaw, hands, skull, and scapula.

Myth: CRMO bone lesions are always symptomatic.

Reality: One common mistake made in working up children with a single symptomatic sterile osteolytic lesion is the failure to look for asymptomatic disease at other sites. A reasonable algorithm for imaging in this disorder is as follows:

1. Plain radiographs of symptomatic lesions.
2. Bone scan to identify asymptomatic lesions.
3. Radiography for all lesions seen on bone scan.
4. Magnetic resonance imaging for any lesions that need additional documentation of the disease extent and for lesions seen on bone scan that are not detectable on plain film.

Pearl: Primary intraosseous lymphoma can mimic CRMO.

Comment: Given that glucocorticoids are a reasonable treatment option for CRMO, one must be very careful not to miss an unusual presentation of lymphoma. Primary multifocal osseous lymphoma is challenging to diagnose because the lymphoma occurs in the bone without the evidence of visceral or lymph node involvement (Sato et al. 2008). The osseous lesions are osteolytic, multifocal, and often involve the long bones. Common sites of bony involvement in primary osseous lymphoma include the femur, tibia, pelvis, and the spine (Sato et al. 2008). These are also common sites of lesions in CRMO. Clues to a more sinister diagnosis of lymphoma include cortical erosion and the involvement of the diaphysis of the long bones.

Glucocorticoids should not be administered before lymphoma has been excluded with certainty. Inappropriate glucocorticoid use can affect survival in lymphoma. When in doubt, re-biopsy should be done.

Myth: Antibiotics have no role in treating CRMO.

Reality: Despite the current dogma that bone lesions in CRMO are sterile, symptomatic improvement associated with azithromycin therapy has been reported (Schilling et al. 2000). One explanation is that CRMO is indeed an infectious disease due to an indolent infectious agent and that azithromycin is helping through its antimicrobial properties. However, microbial signatures have not been identified in bone biopsies taken from active CRMO lesions (Girschick 2007). Another plausible explanation is that azithromycin exerts its benefit through its reported anti-inflammatory properties (Labro 2004). Additional studies are needed to determine the role of azithromycin in treating CRMO.

Pearl: The clavicle is a common site of involvement in CRMO and SAPHO syndrome, but a rare site for infectious osteomyelitis.

Comment: Clinically, CRMO and infectious osteomyelitis can be very difficult to differentiate. In many cases, culture results are unreliable because of empiric antibiotic use before a bone biopsy is obtained. However, clavicular involvement may be a clue that it is inflammatory rather than infectious. Clavicular involvement, rare in infectious osteomyelitis, is relatively common in CRMO (Girschick et al. 1998). Therefore, involvement of the clavicle should raise the suspicion for a noninfectious process such as CRMO or SAPHO.

5.1.6 PAPA

- PAPA syndrome is caused by mutations in the PSTPIP1 gene mapped to chromosome 15q24 and is inherited in an autosomal dominant pattern.
- The most common symptom of PAPA is pyogenic sterile arthritis; other symptoms include pyoderma gangrenosum and cystic acne.
- The arthritis usually presents during childhood with recurrent inflammatory episodes resembling septic arthritis but with sterile cultures.

Pearl: PAPA is an acronym for pyogenic arthritis, pyoderma gangrenosum, and acne.

Comment: PAPA syndrome, which demonstrates an autosomal dominant pattern of inheritance, is caused by missense mutations in the PSTPIP1 gene (chromosome 15q24). Four different mutations have been identified in four Caucasian US families and one Spanish family. The syndrome is characterized by skin lesions and polyarticular arthritis. Skin manifestations include severe cystic acne, pyoderma gangrenosum and sterile abscess formation at injection sites. The arthritis, which involves peripheral joints, presents with recurrent sterile effusions that contain high neutrophil counts.

Periods of arthritis fluctuate throughout the patient's lifetime. Chronic recurrences can lead to joint erosion.

Mutations in PSTPIP1 lead to gains of function. Two in vitro models link the mutations that cause PAPA to the excessive production of IL-1-beta, thereby suggesting that IL-1 inhibition might be an effective treatment strategy (Shoham et al. 2003; Yu et al. 2007). The in vivo function of PSTPIP1 requires further exploration. Treatment for PAPA includes intra-articular and systemic glucocorticoids (Tallon et al. 2006). Case reports show clinical improvement and a decrease in inflammatory markers with either tumor necrosis factor inhibition or anakinra (Cortis et al. 2004; Stichweh et al. 2005; Dierselhuis et al. 2005).

5.1.7 Cherubism

- Cherubism presents with marked, symmetric expansion of the jaw bones resulting in a distinctive chubby cheeked appearance occasionally accompanied by upturned eyes.
- Age of onset is usually between 3 and 5 years of age.
- Bone involvement in cherubism is nearly always confined to the jaw.
- Biopsy of the involved bone reveals fibroblastic stroma and abundant osteoclasts.
- Severe dental problems, including loss of teeth and malocclusion, occur.
- Cherubism is an autosomal dominant disorder. Most cases are associated with mutations in SH3BP2.

Myth: Cherubism is a form of fibro-osseous dysplasia.

Reality: Cherubism is an autosomal dominant disorder with incomplete penetrance that presents with painless jaw swelling (Fig. 5.5) (OMIM reference number 118400). Multiple large osteolytic lesions are seen on radiographs (Fig. 5.6). Bone biopsy reveals dense fibrous connective tissue interspersed with abundant osteoclasts. Mutations in exon 9 of the SH3-binding protein 2 gene are present in majority of the cases (Ueki et al. 2001).

Until recently, cherubism was viewed as a form of bone dysplasia with limited treatment options. However, Ueki et al. used a knock-in mouse model to demonstrate that cherubism is an inflammatory disorder driven by the innate immune system, which is dependent in the presence of tumor necrosis factor (Ueki et al. 2007). Consequently, cherubism is now considered as an autoinflammatory bone disorder (Ferguson et al. 2007; Novack et al. 2007; Ueki et al. 2007). TNF inhibitors are the main approach to treatment.

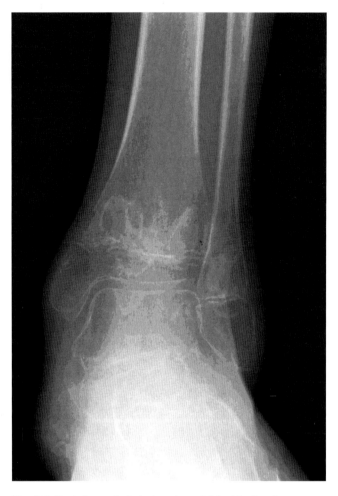

Fig. 5.5 Typical osteolytic lesions in a child with chronic recurrent multifocal osteomyelitis (CRMO). Multiple rounded lacunar shaped osteolytic lesions surrounded by a rim of sclerosis are seen immediately adjacent to the growth plate in the distal fibula and tibia. Additional osteolytic lesions are seen in the dome of the talus and calcaneus. Diffuse osteopenia is present

Pearl: Individuals with cherubism may have extra-gnathic bone lesions.

Comment: The vast majority of patients with cherubism have lesions confined to the jaw. However, several reports have detailed extra-gnathic bone involvement, including involvement of the jaw with the rib, humerus, femur, or tibial disease (Ozkan 2003).

Acknowledgement We would like to thank Dr. Daniel Kastner for sharing his expertise and suggestions for the *myths* and *pearls* in the FMF section.

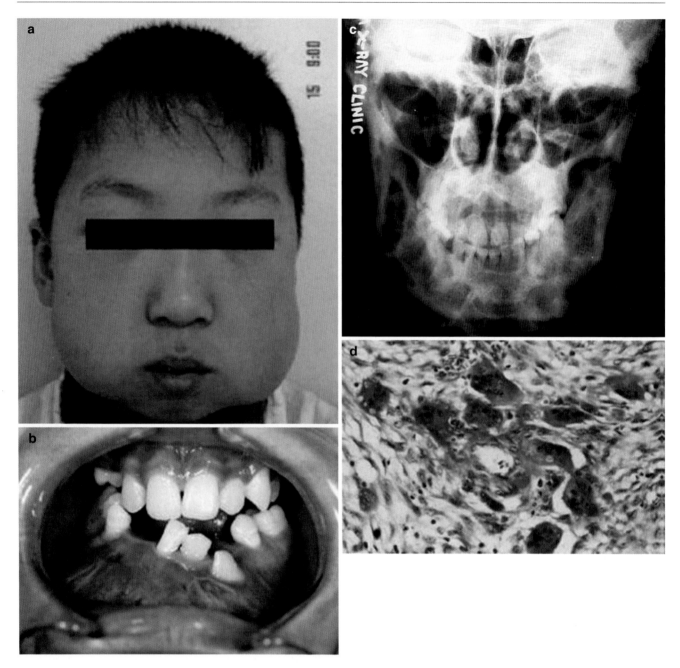

Fig. 5.6 (**a**) *Chubby cheek* appearance due to mandibular enlargement in a boy with cherubism (From Meng et al. (2005). Reprinted with permission from Elsevier). (**b**) Expansion of the mandible in cherubism with resultant dental abnormalities (From Meng et al. (2005). Reprinted with permission from Elsevier). (**c**) This plain film reveals multiple large radiolucent lesions with surrounding sclerosis in the mandible of a female with cherubism (From Jain and Sharma (2006). Reprinted with permission from Springer Science + Business Media). (**d**) Histologic findings in cherubism of multinucleated giant cells in collagen stromal tissue (From Meng et al. (2005). Reprinted with permission from Elsevier)

References

Aganna E, Hammond L, Hawkins PN, et al Heterogeneity among patients with tumor necrosis factor receptor-associated periodic syndrome phenotypes. Arthritis Rheum. 2003;48(9):2632–44

Agostini L, Martinon F, Burns K, McDermott MF, Hawkins PN, Tschopp J. NALP3 forms an IL-1beta-processing inflammasome with increased activity in Muckle-Wells autoinflammatory disorder. Immunity. 2004;20(3):319–25

Aksentijevich I, Galon J, Soares M, et al The tumor-necrosis-factor receptor-associated periodic syndrome: new mutations in TNFRSF1A, ancestral origins, genotype-phenotype studies, and evidence for further genetic heterogeneity of periodic fevers. Am J Hum Genet. 2001;69(2):301–14

Aksentijevich I, Nowak M, Mallah M, et al De novo CIAS1 mutations, cytokine activation, and evidence for geneticheterogeneity in patients with neonatal-onset multisystem inflammatory disease(NOMID): a new member of the expanding family of pyrin-associated autoinflammatory diseases. Arthritis Rheum. 2002 46(12):3340–8

Aksentijevich I, Putnam C, Remmers EF, et al The clinical continuum of cryopyrinopathies: novel CIAS1 mutations in North American patients and a new cryopyrin model. Arthritis Rheum. 2007;56(4): 1273–85

Aksentijevich I, Torosyan Y, Samuels J, et al Mutation and haplotype studies of familial Mediterranean fever reveal new ancestral relationships and evidence for a high carrier frequency with reduced penetrance in the Ashkenazi Jewish population. Am J Hum Genet. 1999;64(4):949–62

Al-Mosawi ZS, Al-Saad KK, Ijadi-Maghsoodi R, et al A splice site mutation confirms the role of LPIN2 in Majeed syndrome. Arthritis Rheum. 2007;56:960–4

Altiparmak MR, Pamuk ON, Pamuk GE, et al Amyloid goitre in familial Mediterranean fever: report on three patients and review of the literature. Clin Rheumatol. 2002;21(6):497–500

Ammouri W, Cuisset L, Rouaghe S, et al Diagnostic value of serum immunoglobulinaemia D level in patients with a clinical suspicion of hyper IgD syndrome. Rheumatology. 2007;46(10):1597–600

Arostegui JI, Solis P, Aldea A, et al Etanercept plus colchicine treatment in a child with tumour necrosis factor receptor-associated periodic syndrome abolishes auto-inflammatory episodes without normalising the subclinical acute phase response. Eur J Pediatr. 2005;164(1):13–6

Ben-Chetrit E, Levy M. Reproductive system in familial Mediterranean fever: an overview. Ann Rheum Dis. 2003;62(10):916–9

Brik R, Litmanovitz D, Berkowitz D, et al Incidence of familial Mediterranean fever (FMF) mutations among children of Mediterranean extraction with functional abdominal pain. J Pediatr. 2001;138:759–62

Cohen SL, Boner G, Shmueli D, et al Cyclosporin: poorly tolerated in familial Mediterranean fever. Nephrol Dial Transplant. 1989; 4(3):201–4

Cortis E, DeBenedetti F, Insalaco A, Cioschi S, Muratori F, D'Urbano LE, Uqazio AG. Abnormal production of tumor necrosis factor (TNF) – alpha and clinical efficacy of the TNF inhibitor etanercept in a patient with PAPA syndrome [corrected]. J Pediatr. 2004;145(6): 851–5

Cuisset L, Drenth JP, Berthelot JM, et al Genetic linkage of the Muckle-Wells syndrome to chromosome 1q44. Am J Hum Genet. 1999;65(4): 1054–9

Delorme N, Drouet M, Thibaudeau A, et al Urticaire au froid. Allergie Et Immunologie. 2002;34(7):255–8

Demirkaya E, Caglar MK, Waterham HR, et al A patient with hyper-IgD syndrome responding to anti-TNF treatment. Clin Rheumatol. 2007;26(10):1757–9

Dierselhuis MP, Frenkel J, Wulfraat NM, et al Anakinra for flares of pyogenic arthritis in PAPA syndrome. Rheumatology. 2005;44: 406–8

D'Osualdo A, Ferlito F, Prigione I, et al Neutrophils from patients with TNFRSF1A mutations display resistance to tumor necrosis factor-induced apoptosis – pathogenetic and clinical implications. Arthritis Rheum. 2006;54(3):998–1008

D'Osualdo A, Picco P, Caroli F, et al MVK mutations and associated clinical features in Italian patients affected with autoinflammatory disorders and recurrent fever. Eur J Hum Genet. 2005;13(3): 314–20

Drenth JP, Haagsma CJ, van der Meer JW. Hyperimmunoglobulinemia D and periodic fever syndrome. The clinical spectrum in a series of 50 patients. International Hyper-IgD Study Group. Medicine (Baltimore). 1994;73(3):133–44

Duffy CM, Lam PY, Ditchfield M, et al Chronic recurrent multifocal osteomyelitis: review of orthopaedic complications at maturity. J Pediatr Orthop. 2002;22:501–5

Eleftheriou G, Bacis G, Fiocchi R, et al Colchicine-induced toxicity in a heart transplant patient with chronic renal failure. Clin Toxicol (Phila). 2008;17:1–4

El-Shanti H, Majeed HA, El-Khateeb M. Familial mediterranean fever in Arabs. Lancet. 2006;367:1016–24

Ferguson PJ, Chen S, Tayeh MK, et al Homozygous mutations in LPIN2 are responsible for the syndrome of chronic recurrent multifocal osteomyelitis and congenital dyserythropoietic anemia (Majeed Syndrome). J Med Genet. 2005;42:551–7

Ferguson PJ, El-Shanti HI. Autoinflammatory bone disorders. Curr Opin Immunol. 2007;19:492–8

Fradkin A, Yahav J, Zemer D, et al Colchicine-induced lactose malabsorption in patients with familial Mediterranean fever. Isr J Med Sci. 1995;31:(10): 616–20

Galon J, Aksentijevich I, McDermott MF, et al TNF receptor-associated periodic syndromes (TRAPS): Mutations in TNFR1 and early experience with Etanercept therapy. Faseb Journal. 2000;14(6): A1150

Gattorno M, Tassi S, Carta S, et al Pattern of interleukin-1beta secretion in response to lipopolysaccharide and ATP before and after interleukin-1 blockade in patients with CIAS1 mutations. Arthritis Rheum. 2007;56(9):3138–48

Gattorno M, Pelagatti MA, Meini A, et al Persistent efficacy of anakinra in patients with tumor necrosis factor receptor-associated periodic syndrome. Arthritis Rheum. 2008a;58(5):1516–20

Gattorno M, Sormani MP, D'Osualdo A, et al A diagnostic score for molecular analysis of hereditary autoinflammatory syndromes with periodic fever in children. Arthritis Rheum. 2008b;58(6):1823–32

Girschick HJ, Krauspe R, Tschammler A, et al Chronic recurrent osteomyelitis with clavicular involvement in children: diagnostic value of different imaging techniques and therapy with non-steroidal anti-inflammatory drugs. Eur J Pediatr. 1998;157:28–33

Goldbach-Mansky R, Dailey NJ, Canna SW, et al Neonatal-onset multisystem inflammatory disease responsive to interleukin-1beta inhibition. N Engl J Med. 2006;355(6):581–92

Goldbach-Mansky R, Shroff SD, Wilson M, et al A pilot study to evaluate the safety and efficacy of the long-acting interleukin-1 inhibitor rilonacept (interleukin-1 Trap) in patients with familial cold autoinflammatory syndrome. Arthritis Rheum. 2008;58(8):2432–42

Hawkins PN, Lachmann HJ, Aganna E, et al Spectrum of clinical features in Muckle-Wells syndrome and response to anakinra. Arthritis Rheum. 2004;50(2):607–12

Hill SC, Namde M, Dwyer A, Poznanski A, et al Arthropathy of neonatal onset multisystem inflammatory disease (NOMID/CINCA). Pediatr Radiol. 2007;37(2):145–52

Hoffman HM, Gregory SG, Mueller JL, Tresierras M, Broide DH, Wanderer AA, Kolodner RD. Fine structure mapping of CIAS1: identification of an ancestral haplotype and a common FCAS mutation, L353P. Hum Genet. 2003;112(2):209–216

Hoffman HM, Mueller JL, Broide DH, et al Mutation of a new gene encoding a putative pyrin-like protein causes familial cold autoinflammatory syndrome and Muckle-Wells syndrome. Nat Genet. 2001a;29(3):301–5

Hoffman HM, Rosengren S, Boyle DL, et al Prevention of cold-associated acute inflammation in familial cold autoinflammatory syndrome by interleukin-1 receptor antagonist. Lancet. 2004;364(9447): 1779–85

Hoffman HM, Throne ML, Amar NJ, et al Efficacy and safety of rilonacept (interleukin-1 Trap) in patients with cryopyrin-associated periodic syndromes: results from two sequential placebo-controlled studies. Arthritis Rheum. 2008;58(8):2443–52

Hoffman HM, Wanderer AA, Broide DH. Familial cold autoinflammatory syndrome: phenotype and genotype of an autosomal dominant periodic fever. J Allergy Clin Immunol. 2001b;108(4):615–20

Hoffmann GF, Charpentier C, Mayatepek E, et al Clinical and biochemical phenotype in 11 patients with mevalonic aciduria. Pediatrics. 1993;91(5):915–21

Houten SM, Kuis W, Duran M, et al Mutations in MVK, encoding mevalonate kinase, cause hyperimmunoglobulinaemia D and periodic fever syndrome. Nature Genetics. 1999;22(2):175–7

Huggins ML, Radford PM, McIntosh RS, et al Shedding of mutant tumor necrosis factor receptor superfamily 1A associated with tumor necrosis factor receptor-associated periodic syndrome: differences between cell types. Arthritis Rheum. 2004;50(8):2651–9

Hull KM, Drewe E, Aksentijevich I, et al The TNF receptor-associated periodic syndrome (TRAPS): emerging concepts of an autoinflammatory disorder. Medicine (Baltimore). 2002;81(5):349–68

Jacobelli S, Andre M, Alexandra JF, et al Failure of anti-TNF therapy in TNF Receptor 1-Associated Periodic Syndrome (TRAPS). Rheumatology (Oxford). 2007;46(7):1211–2

Kallinich T, Haffner D, Niehues T, et al Colchicine use in children and adolescents with familial Mediterranean fever: literature review and consensus statement. Pediatrics. 2007;119(2):e474–83

Kallinich T, Haffner D, Rudolph B, et al "Periodic fever" without fever: two cases of non-febrile TRAPS with mutations in the TNFRSF1A gene presenting with episodes of inflammation or monosymptomatic amyloidosis. Ann Rheum Dis. 2006;65(7):958–60

Kastner D. Familial Mediterranean fever. In: Fauci A, Braunwald E, Kasper D, Hauser SL, Longo DL, Jameson L, Loscalzo J, editors. Harrison's principle of internal medicine. 17th ed. USA: McGraw-Hill; 2008

Kavukçu S, Türkmen M, Eroğlu Y, et al Renal, gastric and thyroidal amyloidosis due to familial Mediterranean fever. Pediatr Nephrol. 1997;11(2):210–2

Kilcline C, Shinkai K, Bree A, et al Neonatal-onset multisystem inflammatory disorder: the emerging role of pyrin genes in autoinflammatory diseases. Arch Dermatol. 2005;141(2):248–53

Labro MT. Macrolide antibiotics: current and future uses. Expert Opin Pharmacother. 2004;5:541–50

Lachmann HJ, Sengul B, Yavuzsen TU, et al Clinical and subclinical inflammation in patients with familial Mediterranean fever and in heterozygous carriers of MEFV mutations. Rheumatology (Oxford). 2006;45:746–50

Leslie KS, Lachmann HJ, Bruning E, et al Phenotype, genotype, and sustained response to anakinra in 22 patients with autoinflammatory disease associated with CIAS-1/NALP3 mutations. Arch Dermatol. 2006;142(12):1591–7

Majeed HA, Al-Tarawna M, El-Shanti H, et al The syndrome of chronic recurrent multifocal osteomyelitis and congenital dyserythropoietic anaemia. Report of a new family and a review. Eur J Pediatr. 2001;160:705–10

Majeed HA, El-Shanti H, Al-Rimawi H, et al On mice and men: an autosomal recessive syndrome of chronic recurrent multifocal osteomyelitis and congenital dyserythropoietic anemia. J Pediatr. 2000;137:441–2

Majeed HA, Kalaawi M, Mohanty D, et al Congenital dyserythropoietic anemia and chronic recurrent multifocal osteomyelitis in three related children and the association with Sweet syndrome in two siblings. J Pediatr. 1989;115:730–4

McDermott MF, Aksentijevich I, Galon J, et al ermline mutations in the extracellular domains of the 55 kDa TNF receptor, TNFR1, define a family of dominantly inherited autoinflammatory syndromes. Cell. 1999;97(1):133–44

Mimouni A, Magal N, Stoffman N, et al Familial Mediterranean fever: effects of genotype and ethnicity on inflammatory attacks and amyloidosis. Pediatrics. 2000;105(5):E70

Minetti EE, Minetti L. Multiple organ failure in a kidney transplant patient receiving both colchicine and cyclosporine. J Nephrol. 2003;16(3):421–5

Neittaanmäki H. Cold urticaria. Clinical findings in 220 patients. J Am Acad Dermatol. 1985;13(4):636–44

Neven B, Callebaut I, Prieur AM, et al Molecular basis of the spectral expression of CIAS1 mutations associated with phagocytic cell-mediated autoinflammatory disorders CINCA/NOMID, MWS, and FCU. Blood. 2004;103(7):2809–15

Novack DV, Faccio R. Jawing about TNF: new hope for cherubism. Cell. 2007;128:15–7

Prieur AM, Griscelli C, Lampert F, et al A chronic, infantile, neurological, cutaneous and articular (CINCA) syndrome. A specific entity analysed in 30 patients. Scand J Rheumatol. 1987;66 Suppl:57–68

Prieur AM. A recently recognised chronic inflammatory disease of early onset characterized by the triad of rash, central nervous system involvement and arthropathy. Clin Exp Rheumatol. 2001;19(1): 103–6

Rynne M, Maclean C, Bybee A, et al Hearing improvement in a patient with variant Muckle-Wells syndrome in response to interleukin 1 receptor antagonism. Ann Rheum Dis. 2006;65:533–4

Saito M, Nishikomori R, Kambe N, Fujisawa A, Tanizaki H, et al Disease-associated CIAS1 mutations induce monocyte death, revealing low-level mosaicism in mutation-negative cryopyrin-associated periodic syndrome patients. Blood. 2008;111(4):2132–41

Samuels J, Aksentijevich I, Torosyan Y, et al Familial Mediterranean fever at the millennium. Clinical spectrum, ancient mutations, and a survey of 100 American referrals to the National Institutes of Health. Medicine (Baltimore). 1998;77(4):268–97

Sato TS, Khanna G, Ferguson PJ. Primary multifocal osseous lymphoma in a child. Pediatr Radiol. 2008;38:1338–41

Schilling F, Wagner AD. Azithromycin: an anti-inflammatory effect in chronic recurrent multifcal osteomyelitis? A preliminary report. Z Rheumatol. 2000;59:352–3

Shinkai K, McCalmont TH, Leslie KS. Cryopyrin-associated periodic syndromes and autoinflammation. Clin Exp Dermatol. 2008;33(1): 1–9

Shoham NG, Centola M, Mansfield E, et al Pyrin binds the PSTPIP1/CD2BP1 protein, defining familial Mediterranean fever and PAPA syndrome as disorders in the same pathway. Proc Natl Acad Sci U S A.. 2003;100(23):13501–6

Siewert R, Ferber J, Horstmann RD, et al Hereditary periodic fever with systemic amyloidosis: is hyper-IgD syndrome really a benign disease? Am J Kidney Dis. 2006;48(3):e41–5

Simon A, Bodar EJ, van der Hilst JC, et al Beneficial response to interleukin 1 receptor antagonist in TRAPS. Am J Med. 2004a;117(3): 208–10

Simon A, Kremer HP, Wevers RA, et al Mevalonate kinase deficiency: Evidence for a phenotypic continuum. Neurol. 2004b;62(6):994–7

Speeg KV, Maldonado AL, Liaci J, et al Effect of cyclosporine on colchicine secretion by the kidney multidrug transporter studied in vivo. J Pharmacol Exp Ther. 1992;261(1):50–5

Stankovic K, Grateau G. Auto inflammatory syndromes: Diagnosis and treatment. Joint Bone Spine. 2007;74:544–50

Stichweh DS, Punaro M, Pascual V. Dramtic improvement of pyoderma gangrenosum with infliximab in a patient with PAPA syndrome. Pediatr Dermatol. 2005;22(3):262–5

Stoffman N, Magal N, Shohat T, et al Higher than expected carrier rates for familial Mediterranean fever in various Jewish ethnic groups. Eur J Hum Genet. 2000;8(4):307–10

Stojanov S, Kastner DL. Familial autoinflammatory diseases: Genetics, pathogenesis and treatment. Curr Opin Rheumatol. 2005;17(5): 586–99

Tallon B, Corkill M. Peculiarities of PAPA syndrome. Rheumatology. 2006;45:1140–3

The French FMF Consortium. A candidate gene for familial Mediterranean fever. Nat Genet. 1997;17(1):25–31

The International FMF Consortium. Ancient missense mutations in a new member of the RoRet gene family are likely to cause familial Mediterranean fever. Cell. 1997;90(4):797–807

Thornton BD, Hoffman HM, Bhat A, Don BR. Am J Kidney Dis. 2007;49:477–81

Touitou I, Sarkisian T, Medlej-Hashim M, et al Country as the primary risk factor for renal amyloidosis in familial Mediterranean fever. Arthritis Rheum. 2007;56(5):1706–12

Ueki Y, Lin CY, Senoo M, et al Increased myeloid cell responses to M-CSF and RANKL cause bone loss and inflammation in SH3BP2 "cherubism" mice. Cell. 2007;128:71–83

Ueki Y, Tiziani V, Santanna C, et al Mutations in the gene encoding c-Abl-binding protein SH3BP2 cause cherubism. Nat Genet. 2001;28:125–6

van der Hilst J, Bodar E, Barron K, et al Follow-up, clinical features, and quality of life in 10.3 patients with HyperImmunoglubulin D syndrome. Clin Exp Rheumatol. 2008;26(2):180

van der Meer JW, Vossen JM, Radl J, et al Hyperimmunoglobulinaemia D and periodic fever: a new syndrome. Lancet. 1984;1(8386): 1087–90

Williamson LM, Hull D, Mehta R, et al Familial Hibernian fever. Q J Med. 1982;1(204):469–80

Yamazaki T, Masumoto J, Agematsu K, et al Anakinra improves sensory deafness in a Japanese patient with Muckle-Wells syndrome, possibly by inhibiting the cryopyrin inflammasome. Arthritis Rheum. 2008;58(3):864–8

Yarom A, Rennebohm RM, Levinson JE. Infantile multisystem inflammatory disease: a specific syndrome? J Pediatr. 1985;106(3): 390–6

Yildiz A, Akkaya V, Kiliçaslan I, et al Cardiac and intestinal amyloidosis in a renal transplant recipient with familial Mediterranean fever. J Nephrol. 2001;14(2):125–7

Yu JW, Fernandes-Alnemri T, Datta P, et al Pyrin activates the ASC pyroptosome in response to engagement by autoinflammatory PSTPIP1 mutants. Mol Cell. 2007;28:214–227

Meng XM et al. Clinicopathologic study of 24 cases of cherubism. Int J Oral Maxillofac Surg. 2005;34:350–6

Jain V, Sharma R. Radiographic, CT and MRI features of cherubism. Pediatr Radiol. 2006;36(10):1099–104

Juvenile Spondyloarthropathy

David A. Cabral and Shirley M. L. Tse

6.1 Overview

> Juvenile spondyloarthropathy includes both differentiated and undifferentiated forms. The differentiated forms include juvenile ankylosing spondylitis, reactive arthritis, psoriatic arthritis, and arthritis with inflammatory bowel disease.

> Enthesitis-related arthritis (ERA) is now the preferred term for undifferentiated forms of juvenile spondyloarthropathy.

> Most juvenile spondyloarthropathy patients present with asymmetric oligoarthritis involving the knee, hip, ankle, tarsal, metatarsophalangeal, or foot interphalangeal joints.

> Enthesitis – pain, tenderness, and swelling at the site of attachment of tendon, ligament, or fascia to bone – is the most common feature of juvenile spondyloarthropathy. The frequency of this finding has led to the term "enthesitis-related arthritis" (ERA).

> Monoarthritis of one of these joints, particularly one of the large ones, is also common disease presentation.

> Axial involvement seldom begins less than 5 years after the clinical onset of juvenile spondyloarthropathy.

> Some patients with ERA are at high risk of developing ankylosing spondylitis. These include males, patients who are HLA-B27 (human leukocyte antigen B27) positive, and those with early arthritis of the hips, ankles, or sacroiliac joints.

> Acute anterior uveitis and inflammatory bowel disease are common extraarticular manifestations of ERA.

Myth: Children with juvenile spondyloarthropathy – by definition – have inflammatory disease of the back and sacroiliitis.

Reality: Most children with a juvenile spondyloarthropathy do not have the archetypal ankylosing spondylitis that occurs in adults. Although many children with a "spondyloarthropathy" ultimately develop classical sacroiliitis and back disease, their initial manifestations are usually a peripheral joint arthritis and either enthesitis or a constellation of other associated features (e.g., acute anterior uveitis).

Patients with juvenile idiopathic arthritis (JIA) who are at high risk of developing ankylosing spondylitis in the future are described by the JIA subcategory of "enthesitis-related arthritis" (ERA) (Petty et al. 1998, 2004). The diagnostic features of ERA are shown in Table 6.1.

Adolescents with ERA may have back symptoms but often lack radiologic evidence of inflammatory disease. The evolution of ERA to back and sacroiliac disease that is radiologically evident generally occurs in the late teens or when the patient is in his/her 20s.

Pearl: Most cases of spondyloarthropathy that present in childhood do so in an "undifferentiated" manner.

Comment: Many adult patients with non-rheumatoid inflammatory arthropathy are at risk of developing axial arthritis; yet do not fulfill criteria for a traditional spondyloarthropathy initially. The generic diagnosis of "spondyloarthropathy" has been used to describe these adult patients with "early" or "undifferentiated" disease (Amor et al. 1990; Dougados et al. 1991).

The same is true for children with inflammatory arthropathy, a large majority of who present with "undifferentiated" spondyloarthropathy syndromes, but ultimately develop axial arthritis (Cabral et al. 1992; Flato et al. 1998; Jacobs et al. 1982; Rosenberg and Petty 1982). A variety of terms have been used to describe children with these pediatric spondyloarthropathies who are recognized as being at high risk of developing axial arthritis (Table 6.2).

The most recently proposed nomenclature for classifying pediatric chronic arthritis has encapsulated all of these syndromes in a subset of JIA described as ERA (Petty et al. 1998, 2004).

Myth: HLA-B27 is a good screening test for juvenile spondyloarthropathy.

Reality: HLA-B27 (human leukocyte antigen B27) is a class I surface antigen encoded by the B locus in the major

J. H. Stone (ed.), *A Clinician's Pearls and Myths in Rheumatology,*
DOI:10.1007/978-1-84800-934-9_6, © Springer Science + Business Media B.V. 2009

Table 6.1 Diagnostic features of ERA (adapted from Petty et al. 2004)

1. Arthritis *and* enthesitis or
2. Arthritis *or* enthesitis with at least two of the following:
   - Sacroiliac joint tenderness or inflammatory lumbosacral pain
   - HLA-B27 antigen positivity
   - Onset of arthritis in a male after 6 years of age
   - Acute (symptomatic) anterior uveitis
   - Family history in a first degree relative of ankylosing spondylitis, ERA, sacroiliitis with inflammatory bowel disease, reactive arthritis, or acute anterior uveitis

Diagnostic exclusion criteria:
   - Rheumatoid factor
   - Features of systemic arthritis
   - Psoriasis in the patient or in a first-degree relative

Table 6.2 Diagnostic syndromes used to describe juvenile spondyloarthropathies

- Seronegative enthesopathy and arthropathy (SEA syndrome)
- Pauciarticular onset JRA* type II
- Late-onset pauciarticular juvenile chronic arthritis (LOPA)
- HLA-B27-associated arthropathy and enthesopathy syndrome
- ERA

histocompatibility complex (MHC). HLA-B27 occurs in about 90% of patients with ankylosing spondylitis and perhaps 75% of children with ERA. The frequency of HLA-B27 varies considerably in different populations. As examples, the frequency of this antigen is as low as 0.1% in the Japanese population but as high as 24% among Laplanders.

As with adults, HLA-B27 is not a good screening test in pediatric patients who do not have complaints that are reasonably specific for ERA. HLA-B27 occurs in about 8% of the Caucasian population. However, only about 10% of HLA-B27-positive individuals develop ankylosing spondylitis, and 10% of patients with ankylosing spondylitis are HLA-B27 negative.

For children who have documented arthritis or enthesitis, the presence of HLA-B27 is useful in classifying the type of arthritis as ERA.

Pearl: Enthesitis is the most common defining clinical feature of juvenile spondyloarthropathy.

Comment: Enthesitis refers to inflammation – pain, tenderness, and swelling – at the enthesis, the site of attachment of tendon, ligament, or fascia to bone. Enthesitis, the most common clinical feature of ERA, occurs more frequently in children who have classically-defined ankylosing spondylitis than it does in adults with that disorder (Burgos-Vargas 1989; Gensler et al. 2008). Enthesitis is not unique to ERA in children, and is detected occasionally among children with other disorders, particularly psoriatic arthritis but also systemic lupus erythematosus (Cabral et al. 1992).

Pearl: Children rarely present with back pain from spondyloarthropathy in the first decade of life.

Comment: Orthopedic, traumatic, infectious, and malignant disorders are much more likely in children than are idiopathic inflammatory conditions such as ERA or ankylosing spondylitis. In particular, pre-pubertal children with ERA virtually never present with back arthritis. Bone infections, discitis, and malignancies such as neuroblastoma are the major diagnostic considerations in that setting. In the older child or youth, Scheuerman's disease (juvenile osteochondrosis of the spine), spondylolisthesis, scoliosis, and trauma are other important considerations.

Some data suggest that Hispanic children and pediatric patients with inflammatory bowel disease have axial arthritis of earlier onset than do pediatric patients with other forms of rheumatic disease (Burgos-Vargas 1989).

Pearl: Tarsitis is a characteristic feature of spondyloarthropathy in children, but occurs in only a minority of patients.

Comment: Tarsitis presents as tenderness and swelling of the mid-foot (Fig. 6.1). This clinical manifestation of pediatric spondyloarthropathy is probably caused by the combination of synovitis, enthesitis, tenosynovitis, and bursitis. It is a characteristic, albeit uncommon, feature of juvenile spondyloarthropathy. Tarsitis may occur early in the disease course (Burgos-Vargas, 1991).

The finding of tarsitis is a clue to look for other features that suggest either ERA or juvenile ankylosing spondylitis. Tarsitis can occur with other forms of JIA, especially the polyarthritis variant, but usually develops later in the disease course as an "extension" of ankle disease.

Pearl: ERA should be considered in the differential diagnosis of Osgood–Schlatter's disease.

Comment: Children diagnosed with ERA may have a previous history of Osgood–Schlatter's disease (osteochondrosis of the tibial tuberosity). The insertion of the patellar tendon to the tibial tubercle is a common site of enthesitis in children with ERA, and may be difficult to distinguish clinically from Osgood–Schlatter's disease.

Osgood–Schlatter's disease is more common than ERA, but ERA should be considered carefully if there is concurrent arthritis, a family history of spondyloarthropathy, or enthesitis at other sites typical of ERA: behind of the heel (at the insertion of the Achilles tendon to calcaneus), beneath the heel (at the insertion of the plantar fascia to calcaneus), and beneath the metatarsal heads.

Myth: Enthesitis requires early, aggressive pharmacologic intervention.

Reality: Untreated enthesitis does not usually lead to permanent functional bony destruction in the same way that

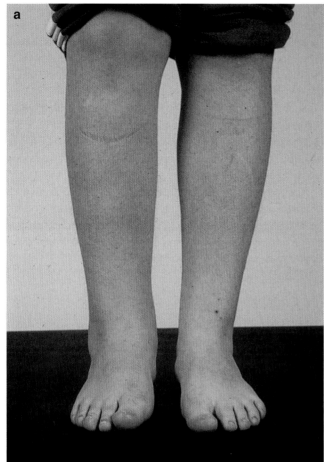

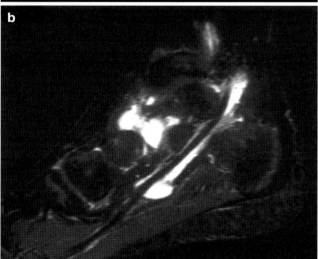

Fig. 6.1 Tarsitis shown clinically in the right foot (**a**) and using MRI (**b**)

Severe cases may be difficult to treat, but initial therapy should include simple analgesics, nonsteroid antiinflammatory drugs (NSAIDs), and physical interventions such as improved footwear and custom-made, semi-rigid orthotics. Insightful podiatric care can redistribute the weight from sites of painful enthesitis and provide cushioning at the tender sites. Heel lifts alleviate stress in the retrocalcaneal area and the knee. Low-dose prednisone is effective in patients when enthesitis persists despite these interventions.

Myth: Inflammatory enthesitis is the most common cause of pain behind the heel and under the feet in children.

Reality: Children who present with foot pain usually have activity-related issues, mechanical problems, or both, rather than inflammatory enthesitis. Flat feet and non-supportive footwear are common. Children with flat feet often complain of pain in the summer, when their levels of physical activity are increased and they wear flat sandals or "flip-flops".

Sever's disease, also known as calcaneal apophysitis, is another diagnostic possibility in the older child who presents with pain behind the heel. Sever's disease is caused by inflammation that arises from overuse and repetitive microtrauma of growth plates of the calcaneus. (It is, essentially, Osgood–Schlatter's disease of the heel.)

Pearl: Buttock pain in a patient with childhood spondyloarthropathy is usually not caused by sacroiliitis.

Comment: When assessing the clinical features of juvenile spondyloarthropathy, clinicians should inquire about the presence of buttock pain. This pain can be exacerbated by activity or noted when sitting on a hard bench or chair. In adults with ankylosing spondylitis, this pain in this area is usually attributed to sacroiliitis. In children, however, sacroiliitis is not an early feature of the disease. Rather, enthesitis involving the ischial tuberosity is the usual cause of buttock pain. Enthesitis of the ischial tuberosity can be particularly painful when sitting.

Myth: Sacroiliitis can only be detected by ordering a radiograph of the pelvis.

Reality: Sacroiliitis can be suspected or confirmed by either physical examination or imaging. Positive clinical signs include pain elicited on direct palpation of the sacroiliac joint or stress maneuvers of the sacroiliac joints (Figs. 6.1 and 6.2).

Imaging techniques available to detect sacroiliitis include radiographs, bone scans, computed tomography (CT), and magnetic resonance imaging (MRI). Radiographic sacroiliitis in children often presents as "pseudo-widening" of the sacroiliac joint. Subsequent changes include sclerosis, erosions, narrowing, and ankylosis (Bennett 1967).

Radiographic evidence of sacroiliitis typically lags behind the clinical signs and MRI findings. Bone scans may not be

arthritis does. As a result, aggressive pharmacological therapies with second- or third-line antirheumatic drugs may not be necessary. The natural history of enthesitis involving the lower limbs in children is that it tends to improve or disappear with age. Nevertheless, enthesitis can be quite debilitating in some patients. As an example, some are unable to walk because of inferior heel pain.

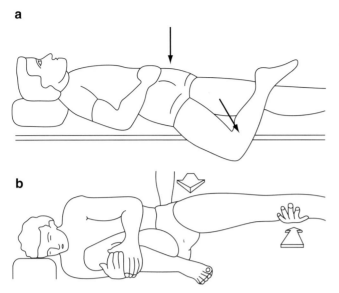

Fig. 6.2 Physical examination maneuvers designed to detect sacroiliitis (**a**) Patrick or FABER test: The patient lies supine and the ankle is placed on the contralateral straight leg. Passive pressure is exerted onto the ipsilateral thigh/knee resulting in flexion, abduction, and external rotation of the hip. Ipsilateral sacroiliac joint region tenderness is elicited in the presence of sacroiliitis. (**b**) Mennell's Sign: The patient is positioned on his or her side and asked to flex the hip on the lower side to the maximum extent. The examiner then extends the patient's upper hip by drawing back patient's upper knee with a slight jerk and presses a hand against the patient's sacrum. Pain in the upper side is consistent with sacroiliitis in the upper sacroiliac joint

helpful in the detection of sacroiliitis in children because the differentiation of sacroiliitis from the growth plate within the pelvis is difficult. CT scans have the significant drawback of high radiation exposure to the pelvic region. MRI has the advantages of high sensitivity and the absence of ionizing radiation, but is (of course) expensive.

Pearl: Extra-articular manifestations of juvenile spondyloarthropathy frequently include the gut and the eye.

Comment: The most common extra-articular manifestations of juvenile spondyloarthropathy are inflammatory bowel disease (IBD) and acute, symptomatic uveitis. Up to 80% of children with juvenile spondyloarthropathy have nonspecific IBD (Mielants et al. 1991, 1993; Cabral et al. 1992).

Many extra-articular manifestations that are reported in adult spondyloarthropathy are less common in children. As examples, cardiac conduction abnormalities, aortic valvular insufficiency, apical fibrosis of the lungs, urethritis, circinate balanitis, and atlanto-axial subluxation are only observed rarely in juvenile spondyloarthropathy.

Myth: Pediatric patients with IBD eventually develop spondylitis.

Reality: Peripheral arthritis, sacroiliitis, and spinal disease can be present at the onset of gut symptoms in children with

IBD. These symptoms can also develop after the onset of gastrointestinal complaints. The activity of peripheral arthritis in these patients correlates well with the activity of bowel inflammation in about half of pediatric patients with IBD. However, the arthritis of IBD in this setting tends to be short-lived, responsive to therapy, and non-erosive.

Sacroiliitis and spondylitis are less common than peripheral arthritis among pediatric patients with IBD, but both are more likely to occur in the setting of HLA-B27 positivity. In addition, sacroiliitis and spondylitis often follow courses that are independent of IBD flares.

The pattern of peripheral arthropathy in children with IBD who ultimately develop a spondyloarthropathy is similar to that of patients with ERA. The most common features are an asymmetric, large-joint, oligoarthritis involving lower extremities, frequently associated with enthesitis.

Myth: Patients with juvenile spondyloarthropathy generally "outgrow" their arthritis.

Reality: Remission in children with juvenile spondyloarthropathy occurs in between 15 and 45% of cases, and appears to have the highest likelihood among patients classified as having "undifferentiated" spondyloarthropathies (Flato et al. 1998, 2006; Minden et al. 2002). However, the majority of patients with undifferentiated juvenile spondyloarthropathy progress to ankylosing spondylitis if followed for sufficient lengths of time (Burgos-Vargas 1989; Cabral et al. 1992; Minden et al. 2002; Flato et al. 2006).

The development of axial disease is most likely in patients who are HLA-B27 positive, who demonstrate hip arthritis at an early stage of disease, and who are older than eight years of age at presentation. Screening and early therapy for axial involvement are especially important in patients with these characteristics.

Myth: Juvenile spondyloarthropathy only occurs in boys.

Reality: The prevalence of spondyloarthropathy is indeed higher among boys, particularly before puberty. However, the proportion of girls with juvenile spondyloarthropathy increases with age. Over time, the percentage of cases that occur in females is approximately equal to that in males. Moreover, some data suggest that girls with juvenile spondyloarthropathy have worse outcomes (Stone et al. 2005). Thus, the notions that juvenile spondyloarthropathy is primarily a disease of boys and that boys have more severe disease than girls both appear untrue.

Pearl: Regular eye examinations are required for some subsets of patients with JIA, but not patients with juvenile spondyloarthropathy.

Comment: Patients with juvenile spondyloarthropathy are at risk for an acute anterior uveitis (iritis). In contrast to the chronic, asymptomatic uveitis that is observed in pauciarticular JIA, the

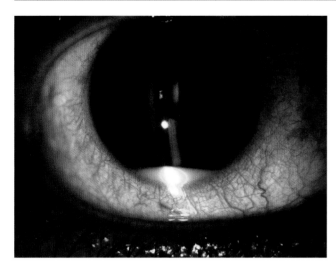

Fig. 6.3 Patient with acute exacerbation of HLA-B27 associated iritis and hypopyon (Figure courtesy of Dr. George Papaliodis)

acute anterior uveitis that complicates juvenile spondyloarthropathy is associated with photophobia, blurred vision, and a red eye (Fig. 6.3).

Because the ocular disease of juvenile spondyloarthropathy is highly symptomatic, most patients do not need more than the recommended ophthalmology follow-up for children unless they have symptomatic eye disease. This normally means eye examinations every 6 to 12 months (Cassidy et al. 2006).

Pearl: Tumor necrosis factor (TNF) inhibitors are effective for both the arthritis and enthesitis of juvenile spondyloarthropathy.

Comment: Currently, there are no effective therapies for the axial disease (spine or sacroiliac) in juvenile spondyloarthropathy. Treatment with NSAIDs and glucocorticoids may provide symptomatic improvement, but do not alter axial disease progression. Disease-modifying antirheumatic drugs such as sulfasalazine and methotrexate are also ineffective for axial disease.

High levels of TNF are identified at the sites of synovitis and enthesitis in adults and children with spondyloarthropathies. Treatment with TNF inhibitors such as etanercept or infliximab has led to clinical and radiologic improvement in juvenile spondyloarthropathy in both short- and long-term studies (Henrickson and Reiff 2004; Schmeling and Horneff 2004; Tse et al. 2005, 2006, 2007; Burgos-Vargas et al. 2007). Specifically, the arthritis (peripheral and axial), enthesitis, and inflammatory markers all improved and demonstrated sustained responses over time.

AntiTNF agents in juvenile spondyloarthropathy are associated with clinical and radiographic (MRI) improvement in the peripheral and axial joints. Because axial involvement is rare early in the disease course and does not present usually until the second or third decade of life, it remains unclear if TNF inhibition will prevent syndesmophyte formation and spinal fusion later in the disease course.

References

Amor B, Dougados M, Mijiyawa M. Criteres de classification des spondyloarthropathies. Rev Rhum Mal Osteoartic 1990; 57:85–89

Bennett PH. B. T. New York symposium on population studies in the rheumatic diseases: New diagnostic criteria. Bull Rheum Dis 1967; 17:453–458

Burgos-Vargas R. Ankylosing tarsitis: Clinical features of a unique form of tarsal disease in the juvenile-onset spondyloarthropathies. Arthritis Rheum 1991; 34(Suppl):D196

Burgos-Vargas R, Clark P. Axial involvement in the seronegative enthesopathy and arthropathy syndrome and its progression to ankylosing spondylitis. J Rheumatol 1989; 16(2):192–197

Burgos-Vargas R, Naranjo A, Castillo J, Katona G. Ankylosing spondylitis in the Mexican Mestizo: Patterns of disease according to age at onset. J Rheumatol 1989; 16:186–191

Burgos-Vargas RC, Gutierrez-Suarez R, Vazquez-Mellado J. Efficacy, safety, and tolerability of Infliximab in Juvenile-onset Spondyloarthropathies (JO-SpA): Results of the three-month, randomized, double-blind, placebo-controlled trial phase. Arthritis Rheum 2007; 56(9S):319

Cabral, DA, Oen KG, et al SEA syndrome revisited: A longterm followup of children with a syndrome of seronegative enthesopathy and arthropathy. J Rheumatol 1992; 19(8):1282–1285

Cassidy J, Kivlin J, et al Ophthalmologic examinations in children with juvenile rheumatoid arthritis. Pediatrics 2006; 117(5):1843–1845

Dougados M, van der Linden S, et al The European Spondylarthropathy Study Group preliminary criteria for the classification of spondylarthropathy. Arthritis Rheum 1991; 34(10):1218–1227

Flato B, Aasland A, et al Outcome and predictive factors in juvenile rheumatoid arthritis and juvenile spondyloarthropathy. J Rheumatol 1998; 25(2):366–375

Flato B, Hoffmann-Vold AM, et al Long-term outcome and prognostic factors in enthesitis-related arthritis: A case–control study. Arthritis Rheum 2006; 54(11):3573–3582

Gensler LS, Ward MM, Reveille JD, Learch TJ, Weisman MH, Davis Jr. JC. Clinical, radiographic, and functional differences between juvenile-onset and adult-onset ankylosing spondylitis: Results from the PSOAS cohort. Ann Rheum Dis 2008; 67:233–237

Henrickson M, Reiff A. Prolonged efficacy of etanercept in refractory enthesitis-related arthritis. J Rheumatol 2004; 31(10):2055–2061

Jacobs JC, Berdon ED, Johnston WE. HLA-B27-associated spondyloarthritis and enthesopathy in childhood: Clinical, pathologic, and radiographic observations in 58 patients. J Pediatr 1982; 100: 521–528

Mielants H, Veys EM, et al Gut inflammation in the spondyloarthropathies: Clinical, radiologic, biologic and genetic features in relation to the type of histology. A prospective study. J Rheumatol 1991; 18(10):1542–1551

Mielants H, Veys EM, et al Gut inflammation in children with late onset pauciarticular juvenile chronic arthritis and evolution to adult spondyloarthropathy–a prospective study. J Rheumatol 1993; 20(9): 1567–1572

Minden K, Niewerth M, et al Long-term outcome in patients with juvenile idiopathic arthritis. Arthritis Rheum 2002; 46(9):2392–2401

Petty RE, Southwood TR, et al Revision of the proposed classification criteria for juvenile idiopathic arthritis: Durban, 1997. J Rheumatol 1998; 25(10):1991–1994

Petty RE, Southwood TR, et al International league of associations for rheumatology classification of juvenile idiopathic arthritis: Second revision, Edmonton, 2001. J Rheumatol 2004; 31(2):390–392

Rosenberg AM, Petty RE. A syndrome of seronegative enthesopathy and arthropathy in children. Arthritis Rheum 1982; 25(9):1041–1047

Schmeling H, Horneff G. Infliximab in two patients with juvenile ankylosing spondylitis. Rheumatol Int 2004; 24(3):173–176

Stone M, Warren RW, et al Juvenile-onset ankylosing spondylitis is associated with worse functional outcomes than adult-onset ankylosing spondylitis. Arthritis Rheum 2005; 53(3):445–451

Tse SM, Burgos-Vargas R, et al Anti-tumor necrosis factor alpha blockade in the treatment of juvenile spondylarthropathy. Arthritis Rheum 2005; 52(7):2103–2108

Tse SM, Laxer RM, et al Radiologic improvement of juvenile idiopathic arthritis-enthesitis-related arthritis following anti-tumor necrosis factor-alpha blockade with etanercept. J Rheumatol 2006; 33(6):1186–1188

Tse SML, Burgos-Vargas R, O'Shea F, Inman R, Laxer R. Long term outcome of anti-TNF therapy in juvenile spondyloarthropathy. Arthritis Rheum 2007; 56(9S):898

Ankylosing Spondylitis

7

Juergen Braun and David Tak Yan Yu

7.1 Overview of Ankylosing Spondylitis

> Ankylosing spondylitis (AS) is the prototypical form of the spondyloarthritides, a group of disorders that involves inflammation of the sacroiliac joints, spine, joints, and entheses, as well as extraspinal lesions of the eye, bowel, and heart.

> Human leukocyte antigen (HLA) B27 is a strong genetic risk factor for AS. However, this gene is neither necessary nor sufficient to cause the disease. Other recently recognized genes are also involved in the pathophysiology of this condition.

> The principal musculoskeletal lesions of AS are sacroiliitis, spondylitis, synovitis, and enthesitis. Enthesitis consists of inflammation at the site of tendinous insertions into bone.

> Sacroiliitis causes inflammatory back pain often localized to the buttocks that can be uni- or bilateral and typically alternates between the left and right side.

> Spondylitis begins characteristically in the lumbosacral region and proceeds cephalad.

> The most common extraspinal joints involved are the hips, knees, ankles, and metatarsophalangeal joints. The pattern of arthritis is typically an asymmetric oligoarthritis that involves the large joints of the lower extremities.

> Acute anterior uveitis usually occurs in one eye at a time, although either eye can be involved in any given episode. Patients usually present with a red, painful, photophobic eye.

Myth: AS is a rare disease.

Reality: AS, the most common subtype of spondyloarthritis, has a prevalence in the range of 0.3–0.5% (Braun and Sieper 2007). The group of spondyloarthritides as a whole has a prevalence that is approximately as high as that of rheumatoid arthritis (RA) (Saraux et al. 2005). The prevalence of spondyloarthritis among patients who present to general practitioners with chronic back pain that has persisted for more than 3 months is on the order of 5% (Underwood and Dawes 1995).

Myth: AS is a benign disease with a relatively good prognosis.

Reality: An oft-quoted study that examined military veterans with AS is partly responsible for this myth (Carette et al., 1983). However, that study was characterized by a high loss to follow-up. Contrary to this Myth as stated, many patients who were tracked for a long period developed severe functional restrictions. Other studies indicate that at least one third of patients with AS have severe courses characterized by significant pain and disability (Zink et al. 2000). These morbidities have substantial implications for family life and occupation (Ward et al. 2008).

Myth: Only males get AS.

Reality: Older textbooks of rheumatology reported the male predominance in AS to be as high as 16:1. However, a more accurate estimation of the male:female ratio is on the order of 2:1. Besides numbers, some true differences do appear between male and female patients with AS. For example, male patients are more likely to have syndesmophytes and bony ankylosis than females with the disease (Rudwaleit et al. 2009a).

Myth: Inflammatory back pain is such a highly specific symptom that it is nearly diagnostic of AS or some form of spondyloarthritis.

Reality: Inflammatory back pain is a hallmark of AS. However, it is present in only about 70% of patients with established disease. In addition, up to 30% of patients with back pain due to other causes also report symptoms compatible with an inflammatory etiology. Thus, additional history that supplements symptoms compatible with inflammatory back pain is required to make the diagnosis. Such additional information might include a good response to NSAIDs, positivity for HLA-B27, an elevated C-reactive protein, other features of spondyloarthritis such as uveitis, psoriasis, and colitis, and compatible findings on imaging studies of the sacroiliac joints. New criteria for inflammatory back pain (Rudwaleit et al. 2006) and axial SpA (Rudwaleit et al. 2009b, c) have been proposed recently.

J. H. Stone (ed.), *A Clinician's Pearls and Myths in Rheumatology,*
DOI:10.1007/978-1-84800-934-9_7, © Springer Science + Business Media B.V. 2009

Myth: All patients with AS are HLA-B27 positive.

Reality: Although HLA-B27 is clearly the strongest genetic factor involved in the pathogenesis of AS, it is neither necessary nor sufficient to cause the disease. The risk contributed by HLA B27 is about 50% of the total risk attributed to genes. Other genetic factors such as the IL-23 receptor and ERAP-1 have been discovered recently (Wellcome Trust Nature Genetics 2007). Environmental factors may also play a role, albeit a less important one. Firmly linked environmental factors have been identified for only a subgroup of SpA, namely, patients with reactive arthritis (see Chap. 9).

The relative frequency of HLA-B27 varies across different populations. More than 40 HLA-B27 subtypes exist. At least two subtypes are not associated with AS. These are HLA-B2706 found in Thailand (Lopez-Larrea et al. 2002) and HLA-B2709 found in Sardinia. In Western countries, it is generally not useful to determine HLA B27 subtypes. Caucasians usually carry the HLA B2705 subtype, which is known to be associated with the disease. A substantial number of patients who have clinical features compatible with AS, but who lack HLA-B27 actually have psoriasis or inflammatory bowel disease.

Myth: HLA-B27 is not useful for the diagnosis of AS.

Reality: In certain populations, including the Caucasians of North America and Western Europe and most of the populations in China and India, HLA-B27 is present in at least 90% of patients with AS but among less than 10% of the general population.

The utility of HLA-B27 in diagnosing AS and SpA is because, in a patient who presents with lower back pain of greater than 3 months' duration, the likelihood of an SpA increases tenfold if HLA-B27 is present (Braun et al. 1998). In general, the pretest probability of having the disease matters. The higher the suspicion of AS before the test, the greater the posttest probability of a positive result (Fig. 7.1) (Brown 2007). However, its contribution to clinical diagnosis is greatest in early disease, the time at which patients often do not have definitive radiographic signs. Accordingly, a negative test for HLA-B27 largely decreases the likelihood for AS and SpA.

Thus, if HLA-B27 genotyping is used in an appropriate clinical circumstance, a positive result contributes significantly to the diagnostic evaluation. Therefore, HLA B27 testing has become an important item in the new classification criteria for axial SpA (Rudwaleit et al. in press (b)).

Myth: All patients with AS have elevated C-reactive protein (CRP) levels.

Reality: This unfortunate but widely espoused myth frequently leads to diagnostic delays. Only one half of all patients with AS have elevated CRP levels (Spoorenberg et al. 1999). However, among the sizeable subset of patients who have

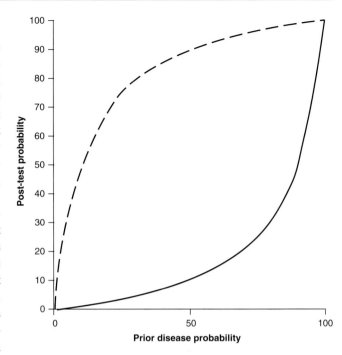

Fig. 7.1 The relationship between pretest probability to posttest probability for HLA-B27 determinations (Reproduced from Brown 2007, with permission from Wiley-Blackwell)

elevated CRP levels at baseline, these levels usually fall dramatically once TNF inhibition is begun (Braun et al. 2002).

A low CRP level does not necessarily predict that the patient will respond poorly to TNF inhibition. If sufficient doses of NSAIDs do not lead to an adequate clinical response, a trial of a TNF inhibitor is indicated.

Myth: Measurement of CRP levels is the only way to assess disease activity in AS.

Reality: The clinical standard to assess disease activity in AS is the BASDAI (see below). The items "pain" and "morning stiffness" are considered especially relevant in this regard. However, magnetic resonance imaging (MRI) has emerged as an important tool that has the capacity to localize spinal inflammation rather exactly (Fig. 7.2) (Braun 2002). MRI is also useful in quantifying the extent of spondylitis before and after anti-TNF therapy (Braun 2006a).

Myth: Function in AS is mainly determined by ankylosis.

Reality: As shown in a recent study (Landewé 2009), disease activity and structural damage both contribute independently to functional decline in patients with AS. This information is highly relevant for determining patients' prognosis for functional recovery and informs management decisions.

Pearl: Remember to exclude inflammatory bowel disease in a patient with AS/SpA.

Comment: The clinical features of AS overlap substantially with those of inflammatory bowel disease. Patients with

Fig. 7.2 Patient with AS, spondylitis, and structural changes (**a**) chronic structural changes (**b**) active lesions

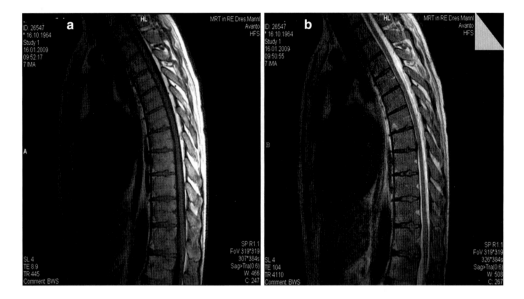

symptoms such as elevated stool frequency and unexplained abdominal pain should undergo endoscopy. A low threshold for endoscopy should also be maintained in patients who are HLA-B27 negative. This is because, among patients with inflammatory bowel disease who have symptoms of SpA, only approximately 50% are HLA-B27 positive. This contrasts with the situation with AS, a population of patients in whom the great majority are HLA-B27 positive.

A reorientation of the diagnosis to inflammatory bowel disease alters the entire therapeutic strategy for a patient with joint symptoms. TNF blockers such as infliximab and adalimumab are also approved for Crohn's disease, but additional therapeutic measures may also be important.

Myth: Because all patients with AS have sacroiliitis, the diagnosis is generally quite straightforward.

Reality: The 1984 New York classification criteria for AS (van der Linden et al. 1984) are useful for the purpose of classification and diagnosis in patients with long-standing disease, but not in patients with early disease. This is because the sensitivity of structural changes within the sacroiliac joints is high among patients with established disease, but low (approximately 20%) in patients with early SpA.

New criteria under development for the diagnosis of AS include HLA-B27 positivity and findings on MRI studies. These new criteria are likely to resolve most issues related to an early diagnosis of axial SpA. Importantly, several parameters are required in order for the diagnosis to be classified as secure (Table 7.1) (Rudwaleit et al. b, c).

In the discipline of rheumatology, criteria sets seldom obviate the need for astute clinical judgement.

Myth: The radiographic pattern of sacroiliac changes is clinically relevant because it helps differentiate among the different forms of spondyloarthritis.

Table 7.1 Preliminary criteria for the diagnosis of ankylosing spondylitis

ASAS classification criteria for SpA

In patients with ≥3 months back pain and age at onset < 45 years	In patients with peripheral symptoms ONLY

Sacroiliitis on imaging plus ≥1 SpA feature	OR	HLA-B27 plus ≥2 other SpA features	Arthritis or enthesitis or dactylitis plus

SpA features
– IBP
– arthritis
– enthesitis heel
– uveitis
– dactylitis
– psoriasis
– Crohn's/colitis
– good response to NSAIDs
– family history for SpA
– HLA-B27
– elevated CRP

≥1 SpA features
– Uveitis
– psoriasis
– Crohn's/colitis
– Preceding infection
– HLA-B27

OR

≥2 SpA features
– Arthritis
– enthesitis
– Dactylitis
– amily history for SpA
– Sacroiliitis on imaging

Reality: Structural changes in the sacroiliac joints occur in approximately 95% of patients with AS. In contrast, only about 30% of patients with psoriatic SpA and an even smaller percentage of those with reactive arthritis develop sacroiliitis. Thus, AS is much more prevalent than other forms of axial SpA.

Whereas the sacroiliitis in AS is typically bilateral (at least in advanced stages of disease), sacroiliac joint inflammation in PsA and ReA is often unilateral and asymmetric (Muche et al. 2003). However, the full clinical picture and an accurate determination of symptoms and signs of inflammation in all joints (and skin, eyes, and gastrointestinal tract) is crucial. In the early diagnosis of sacroiliitis, MRI is clearly the study of choice.

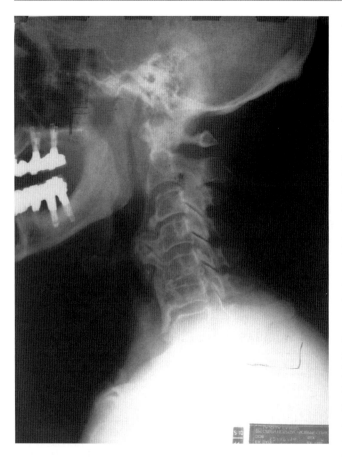

Fig. 7.3 Lateral view of the cervical spine in a patient with ankylosing spondylitis. Note the slender and vertical characters of the bony briges between the anterior aspects of the vertebrae (Figure courtesy of Dr. Thomas Learch, Cedar Sinai Medical Center, Los Angeles)

A patient with cutaneous psoriasis and definite structural changes in the sacroiliac joints is usually diagnosed more appropriately as AS associated with psoriasis. Structural changes in the sacroiliac joints of patients with reactive arthritis are relatively rare.

Pearl and Myth: The nature of syndesmophytes differs across the subtypes of spondyloarthritis.

Comment: The syndesmophytes of AS are usually symmetric, delicate, and vertical— at least in about 90% of the patients (Fig. 7.3). In contrast, the syndesmophytes of patients with psoriasis are often bulky, asymmetric, and tend to protrude laterally before progressing vertically.

Although this fine point is correct from the standpoint of diagnosis, it makes little difference now in most circumstances with regard to treatment. Regardless of the radiologic appearance of their syndesmophytes, the back pain symptoms of patients with AS, psoriatic arthritis, or inflammatory bowel disease all respond well to TNF inhibitors.

Myth: Syndesmophytes are distinguished easily from the osteophytes associated with degenerative arthritis of the spine.

Reality: Advanced cases of AS are difficult to distinguish from diffuse idiopathic skeletal hyperostosis (DISH). One study of patients with AS, who had a mean disease duration of approximately 12 years, indicated that more than 10% of all spinal osteophytes detected had the radiologic appearance of degenerative osteophytes. The cutoff used in that study was a 45° growth angle (Baraliakos et al. 2007b).

There are two potential causes of difficulty in parsing the etiology of syndesmophytes. First, patients with AS may develop degenerative spinal changes secondary to those induced by inflammation. Second, not all syndesmophytes follow the same rules, and they may have a less than classic appearance. There is evidence that the detection of syndesmophytes by MRI is difficult (Braun 2002). Radiography remains the gold standard for syndesmophyte characterization.

Pearl: Remember to consider DISH before diagnosing advanced AS.

Comment: Many patients with late-stage AS are recognizable easily by their posture. They have a forward stooping of the neck, a high dorsal kyphosis, a rounding of the shoulders, loss of the normal lumbar lordosis, wasting of the buttocks muscles, flattening of the chest, and ballooning of the abdomen (Olivieri et al. 2007). Before rendering the diagnosis of AS on this posture alone, however, clinicians should consider an alternative diagnosis that can cause the identical postural changes: diffuse idiopathic skeletal hyperostosis, commonly known as DISH or Forestier's disease (Mader 2008).

Physical examination maneuvers alone cannot distinguish DISH from AS. The range of motion in the cervical and lumbar spines can be limited to similar extents in these two conditions. In addition, patients with DISH have similar decreases in their chest expansions and in the ranges of motion at the shoulders and hips. Patients with DISH may complain of spinal pain, but their history of back pain starts usually later than in AS, and the initial localization is different.

Patients with both DISH and AS develop bony bridges between their vertebral bodies. The key to differentiating these disorders is that these bony bridges have different radiologic appearances:

- DISH leads to ossification of the anterior longitudinal ligament of the spine. These changes are frequently described as "exuberant" or "flowing" mantles along the anterior and anterolateral aspects of the vertebrae (Fig. 7.4).
- In AS, the bony bridges between the vertebrae are vertical and much more slender, involving the outer margin of the annulus fibrosus (see Fig. 7.3).

The other radiological feature that distinguishes AS from DISH, sometimes more reliably, is the presence of erosions within the sacroiliac joints of patients with AS. Sacroiliac joint erosions are present invariably among patients with AS who have significant radiological involvement of the spine.

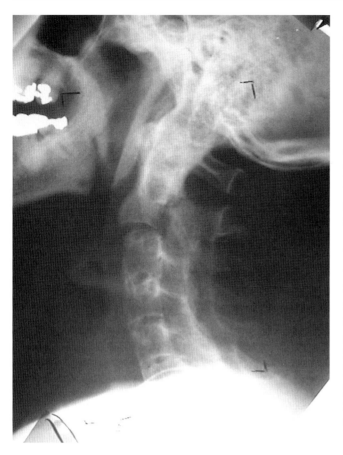

Fig. 7.4 Lateral view of the cervical spine in a patient with DISH. Note the exuberant appearance of the ossification along the anterior margins of the vertebrae (Figure courtesy of Dr. Thomas Learch, Cedar Sinai Medical Center, Los Angeles)

Sacroiliac joint erosions tend to occur first on the iliac side of the joint.

Sacroiliac joint erosions do not occur in DISH, but the sacroiliac joints are obscured in some patients by sacroiliac capsular bridging. In such cases, computed tomography may be required to differentiate AS from DISH. However, this is a largely academic question that has usually no therapeutic consequences.

HLA-B27 is present in a subtantially higher percentage of patients with AS compared with patients with DISH. However, the coexistence of not only HLA-B27 positivity and DISH but also AS and DISH has been reported (Maertens et al. 1992).

Myth: AS is caused by Klebsiella or some other species of bacteria.

Reality: The concept that bacterial infections in the urogenital tract, gastrointestinal tract, and other sites can trigger a noninfectious inflammatory arthritis stems from the strong association that exists between certain pathogens and reactive arthritis (Chapter 9). Reactive arthritis shares some features with other SpA.

The hypothesis that Klebsiella infections cause some cases of AS was put forth in the 1970s and 1980s on the basis of two arguments:

- The potential for molecular mimicry between Klebsiella species and HLA B27
- The reportedly high prevalence of antiKlebsiella antibodies in AS.

The functional relevance of the molecular similarity between Klebsiella species and HLA B27 has never been proven. In addition, the serologic findings are probably attributable to silent gut inflammation, possibly enhanced by NSAID use, rather than a true pathogenetic mechanism.

Putative links between AS and Chlamydia species or other bacteria that can cause clinically inapparent inflammation within the urogenital tract have been proposed, but the data for such associations are not convincing. Extensive polymerase chain reaction studies have provided evidence for small amounts of bacterial DNA in the joints of patients with reactive arthritis but not of those with AS (Braun et al. 2007a, b). However, it is altogether much more probable that the cellular immune reaction to bacterial antigens is of greater pathophysiological importance than the presence of bacteria—especially since they have also been detected in the joints of healthy individuals.

Although several interesting ideas have been followed, the pathogenesis of AS has still not been fully elucidated. The genetic contribution seems to be rather dominant, explaining at least 80% of the pathogenesis.

Myth: AS is difficult to treat.

Reality: This was true–painfully true–until the era of TNF inhibitors (Braun 2002). Assuming that patients have access to appropriate anti-TNF regimens, most respond very well to this intervention. Of note, there is some evidence that these agents work even better in SpA than in RA (Heiberg et al. 2008).

NSAIDs remain the standard first-line therapy for AS (Zochling et al. 2006). TNF inhibition, on the other hand, is the standard of care for patients who have persistently high disease activity despite optimal NSAID regimens. In contrast to the situation with RA, in which methotrexate remains the cornerstone of therapy even if a biologic agent is employed simultaneously (see Chap. 1), methotrexate and other synthetic DMARDs have extremely limited roles in the treatment of AS.

Pearl: Doses of NSAIDs must be optimized.

Comment: NSAIDs should be employed in at the highest approved dose when treating AS. NSAIDs with longer half lives may be more effective than those with shorter half lives, particularly in providing pain relief through the night. If a particular, NSAID has not demonstrated sufficient therapeutic effect within 1 week, another NSAID should be prescribed (Song et al. 2008).

The potential for gastrointestinal, renal, and cardiovascular adverse effects must always be considered when using NSAIDs and weighed against the possible adverse effects of TNF inhibitors.

Pearl: Elevated acute phase reactants in a patient with AS do not imply that glucocorticoids will be an effective treatment.

Comment: The systemic use of glucocorticoids is not recommended in AS, in contrast to RA. Clinical experience in AS indicates that only high doses of glucocorticoids (too high) are effective for the spinal disease in AS, and even then only in some patients. Greater efficacy of glucocorticoids may be anticipated for patients with a predominantly peripheral arthritis, but even this has not been tested adequately. The clinical judgement of AS experts is that comparable doses of glucocorticoids are far less likely to be effective in AS than in RA.

Pearl: Injectable glucocorticoid preparations are effective in patients with isolated sacroiliitis, monoarthritis or oligoarthritis of peripheral joints, or enthesitis.

Comment: Although oral glucocorticoids are generally ineffective in AS, clinical anecdotes suggest that intraarticular injections provide clinical relief for up to 9 months in many patients. Computed tomography-guided injections may be necessary for the sacroiliac joints, especially if sacroiliitis is the predominant clinical problem (Braun et al. 1996).

Pearl: Methotrexate definitely does not work for axial disease.

Comment: Although methotrexate has been used for this indication for a long time, there is no evidence (not even a hint) that this agent is effective for the spinal inflammation of AS (Haibel et al. 2007). There is also no evidence that the addition of methotrexate to a TNF inhibitor regimen potentiates the effect of the biologic agent (Breban et al. 2008). In theory, methotrexate might prevent the formation of human antichimeric antibodies in patients treated with infliximab, but this has not been demonstrated to be relevant in patients with AS.

Pearl: Consider sulfasalazine in patients with relatively mild disease, but don't hesitate to prescribe anti-TNF therapy in patients with persistently active disease.

Comment: Some studies indicate a limited effect of sulfasalazine for patients with active peripheral and axial disease, especially in early stages (Braun 2006b). However, this does not imply that sulfasalazine must be prescribed before resorting to an anti-TNF agent. Patients with persistently active disease should receive a TNF inhibitor early in their disease course (Zochling et al. 2006).

Myth: TNF blockers are useful only in patients with AS before their spines become fused.

Reality: Most of the phase III studies on the use of TNF blockers have not included patients with total ankylosis of the spine.

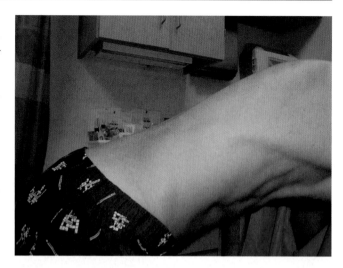

Fig. 7.5 A patient with severe ankylosis of the spine from long-standing, untreated ankylosing spondylitis. The patient had a serum C-reactive protein level of 62.4 mg/dL (normal < 8.0 mg/dL) and an erythrocyte sedimentation rate of 132 mm/h (normal < 20 mm/h). He responded dramatically to infliximab, with pronounced symptom relief and a swift normalization of his acute phase reactants

A prevalent myth holds that as the spine becomes ankylosed, the degree of inflammation also subsides, such that patients' symptoms become much less responsive to antiinflammatory therapies. The response of the patient whose spine is shown Fig. 7.5 to infliximab repudiates this myth strongly.

The only phase III TNF blocker study that included some patients with AS with complete spinal ankylosis ($n = 11$) was a multicenter trial involving 315 patients that compared adalimumab with placebo (Van der Heijde et al. 2006). Among these patients, three of the six who were treated with adalimumab demonstrated significant clinical responses. In contrast, none of the five patients who received placebo were responders. Hence, TNF blockers can be considered even in patients with very late stages of the AS, especially if NSAIDs and other analgesics are poorly tolerated or not efficacious.

This is in agreement with immunohistological studies showing that even at a late stage of ankylosis, significant inflammatory changes still exist in the spine (Appel 2006; Neidhart et al. 2008).

Myth: TNF blockers can arrest the progression of AS.

Reality: The reverse side of the myth discussed earlier is the misconception that TNF inhibitors should be used early in patients with AS, even those with mild disease, because they will arrest the progression of structural damage. One of the major problems in trying to test this hypothesis is that AS progresses at a slower rate compared with that of RA. At least 2 years are required in AS to detect significant radiologic changes using the best available scoring system, the mSASSS. In this era, it is not ethical to put patients on placebo for a period that long.

Because of this limitation, radiological progression in patients on TNF blockers can be compared only with baseline observations of the same cohort or alternately to data of cohorts collected before use of biologics. Using either method of comparison, neither infliximab nor etanercept has shown significant effects on radiological progression (Baraliakos et al. 2007a; Van der Heijde et al. 2008). This is not surprising, because the process of bone remodeling responsible for ankylosis may be partly independent of that of inflammation (Baraliakos et al. 2008). Etanercept, which suppresses the symptoms of AS effectively, does not suppress ankylosis in an animal model of enthesitis (Lories et al. 2007). The optimal approach to suppressing bone remodeling is a major current focus of AS research.

Myth: The concomitant use of methotrexate enhances the utility of TNF blockers in patients with AS.

Reality: In a randomized trial, patients with AS received either the combination of infliximab and methotrexate or infliximab and placebo (Breban et al. 2008). No additional effect of MTX was found. In another study, there was no synergistic effect of methotrexate plus a TNF inhibitor on MRI progression of disease (Li et al. 2008).

Not all patients with AS respond dramatically to their first TNF inhibitor. In practice, if a patient with AS responds poorly to one TNF blocker, it is probably more useful to switch to another TNF blocker than to add methotrexate (Coates et al. 2008).

Pearl: Remind the patient regularly that physiotherapy and exercise are as important as the use of medications designed to inhibit inflammation.

Comment: Patients (and clinicians) sometimes place too much faith on the pharmacological side of therapy. Regular physiotherapy and exercise are also critical features of the therapy for patients with AS. These measures improve and maintain muscle strength over time and contribute to the preservation of proper posture.

Pearl: Talk to the patient about the increased cardiovascular risk associated with systemic inflammatory disorders and explain the detrimental effects of smoking on the disease.

Comment: Patients with AS have an increased cardiovascular risk because of the chronic inflammation. Moreover, smoking is a risk factor for poor clinical outcomes. Patients should understand the importance of pursuing healthful lifestyles and modifying risk factors for cardiovascular disease.

Pearl: Check bone mineral density in time and measure it at the right location.

Comment: Approximately half of all patients with AS have abnormal bone mineral density levels. The risk of pathologic fractures among patients with AS is increased several fold compared with healthy controls. The treatment of osteopenia and osteoporosis has not been studied in AS, but reasonable approaches to this problem include calcium (1,500 mg of elemental calcium per day) and vitamin D, as well as bisphosphonates if appropriate. Some data indicate that bisphosphonates have a favorable effect on other disease outcomes (Maksymowych et al. 2002).

Bone mineral density measurements at the lumbar spine in patients with syndesmophytes are not useful because the measurements will be falsely high (Karberg et al. 2005).

Pearl: Talk to the patient with a physically demanding job about the future of his employment.

Comment: A physically demanding profession is associated with a poor AS outcome in terms of both structural and functional damage (Ward et al. 2008). Patients with AS should be advised of the potential wisdom of selecting different types of work if their current occupations bring significant physical demands.

Pearl: Systematic assessments of disease activity are crucial to the longitudinal management of AS.

Comment: Standardized and validated assessments are increasingly the standard of care for the management of patients with RA. Similarly, measuring the degree of disease activity is also crucial to the management of AS. It helps physicians to decide on what particular therapies to initiate. Once a therapy is initiated, disease activity assessment is required to monitor response. However, assessing disease activity in AS is more difficult than that in RA because of several factors: there are very few if any swollen joints to count; the correlation with acute phase reactants is often poor; and radiographic changes are comparatively slow.

Partly because of our ignorance on the factors that cause the symptoms and disability of AS, the instruments we use to measure disease activity are rather artificial and not based on the pathophysiology of the disease. For drug trials and for consideration of TNF blocker treatment, a frequently recommended method is the Bath AS Disease Activity Index (BASDAI) (Garrett et al. 1994). The BASDAI is available at http://www.basdai.com/ and is illustrated in Table 7.2.

For patients with established AS, the BASDAI scores are rather stable when studied over a period as long as 5 years (Robertson and Davis 2004). BASDAI scores have been used to assist in making decisions about whether or not TNF inhibitors should be employed in a patient with AS. A BASDAI score >4.0 has been felt to justify TNF inhibitor use (Braun et al. 2005; Henderson and Davis 2006). Most clinical trials of TNF blockers in AS have used this cutoff as one of the entry criteria.

An obvious drawback of the BASDAI is that the parameters are dependent entirely upon subjective patient-based

Table 7.2 Calculating the Bath Ankylosing Spondylitis Disease Activity Index (BASDAI)

• How would you describe the overall level of fatigue/tiredness you have experienced?
• How would you describe the overall level of AS neck, back or hip pain you have had?
• How would you describe the overall level of pain/swelling in joints other than neck, back or hips you have had?
• How would you describe the overall level of discomfort you have had from any areas tender to touch or pressure?
• How would you describe the overall level of morning stiffness you have had from the time you wake up?
• How long does your morning stiffness last from the time you wake up? The scale of the duration of morning stiffness ranges from the minimum score of 0 h to the maximum score of 2 or more hours.

Calculating the mean BASDAI score:

Patients are requested to provide a score for six questions regarding their conditions in the preceding week. The scoring can be accomplished either on a visual analogue scale or in a numerical scale ranging from 0 to 10.

Because questions five and six both address the symptom of morning stiffness, their scores are averaged and then added to the sum of the other four questions. The total of these five items are then divided by 5 to derive the mean BASDAI score.

evaluations. Alternative strategies for measuring disease activity in AS have been proposed (Spoorenberg et al. 2005; Dougados et al. 2008; Maksymowych et al. 2007).

References

Appel H, Kuhne M, Spiekermann S, Ebhardt H, Grozdanovic Z, Kohler D, et al Immunohistologic analysis of zygapophyseal joints in patients with ankylosing spondylitis. Arthritis Rheum 2006; 54(9):2845–2851

Baraliakos X, Listing J, Brandt J, Haibel H, Rudwaleit M, Sieper J, et al Radiographic progression in patients with ankylosing spondylitis after 4 yrs of treatment with the anti-TNF-alpha antibody infliximab. Rheumatol (Oxford) 2007a; 46(9):1450–1453

Baraliakos X, Listing J, Rudwaleit M, Haibel H, Brandt J, Sieper J, Braun J. Progression of radiographic damage in patients with ankylosing spondylitis - Defining the central role of syndesmophytes. Ann Rheum Dis 2007; 66(7):910–5

Baraliakos X, Listing J, Rudwaleit M, Sieper J, Braun J. The relationship between inflammation and new bone formation in patients with ankylosing spondylitis. Arthritis Res Ther 2008 Sep 1; 10(5):R104

Braun J, Sieper J. Ankylosing spondylitis. Lancet 2007; 369:1379–1390

Braun J, Bollow M, Seyrekbasan F, et al Computed tomography guided corticosteroid injection of the sacroiliac joint in patients with spondyloarthropathy with sacroiliitis: Clinical outcome and followup by dynamic magnetic resonance imaging. J Rheumatol 1996; 23(4): 659–664

Braun J, Tuszewski M, Ehlers S, et al Nested polymerase chain reaction strategy simultaneously targeting DNA sequences of multiple bacterial species in inflammatory joint diseases. II. Examination of sacroiliac and knee joint biopsies of patients with spondyloarthropathies and other arthritides. J Rheumatol 1997a; 24(6):1101–1105

Braun J, Tuszewski M, Eggens U, et al Nested polymerase chain reaction strategy simultaneously targeting DNA sequences of multiple

bacterial species in inflammatory joint diseases. I. Screening of synovial fluid samples of patients with spondyloarthropathies and other arthritides. J Rheumatol 1997b; 24(6):1092–1100

Braun J, Bollow M, Remlinger G, et al Prevalence of spondylarthropathies in HLA-B27 positive and negative blood donors. Arthritis Rheum 1998; 41(1):58–67

Braun J, Brandt J, Listing J, et al Treatment of active ankylosing spondylitis with infliximab - a double-blind placebo controlled multicenter trial. Lancet 2002; 359:1187–1193

Braun J, Davis J, Dougados M, Sieper J, van der Linden S, van der Heijde D. First update of the international ASAS consensus statement for the use of anti-TNF agents in patients with ankylosing spondylitis. Ann Rheum Dis 2005 Aug 11 [Epub ahead of print]

Braun J, Landewe R, Hermann KG, Han J, Yan S, Williamson P, van der Heijde D. Major reduction in spinal inflammation in patients with ankylosing spondylitis after treatment with infliximab: Results of a multicenter, randomized, double-blind, placebo-controlled magnetic resonance imaging study. Arthritis Rheum 2006a; 54(5):1646–1652

Braun J, Zochling J, Baraliakos X, et al Efficacy of sulfasalazine in patients with inflammatory back pain due to undifferentiated spondyloarthritis and early ankylosing spondylitis: A multicentre randomized controlled trial. Ann Rheum Dis 2006b

Breban M, Ravaud P, Claudepierre P, et al Maintenance of infliximab treatment in ankylosing spondylitis: Results of a one-year randomized controlled trial comparing systematic versus on-demand treatment. Arthritis Rheum 2008; 58(1):88–97

Brown MA. Human leukocyte antigen-B27 and ankylosing spondylitis. Int Med J 2007; 37:739–740

Carette S, Graham D, Little H, Rubenstein J, Rosen P. The natural disease course of ankylosing spondylitis. Arthritis Rheum 1983; 26(2):186–190

Coates LC, Cawkwell LS, Ng NW, et al Real life experience confirms sustained response to long-term biologics and switching in ankylosing spondylitis. Rheumatology (Oxford) 2008; 47(6):897–900

Dougados M, Luo MP, Maksymowych WP, et al Evaluation of the patient acceptable symptom state as an outcome measure in patients with ankylosing spondylitis: Data from a randomized controlled trial. Arthritis Rheum 2008; 59(4):553–560

Garrett S, Jenkinson T, Kennedy LG, et al A new approach to defining disease status in ankylosing spondylitis: The bath ankylosing spondylitis disease activity index. J Rheumatol 1994; 21(12):2286–2291

Haibel H, Brandt HC, Song IH, et al No efficacy of subcutaneous methotrexate in active ankylosing spondylitis: A 16-week open-label trial. Ann Rheum Dis 2007; 66(3):419–421

Heiberg MS, Koldingsnes W, Mikkelsen K, et al The comparative one-year performance of anti-tumor necrosis factor alpha drugs in patients with rheumatoid arthritis, psoriatic arthritis, and ankylosing spondylitis: Results from a longitudinal, observational, multicenter study. Arthritis Rheum 2008; 59(2):234–240

Henderson C, Davis JC. Drug insight: Anti-tumor-necrosis-factor therapy for ankylosing spondylitis. Nat Clin Pract Rheumatol 2006; 2(4):211–218

Karberg K, Zochling J, Sieper J, Felsenberg D, Braun J. Bone loss is detected more frequently in patients with ankylosing spondylitis with syndesmophytes. J Rheumatol 2005; 32(7):1290–1298

Landewé R, Dougados M, Mielants H et al Physical function in ankylosing spondylitis is independently determined by both disease activity and radiographic damage of the spine. Ann Rheum Dis 2009; 68(6):863–7

Li EK, Griffith JF, Lee VW, et al Short-term efficacy of combination methotrexate and infliximab in patients with ankylosing spondylitis: A clinical and magnetic resonance imaging correlation. Rheumatology (Oxford) 2008 Sept; 47(9):1358–1363 [Epub 2008 Jun 23]

Lopez-Larrea C, Sujirachato K, Mehra NK, et al HLA-B27 subtypes in Asian patients with ankylosing spondylitis. Evidence for new associations. Tissue Antigens 1995; 45(3):169–176

Lories RJ, Derese I, de Bari C, Luyten FP. Evidence for uncoupling of inflammation and joint remodeling in a mouse model of spondylarthritis. Arthritis Rheum 2007; 56(2):489–497

Mader R. Diffuse idiopathic skeletal hyperostosis: Time for a change. J Rheumatol 2008; 35(3):377–379

Maertens M, Mielants H, Verstraete K, Veys EM. Simultaneous occurrence of diffuse idiopathic skeletal hyperostosis and ankylosing spondylitis in the same patient. J Rheumatol 1992; 19(12):1978–1983

Maksymowych WP, Jhangri GS, Fitzgerald AA, et al A six-month randomized, controlled, double-blind, dose-response comparison of intravenous pamidronate (60 mg versus 10 mg) in the treatment of nonsteroidal antiinflammatory drug-refractory ankylosing spondylitis. Arthritis Rheum 2002; 46(3):766–773

Maksymowych WP, Richardson R, Mallon C, et al Evaluation and validation of the patient acceptable symptom state (PASS) in patients with ankylosing spondylitis. Arthritis Rheum 2007; 57(1):133–139

Muche B, Bollow M, François RJ, Sieper J, Hamm B, Braun J. Which anatomical structures are involved in early and late sacroiliitis in spondylo¬arthritis – a detailed analysis by contrast enhanced magnetic resonance imaging. Arthritis Rheum 2003; 48(5):1374–1384

Neidhart M, Baraliakos X, Seemayer C, et al Expression of cathepsin K and MMP-1 indicate persistent osteodestructive activity in longstanding ankylosing spondylitis. Ann Rheum Dis 2008 Aug 4 [Epub ahead of print]

Olivieri I, D'Angelo S, Cutro MS, et al Diffuse idiopathic skeletal hyperostosis may give the typical postural abnormalities of advanced ankylosing spondylitis. Rheumatology (Oxford) 2007; 46(11):1709–1711

Robertson LP, Davis MJ. A longitudinal study of disease activity and functional status in a hospital cohort of patients with ankylosing spondylitis. Rheumatology (Oxford) 2004; 43(12):1565–1568

Rudwaleit M, Metter A, Listing J, Sieper J, Braun J. Inflammatory back pain in ankylosing spondylitis - a reassessment of the clinical history for classification and diagnosis. Arthritis Rheum 2006; 54(2):569–578

Rudwaleit M, Haibel H, Baraliakos X et al. The early disease stage in axial spondylarthritis: results from the German Spondyloarthritis Inception Cohort. Arthritis Rheum 2009a; 60(3):717–27

Rudwaleit M, Landewé R, van der Heijde D et al The development of Assessment of SpondyloArthritis international Society classification criteria for axial spondyloarthritis (part I): classification of

paper patients by expert opinion including uncertainty appraisal. Ann Rheum Dis 2009b; 68(6):770–6

Rudwaleit M, van der Heijde D, Landewé R et al The development of Assessment of SpondyloArthritis international Society classification criteria for axial spondyloarthritis (part II): validation and final selection. Ann Rheum Dis 2009c; 68(6):777–83

Saraux A, Guillemin F, Guggenbuhl P, et al Prevalence of spondyloarthropathies in France: 2001. Ann Rheum Dis 2005; 64(10):1431–1435

Song IH, Poddubnyy DA, Rudwaleit M, Sieper J. Benefits and risks of ankylosing spondylitis treatment with nonsteroidal antiinflammatory drugs. Arthritis Rheum 2008; 58(4):929–938

Spoorenberg A, van der Heijde D, de Klerk E, et al Relative value of erythrocyte sedimentation rate and C-reactive protein in assessment of disease activity in ankylosing spondylitis. J Rheumatol 1999; 26(4):980–984

Spoorenberg A, van Tubergen A, Landewe R, et al Measuring disease activity in ankylosing spondylitis: Patient and physician have different perspectives. Rheumatology (Oxford) 2005; 44(6):789–795

Underwood MR, Dawes P. Inflammatory back pain in primary care. Br J Rheumatol 1995; 34(11):1074–1077

van der Heijde D, Kivitz A, Schiff MH, et al Efficacy and safety of adalimumab in patients with ankylosing spondylitis: Results of a multicenter, randomized, double-blind, placebo-controlled trial. Arthritis Rheum 2006; 54(7):2136–2146

van der Heijde D, Landewe R, Einstein S, et al Radiographic progression of ankylosing spondylitis after up to two years of treatment with etanercept. Arthritis Rheum 2008; 58(5):1324–1331

van der Linden S, Valkenburg HA, Cats A. Evaluation of diagnostic criteria for ankylosing spondylitis. A proposal for modification of the New York criteria. Arthritis Rheum 1984; 27(4):361–368

Ward MM, Reveille JD, Learch TJ, Davis JC Jr, Weisman MH. Occupational physical activities and long-term functional and radiographic outcomes in patients with ankylosing spondylitis. Arthritis Rheum 2008; 59(6):822–832

Zink A, Braun J, Listing J, Wollenhaupt J. Disability and handicap in rheumatoid arthritis and ankylosing spondylitis–results from the German rheumatological database. German Collaborative Arthritis Centers. J Rheumatol 2000; 27(3):613–622

Zochling J, van der Heijde D, Burgos-Vargas R, et al ASAS/EULAR recommendations for the management of ankylosing spondylitis. Ann Rheum Dis 2006 Aug 26 [Epub ahead of print]

Psoriatic Arthritis

8

Christopher Ritchlin, Elinor Mody, Philip Mease,
and Dafna D. Gladman

8.1 Overview of Psoriatic Arthritis

> Psoriatic arthritis (PsA) is a distinctive category of inflammatory arthritis that complicates cutaneous psoriasis.

> The prevalence of PsA in the general population is estimated to be between 0.3% and 1%, only slightly less common than that of rheumatoid arthritis (RA).

> PsA is one of the "seronegative spondyloarthropathies", along with ankylosing spondylitis (AS), reactive arthritis, and the arthropathy of inflammatory bowel disease. As a seronegative disorder, PsA is not associated with autoantibodies such as rheumatoid factor or antibodies to cyclic citrullinated peptides.

> A variety of clinical patterns of PsA are recognized: distal joint disease, oligoarthritis, a symmetrical polyarthritis that resembles RA, and spondylitis. Some patients present with combinations of these features: e.g., oligoarthritis plus spondylitis.

> These clinical patterns are not necessarily stable over time. For example, distal joint disease can evolve into polyarthritis.

> The most common pattern of joint involvement at presentation is an asymmetric oligoarthritis. This pattern accounts for about 70% of PsA cases.

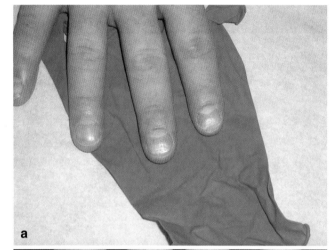
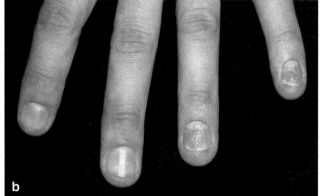
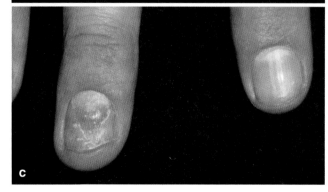

Fig. 8.1 Nail changes in psoriasis (**a**) Nail pitting (**b**) Onycholysis. Note that some fingernails are affected and others are not (**c**) A close-up of onycholysis (figures courtesy of Dr. John Stone)

Myth: PsA is RA with psoriasis.

Reality: The principal differences between PsA and RA are summarized in Table 8.1. Cutaneous psoriasis occurs in up to 3% of the population, and RA in about 1%. Thus, the co-occurrence of psoriasis and RA is expected in about three people in 10,000. Nail lesions, particularly onycholysis and more than 20 nail pits per person, are associated with PsA (Fig. 8.1a and 8.1b) (Eastmond andWright 1979). The presence of nail pits not only helps distinguish PsA from RA in some circumstances, it also identifies patients with psoriasis who are more likely to develop PsA, particularly arthritis of the distal interphalangeal (DIP) joints (Fig. 8.2) (Gladman et al. 1986).

J. H. Stone (ed.), *A Clinician's Pearls and Myths in Rheumatology,*
DOI:10.1007/978-1-84800-934-9_8, © Springer Science + Business Media B.V. 2009

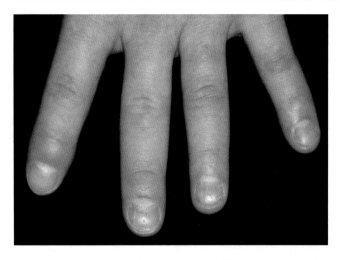

Fig. 8.2 DIP joint arthritis in PsA (note the DIP joint of the index finger). This patient also had nail pitting. DIP involvement and nail pitting often occur together in PsA (figure courtesy of Dr. John Stone)

Table 8.1 Contrasts between PsA and RA

Disease feature	PsA	RA
Nail lesions	Pitting	Bywaters' lesions
	Onycholysis	Splinter hemorrhages
Joint pattern in hands and wrists	Asymmetry	Symmetry
	DIP involvement common	MCPs/PIPs/DIPs
	"Ray" pattern	Ulnar styloid involvement
	Dactylitis ("sausage" digits)	
Spinal disease	Syndesmophytes	C1–C2 involvement
Eye disease	Anterior and posterior uveitis	Episcleritis
		Keratoconjunctivitis
		Scleritis
		Peripheral ulcerative keratitis
Other extra-articular features	Cutaneous psoriasis	Nodules
	Bluish discoloration over joints	Interstitial lung disease
	Enthesitis	Pericarditis
	Urethritis	Systemic vasculitis
	Inflammatory bowel disease	

PsA is not associated with atlanto-axial subluxation (C1–C2), the classic form of spinal involvement in RA. About half of all PsA patients have some degree of spinal inflammation (Gladmann 2007), but PsA in the cervical spine usually manifests itself as syndesmophytes rather than erosions of the dens (C2).

PsA affects males and females almost equally. This contrasts with RA, in which a predilection for women exists. Patients with PsA often have a bluish–purplish discoloration over their inflamed joints (Jajic 2001), a finding that is not common in RA. Patients with PsA generally have less joint tenderness than patients with RA and are also less likely to have secondary fibromyalgia (Buskila et al. 1992).

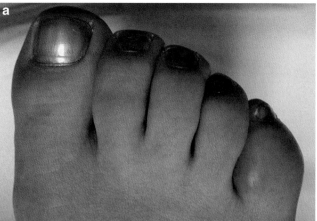

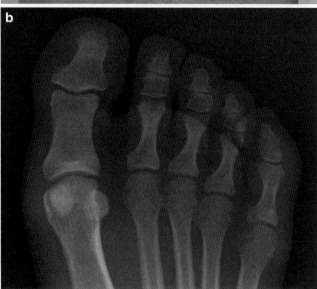

Fig. 8.3 Dactylitis: A "Sausage Digit" in PsA (**a**) A 21-year-old woman presented with sudden onset of pain and swelling in the right fifth toe, but denied pain in other joints. She had a small patch of scalp psoriasis. (**b**) A radiograph of the right fifth toe taken 3 months after presentation revealed fusion of the DIP joint (with kind permission from the american college of Rheumatology)

Pearl: PsA tends to occur in a "ray" distribution.

Comment: PsA has a tendency to affect all joints in a particular digit: e.g., the MCP (metacarpophalangeal), PIP (proximal interphalangeal), and DIP joints of a finger (Fig. 8.3). This is termed dactylitis (from the Greek word "daktyos" for finger), but known more colloquially as a "sausage digit" (Brockbank et al. 2005). The sausage appearance of the affected digit likely results from the involvement not only of the joints by synovitis, but also by tenosynovitis, particularly of flexor tendons. Even though all of the joints in one finger might be affected by PsA, the adjacent fingers can be entirely free of arthritis.

In some patients, dactylitis becomes chronic such that the finger remains swollen but is no longer painful or red. Chronic dactylitis may respond less well to anti-inflammatory therapies, which may need to be modified accordingly.

Pearl: Enthesitis can help differentiate PsA from RA.

Comment: Forty percent of patients with PsA have enthesitis or inflammation at insertion of tendons into bones (Fig. 8.4) (Fernández-Sueiro et al. 2007). This feature is atypical of RA and strongly suggests the presence of a seronegative spondyloarthropathy. The most common sites of enthesitis in PsA are the plantar fascia, the Achilles tendon, the insertions of tendons at the knees and shoulders, and in the pelvic bones. The finding of enthesitis in association with cutaneous psoriasis is sufficient for the diagnosis of PsA.

Pearl: PsA and RA have distinctive extra-articular features.

Comment: Rheumatoid nodules do not occur in PsA. Indeed, if a patient with a diagnosis of PsA has a rheumatoid nodule, the diagnosis should be called into question. Other extra-articular features of PsA and RA also contrast strikingly: urethritis and inflammatory bowel disease symptoms are common in PsA, but interstitial lung disease, myocarditis, and pericarditis are far more characteristic of RA. The extra-articular differences are highlighted most often in the eye, where anterior and less commonly posterior uveitis typifies PsA but episcleritis, scleritis, keratitis, and keratoconjunctivitis are much more likely to complicate RA.

Pearl: Inflammatory arthritis in PsA can occur before cutaneous psoriasis has become evident.

Comment: About 25% of patients with cutaneous psoriasis develop PsA. The majority of patients with PsA have psoriasis either simultaneously or before the onset of arthritis. However, about 15% of PsA patients have arthritis that precedes their cutaneous disease. In those patients, the pattern of joint involvement is critical to arriving at the correct diagnosis. PsA

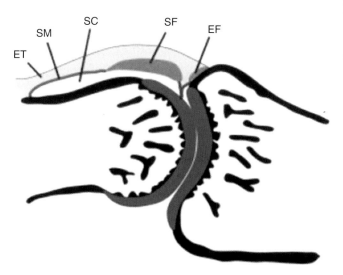

Fig. 8.4 Schematic representation of the synovial entheseal complex (SEC). An SEC of an extensor tendon (ET) in an interphalangeal joint, as seen in a sagittal section of a finger. The synovium lines the deep surface of the tendon except in the region of the sesamoid fibrocartilage (SF) that, in a flexed finger, is compressed against articular cartilage. SM = synovial membrane; *SC*=synovial cavity; *EF*=enthesis fibrocartilage (from McGonagle 2007. With kind permission from Wiley)

affects the DIP joints of the hands and feet; i.e., the joints that are not usually affected by RA. Furthermore, the distribution of joint disease in PsA tends to be asymmetric, but RA is characteristically symmetric, with a tendency to involve the MCP and PIP joints bilaterally (Gladman 1987).

Myth: There is a direct relationship between the activity of skin and joint disease in PsA.

Reality: Some investigators suggest that there is a relationship between the severity of psoriasis and the prevalence of PsA; i.e., the more severe the skin disease, the higher the likelihood of inflammatory joint disease (Gelfand et al. 2005). However, once a patient has developed PsA, there does not appear to be a direct relationship between the flares of skin and joint disease (Jones et al. 1994; Cohen et al. 1999; Elkayam et al. 2000).

Some medications employed by rheumatologists exacerbate cutaneous psoriasis. These include non-steroidal anti-inflammatory drugs and glucocorticoids. Moreover, not all disease-modifying antirheumatic drugs (DMARDs) used potentially by rheumatologists to treat joint disease are effective for skin disease, nor are all therapies for cutaneous psoriasis efficacious in PsA. When cutaneous psoriasis is severe and fails to respond to treatments directed primarily toward the arthritis, consultation and co-management with a dermatologist is appropriate.

Myth: PsA is AS with psoriasis.

Reality: PsA and AS are both seronegative spondyloarthropathies. The seronegative spondyloarthropathies affect the spine and share a number of extra-articular manifestations (Helliwell 2004). About 10% of patients with AS have psoriasis, but important clinical and radiologic differences exist between these disorders (Gladman 1998).

Moll and Wright described a number of different patterns of joint disease in PsA, including an arthritis that resembles RA (symmetrical, polyarticular, small joint), DIP-joint predominant, oligoarticular, spondylitis, and arthritis mutilans (Moll and Wright 1973). These categories encompass both peripheral and axial joint involvement. The majority of PsA patients have peripheral disease, and about 50% have spondylitis. Less than 5% of patients with PsA have isolated spondylitis.

Although the types of extra-articular manifestations observed in PsA and AS are similar, their frequencies differ substantially. The most obvious example, of course, is the skin, whereas essentially 100% of patients with PsA have cutaneous psoriasis and more than 80% have nail lesions; only 10% of AS patients have psoriasis. Iritis (anterior uveitis) occurs in more than 30% of AS patients but in a far lower percentage of PsA patients. Urethritis is more common in AS than PsA.

Pearl: Spinal involvement presents later in life in PsA than it does in AS.

Comment: Patients with AS present with back pain in their late teens or early 20s. In contrast, those with psoriatic spondylitis seldom present before their 30s or 40s. Moreover, the presenting feature of spondylitis in PsA is limitation of movement rather than back pain (Gladman 2009). Just as the peripheral arthritis of PsA is less symptomatic than that of RA, so too is the spinal disease of PsA less symptomatic than that of AS (Gladman et al. 1993; Helliwell et al. 1998; O'Shea et al. 2006). Patients with PsA demonstrate more spinal mobility on average than do AS patients, perhaps because the syndesmophytes in PsA are asymmetric, allowing for a greater preservation of spinal mobility.

Myth: PsA is a mild disease that does not require aggressive intervention.

Reality: This notion was prevalent following the early descriptions of PsA (Shbeeb et al. 2000). Wright observed that PsA tends to be less severe than RA (Wright 1959). A subsequent study reported less mortality and greater functional capacity among PsA patients compared with RA (Coulton et al. 1989).

More recent studies have confirmed the high prevalence of severe, destructive, and disabling disease in PsA, and an increased mortality risk for patients with this diagnosis (Gladman 2007; Sokoll and Helliwell 2001; McHugh et al. 2003; Kane et al. 2003; Queiro-Silva et al. 2003; Bond et al. 2007; Ali et al. 2007). A large proportion of PsA patients develop joint erosions and disability within the first 2 years of disease. In many patients, particularly those with the aptly named "arthritis mutilans," PsA is a more severe disease even than is RA. Early, aggressive treatment of PsA may prevent untoward outcomes (Kane et al. 2003; Ali et al. 2007).

Myth: PsA is basically a disease of skin and joints.

Reality: PsA patients are at an increased risk of both coronary artery disease and the metabolic syndrome, as are patients with RA and systemic lupus erythematosus (Bruce et al. 2000; Gladman et al. 2008; Eder et al. 2008; Tam et al. 2008a, b). Some data suggest that the underlying inflammatory milieu in PsA is responsible for these co-morbidities (Tam et al. 2008a, b).

References

Ali Y, Tom BDM, Schentag CT, Farewell VT, Gladman DD. Improved survival in psoriatic arthritis (PsA) with calendar time. Arthritis Rheum 2007; 56:2708–2714

Bond SJ, Farewell VT, Schentag CT, Gladman DD. Predictors for radiological damage in Psoriatic Arthritis: Results from a single centre. Ann Rheum Dis 2007; 66:370–376

Brockbank J, Stein M, Schentag CT, Gladman DD. Dactylitis in psoriatic arthritis (PsA): A marker for disease severity? Ann Rheum Dis 2005; 62:188–190

Bruce IN, Schentag C, Gladman DD. Hyperuricemia in psoriatic arthritis (PsA) does not reflect the extent of skin involvement. J Clin Rheumatol 2000; 6:6–9

Buskila D, Langevitz P, Gladman DD, Urowitz S, Smythe H. Patients with rheumatoid arthritis are more tender than those with psoriatic arthritis. J Rheumatol 1992; 19:1115–1119

Cohen, MR, Reda, DJ, Clegg, DO. Baseline relationships between psoriasis and psoriatic arthritis: Analysis of 221 patients with active psoriatic arthritis. J Rheumatol 1999; 26:1752–1756

Coulton BL, Thomson K, Symmons DP, Popert AJ. Outcome in patients hospitalised for psoriatic arthritis. Clin Rheumatol 1989; 8:261–265

Eastmond CJ, Wright V. The nail dystrophy of psoriatic arthritis. Ann Rheum Dis 1979; 38:226–228

Eder L, Zisman D, Barzilai M, Laor A, Rahat M, Rozenbaum M, et al Subclinical atherosclerosis in psoriatic arthritis: A case-control study. J Rheumatol 2008; 35:877–782

Elkayam O, Ophir J, Yaron M, Caspi D. Psoriatic arthritis: Interrelationships between skin and joint manifestations related to onset, course and distribution. Clin Rheumatol 2000;19: 301–305

Fernández-Sueiro JL, Willisch A, Pinto J, et al Prevalence and location of enthesitis in ankylosing spondylitis and psoriatic arthritis. Ann Rheum Dis 2007; 66(Suppl II):99

Gelfand JM, Gladman DD, Mease PJ, et al Epidemiology of psoriatic arthritis in the United States population. J Amer Acad Dermatol 2005; 53:573–577

Gladman DD. Clinical aspects of spondyloarthropathies. Am J Med Sci 1998; 316:234–238

Gladman DD. Axial disease in psoriatic arthritis. Curr Rheumatol Rep 2007; 9:455–460

Gladman DD, Anhorn KB, Schachter RK, Mervart H. HLA antigens in psoriatic arthritis. J Rheumatol 1986; 13:586–592

Gladman DD, Shuckett R, Russell ML, Thorne JC, Schachter RK. Psoriatic arthritis - clinical and laboratory analysis of 220 patients. Quart J Med 1987; 62:127–141

Gladman DD, Brubacher B, Buskila D, Langevitz P, Farewell VT. Differences in the expression of spondyloarthropathy: A comparison between ankylosing spondylitis and psoriatic arthritis. Genetic and gender effects. Clin Invest Med 1993; 16:1–7

Gladman DD, Farewell VT, Husted J, Wong K. Mortality studies in psoriatic arthritis. Results from a single centre. II. Prognostic indicators for mortality. Arthritis Rheum 1998; 41:1103–1110

Gladman DD, Ang M, Su L, Tom BDM, Schentag CT, Farewell VT. Cardiovascular morbidity in psoriatic arthritis (PsA). Ann Rheum Dis Online. Accessed December 8, 2008

Gladman DD, Helliwell PS, Mease PJ. GRAPPA at the European League Against Rheumatism (EULAR) 2008. J Rheumatol 2009; 36:656–658

Helliwell PS. Relationship of psoriatic arthritis with the other spondyloarthropathies. Curr Opin Rheumatol 2004; 16:344–349

Helliwell PS, Hickling P, Wright V. Do the radiological changes of classic ankylosing spondylitis differ from the changes found in the spondylitis associated with inflammatory bowel disease, psoriasis, and reactive arthritis? Ann Rheum Dis 1998; 57:135–140

Jajic J. Blue-coloured skin over involved joints in psoriatic arthritis. Clin Rheumatol 2001; 20:304–305

Jones SM, Armas JB, Cohen MG, et al Psoriatic arthritis: Outcome of disease subsets and relationship of joint disease to nail and skin disease. Br J Rheumatol 1994; 33:834–839

Kane D, Stafford L, Bresniham B, Fitzgerald O. A prospective, clinical and radiological study of early psoriatic arthritis: an early synovitis clinic experience Rheumatol 2003; 42:1460–1468

McGonagle, D. The concept of a synovio-enthesial complex and its implications for understanding joint inflammation and damage in psoriatic arthritis and beyond. Arthritis Rheum 2007; 56:8

McHugh NJ, Balachrishnan C, Jones SM. Progression of peripheral joint disease in psoriatic arthritis: A 5-yr prospective study. Rheumatology (Oxford) 2003; 42:778–783

Moll JM, Wright V. Psoriatic arthritis. Semin Arthritis Rheum 1973; 3:55–78

O'Shea FD, Chandran V, Toloza SMA, Schentag CT, Inman RD, Gladman DD. Does axial disease exhibit a different phenotype in primary ankylosing spondylitis versus psoriatic arthritis? Arthritis Rheum 2006; 54:4091

Queiro-Silva R, Torre-Alonso JC, Tinture-Eguren T, et al A polyarticular onset predicts erosive and deforming disease in psoriatic arthritis. Ann Rheum Dis 2003; 62:68–70

Shbeeb M, Uramoto KM, Gibson LE, O'Fallon WM, Gabriel SE. The epidemiology of psoriatic arthritis in Olmsted County, Minnesota, USA, 1982–1991. J Rheumatol 2000; 27:1247–1250

Sokoll KB, Helliwell PS. Comparison of disability and quality of life in rheumatoid and psoriatic arthritis. J Rheumatol 2001; 28: 1842–1846

Tam LS, Shang Q, Li EK, Tomlinson B, Chu TT, Li M, et al Subclinical carotid atherosclerosis in patients with psoriatic arthritis. Arthritis Rheum 2008a; 59:1322–1331

Tam LS, Tomlinson B, Chu TT, et al Cardiovascular risk profile of patients with psoriatic arthritis compared to controls–the role of inflammation. Rheumatology (Oxford) 2008b; 47:718–723

Wright V. Rheumatism and psoriasis a re-evaluation. Am J Med 1959; 27:454–462.

Reactive Arthritis

Robert D. Inman and Andrew Keat

9.1 Overview of Reactive Arthritis

> In reactive arthritis (ReA), exposure to an infectious agent leads to the development of an inflammatory arthritis and other characteristic clinical findings. However, this syndrome occurs in the absence of an ongoing infectious process.

> About 50% of ReA and undifferentiated oligoarthritis cases can be attributed to a specific pathogen by a combination of culture and serology. The predominant organisms are *Chlamydia*, *Salmonella*, *Shigella*, *Yersinia*, and *Campylobacter* species.

> The frequency of ReA following exposure to potential etiologic agents is between 3% and 10%.

> ReA characteristically involves the joints of the lower extremities in an asymmetric, oligoarticular pattern.

> The presence of HLAB27 increases disease susceptibility, but is neither sufficient nor necessary for ReA to occur. Individuals who are HLA-B27 positive tend to have more severe and longer episodes of ReA.

> A dactylitis ("sausage digit") pattern of arthritis in the feet is typical of ReA, as it is of psoriatic arthritis. ReA has a predilection for joints of the lower extremities, usually in an asymmetric, oligoarticular pattern.

> Enthesopathy and anterior uveitis often occur in ReA.

> Cutaneous manifestations of ReA include:
>   – Oral ulcers, typically painless
>   – Nail dystrophy
>   – Keratoderma blenorrhagicum, a papulosquamous rash that affects the palms and soles
>   – Circinate balanitis, characterized by shallow ulcers on the glans or the shaft of the penis

Pearl: Always consider ReA when confronted with monoarthritis in a young adult.

Comment: ReA most often affects adults between 18 and 40 years of age. This disorder presents as an oligoarthritis, with pain and swelling only a few joints (often only one). The knee, ankle, or one of the metatarsophalangeal joints is usually affected first (Fig. 9.1). When the patient is a child, ReA must be distinguished from juvenile idiopathic arthritis, particularly the oligoarticular form. Among adult patients, ReA must be differentiated from microcrystalline disorders. Septic arthritis must always be considered and excluded in any patient who presents with a monoarthritis.

Symptoms of ReA may develop before other features of the infection that triggered the inflammation become apparent. Thus, a clear history relating to other features of a spondyloarthropathy (past or present) and exposure to and symptoms of *genitourinary* (GU) or enteric infection should be sought.

Pearl: Acute ReA may mimic septic arthritis.

Comment: Most often ReA is associated with relatively mild systemic symptoms and characteristic multi-site disease. In a

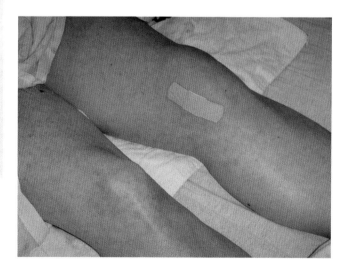

Fig. 9.1 Monoarthritis of the left knee in a patient with post-streptococcal ReA (figure courtesy of Dr. John Stone)

few patients, however, monoarthritis is associated with high fever and marked malaise. Yersiniosis and salmonellosis are particularly likely to be associated with such systemic features. Septic arthritis may occur in Campylobacter and Salmonella infections. The culture of organisms from a joint indicates treatment for a septic arthritis, even if other clinical features are highly consistent with ReA.

Pearl: The only way to differentiate definitively between ReA and septic arthritis is through culture of the synovial fluid.

Comment: Certain organisms, e.g., Yersinia and Salmonella, can cause both septic arthritis and ReA. Thus, sampling and culture of the synovial fluid is mandatory in the assessment of a patient with possible ReA. Differentiating gonococcal arthritis from post-GU ReA is a common challenge in this regard. Recall that joint cultures for Neisseria gonococcus are frequently negative, even in the setting of disseminated gonococcal infection. This heightens the difficulty in discriminating between gonococcal infections and ReA.

Myth: ReA responds to antibiotic therapy.

Reality: Despite the role of infections in triggering ReA, cultures of synovial fluid are sterile. There is no evidence that antibiotics alter the long-term course of ReA that follows a gastrointestinal infection, and no indication that long-term treatment with antibiotics is effective for shortening episodes of ReA. There remains some uncertainty about the impact of antibiotics on the course of ReA after an infection of the GU tract caused by *Chlamydia*. However, no compelling data support the prolonged use of antibiotics beyond the course required to eradicate the inciting infection (Hamdulay et al. 2006).

Pearl: Dysuria and a genital rash can follow gastrointestinal infections as well as GU infections.

Comment: When GU complaints occur concurrently with an inflammatory arthritis, clinicians may assume that a sexually-transmitted disease has been the inciting event. However, urethritis is perfectly compatible with the syndrome of ReA that follows a gastrointestinal infection (Ahvonen et al. 1969), and circinate balanitis may occur without an antecedent infection of the urogenital tract. A sexually-transmitted disease need not be invoked to explain GU features.

Pearl: The enthesitis of ReA can be the dominant feature of the disease.

Comment: Enthesitis, particularly Achilles tendonitis and plantar fasciitis, can be profoundly disabling in the acute phase. Always examine patients with suspected ReA standing, to search for Achilles' tendonitis (Fig. 9.2). Enthesitis overshadows inflammatory joint symptoms in some patients.

Myth: Post-streptococcal ReA is really acute rheumatic fever.

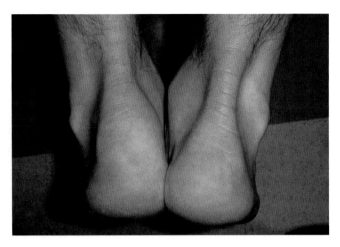

Fig. 9.2 Left Achilles' tendon swelling, consistent with a ReA-related enthesopathy (figure courtesy of Dr. John Stone

Reality: In adult patients, post-streptococcal ReA is not accompanied by carditis, chorea, erythema marginatum, or subcutaneous nodules (Barash et al. 2008). Post-streptococcal ReA and acute rheumatic fever are two different entities. The implications of this are significant; for example, long-term antibiotic prophylaxis is not indicated in adults with post-streptococcal ReA.

Pearl: No inflammation, no ReA!

Comment: ReA is an inflammatory condition associated with genuine signs of joint or enthesial swelling. Tenderness or aching in the joints or periarticular tissues without hard signs of inflammation is not sufficient for the diagnosis. Similarly, non-specific urethral symptoms in men must not be attributed to ReA if they are not associated with musculoskeletal symptoms that are incompatible with ReA. No inflammation, no ReA.

Myth: HLA-B27 typing is a helpful diagnostic test for ReA.

Reality: About 50% of people with ReA carry the HLA-B27 gene, with the figure being somewhat higher in certain populations. Thus, negative HLA-B27 genotyping does not exclude the diagnosis of ReA. The diagnosis must be founded upon compatible clinical features and compelling evidence of an infection.

Pearl: The presence or absence of HLA-B27 affects clinical disease phenotype.

Comment: HLA-B27 positivity is typical of patients who have persistent disease and is nearly universal among patients with ReA and uveitis. In addition, 90% of patients with radiographic evidence of sacroiliitis are HLA-B27 positive.

In patients with ReA in sub-Saharan Africa, an aggressive form of disease is observed. These patients are generally HLA-B27 negative, but often are infected with the human immunodeficiency virus (Leirisalo-Repo 1998).

Myth: When ReA is suspected, examination of the joint fluid by PCR may reveal the infectious cause.

Reality: Inflamed joints contain a wide range of bacterial proteins and some bacterial DNA. Some studies have revealed specific bacterial DNA (Hannu et al. 2006) and even RNA, indicating probable viability of the bacteria presumed to have caused the arthritis (Hannu et al. 2006). However, bacterial DNA from many different genera have been identified within joint material (Kempsell et al. 2000), and it remains unclear how (or if) to ascribe causality to any of these findings. This is an exciting space to be watched, but not a helpful clinical test.

Pearl: The uveitis of ReA is anterior, unilateral, and highly symptomatic.

Comment: ReA is associated with an anterior uveitis that tends to afflict one eye at a time. The contralateral eye may be involved in a subsequent disease flare. The finding of concurrent bilateral disease or disease in the posterior pole of the eye strongly invokes other diagnoses, e.g., sarcoidosis or Behcet's disease.

Patients with the anterior uveitis of ReA have pronounced photophobia, eye pain, ocular erythema, and tearing. Shining a flashlight in the contralateral (uninvolved) eye leads to pain in the involved eye because of the consensual light response, which leads to pupillary narrowing in the inflamed eye and an increase in ocular discomfort. In addition to topical glucocorticoid eye drops, a mydriatic agent is essential to dilate the involved eye and prevent the formation of synechiae between the pupil and the lens.

Pearl: An episode of ReA may be followed by a prolonged period of non-inflammatory arthralgia.

Comment: Most episodes of ReA resolve within 12 months (Keat 1983), but the persistence of symptoms following an episode of inflammatory disease is not uncommon in ReA. The explanation for this phenomenon is not clear though it may be a source of great anxiety for patients. Indeed, a psychological element may complicate the clinical picture, requiring great reassurance from the clinician. If all evidence of inflammation has resolved, there is no role for antibiotic treatment or disease-modifying antirheumatic drugs (DMARDs).

Pearl: Recurrence of ReA is common.

Comment: Recurrence of sexually-acquired ReA is common (Colmegna et al. 2004). About 50% of such patients suffer subsequent episodes. In contrast, recurrence after enteric infection is uncommon. Patients should be advised about the risk of re-infection leading to recurrence of arthritis and about specific precautions for avoiding re-infection.

The precise role of repeated infections in precipitating recurrences of ReA is not clear. Additional genital tract infections may be associated with recurrent ReA, but re-infection with enteric bacteria – even when of the same species as that which caused the initial episode – does not always lead to a recurrence of ReA.

Myth: ReA is precipitated only by gastrointestinal and GU infections.

Reality: The commonly recognized arthritogenic pathogens are *Salmonella, Shigella, Campylobacter, Yersinia,* and *Chlamydia.* However, ReA may occur after infection by any portal of entry, and may be caused by a large number of other organisms, as well. As an example, cases of ReA following *Clostridium difficile* infections are well described.

In some patients whose clinical features are consistent with ReA, there is no antecedent history of infection. This suggests that this syndrome can result either from subclinical infections or from other environmental (non-infectious) triggers.

Myth: The interval between antecedent infection and ReA is 1 week or less.

Reality: Although an interval of 1–2 weeks after the inciting infection is typical for the appearance of ReA, this time period extends up to 4 weeks. Patients with joint symptoms and other clinical features compatible with ReA must therefore be queried closely about more "remote" occurrences of infections.

Myth: ReA is a chronic disease similar to rheumatoid arthritis.

Reality: ReA usually consists of either a single attack that runs its course within a matter of months or recurrent episodes of arthritis that last weeks to months between longer periods of remission. A chronic, destructive, disabling arthritis evolves in only a minority of patients.

Pearl: Not all inflammatory back pain symptoms in ReA are caused by spondylitis, sacroiliitis, or both.

Comment: Some symptoms of low back pain in ReA are caused by enthesitis that involves the pelvic girdle. The pelvis, in addition to the Achilles tendon and the plantar fascia, is another common site of involvement by enthesopathy. Unrelated, non-inflammatory causes of back pain should not be overlooked even during an episode of ReA.

Myth: DMARDs should be avoided in ReA.

Reality: The typical course of ReA is a period of greatest joint activity over 8–12 weeks. Most patients respond satisfactorily to sustained doses of NSAIDs. If the symptoms are not controlled adequately or if the course is more protracted, methotrexate or sulfasalazine can be added to the NSAID regimen. Intra-articular glucocorticoid injections can be of symptomatic benefit.

There is little published experience with the use of biologic agents in chronic refractory ReA. However, given the efficacy of tumor necrosis factor inhibition in the treatment of several related disorders, e.g., ankylosing spondylitis, psoriatic arthritis, and inflammatory bowel disease, this approach is reasonable for patients with highly symptomatic, persistent ReA.

Pearl: The appearance of circinate balanitis differs according to whether or not the patient is circumcised.

Comment: If the male is uncircumcised, the lesions of circinate balanitis can appear as multiple, serpiginous, shallow ulcers on the glans or shaft of the penis. These lesions often have raised borders. In circumcised males, circinate balanitis can appear as dry, hyperkeratotic plaques that are reminiscent of psoriasis.

Pearl: If the arthritis of ReA persists beyond the time usually associated with this condition, consider whether the patient might have psoriatic arthritis instead.

Comment: The clinical features of ReA overlap significantly with those of many patients with psoriatic arthritis. As examples:

- Asymmetric, oligoarticular patterns of joint disease are present in both ReA and psoriatic arthritis.
- Keratoderma blenorrhagicum, a finding associated with ReA, cannot be distinguished histologically from pustular psoriasis.
- The fingernails and toenails in ReA can become thickened and develop subungual debris and onychodystrophy. However, nail pitting in a patient with inflammatory joint disease clearly favors psoriatic arthritis as the underlying diagnosis.

Pearl: Preventing a recurrence of ReA is influenced more by advice than antibiotics.

Comment: Safe sex practice is sound advice for all sexually-active individuals. Among patients with a history of ReA following a GU infection, such advice should be reinforced with particular vigor. Similarly, for patients who have had episodes of ReA following enteric infections, extra precaution with regard to local food and hygiene should be exercised when traveling to locales where enteric pathogens are common.

Pearl: Post-diarrheal arthritis should always occasion a search for gastrointestinal pathogens.

Comment: The new onset of joint pain in the setting of diarrhea may indeed herald a case of inflammatory bowel disease with accompanying arthritis. However, infectious diarrhea from bacteria, parasites, or toxins must be excluded definitively as the first priority. Sending stool specimens for fecal leukocytes, cultures, ova and parasites, and Clostridium difficile toxin assays are critical in this evaluation.

Pearl: Gonococcal arthritis and ReA are different.

Comment: The term "gonococcal arthritis" refers to a septic arthritis, often part of a syndrome of persistent gonococcemia in which primary infection with Neisseria gonorrhea disseminates widely, leading to low-grade fevers, sparse skin lesions, and septic arthritis. The primary infection is usually but not always in the genital tract. The disease responds to appropriate antimicrobial therapy.

The problem arises when aseptic arthritis arises in an individual who also has gonococcal infection. It is unclear whether *Neisseria gonorrhea* is a true initiator of ReA, but the prevailing view is that in this circumstance the gonococcal infection is accompanied by an additional simultaneous non-gonococcal infection and it is this that provokes the arthritis.

Pearl: Attempting to identify the presumed causal infection may be very helpful.

Comment: Frequently the diagnosis of ReA is made (accurately) on evidence of infection – e.g., diarrhea or urethritis – without identification of a specific bacterial pathogen. Because the precise causal link between the bacterium and the arthritis is unknown, this is not a great problem. However, if there is an infection, knowing its cause or excluding some potential etiologies is valuable. A patient who develops severe ReA after bacterial diarrhea associated with ingestion of particular food may be an "index case" that explains a pattern of food-borne illness within a community. Moreover, the diagnosis of chlamydial urethritis offers the opportunity to treat this infection in the patient's sexual partners, who may or may not be symptomatic.

References

Ahvonen P, Sievers K, Aho K. Arthritis associated with *Yersinia enterocolitica* infection. Acta Rheumatol Scand 1969; 15(3):232–253

Barash J, Mashiach E, Navon-Elkan P, et al Differentiation of post-streptococcal reactive arthritis from acute rheumatic fever. J Pediatrics 2008; 153:696

Colmegna I, Cuchacovich R, Espinosa LR. HLA-associated reactive arthritis: Pathogenic and clinical considerations. Clin Microbiol Rev 2004; 17:348–369

Hamdulay SS, Glynne SJ, Keat A. When is arthritis reactive? Postgrad Med J 2006; 82(969):446–453

Hannu T, Inman R, Granfors K, Leirisalo-Repo M. Reactive arthritis or post-infectious arthritis? Best Pract Res Clin Rheumatol 2006; 20 (3):419–433

Keat A. Reiter's syndrome and reactive arthritis in perspective. N Engl J Med 1983; 29;309(26):1606–1615

Kempsell KE, Cox CJ, Hurle M, et al Reverse transcriptase-PCR analysis of bacterial rRNA for detection and characterization of bacterial species in arthritis synovial tissue. Infect Immun 2000; 68(10): 6012–6026

Leirisalo-Repo M. Prognosis, course of diseases and treatment of the spondyloarthropathies. Rheum Dis Clin N Amer 1998; 24:737–751

Systemic Sclerosis (Scleroderma) and Raynaud's Phenomenon

10

Janet E. Pope, Philip J. Clements, Daniel E. Furst, Laura K. Hummers, Dinesh Khanna, Maureen D. Mayes, Thomas Medsger, James Seibold, and Virginia Steen

10.1 Overview of Systemic Sclerosis

> Systemic sclerosis (scleroderma; SSc) is a chronic connective tissue disease characterized by inflammation within, and fibrosis of, the skin, vascular abnormalities, visceral damage, and the production of autoantibodies.
> SSc is divided generally into limited and diffuse forms, based on the extent of skin involvement.
> A group of conditions known as "localized" scleroderma, which includes morphea, linear scleroderma, and en coup de sabre, is discussed in the chapter on Scleroderma Mimickers (Chap. 11).
> Diffuse SSc has a greater extent of skin involvement and is more likely to be associated with renal crisis, pulmonary fibrosis, and cardiomyopathy. Patients with diffuse SSc have a higher mortality rate.
> Pulmonary disease remains a major source of morbidity and mortality for patients with SSc. Patients with limited SSc are predisposed to the development of pulmonary arterial hypertension (PAH). Those with diffuse SSc are predisposed to interstitial fibrosis.
> Autoantibody profiles can predict to a certain extent the types of organ involvement that can be expected in SSc.
> Raynaud's phenomenon (RP) is characterized by vasospasm of the digital arteries that leads to well-demarcated pallor with cyanosis and rubor.
> RP is essentially universal among patients with SSc and is the first symptom in a large majority of patients.
> Primary RP is often mild enough not to require treatment; however, with secondary RP from SSc, there is not only vasospasm but also fixed blood vessel problems with luminal narrowing, so the ischemia can be more severe.
> Complications of RP in SSc can include digital ulcers often leading to infection and amputation causing pain and functional disability.
> Diffuse SSc often presents with puffiness of the hands associated with pain, in a way that can mimic rheumatoid arthritis. RP often occurs around the time of development of puffy hands in diffuse SSc.

10.1.1 Raynaud's Phenomenon and Digital Ischemia

Pearl: Skin induration that spares the fingers and is not associated with RP is not SSc.

Comment: The diagnosis of RP is made when a patient provides a history of acral skin color changes precipitated by cold or emotional distress.

Pearl: The timing of the first development of Raynaud's phenomenon and of the onset of other SSc features differs according to whether the patient has limited or diffuse SSc.

Comment: RP and the skin changes of early diffuse SSc often occur closely together in time. In contrast, RP may be evident years before other features of limited SSc are manifest.

Pearl: Those who develop RP later in life (age >40) are more apt to have secondary RP.

Comment: RP that begins in childhood, during the teen years, or in the patient's 20s, when it is most likely to be primary RP in the absence of overt connective tissue disease symptomotology. When trying to determine if a patient has a secondary cause of RP, essential points on the physical examination are swollen fingers and the presence of dilated capillaries in the finger nailbeds, either of which points to a secondary cause of RP. A positive antinuclear antibody (ANA) assay is also instructive; particularly if an anticentromere pattern is present on immunofluorescence (Fig. 10.1) or if additional testing identifies a common connective tissue disease autoantibody such as those directed against the Ro, La, Sm, or RNP antigens. However, most RP is primary and not associated with an underlying condition (Pope 2007; Hirschl et al. 2006; Luggen et al. 1995).

Myth: All calcium channel blockers are equally effective for the treatment of RP.

Reality: Only the dihydropyridine class of calcium channel blockers (nifedipine, amlodipine, felodipine) offers significant benefit in treating RP. These agents have a stronger peripheral vasodilatory action when compared with other

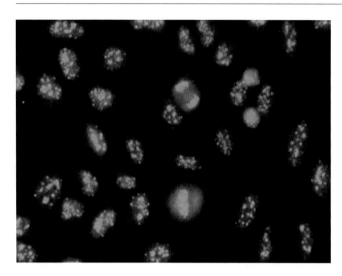

Fig. 10.1 Anti-centromere pattern of immunofluorescence on antinuclear antibody testing. If this pattern is present, a specific anticentromere antibody assay does not need to be performed

calcium channel blockers. Diltiazem and verapamil provide only limited benefit and should play no role in therapy (Thompson et al. 2001).

Pearl: Calcium channel blockers in SSc reduce the number of RP attacks.

Comment: The best studied treatment class for RP is the dihydropyridine calcium channel blockers. The usual benefit is on the order of a 30% reduction in attack frequency. Most randomized controlled trials of these agents have shown no improvement in attack severity, but the doses employed in most studies have been low (Thompson et al. 2001). Calcium channel blockers can be prescribed on either a regular or an as needed basis. Side effects of calcium channel blockers are common and often limit the dose that can be used.

Pearl: Clinical indicators provide clues to the likelihood of secondary RP.

Comment: Leading clinical indicators of secondary RP are shown in Table 10.1. Longitudinal prospective studies of patients presenting with RP suggest that abnormal nailfold capillary at baseline is the strongest predictor of the development of a defined connective tissue disease in the future (Pavlov-Dolijanović et al. 2006).

Table 10.1 Leading clinical indicators of secondary Raynaud's phenomenon

Age of onset >40 years
Males presenting at any age
Presence of antinuclear antibodies (at a titer greater than 1:160) (Pope 2003a)
Presence of abnormal nailfold capillaries (Pope 2003a; Herrick 2005)

Pearl: Nailfold capillary examination is easily performed in a standard examination room.

Comment: The only tool that is required is a standard ophthalmoscope. Microscope immersion oil enhances the technique, but surgical lubricating jelly can be substituted if immersion oil is not available. The oil is placed at the nailfold and the ophthalmoscope is set at +40 diopters, the highest magnification, which is equivalent to magnifying the skin by a factor of 10. To bring the nailfold capillaries into focus, the examiner does not adjust the ophthalmoscope but rather moves his or her head toward or away from the finger under examination. The presence of dilated capillary loops or areas of capillary dropout are indicative of an underlying connective tissue disease (most often SSc). Some capillaries at the nailbed are seen on the cuticle and can even be observed by the naked eye.

Myth: Dilated capillary loops are observed only in patients with SSc.

Reality: Nailfold capillary loop dilations are characteristic of a number of connective tissue disorders, including lupus, dermatomyositis, and even (occasionally) rheumatoid arthritis (Fig. 10.2) (Pope et al. 2008). However, this finding is most common in SSc. Nailfold capillary abnormalities usually occur early in the patient's disease course and drop out or disappear over time, perhaps an indication of the progression of an obliterative vasculopathy that is present in some patients with SSc.

Myth: The disappearance of dilated capillaries is a good thing.

Reality: The vasculature in SSc becomes more abnormal over time and often eventually no dilated capillaries are seen at the nailbeds. This is because of the "dropout" of vasculature that

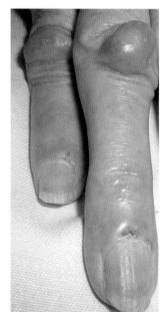

Fig. 10.2 A patient with a history of decades of seropositive rheumatoid arthritis developed Raynaud's phenomenon, dilated capillaries at the nailbeds, and sclerodactyly distal to the proximal interphalangeal joints

occurs over time with this disorder. An inverse correlation exists between the extent of nailfold changes detected by videocapillaroscopy and the duration of both RP symptoms and the time since diagnosis of SSc (Cutolo et al. 2004). Enlarged and giant capillaries, at times with hemorrhages, are the earliest pattern observed. Loss of capillaries, ramified capillaries, and vascular architectural disorganization are increased in later disease (Cutolo et al. 2004; Meli et al. 2006).

Myth: Cyanosis correlates with ischemia.

Reality: Cyanosis occurs when blood is stagnant and deoxygenation occurs. An intact nutritional blood supply can exist even in the presence of cyanosis. This fact is evidenced by the lack of ischemic pain and the finding of intact capillary refill that generally accompanies cyanosis. Many patients have completely asymptomatic episodes of cyanosis. Ischemic pain and diminished capillary refill with or without evidence of tissue damage are signs of ongoing ischemia and require immediate action to try and improve flow.

Myth: Ulcerations that occur overlying the dorsum of the PIP and MCP joints are ischemic in nature and should be managed with aggressive vasodilator therapy.

Reality: Digital tip ulcerations are related mostly to the absence of blood flow to the distal finger. In contrast, the lesions that occur over the dorsal surfaces of the PIP and MCP joints are multifactorial in nature. Patients who develop these lesions typically have significant skin thickening in their fingers, usually accompanied by more widespread cutaneous changes characteristic of diffuse SSc.

The hand joints in such patients have a tendency to become contracted and prone to minor trauma. The skin overlying the joint is atrophic and dry because of damage of sebaceous glands that increases the sensitivity to minor trauma and irritation. The overall blood flow in the fingers is reduced. Management of these lesions requires a multi-faceted approach with topical antimicrobial therapy, protection of the area (bandaging) when minor trauma is more likely, vasodilator therapy, and good skin care practice (moisturizer and emollient therapy).

Pearl: SSc patients can lose padding on their feet, just as they do on their fingertips.

Comment: Digital pulp loss in the fingertips is characteristic of SSc. SSc patients can also develop thinned padding on the soles of the feet, which makes it uncomfortable to walk in bare feet (Fig. 10.3). Loss of connective tissues on the sole of the foot tends to occur in the distal portions.

Pearl: Extrusion of digital tip calcium deposits is a challenging mimicker of infected ulcerations.

Comment: Subcutaneous calcinosis frequently occurs at sites of minor trauma and pressure, such as the extensor surfaces of the forearms and the fingertips. These deposits can erupt through the skin, leading to a purulent-appearing discharge. This lesion is often mistaken for a digital tip ulceration that has become secondarily infected. A pocket of subcutaneous calcinosis can often also be accompanied by erythema, particularly as new deposit occurs, further confusing the picture.

Calcinosis should be suspected when an SSc patient presents with spontaneous development of a draining lesion of the fingertip in the absence of ischemic pain and any history of previous digital ulcerations. Some patients describe a chalky discharge. Plain radiographs can confirm the presence of calcium (Fig. 10.4a, b). Recognition of this complication can help distinguish an infected digital ulcer from the drainage of calcinosis. The extrusion of an area of calcinosis is accompanied normally by the relief of discomfort.

Pearl: Acro-osteolysis in SSc can mimic "clubbing" and may be a manifestation of peripheral vascular disease rather than pulmonary disease.

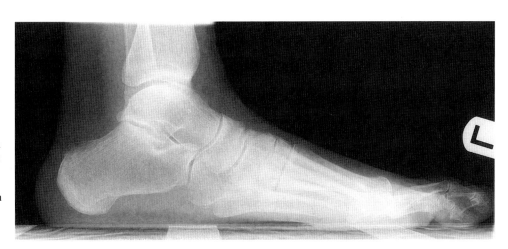

Fig. 10.3 Diminished fat pads on the feet. Scleroderma patients can lose padding on their feet, just as they do on their fingertips. This makes it uncomfortable to walk in bare feet. Note loss of connective tissues on the sole, especially distally

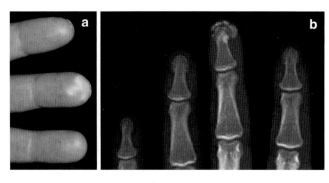

Fig. 10.4 (**a**) Fingertips in a patient with scleroderma. The middle finger shown (the third digit) has a calcium deposit in the pulp of the finger. The patient presented with intense pain in the digit that was exacerbated by dorsiflexion. A digital pit is also present in the second digit, positioned superiorly to the third digit in this photograph. (**b**) Radiograph revealing calcinosis of the third digit (Figures courtesy of Dr. John Stone)

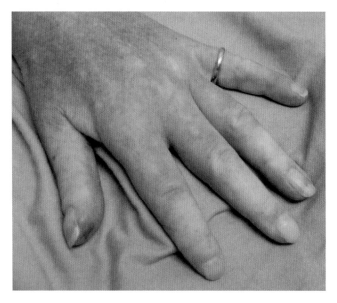

Fig. 10.5 The second and third fingertips have lost pulp. There is a healed ulcer on the thumb (volar side) (Figure courtesy of Dr. John Stone)

Comment: Pseudo-clubbing can occur when a patient develops osteolysis of the distal digital tuft (Fig. 10.5). This process may be completely painless, or may be associated with chronic ischemia.

10.1.2 Diagnosis

Myth: As a "connective tissue disorder," SSc is usually associated with an elevated erythrocyte sedimentation rate.

Reality: On the contrary, even in the setting of significant end-organ involvement in SSc, the ESR is often entirely normal. This stands in stark contrast to other connective tissue disorders, in which the acute phase reactants are usually elevated (often strikingly so).

Despite the often normal ESR in SSc, the ANA titer is typically sky-high. Few if any disease entities lead to higher ANA titers than does SSc.

Myth: Sclerodactyly distal to the metacarpophalangeal (MCP) joints usually indicates a diagnosis of SSc.

Reality: Sclerodactyly distal to the MCP joints without any proximal skin involvement can occur in many other conditions such as in diabetes, other connective tissue diseases, and rheumatoid arthritis. It is not specific for SSc.

Pearl: Scleroderma can mimic rheumatoid arthritis in its presentation.

Comment: Scleroderma can present with arthralgias and diffusely swollen hands, frequently leading to the diagnosis of an undifferentiated polyarthropathy or even rheumatoid arthritis.

10.1.3 Autoantibodies and Disease Phenotypes

Myth: Anti-centromere antibodies are the principal SSc autoantibodies that are linked to pulmonary hypertension.

Reality: Anti-centromere antibodies are the classic marker for limited SSc (formerly called the CREST syndrome, an acronym for *c*alcinosis, *R*aynaud's phenomenon, *e*sophageal dysmotility, *s*clerodactyly, and *t*elangiectasias). The limited SSc disease subset is a population of patients generally considered to be at the highest risk for the development of PAH. However, the presence of anti-centromere antibodies is not a predictor of pulmonary hypertension within the limited SSc population (Steen et al. 1984).

Limited SSc patients with a nucleolar staining pattern on their ANA, typically caused by antibodies to either the U3-RNP or the Th/To antigen, are at an increased risk for PAH (Fig. 10.6) (Steen 2005). Patients with anti-topoisomerase-3 antibodies are predisposed to the development of pulmonary fibrosis. When their interstitial lung disease is severe, patients with anti-topoisomerase-3 antibodies often develop pulmonary hypertension that is secondary to fibrosis. Patients with diffuse SSc can also develop the primary vasculopathy that leads to severe PAH, particularly if they have U3RNP autoantibodies (Sacks et al. 1996). Because pulmonary hypertension can occur in either major disease subset of SSc, the risk of this complication should be stratified by serologic phenotypes rather than clinical classification schemes.

Myth: Autoantibodies in SSc are epiphenomena.

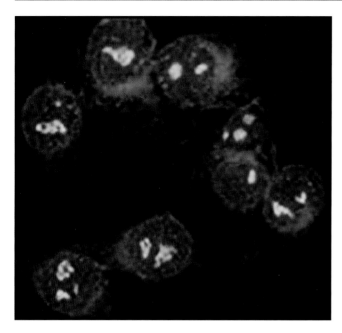

Fig. 10.6 Immunofluorescence assay for antinuclear antibodies demonstrating a nucleolar pattern of immunofluorescence

Reality: The pathways through which at least some SSc autoantibodies exert direct deleterious effects remain to be elucidated fully, but as described elsewhere in this chapter there is abundant evidence that specific autoantibodies correlate with particular clinical features. As an example, the topoisomerase I (Scl70) autoantibody promotes interstitial lung disease in a genetically predisposed animal model (Kuwana et al. 2001). These autoantibodies are also linked strongly to the risk of developing interstitial lung disease. Another autoantibody, directed against RNA polymerase III, is associated with a high risk of the development of scleroderma renal crisis. Finally, anticentromere antibodies are linked tightly to the limited SSc phenotype.

Thus, at a minimum, autoantibody profiles in patients with SSc are helpful in identifying the probably evolution of clinical phenotypes. Mechanistic proof of the pathways

through which these autoantibodies operate and interact with other elements of the immune system requires further study.

Pearl: Antibodies to RNA polymerase are associated with scleroderma renal crisis.

Comment: Autoantibodies are increasingly being recognized to be associated with specific phenotypic manifestations of rheumatic disease. Antibodies to RNA polymerase are a significant risk factor for scleroderma renal crisis. Some patients with scleroderma renal crisis (with or without anti-RNA polymerase antibodies) present with microangiopathic hemolytic anemia, mimicking thrombotic thrombocytopenic purpura. Other examples of the associations between autoantibodies and clinical manifestations of SSc are shown in Table *10.2*.

Pearl: Anticentromere antibody, an autoantibody associated with good survival, virtually never occurs in diffuse SSc.

Comment: Patients with diffuse SSc may have antibodies to topoisomerase I (Scl-70), RNA polymerase, and a number of other antigens, but virtually never possess anticentromere antibodies. Ten-year survival rates for patients with anticentromere antibodies are on the order of 93%, compared with 66% for patients with anti-Scl70 antibodies (Kuwana et al. 1994).

Pearl: SSc can overlap with other CTDs, so treat what is treatable.

Comment: SSc is commonly associated with Sjögren's syndrome and less often occurs in overlap combinations with clinical features of systemic lupus erythematosus, inflammatory myopathy, or rheumatoid arthritis. Remember to treat what is treatable. Some clinicians believe that Sjögren's syndrome is associated with (as opposed to "secondary to") SSc. There are reports of patients whose clinical features are similar to those of primary Sjögren's syndrome who also appear to have "incidentally" mild cases of SSc (Pope 2002; Salliot et al. 2007).

Pearl: Men are more likely to have diffuse SSc if they get SSc.

Table 10.2 Systemic sclerosis: Associations of phenotypic features with specific autoantibodies (Steen 2005)

Autoantibody	Staining pattern	Disease	Organ manifestations
ANA			
	Nucleolar	Scleroderma	
	Centromere	Limited scleroderma	Pulmonary hypertension
Anti-topoisomerase 1 (Scl-70)	Speckled or homogeneous	Diffuse scleroderma	Renal crisis; pulmonary fibrosis
Anti-U1-RNP		Limited scleroderma	Severe GI involvement
Anti-U3-RNP (fibrillarin)	Nucleolar	Scleroderma and mixed connective tissue disease	Pulmonary fibrosis; Severe GI involvement
Anti-PM/Scl	Nucleolar	Scleroderma/polymyositis overlap	Inflammatory myopathy; Pulmonary fibrosis; Severe GI involvement
Anti-RNA polymerase	Scleroderma		Renal crisis; *Decreased* frequency of lung disease

Comment: Although SSc is more common in women than in men – up to 87% of SSc patients are women – SSc in males is likely to be diffuse in nature. The ratio of limited to diffuse disease among female SSc patients has been estimated to be 2:1. In contrast, the ratio of limited to severe disease among male SSc patients is 1:2. Thus, if a man has SSc he is more likely to have diffuse disease. A woman is more likely to have limited disease (Walker et al. 2007; Al-Dhaher et al. 2008).

Pearl: Most major organ involvement in diffuse SSc also occurs early in the disease course (within the first 5 years).

Comment: Interstitial lung disease (Fig. 10.7), scleroderma renal crisis, and scleroderma cardiomyopathy, all of which are features of diffuse SSc, usually begin within the first 5 years but can recur or worsen over time. Severe organ involvement in SSc patients with diffuse SSc most often occurs early in the course of the disease (Steen 2000; Al-Dhaher et al. 2008). This is not necessarily true for PAH, typically a complication of limited SSc, which can develop at any time.

Pearl: There is more pigmentation in patients with diffuse SSc as opposed to limited SSc.

Comment: SSc can be associated with either hyper- or hypopigmentation, and sometimes both are found in the same patient (Fig. 10.8). Hyperpigmentation can be caused by either increased numbers of melanocytes within the skin of patients with SSc, but can also be a function of postinflammatory hyperpigmentation. Pigmentary changes are more common in patients with diffuse SSc than in those with limited SSc. Some patients with diffuse disease have a strikingly tanned appearance and smooth skin, because skin affected by SSc tends to lose its appendages. As the cutaneous features of SSc improve over time as they often do, there may be a regrowth of hair on the patient's extremities (Pope et al. 1996). Pigmentary changes are slower to resolve.

Pearl: The Health Assessment Questionnaire Disability Index (HAQ-DI) is useful in SSc.

Comment: Because of its multi-organ system nature, SSc normally has a substantial impact on patients' function and quality of life. The Health Assessment Questionnaire Disability Index (HAQ-DI) is one of the most commonly used health related quality of life (HRQoL) measures in SSc (Khanna 2006). This index has been validated for use in SSc patients (Merkel et al. 2002; Poole et al. 1995; Steen and Medsger 1997b). The HAQ-DI is usually higher in diffuse SSc than in limited disease.

Pearl: Most men with SSc have erectile dysfunction.

Comment: Erectile dysfunction can occur early in the disease course of SSc. Male patients suffering from erectile dysfunction who also have RP should be queried and examined for other clinical features of SSc.

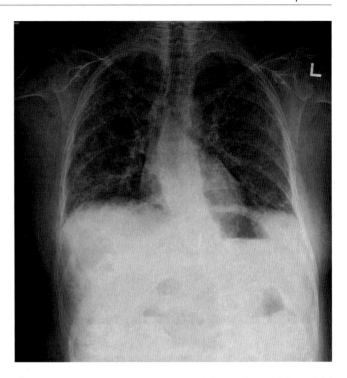

Fig. 10.7 Posteroanterior chest radiograph in a patient with interstitial lung disease secondary to scleroderma. The radiograph reveals severe scarring and very small lung volumes

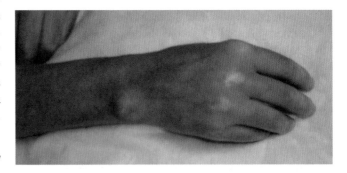

Fig. 10.8 Photograph of a patient with both hyperpigmentation and hypopigmentation secondary to scleroderma. The "tanned" skin is actually hyperpigmentation secondary to scleroderma. The hypopigmentation over the metacarpophalangeal joints is also a result of skin inflammation

Pearl: The strongest epidemiologic risk factor for SSc is a family history of the disease.

Comment: The prevalence of SSc in the US population is 0.026%. This compares with prevalence in the families of patients with SSc that is on the order of 1.6% (Arnett et al. 2001).

Pearl: Many SSc patients have depression. Recognize and treat it.

Comment: Many chronic diseases associated with pain and fatigue are accompanied by depression. However, in SSc, patients also often suffer from significant changes in appearance over time. This constitutes an additional "issue" for patients, and for many their altered appearance has a substantial impact on mood. The estimate of depression in SSc is higher than that of comparative population estimates and may be higher than many other chronic diseases such as heart and lung diseases (Hudson et al. 2009).

Myth: Patients with limited SSc do not develop significant internal organ disease.

Reality: Although limited SSc has a better overall prognosis than does diffuse disease, some individuals with limited SSc develop severe pulmonary hypertension or profound gastrointestinal hypomotility. A subset of patients with limited SSc also develops pulmonary fibrosis, a complication usually associated with diffuse SSc.

Monitoring for pulmonary hypertension in limited SSc includes periodic echocardiography with confirmation by right heart catheterization in those individuals with elevated right ventricular systolic pressures. Exercise echocardiography and exercise pulmonary function tests may also have a role in detecting incipient pulmonary hypertension.

Pearl: The new onset of pruritus in a patient with SSc can be an early symptom of primary biliary cirrhosis (PBC).

Comment: Intense pruritus is sometimes experienced by patients with new-onset SSc, particularly those with diffuse disease. The pruritus, probably caused by cutaneous inflammation accompanied by mast cells and histamine elevations in the skin (Pope et al. 1996), commonly subsides once the skin thickening has become established.

In contrast, the new onset or recurrence of pruritus in an otherwise stable SSc patient might herald the presentation of PBC. PBC occurs almost exclusively among patients with limited SSc rather than diffuse SSc, and also develops in a minority of patients with Sjögren's syndrome (Pope and Thompson 1999). The first laboratory indication of PBC is usually an elevation of the alkaline phosphatase that occurs in the absence of serum transaminase increases. Antimitochondrial antibodies (AMA) are present in most but not all patients with SSc who have PBC. The early diagnosis of PBC is important, because ursodiol can delay or prevent the development of cirrhosis (Rigamonti et al. 2006).

10.1.4 Skin Disease

Myth: Patients with SSc have a difficult time keeping their nails clean.

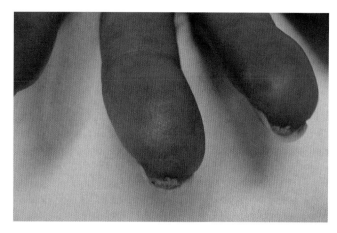

Fig. 10.9 Pterygium inversum unguis. This finding gives the fingernails of patients with SSc an "unclean" appearance (Courtesy of Dr. Fredrick Wigley)

Reality: Patients with SSc often develop a condition known as pterygium inversum unguis (Fig. 10.9), a distal extension of the hyponychial (subungual) tissue that is anchored to the undersurface of the nail.

Myth: Telangiectasias are uncommon in diffuse SSc.

Reality: In the 1970s, the term "CREST syndrome" was used to describe patients with SSc who had most or all the following constellation of symptoms: C – calcinosis, R – Raynaud phenomenon, E – esophageal dysmotility, S – sclerodactyly, and T – telangiectasias. CREST patients were considered to have skin thickening restricted to their distal extremities and occasionally their faces, and distinctions were drawn between this disease subset and patients with diffuse SSc. Although differences clearly exist between patients who fit the CREST phenotype and those with diffuse SSc, it has been noted that many patients with diffuse SSc demonstrate many or all of the features of CREST, particularly later in the course of their illness when diffuse skin changes have softened (Furst et al. 1984). For this reason, the term CREST syndrome has been replaced by the preferred "limited cutaneous involvement."

Pearl: The rate of skin thickness progression is a useful clinical tool.

Comment: A rapid rate of skin thickness progression in diffuse SSc identifies patients at increased risk for new major internal organ involvement and death. When calculated either at the first visit from onset of skin thickening or between the second and third visits using the modified Rodnan skin score, a rapid rate is associated with an increased frequency and earlier appearance of interstitial lung disease, cardiac dysfunction, renal involvement, and higher mortality (Perera et al. 2007; Shand et al. 2007).

Myth: Skin of normal thickness in SSc is unaffected.

Reality: Although the clinical assessment of skin thickness at different anatomical sites is helpful in classifying SSc patients, the Rodnan skin score is in reality a fairly blunt instrument. Many patients with limited cutaneous involvement have widespread cutaneous hyper- and hypopigmentation, signifying that melanocytes are either over- or understimulated in areas without apparent skin thickening. In immunohistochemical studies of clinically involved and uninvolved skin in diffuse SSc, both contained markers of endothelial and fibroblastic activation compared with controls (Claman et al. 1991). Thus, it is likely that all skin is affected by the disease process, even if it appears to be normal clinically by palpation (Pope et al. 1996).

Pearl: After 2–5 years, skin tightening in diffuse SSc often regresses somewhat but internal organs can continue to worsen.

Comment: In patients with diffuse SSc who were participants in a clinical trial, the mean skin score remained stable for the first 12 months but decreased significantly at both 24 and 36 months. Among patients with limited SSc, however, the skin score did not change significantly over 3 years.

Although the involved skin in diffuse SSc often displays softening by 5 years of disease duration, progression of the disease in internal organs (e.g., the lung) can progress even as the skin softens over time. The rapid progression of skin disease in diffuse SSc is an ominous sign. However, improvement in the skin score does not equate to a lack of disease progression within internal organs (Clements et al. 1993; Perera et al. 2007; Steen and Medsger 2001).

Myth: Scleroderma skin often normalizes over time.

Reality: Skin thickness measured by the modified Rodnan method at a given anatomic site, e.g., forearm, can regress over time from 2+ (moderate thickening) to 0 (no thickening). However, skin biopsies from later phases of the disease do not show normal skin but rather thinning (atrophy) of the dermis and "tethering," i.e., increased attachment of the dermis to the underlying subcutaneous tissue (Clements et al. 2004).

Pearl: Skin thickening that precedes RP predicts subsequent events.

Comment: RP is the first clinical manifestation in more than half of all SSc patients. However, skin thickening precedes RP in a minority of SSc patients (25%), where such individuals were at higher risk of developing diffuse SSc (79 vs. 45%; p = 0.0001) and renal crisis (9 vs. 3%, p = 0.0001) compared with those whose RP came before thickening of the skin (Medsger 2009).

10.1.5 Gastrointestinal Involvement

Pearl: All patients with SSc should be treated with therapy designed to suppress acid production by the stomach.

Comment: Severe esophageal disease may be subclinical in patients with SSc. Consequently, empiric treatment with a proton pump inhibitor should be employed in all patients with SSc because such therapy can prevent stricture formation, aspiration pneumonitis, and Barrett's esophagus (Ebert 2006).

Pearl: SSc patients are prone to a host of dental problems.

Comment: Oral hygiene is compromised in SSc for several reasons. The frequent findings of a small oral aperture from mouth furrowing and decreased hand function conspire to make holding a toothbrush a challenge. Xerostomia caused by coexistent Sjögren's syndrome or fibrosis of the salivary glands, acid reflux (GERD) (Fig. 10.10), and the use of medications that alter oral hygiene unfavorably (e.g., nonsteroidal antiinflammatory drugs or glucocorticoids) also complicate dental care. SSc patients should therefore have frequent, regular visits to the dentist.

Myth: Gastric antral vascular ectasia is a rare complication of SSc.

Reality: More than 90% of SSc patients have gastrointestinal dysfunction, with problems that range in severity and include dysphagia, reflux, small bowel overgrowth, gastroparesis, rectal incontinence, pseudodiverticuli, and a dilated esophagus (Fig. 10.11) (Marie 1996). Gastric antral vascular ectasia (GAVE, watermelon stomach) (Fig. 10.12) is a common finding on endoscopy in patients with early diffuse SSc. GAVE is an infrequent finding in the non-SSc population and some gastroenterologists are unfamiliar with this entity, particularly in its early or developing phase. The most common features of this disorder relate to the gradual

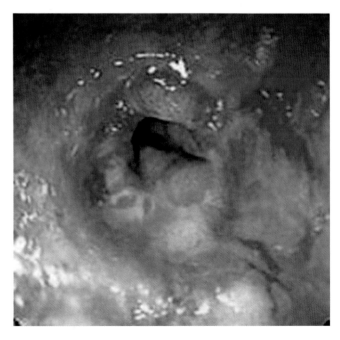

Fig. 10.10 Gastroesophageal reflux disease (GERD) with esophagitis near the lower esophageal sphincter in a patient with scleroderma

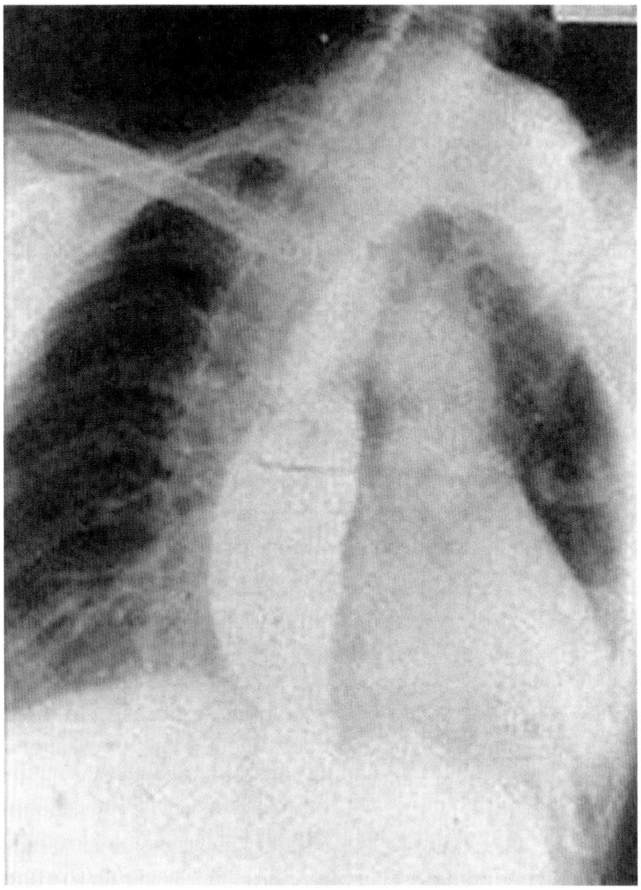

Fig. 10.11 Dilated esophagus in scleroderma, as seen on a barium swallow

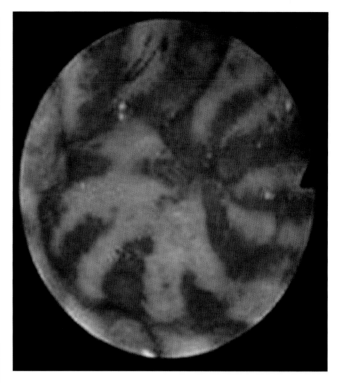

Fig. 10.12 Gastric antral vascular ectasia ("watermelon stomach") in a patient with scleroderma

development of iron deficiency anemia. Upper endoscopy may not show an obvious bleeding site as the ectatic blood vessels ooze blood on an intermittent basis. Therapy for GAVE includes laser coagulation. More than one session may be required (Calamia et al. 2000; Shibukawa et al. 2007).

Pearl: Abdominal bloating, early satiety, gas, and constipation that alternates with intermittent diarrhea might be related to small bowel overgrowth.

Comment: Patients can be diagnosed with small bowel overgrowth by the history alone. No additional investigations such as a hydrogen breath test are necessary in most cases. This underdiagnosed problem can have a substantial impact on patients' quality of life and should be treated if symptomatic. Empiric courses of therapy are reasonable to undertake without diagnostic testing if the history is sufficiently compelling. Intermittent antibiotics can be highly effective and may need to be cycled. The most commonly used antibiotics are amoxicillin, ciprofloxacin, tetracycline, erythromycin, and metronidazole. Promotility agents such as metaclopromide, domperidone, and erythromycin can also be helpful.

Pearl: Malnutrition may occur in SSc.

Comment: Malnutrition should be suspected if there is marked weight loss or a low serum albumin. If severe dysphagia necessitates consideration of tube feeding, a jejunal tube is preferable to a gastric tube because of the high likelihood of significant gastroesophageal reflux. Total parenteral nutrition may be needed in some patients. Features associated with SSc malnutrition are weight loss, anorexia, diarrhea, history of bloating, a low serum albumin level, and a distended abdomen on physical examination.

Pearl: Proton pump inhibitors should be taken before a meal in patients with severe gastroesophageal reflux disease (GERD).

Comment: Proton pump inhibitors (PPIs) work better on an empty stomach. The PPI dose may need to be doubled or increased even further beyond approved doses. Raising the head of the bed at night, no food after supper time, and the addition of other prokinetic agents may help to reduce GERD. Individual triggers of GERD such as alcohol, caffeine, chocolate, and mint should be avoided if they worsen symptoms.

10.1.6 Interstitial Lung Disease

Pearl: Most declines in patients' forced vital capacity (FVC) occur during the first 4–6 years after the onset of symptoms attributable to SSc.

Comment: Steen et al. assessed 890 patients with SSc, 13% of whom (n = 116) developed severe restrictive lung disease with an FVC ≤ 50% predicted (Steen et al. 1994). Among those 116 patients, 55 (48%) with severe restrictive disease had two sets of pulmonary function tests during the first 5 years after diagnosis. The FVC% predicted declined by 32% per year in the first 2 years of illness, 12% in years 2–4, and only 3% during years 4–6 of disease. These observational data suggest that only a minority of SSc patients develop severe restrictive disease and that the greatest decline occurs in the first 4–6 years after onset of SSc symptoms.

Similar observational data from Greece also suggested that the 10% of patients who are destined to have major declines, most of the change occurs early in disease (Plastiras et al. 2006).

Pearl: The interstitial lung disease in SSc usually occurs at the bases.

Comment: Interstitial lung disease or pulmonary fibrosis in SSc is found primarily in the lung bases bilaterally, but the process can extend beyond this area to involve all regions of the lungs. In patients with atypical patterns of pulmonary disease, aspiration caused by incompetence of the lower esophageal sphincter should be considered.

Myth: Interstitial lung disease does not occur in patients with limited SSc.

Reality: The community perception of interstitial lung disease in SSc is that this complication occurs almost exclusively in patients with diffuse cutaneous SSc. A recent example of how this bias could influence the care of SSc patients with interstitial lung disease was a randomized controlled trial that compared bosentan therapy to placebo in interstitial lung disease: patients with limited SSc were excluded from that study. Yet approximately 40% of SSc patients who have an FVC that is less than 75% of predicted – the definition of interstitial lung disease in some studies – have limited SSc (Steen et al. 1994).

In the Scleroderma Lung Study (Tashkin et al. 2006), approximately 40% of the 158 patients enrolled had limited SSc. The lung physiology of these patients was not different from that of patients with diffuse SSc at baseline. Moreover, the limited SSc subset actually had more extensive fibrotic changes at baseline, as assessed by high-resolution computed tomograms of the chest. Most importantly, the course of interstitial lung disease in the two patient subsets did not differ over 24 months.

Myth: Data from bronchoalveolar lavage in patients with SSc predict the response of interstitial lung disease to treatment.

Reality: The finding of increased neutrophils or eosinophils in bronchoalveolar lavage (BAL) fluid has been considered to be predictive of a deteriorating course in lung physiology in patients with SSc (White et al. 2000; Silver et al. 1990; Behr et al. 1996; Witt et al. 1999). However, more recent reports suggest that the percentage of neutrophils and eosinophils in BAL fluid does not predict FVC declines (Goh et al. 2007; Strange et al. 2008). Goh et al. reported their analysis of data drawn from a prospective longitudinal study. Strange et al. analyzed findings from the Scleroderma Lung Study. In that latter analysis, the presence of an abnormal BAL did not add to the information obtained from pulmonary function tests and high-resolution computed tomography of the chest (Fig. 10.13) in the prediction of treatment response.

Myth: The use of glucocorticoids in interstitial lung disease associated with SSc has a sound scientific basis.

Reality: The American Thoracic Society and European Respiratory Society issued an International Consensus Statement that addressed the use of glucocorticoids in interstitial lung disease in 2000 (American Thoracic Society 2000). To quote the statement: "Despite their ubiquitous use, no prospective, randomized, double-blind, placebo-controlled trial has evaluated the efficacy of glucocorticoids in the treatment of idiopathic pulmonary fibrosis. In three trials that compared glucocorticoids with no treatment, none of the untreated patients with IPF improved." Thus, as in

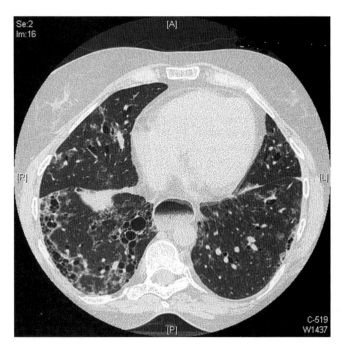

Fig. 10.13 Computed tomographic scan in scleroderma, showing interstitial lung disease (ILD). The ILD in SSc typically involves the bases but can be widespread. If pulmonary changes spare the bases, one should think of aspiration or other reasons. This high-resolution computed tomography scan is from a woman with "scleroderma lung," characterized by marked honeycombing. She has only 30% lung capacity and is on oxygen. The imaging study shows scarring, traction fibrosis, and honeycombing

many inflammatory conditions associated with autoimmunity, the benefit of treatment with immunosuppression is inferred from the outcomes of patients whose natural history unfolds without an intervention.

A more recent article stated: "Treatment of IPF has not been shown to influence outcomes." Therapeutic options are limited and usually ineffectual. Glucocorticoids and immunosuppressive or cytotoxic agents have been used to treat idiopathic pulmonary fibrosis and usual interstitial pneumonitis, but benefit has not been established" (Lynch et al. 2006). The International Consensus Statement of the American Thoracic Society and European Respiratory Society concluded that "no data exist that adequately document that any of the current treatment approaches improves survival or the quality of life for patients with IPF. Nonetheless, given the poor prognosis associated with idiopathic pulmonary fibrosis/usual interstitial pneumonitis, physicians may offer treatment in patients with severe or progressive disease."

In this context, the International Consensus Statement advocated an empirical trial of either azathioprine or cyclophosphamide alone or combined with low-dose glucocorticoids. These recommendations reflect expert opinion, but have not been validated. In addition, the recommendations apply to interstitial lung disease in general rather than to the specific entity of SSc. Thus, the use of glucocorticoids in SSc is still based on "eminence" rather than "evidence." In the Scleroderma Lung Study, glucocorticoid use was limited to a maximum prednisone dose of 10 mg/day (Tashkin et al. 2006).

In summary, there is no firm scientific evidence that glucocorticoids have a place in the treatment of interstitial lung disease, especially in the interstitial lung disease associated with SSc.

Pearl: Cyclophosphamide has a modest effect on forced vital capacity, function, and dyspnea in interstitial lung disease associated with SSc.

Comment: Two randomized, double-blind, placebo-controlled trials of cyclophosphamide have shown modest but real efficacy in the treatment of SSc-related interstitial lung disease. One study compared oral cyclophosphamide (2 mg/kg, rounded to the nearest 25 mg) against placebo for 1 year, followed by a 1 year period of untreated observation (Tashkin et al. 2006). Among the 158 patients, 79 were assigned to cyclophosphamide and 79 to placebo. At the end of the year of treatment, the mean FVC among the cyclophosphamide-treated patients was only about 3% higher than that of the placebo-treated patients (p = 0.03). When stratified into patients whose baseline FVCs were less than 70% of predicted, the differences at 1 year were somewhat greater (6.8%).

It is worth noting that baseline fibrosis as demonstrated by high-resolution computed tomography was associated with a better response to cyclophosphamide than was the finding of a "ground glass" appearance or "active alveolitis" on BAL. In addition, physical function, vitality, and dyspnea all improved in a clinically meaningful ways among the cyclophosphamide-treated patients compared with the placebo group, as did skin findings.

The other study examined 6 months of pulse intravenous cyclophosphamide (600 mg per meters-squared) followed by azathioprine (2.5 mg/kg/day, maximum 200 mg/day) for 6 months versus placebo cyclophosphamide followed by placebo azathioprine (Hoyles et al. 2006). This study was substantially smaller than the Scleroderma Lung Study, with a total of only 46 patients. The cyclophosphamide group had a 4% improvement in FVC when compared with the placebo group. Although the difference was not statistically significant – $p = 0.08$ – the results were consistent with those of the larger study.

One understandable criticism of these studies is that the improvement in FVC was small, albeit statistically significant. However, given the clinically important differences in patient-derived measures such as dyspnea and function, cyclophosphamide appears to have a modest but real effect in the interstitial lung disease associated with SSc. There remains ample room for improvement.

Pearl: One year of oral cyclophosphamide has effects that last long after the medication has been discontinued.

Comment: The perception is that cyclophosphamide has very dangerous long-term consequences and that it is therefore prudent to stop the medication after 6 months to a year. So what happened in the second year of the Scleroderma Lung Trial, when patients were followed on no medications after stopping cyclophosphamide? In fact, the FVC in the group of patients treated previously with cyclophosphamide continued to improve for 6 months, while the FVC in the placebo treated group remained stable or decreased slightly. By 18 months the differences in FVC between the two treatment groups actually increased to about 6.8% (Tashkin et al. 2007). Thereafter, the FVC in the cyclophosphamide group declined rapidly so that by 24 months, the two treatment groups were equivalent by this measure. Other outcomes tended to remain stable after the year of cyclophosphamide therapy so that whatever difference occurred at 12 months remained that way for 18 and even 24 months, including dyspnea scores, function, and skin score.

Pearl: Cyclophosphamide therapy is well-tolerated during 1 year of treatment.

Comment: When cyclophosphamide is used in large doses to treat cancer, there are numerous and important toxicities, ranging from severe stomatitis through hair loss to bone marrow suppression, bleeding, infection, and possible cancer. The toxicities of relatively low-dose cyclophosphamide regimens, as used in the oral cyclophosphamide study by Tashkin et al. and Hoyles et al. are significantly lower over the short term (Tashkin et al. 2006; Hoyles et al. 2006).

The adverse effects reported in the Scleroderma Lung Trial were strikingly fewer than those observed in the Wegener's Granulomatosis Etanercept Trial (WGET Research Group 2005), a study of comparable size in which the majority of patients received oral cyclophosphamide in addition to the investigational treatment or placebo (WGET Research Group 2002). The major difference in the experience of these two clinical trials may be that the Scleroderma Lung Trial used far lower doses of glucocorticoids.

Pearl: In a patient with SSc-interstitial lung disease, GERD may be a contributing factor to the signs and symptoms of lung involvement.

Comment: GERD affects approximately 90% of patients with SSc. Previous studies have shown an association between GERD and SSc-related interstitial lung disease (Marie et al. 2001; Lock et al. 1997). GERD has been implicated as one of inciting factors for SSc-related interstitial lung disease due to repeated microaspirations of acid gastric contents in the lungs. In a recent study, severity of esophageal manometric changes was associated with higher prevalence of interstitial lung disease (57% with severe involvement versus 18% without involvement) on high-resolution computed tomography (Marie et al. 2001). At 2-year follow-up, patients with severe esophageal motor impairment had a greater decline in DLCO (−16% of the predicted value) when compared with those without any manometric changes (+1% predicted). However, other authors have failed to show this association. In other respiratory disorders (e.g., asthma), treatment of GERD improves symptoms and PFT parameters.

In summary, patients with SSc and early interstitial lung disease should be managed aggressively with antireflux measures (e.g., elevating the head of the bed, not eating for several hours before bedtime), proton-pump inhibitors, antacids, and prokinetic therapy.

Pearl: Certain baseline clinical, physiological, and radiological variables inform the treatment of SSc-related interstitial lung disease.

Comment: The performance of pulmonary function tests with DLCO measurement every 6–12 months for the first 5 years after the onset of symptoms or signs attributable to SSc is a reasonable approach to longitudinal management. Which SSc patients should be offered treatment for interstitial lung disease? Several categories of patients are good candidates for treatment:

- Patients whose FVC has declined at least 7% within 6 months of the last measurement.
- Patients whose FVC is less than 70% predicted at the time of presentation may also benefit from therapy.

- Patients who have at least moderate fibrosis on baseline high-resolution computed tomography scans of the chest. "Moderate" had been defined variably across studies, e.g., more than 20% lung involvement in one study and at least 25% of six lobes in another.

Debatable points within clinical practice now are the wisdom of treating patients who have had more than 6 years of SSc and the appropriateness of treating patients who have no dyspnea.

Myth: Patients with SSc and significant interstitial lung disease always have Velcro crackles.

Reality: The physical and radiological examination is not always concordant. Most but not all patients with significant interstitial lung disease in SSc have crackles on auscultation. The breath sounds may be quiet or even normal in patients with interstitial lung disease. Thus, pulmonary function tests and chest radiographs should be ordered in patients with SSc who complain of dyspnea.

10.1.7 Pulmonary Arterial Hypertension

Myth: Echocardiography can diagnose PAH in SSc.

Reality: Although following Doppler echocardiograms regularly to estimate the pulmonary artery pressure using the tricuspid regurgitant jet, right heart catheterization is essential to confirm the diagnosis and exclude other pathological entities (Arcasoy 2003). Echocardiograms give both false-negative and (more likely) false-positive results.

Myth: PAH occurs late in SSc.

Reality: PAH often occurs among limited SSc patients who are older, i.e., they have had longstanding disease or disease that was subclinical for years before the diagnosis was made. In contrast, among patients with diffuse, SSc, PAH can occur at any age or duration of disease. Thus, regular monitoring for PAH by routine echocardiography is important (Al-Dhaher et al. 2008).

Pearl: An FVC%/DLCO% ratio of greater than 1.8 is a helpful predictor for patients at increased risk for PAH, regardless of the mechanism of PAH.

Comment: A falling DLCO occurs well in advance of PAH in some patients. PAH causes impaired gas exchange, which is reflected by low DLCO measurements. Isolated PAH in SSc is strongly associated with a marked increase in the ratio of the percentage predicted FVC to the percentage predicted DLCO, i.e., the FVC%/DLCO% ratio (Fig. 10.14). In patients with classic PAH related to SSc, interstitial lung disease is minimal but impaired gas exchange secondary to pulmonary

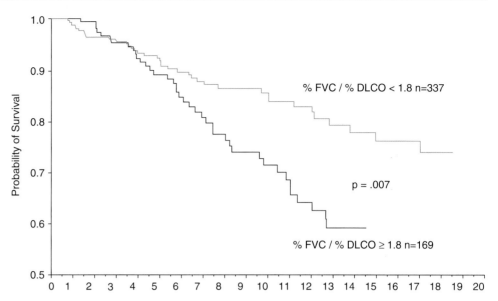

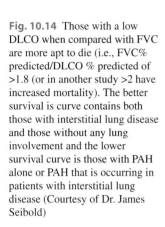

Fig. 10.14 Those with a low DLCO when compared with FVC are more apt to die (i.e., FVC% predicted/DLCO % predicted of >1.8 (or in another study >2 have increased mortality). The better survival is curve contains both those with interstitial lung disease and those without any lung involvement and the lower survival curve is those with PAH alone or PAH that is occurring in patients with interstitial lung disease (Courtesy of Dr. James Seibold)

vascular injury is the rule. The significant intimal proliferation of the pulmonary vessels leads to a marked decrease in the DLCO. This typically develops over many years and leads to a high FVC%/DLCO% ratio (Steen 2003a).

A high FVC%/DLCO% ratio has also been observed in patients who have a low FVC because of interstitial lung disease. A disproportionately low DLCO in this setting implies injury to both the pulmonary vasculature as well as to the alveolar diffusing surface. Thus, the FVC%/DLCO% ratio is high in this setting. Many of these patients have only moderate fibrosis and have not been hypoxic, so their pulmonary hypertension is more likely to be vascular than to be related to parenchymal lung disease. However, even the patients with severe fibrosis, hypoxia, and secondary pulmonary hypertension can have a severe decrease in the DLCO and a high ratio (Steen et al. 2007).

Myth: A reduced 6 min walk is reflective of pulmonary hypertension in SSc.

Reality: The 6 min walk test (6MWT) is a standardized measure of submaximal exercise capacity that has served as the primary measure of outcome in studies of PAH. The 6MWT has never been validated fully in SSc. However, a variety of data suggest that many nonpulmonary aspects of SSc contribute affect the 6MWT, thereby blunting the ability of the 6MWT to discriminate between pulmonary issues and other SSc-associated problems as a cause of an abnormal 6MWT.

Many factors can influence the distance walked: sources of variability in test conduct, training effect, technician experience, subject encouragement, medication, supplemental oxygen, other activities on day of testing, deconditioning, and the effect of musculoskeletal conditions. Investigators have studied exercise capacity in SSc patients with and without pulmonary involvement. In one study, 18

women with SSc were studied by bicycle ergometer (Morelli et al. 2000). The results indicated a marked limitation of exercise performance among SSc patients when compared with normal controls. Patients with baseline pulmonary hypertension had an even further decrease in exercise performance compared with SSc patients who did not have elevations in their baseline pulmonary pressures. More recently, patients with SSc judged to be free of both cardiac and pulmonary disease were confirmed to have reduced VO_2 peak but also a reduced metabolic equivalent at VO_2 peak (De Oliviera et al. 2007). Although not directly measured, this infers that muscle perfusion is an unrecognized influence on exercise capacity in SSc.

The 6MWT may be helpful to measure change in short term intervention for a specific problem (i.e., pulmonary fibrosis, pulmonary hypertension, myopathy), but further validation studies need to be done in SSc.

Myth: SSc patients with significant PAH will report dyspnea.

Reality: SSc patients adapt often to PAH, as this condition is sometimes slow in onset. They complain of dyspnea less often than do patients with idiopathic PAH. Questions such as "Has your breathing changed over the last year?" might be more useful than "Are you short of breath?" Other useful queries are "Can you carry in the groceries from the car?"; "If not, what stops you (Pain? Poor hand function? Dyspnea?)"; "How many flights can you climb?"; and "Does breathing worsen if you go outside in the cold?" (Mathai et al. 2009).

Myth: All patients with elevated pulmonary artery pressures demonstrated by echocardiography will progress to PAH.

Reality: Echocardiography estimates the pulmonary arterial pressure and often overestimates it. In addition, upon follow-up of patients with an elevated pulmonary artery systolic pressure >35 mmHg on echocardiogram, 65% did not progress over the next 3 years. In addition, most studies of SSc patients show that 25% have echocardiograms that suggest an elevated pulmonary artery pressure, but only 10–15% have PAH that is class III or greater PAH (Steen 2005; Arcasoy 2003; Pope 2005a).

Myth: A normal echocardiogram in SSc excludes PAH.

Reality: Although there are more false-positive echocardiograms in the estimation of pulmonary artery pressure than false-negative ones, there are some patients in whom an estimate of the pulmonary artery pressure cannot be obtained because no tricuspid regurgitation is evident. Accurate echocardiographic measurements are operator-dependent and can vary according to the precise placement of the probe. Thus, if PAH is suspected but the echocardiogram does not appear to support this diagnosis, other procedures need to be considered: right heart catheterization; a magnetic resonance imaging study of the heart, or exercise echocardiography. In addition, one should also consider the possibility that a falling PA pressure in a patient with severe PAH may indicate a failing right ventricle (Arcasoy 2003).

Pearl: A pericardial effusion in SSc is often related to PAH.

Comment: Obstruction of drainage of the heart can cause a pericardial effusion when the right-sided heart pressures are high, such as in PAH. The presence of a moderate to large pericardial effusion in SSc is usually a poor prognostic sign (Thompson and Pope 1998).

10.1.8 Cardiac Disease

Pearl: Treat congestive heart failure from a cardiomyopathy in SSc the same way you would treat other cardiomyopathies.

Comment: Cardiac involvement in SSc is a major cause of death, but it can be subtle and is often under-recognized. Diastolic dysfunction is particularly common in SSc. The treatments for congestive heart failure in SSc are the same as those employed for this condition in other settings: angiotensin converting enzyme (ACE) inhibitors, diuretics, and beta blockers. Attention to traditional cardiac risk factors such as hypertension, smoking, and hyperlipidemia is also important. Patients with SSc are not immune to atherosclerosis or ischemic cardiomyopathy (Steen 2000).

10.1.9 Scleroderma Renal Crisis

Myth: Scleroderma renal crisis occurs only in patients with diffuse SSc.

Reality: Scleroderma renal crisis usually occurs in patients with diffuse SSc and is almost never seen in patients who are anticentromere antibody positive. However, scleroderma renal crisis may emerge at a time when the full disease phenotype of the patient is not yet clear and diffuse cutaneous disease is absent. Some who develop scleroderma renal crisis have very early disease with less than a year of symptoms, such as carpal tunnel syndrome, arthritis, fatigue, Raynaud's phenomenon, and swollen fingers or legs, and may have been considered to have undifferentiated connective tissue disease (Steen 2003b). In short, the full disease phenotype may not have emerged at the time scleroderma renal crisis strikes.

Patients with the highest risk for renal crisis are those with an anti-RNA polymerase III antibody (Steen 2005). These patients often do not have Raynaud's phenomenon at the onset of their disease and the ANA may be negative if the assay is performed by ELISA, since RNA polymerase III is not identified by the ELISA ANA assay. In addition, since scleroderma renal crisis occurs (or recurs) late in the illness in almost 20% of patients, diffuse cutaneous skin changes may have remitted. Such patients have a history of severe skin disease and are likely to have significant hand contractures (Fig. 10.15).

Pearl: Scleroderma renal crisis may be the first manifestation of SSc.

Comment: In some patients, nonspecific symptoms and signs such as puffy fingers (Fig. 10.16), Raynaud's phenomenon, and GERD had not yet been recognized as manifestations of SSc when scleroderma renal crisis develops (Steen 2003b). Keen diagnostic acumen and a high degree of suspicion are required to make the diagnosis in this setting.

Myth: Treatment with an ACE inhibitor prevents scleroderma renal crisis.

Reality: ACE inhibitors have changed patient outcomes in scleroderma renal crisis dramatically (Steen 2003b). Scleroderma renal crisis is driven by a rennin-mediated hypertension. Thus, it was anticipated prophylaxis with ACE inhibitors would prevent renal crisis. Unfortunately, this is not the case. Two reviews of patients with renal crisis both demonstrated that patients who received ACE-inhibitors prior to the onset of scleroderma renal crisis actually had worse outcomes when compared with those without previous ACE inhibitor use (Penn et al. 2007; Teixeira et al. 2007).

One explanation for this is that the dose of ACE inhibitors used in patients who are not hypertensive is insufficient to control the excessive outpouring of rennin that occurs acutely from the juxtaglomerular apparatus in scleroderma renal crisis. The acute response may be blunted in such patients, but instead they develop a more chronic, less reversible process. The best outcomes occurred in patients with the highest

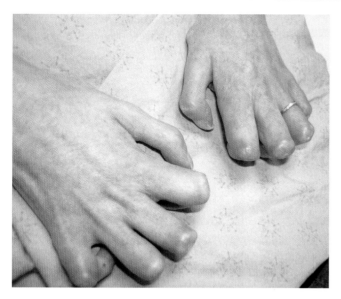

Fig. 10.15 Hand contractures in severe, long-standing diffuse systemic sclerosis. This patient's disease had its onset in childhood

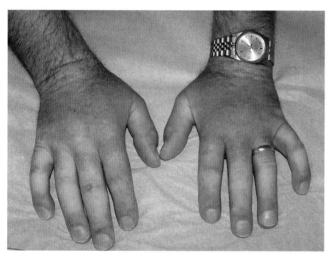

Fig. 10.16 A man with early diffuse systemic sclerosis, demonstrating erythema and puffiness of the hands. The patient also had significant cutaneous pruritus

blood pressure levels but the lowest serum creatinine measurements. These variables may be a function of the acuity of the process.

In summary, although ACE inhibitors can be lifesaving drugs in patients with scleroderma renal crisis, one cannot assume that having the patient on such a medication as prophylaxis or to treat baseline hypertension will prevent the development of this potentially lethal disease complication. Patients with diffuse SSc should be instructed to take their blood pressures regularly and report increases to their doctors.

Myth: Scleroderma renal crisis always presents with hypertension.

Reality: Normotensive cases have been described. A high index of suspicion is required if a decline in renal function is observed in a patient with SSc (Teixeira et al. 2007). SRC is defined as new onset hypertension (occurs in >90%), elevated creatinine (50% at onset of diagnosis of SRC) and microangiopathic hemolytic anemia (50%).

Myth: Once SSc patients go on dialysis, the renal "ballgame" is over.

Reality: ACE inhibition should be continued even in patients who require dialysis because of scleroderma renal crisis. A significant number of such patients are eventually able to discontinue dialysis, even after undergoing renal replacement therapy for many months.

Pearl: If a patient has scleroderma renal crisis, use an ACE inhibitor and ADD any other antihypertensive agent required to control the blood pressure as rapidly as possible.

Comment: Before the introduction of ACE inhibitors, scleroderma renal crisis was the leading cause of death among patients with diffuse SSc (Steen and Medsger 2001, 2003). When prescribing ACE inhibitors in scleroderma renal crisis, it is helpful to use captopril because of its three-times-a-day dosing. However, likely any ACE inhibitor can be used and the dose can and should be increased rapidly to the maximal dose or until adequate blood pressure control is achieved. The ACE inhibitor should never be stopped, even in the face of a rising serum creatinine.

Other antihypertensive can also be added if necessary, but maximizing the ACE inhibitor dose is the chief priority.

Myth: Angiotensin II inhibitors are also useful in the treatment of scleroderma renal crisis.

Reality: Angiotensin II inhibitors do not lead to consistent reductions of bradykinins, in contrast to ACE inhibitors. This is believed to be the reason that angiotensin II inhibitors are less effective in the treatment of scleroderma renal crisis (Steen 2000; Steen and Medsger 2001; Rhew and Barr 2004).

Myth: Low-dose glucocorticoids do not increase the risk of scleroderma renal crisis.

Reality: Glucocorticoids at high dose do appear to increase the risk of scleroderma renal crisis and some data indicated that even low doses of prednisone (e.g., >10 mg/day) increase the risk of scleroderma renal crisis. For this reason, it is wise to avoid the use of glucocorticoids in patients with early diffuse SSc unless an absolute indication for these medications is present (Steen and Medsger 2001).

10.1.10 Musculoskeletal Manifestations

Myth: SSc associated arthritis is not erosive.

Fig. 10.17 This SSc patient has diffuse SSc, with inflammatory arthritis. She had evidence of ankylosis and erosive arthritis at the wrists and a pencil and cup type deformity of the R second MCP. There is distal tuft resorption at many fingertips and a Z deformity (or Boutinneire) at the thumbs. She has periarticular osteopenia. Ulnar styloids have eroded away and architecture of the proximal carpel bones is destroyed

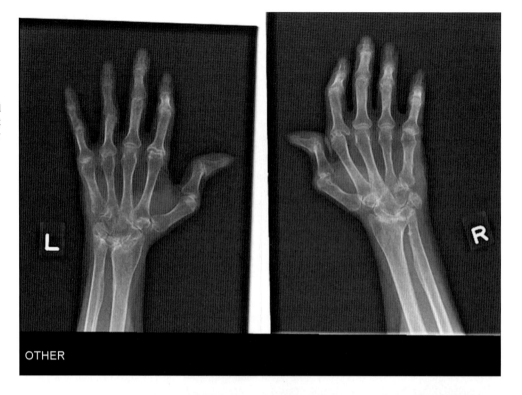

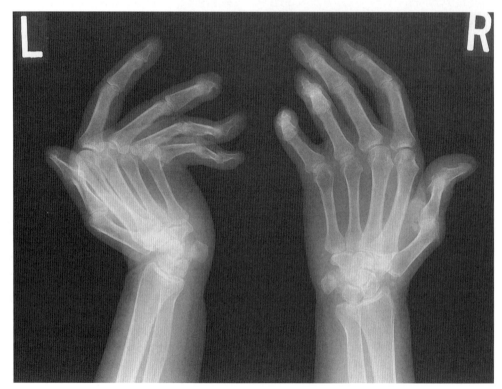

Fig. 10.18 This left-hand dominant SSc patient has subluxed MCPs on dominant hand with MCP inflammatory arthritis. Note loss of distal finger pulp, acro-osteolysis on L third distal phalanx and calcinosis such as distal tip of L thumb

Reality: The arthritis of SSc can be erosive and can mimic a destructive seronegative arthritis (Figs. 10.17 and 10.18) (Pope 2003b, 2005b). However, the more common scenario is that patients with early-onset diffuse SSc have puffy hands and pain that is difficult to localize to joints and refractory to treatment. This discomfort generally improves over several months as other disease features become manifest.

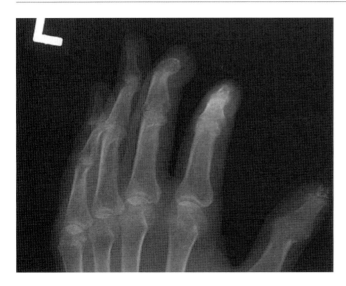

Fig. 10.19 This radiograph shows thumb calcinosis distally. The third distal phalanx is missing and the dip is ankylosed on that finger. In addition the fifth DIP and first IP joints are beginning to ankylose

Pearl: Calcinosis on hand radiographs can be a tip-off to the presence of SSc.

Comment: Figure 10.19 shows distal calcinosis of the thumb. The third distal phalanx is missing and the distal interphalangeal (DIP) joint on that finger is ankylosed. In addition, the fifth DIP and the first interphalangeal joint are beginning to undergo ankylosis.

Pearl: Palpable tendon friction rubs herald an evolution to diffuse SSc.

Comment: Tendon friction rubs result from fibrous tenosynovitis or bursitis and are detected frequently in early diffuse SSc. In patients whose skin thickening is limited at the time of examination, patients with one or more friction rubs have a greater risk of progression to diffuse skin thickening (36 vs. 13%, p = 0.0007) (Steen and Medsger 1997a). Tendon friction rubs are a marker for a poor prognosis and are associated with a increased mortality risk (Medsger 2009).

10.1.11 Peripheral Neuropathy in SSc

Pearl: Aside from unusual cases of compression neuropathies, nervous system involvement is not characteristic of SSc.

Comment: Carpal tunnel syndrome can develop in early SSC because of edema in the skin and subcutaneous tissues. Carpal tunnel syndrome and other compression neuropathies such as trigeminal nerve compression may occur in SSc because of fibrosis, but the latter is uncommon. Other overt

neuropathies such as the pure sensory neuropathy that sometimes occurs in Sjögren's syndrome or the mononeuritis multiplex of vasculitis are notable for their absence in SSc (Lori et al. 1996; Steen et al. 1994; Tashkin et al. 2006; Khanna et al. 2008).

References

Al-Dhaher FF, Pope JE, Ouimet JM. Determinants of morbidity and mortality of systemic sclerosis in Canada. Semin Arthritis Rheum. 2009 (in press)

American Thoracic Society Statement. Guidelines for the six-minute walk test. Am J Respir Care Med. 2002;166:111–7

Arcasoy SM. Echocardiographic assessment of pulmonary hypertension in patients with advanced lung disease. Am J Respir Crit Care Med. 2003;167:735–40

Arnett FC, Cho M, Chatterjee S, et al Familial occurrence frequencies and relative risks for systemic sclerosis (scleroderma) in three United States cohorts. Arthritis Rheum. 2001;44: 1359–62

Behr J, Vogelmeier C, Beinert T, et al Bronchoalveolar lavage for evaluation and management of scleroderma disease of the lung. Am J Respir Crit Care Med. 1996;154:400–6

Calamia KT, Scolapio JS, Viggiano TR. Endoscopic YAG laser treatment of watermelon stomach (gastric antral vascular ectasia) in patients with systemic sclerosis. Clin Exp Rheumatol. 2000; 18(5):605–8

Claman HN, Giorno RC, Seibold JR. Endothelial and fibroblastic activation in scleroderma. The myth of the "uninvolved skin". Arthritis Rheum. 1991;34:1495–501

Clements P, Lauchenbruch P, Furst D, Paulus H. The course of skin involvement in systemic sclerosis over three years in a trial of chlorambucil versus placebo. Arthritis Rheum. 1993;36:1575–9

Clements PJ, Medsger TA Jr, Feghali CA. Cutaneous involvement in systemic sclerosis. In: Clements PJ, Furst DE, editors. Chapter 7 Systemic sclerosis. 2nd ed. Philadelphia, PA: Lippincott Williams and Wilkins; 2004. p. 129–50

Cutolo M, Pizzorni C, Tuccio M, et al Nailfold videocapillaroscopic patterns and serum autoantibodies in systemic sclerosis. Rheumatology (Oxford) 2004;43(6):719–26

De Oliviera NC, dos Santos Sabbag LM, et al Reduced exercise capacity in systemic sclerosis patients without pulmonary involvement. Scand J Rheumatol. 2007;36:458–61

Ebert EC. Esophageal disease in scleroderma. J Clin Gastroenterol. 2006;40:769–75

Furst DE, Saab M, Clements P. Clinical and serological comparison of 17 PSS and 17 CREST syndrome patients for sex, age and matched disease duration. Ann Rheum Dis. 1984;43:794–801

Goh NS, Veeraraghavan S, Desai SR, et al Bronchoalveolar lavage cellular profiles in patients with systemic sclerosis-associated interstitial lung disease are not predictive of disease progression. Arthritis Rheum. 2007;56:2005–12

Herrick A. Pathogenesis of Raynaud's phenomenon. Rheumatology (Oxford) 2005;44(5):587–96

Hirschl M, Hirschl K, Lenz, et al Transition from primary Raynaud's phenomenon to secondary Raynaud's phenomenon identified by diagnosis of an associated disease results of ten years of prospective surveillance. Arthritis Rheum. 2006;54(6):1974–81

Hoyles RK, Ellis RW, Wellsbury J, et al A multicenter, prospective, randomized, double-blind, placebo-controlled trial of corticosteroids and intravenous cyclophosphamide followed by oral azathioprine for the treatment of pulmonary fibrosis in scleroderma. Arthritis Rheum. 2006;54(12):3962–70

Hudson M, Thombs BD, Panopalis P, et al Quality of life in patients with systemic sclerosis compared to the general population and patients with other chronic conditions. J Rheumatol 2009;36:768–72

Khanna D. Health-related quality of life: A primer with a focus on scleroderma. Scleroderma Care Res. 2006;3(2):3–13

Khanna D, Furst DE, Clements PJ, et al Oral cyclophosphamide for active scleroderma lung disease: a decision analysis. Med Decis Making. 2008;28(6):926–37

Kuwana M, Kaburaki J, Okano Y, et al Clinical and prognostic associations based on serum antinuclear antibodies in Japanese patients with systemic sclerosis. Arthritis Rheum. 1994;37(1):75–83

Kuwana M, Feghali CA, Medsger TA Jr, Wright TM. Autoreactive T cells to topoisomerase I in monozygotic twins discordant for systemic sclerosis. Arthritis Rheum. 2001;44:1654–59

Lock G, Holstege A, Lang B, Scholmerich J. Gastrointestinal manifestations of progressive systemic sclerosis. Am J Gastroenterol. 1997;92(5):763–71

Lori S, Matucci-Cerinic M, Casale R, et al Peripheral nervous system involvement in systemic sclerosis: The median nerve as target structure. Clin Exp Rheumatol. 1996;14(6):601–05

Luggen M, Belhorn L, Evans T, Fitzgerald O, Spencer-Green G. The evolution of Raynaud's phenomenon: A longterm prospective study. J Rheumatol. 1995;22(12):2226–32

Lynch JP 3rd, Saggar R, Weigt SS, et al Usual interstitial pneumonia. Semin Respir Crit Care Med. 2006;27(6):634–51

Marie I. Gatrointestinal involvement in systemic sclerosis. Presse Med. 1996;35:1952–65

Marie I, Dominique S, Levesque H, et al Esophageal involvement and pulmonary manifestations in systemic sclerosis. Arthritis Rheum. 2001;45(4):346–54

Mathai SC, Hummers LK, Champion HC, et al Survival in pulmonary hypertension associated with the scleroderma spectrum of diseases: Impact of interstitial lung disease. Arthritis Rheum. 2009;60(2): 569–77

Medsger TA Jr. Unpublished data from the University of Pittsburgh Scleroderma Databank, 2009

Meli M, Gitzelmann G, Koppensteiner R, et al Predictive value of nailfold capillaroscopy in patients with Raynaud's phenomenon. Clin Rheumatol. 2006;25(2):153–8

Merkel PA, Herlyn K, Martin RW, et al Measuring disease activity and functional status in patients with scleroderma and Raynaud's phenomenon. Arthritis Rheum. 2002;46(9):2410–20

Morelli S, Ferrante L, Sgreccia A, et al Pulmonary hypertension is associated with impaired exercise capacity in patients with systemic sclerosis. Scand J Rheumatol. 2000;29:236–42

No authors: American Thoracic Society. Idiopathic pulmonary fibrosis: diagnosis and treatment. International consensus statement. American Thoracic Society (ATS), and the European Respiratory Society (ERS). Am J Respir Crit Care Med. 2000;161:646–64

Pavlov-Dolijanovic S, Damjanov N, Ostojic P, et al The prognostic value of nailfold capillary changes for the development of connective tissue disease in children and adolescents with primary Raynaud's phenomenon: A follow-up study of 250 patients. Pediatr Dermatol. 2006;23(5):437–42

Penn H, Howie AJ, Kingdon EJ, Bunn CC, Stratton RJ, Black CM, et al Scleroderma renal crisis: Patient characteristics and long-term outcomes. QJM 2007;100(8):485–94

Perera A, Fertig N, Lucas M, et al Clinical subsets, skin thickness progression rate, and serum antibody levels in systemic sclerosis patients with anti-topoisomerase I antibody. Arthritis Rheum. 2007; 56:2740–6

Plastiras SC, Karadimitrakis SP, Ziakas PD, et al Scleroderma lung: Initial forced vital capacity as predictor of pulmonary function decline. Arthritis Rheum. 2006;55(4):598–602

Poole JL, Williams CA, Bloch DA, et al Concurrent validity of the Health Assessment Questionnaire disability index in scleroderma. Arthritis Care Res. 1995;8:189–93

Pope J. Scleroderma Overlap Syndromes. Curr Opin Rheumatol. 2002; 14(6):704–10

Pope J. The diagnosis and treatment of Raynaud's phenomenon: A practical approach. Drugs 2007;67(4):517–25

Pope J. Raynaud's phenomenon (primary). Clin Evidence. 2003a;9: 1339–48

Pope J, Lee P, Baron M, Dunne J, Smith D, Docherty PS. The prevalence of elevated pulmonary arterial pressures as measured by echocardiography in a large multi-centre cohort of systemic sclerosis subjects in Canada. J Rheumatol. 2005a;32(7):1273–8

Pope JE. Musculoskeletal involvement in scleroderma. Rheum Dis Clin North Am Scleroderma 2003b May 29:391–408

Pope JE. Other manifestations of mixed connective tissue disease. Rheum Dis Clin North Am. 2005b;31(3):519–33

Pope JE, Thompson A. Antimitochondrial antibodies and their significance in diffuse and limited scleroderma. J Clin Rheumatol. 1999; 5(4):206–9

Pope JE, Shum D, Gottschalk R, et al Increased pigmentation in scleroderma. J Rheumatol. 1996;23:1912–16

Pope JE, Al-Bishri J, Al-Azem H, Ouimet JM. The temporal relationship of Raynaud's phenomenon and features of connective tissue disease in rheumatoid arthritis. J Rheumatol. 2008;35(12):2329–33

Rhew EY, Barr, WG. Scleroderma renal crisis: new insights and developments. Curr Rheumatol. Rep 2004;6(2):129–36

Rigamonti C, Shand LM, Feudjo M, et al Clinical features and prognosis of primary biliary cirrhosis associated with systemic sclerosis. Gut 2006;55(3):388–94

Sacks DG, Okano Y, Steen VD, et al Isolated pulmonary hypertension in systemic sclerosis with diffuse cutaneous involvement: Association with serum anti-U3RNP antibody. J Rheumatol. 1996; 23(4):639–42

Salliot C, Mouthon L, Ardizzone M, et al Sjögren's syndrome is associated with and not secondary to systemic sclerosis. Rheumatology (Oxford) 2007;46(2):321–6

Shand L, Lung M, Nihtyanova S, et al Relationship between change in skin score and disease outcome in diffuse cutaneous systemic sclerosis. Application of a latent linear trajectory model. Arthritis Rheum. 2007;56(7):2422–31

Shibukawa G, Irisawa A, Sakamoto N, et al Gastric antral vascular ectasia (GAVE) associated with systemic sclerosis: Relapse after endoscopic treatment by argon plasma coagulation. Intern Med. 2007;46 (6):279–83

Silver RM, Miller KS, Kinsella, et al Evaluation and management of scleroderma lung disease using bronchoalveolar lavage. Am J Med. 1990;88:470–6

Steen V. Epidemiology of systemic sclerosis. In: Hochberg MC, Silman AJ, Smolen JS, Weinblatt ME, Weisman MH, editors. Rheumatology. Vol. 2. Toronto: Elsevier(Mosby); 2003. p. 1455–61

Steen V. Advancements in diagnosis of pulmonary arterial hypertension in scleroderma. Arthritis Rheum. 2005a;52(12):3698–700

Steen V, Medsger T. Severe organ involvement in systemic sclerosis with diffuse scleroderma. Arthritis Rheum. 2000;43(11):2437–44

Steen VD. Scleroderma renal crisis. Rheum Dis Clin North Am. 2003;29(2):315–33

Steen VD. Autoantibodies in systemic sclerosis. Semin Arthritis Rheum. 2005b;35(1):35–42

Steen VD, Medsger TA Jr. The palpable tendon friction rub: An important physical examination finding in patients with systemic sclerosis. Arthritis Rheum. 1997a;40:1146–51

Steen VD, Medsger TA Jr. The value of the Health Assessment Questionnaire and special patient-generated scales to demonstrate change in systemic sclerosis patients over time. Arthritis Rheum. 1997b;40:1984–91

Steen VD, Medsger TA Jr. Long-term outcomes of scleroderma renal crisis. Ann Intern Med. 2000;133(8):600–3

Steen VD, Ziegler GL, Rodnan GP, Medsger TA Jr. Clinical and laboratory associations of anticentromere antibody in patients with progressive systemic sclerosis. Arthritis Rheum. 1984;27(2):125–31

Steen VD, Conte C, Owens GR, Medsger TA Jr. Severe restrictive lung disease in systemic sclerosis. Arthritis Rheum. 1994;37(9): 1283–9

Steen VD, Lucas M, Fertig N, Medsger TA Jr. Pulmonary arterial hypertension and severe pulmonary fibrosis in systemic sclerosis patients with a nucleolar antibody. J Rheumatol. 2007;34(11):2230–5

Strange C, Bolster MB, Roth MD, et al Bronchoalveolar lavage and response to cyclophosphamide in scleroderma interstitial lung disease. Am J Respir Crit Care Med. 2008;177:91–8

Tashkin DP, Elashoff R, Clements PJ, et al Cyclophosphamide versus placebo in scleroderma lung disease. N Engl J Med. 2006;354(25): 2655–66

Tashkin DP, Elashoff R, Clements PJ, et al Effects of 1-year treatment with cyclophosphamide on outcomes at 2 years in scleroderma lung disease. Am J Respir Crit Care Med. 2007;176(10): 1026–34

Teixeira L, Mahr A, Berezne A, et al Scleroderma renal crisis, still a life-threatening complication. Ann N Y Acad Sci. 2007;1108:249–58

Thompson A, Pope JE. A study of the frequency of pericardial and pleural effusions in scleroderma. Br J Rheumatol. 1998;37: 1320–3

Thompson AE, Shea B, Welch V, et al Calcium Channel Blockers for Raynaud's Phenomenon in Progressive Systemic Sclerosis. Arthritis Rheum. 2001;44(8):1841–7

Walker UA, Tyndall A, Czirjak L, et al Clinical risk assessment of organ manifestations in systemic sclerosis: A report from the EULAR scleroderma trials and research group database. Ann Rheum Dis. 2007;66(6):754–63

WGET Research Group. Design of the Wegener's Granulomatosis Etanercept Trial (WGET). Controlled Clinical Trials. 2002;23: 450–68

WGET Research Group. Etanercept plus standard therapy for Wegener's granulomatosis. N Engl J Med. 2005;352(4):351–61

White B, Moore WC, Wigley FM, et al Cyclophosphamide is associated with pulmonary function and survival benefit in patients with scleroderma and alveolitis. Ann Intern Med. 2000;132:947–54

Witt C, Borges AC, John M, et al Pulmonary involvement in diffuse cutaneous systemic sclerosis: Broncheoalveolar fluid granulocytosis predicts progression of fibrosing alveolitis. Ann Rheum Dis. 1999;58:635–40

Nephrogenic Systemic Fibrosis and Other Scleroderma Mimickers

Mark A. Perazella, Janet E. Pope, and Shawn E. Cowper

11.1 Overview of Nephrogenic Systemic Fibrosis and Other Scleroderma Mimickers

> Nephrogenic systemic fibrosis (NSF) is a systemic fibrosing disorder that mimics systemic sclerosis (scleroderma) and is strongly associated with exposure to gadolinium in the setting of renal insufficiency.

> In addition to the skin, fibrotic changes can occur in the lungs, diaphragm, muscles, heart, and esophagus.

> Both clinical and histopathological findings are required to confirm the diagnosis of NSF.

> No cases of NSF have been described in patients with normal kidney function or mild underlying renal disease.

> The more severe the kidney dysfunction and the higher the dose of gadolinium, the greater is the risk of NSF.

> NSF develops subacutely in most cases. It usually becomes apparent first in the lower extremities with symmetrical edema that may involve the upper extremities. The edema may be associated with erythema, blisters, and bullae. Upon resolution of the edema, the indurated skin is nonpitting and "unpinchable."

> NSF tends to spare the skin of the face, in contrast to both scleroderma and scleromyxedema.

> Yellow scleral plaques are described in many cases of NSF.

> The histopathological features of NSF are consistent with a dermal reaction to injury: fibrocyte-like cells, histiocytes, dermal dendritic cells, scar-like fibrosis, mucin, edema, calcification, and ossification.

> Scleroderma mimickers such as morphea, scleromyxedema, and eosinophilic fasciitis are generally distinguished from scleroderma by their absence of extracutaneous disease, Raynaud's phenomenon, and antinuclear antibodies.

Myth: Nephrogenic systemic fibrosis is the "systemic" form of nephrogenic fibrosing dermopathy.

Reality: "Nephrogenic fibrosing dermopathy" was the first popular name given to a disorder that has carried multiple monikers in its relatively brief lifetime. Other examples are shown in Table 11.1. Nephrogenic systemic fibrosis (NSF) is currently the preferred term, because it reflects the concept that NSF is a systemic disorder and that dialysis is not required for its development (Cowper et al. 2006b).

Myth: NSF develops more commonly in certain subgroups of people, such as women, Caucasians, and the elderly.

Reality: NSF afflicts patients of both genders and all ages and race. In one report from 2008, the age of the patients who had developed NSF ranged from 8 to 87 years (mean 46.4 years). The male:female ratio approximates one. The condition has been reported in Caucasians, Hispanics, African–Americans, and Asians, and described in North and South America, Europe, Australia, and Asia (Cowper 2008)

Myth: NSF is distinguished from other fibrosing disorders primarily by its tendency to involve the skin as opposed to internal organs.

Reality: NSF is a systemic fibrosing disorder in which the most readily recognized clinical manifestations are cutaneous. The description of skin involvement as a primary disease feature led initially to the name of "nephrogenic fibrosing dermopathy" (NFD) for this condition (Cowper et al. 2001). However, in 2003, fibrosis was detected in other organs in an "NFD" patient who died from complications of the disorder and underwent autopsy (Ting et al. 2003; Swaminathan et al. 2008). Fibrotic involvement was discovered in the diaphragm, muscles, heart, and esophagus. In addition, the systemic nature of "NFD" was confirmed by identification of the spindle cells within NFD tissues as bone marrow-derived cells by their CD34/procollagen-1 coexpression with special train (Cowper et al. 2003). This cell,

Table 11.1 Names given to the syndrome now known as nephrogenic systemic fibrosis.

Nephrogenic fibrosing dermopathy
Scleromyxedema-like cutaneous disease in renal dialysis patients
Fibrosing dermopathy of dialysis
Dialysis-associated systemic fibrosis
Scleromyxedema-like fibromucinosis

termed the "circulating fibrocyte," has been implicated as the cell principally responsible for the fibrosing process that characterizes NSF.

Numerous other reports have confirmed the occurrence of fibrosis within systemic organs, including the lungs, kidneys, and other tissues. Thus, NSF must be distinguished from other fibrosing disorders by the combination of clinical features and histopathological findings. Clinical features that help differentiate NSF from other disorders are:

- Its tendency to spare the skin of the face, in contrast to both scleroderma and scleromyxedema.
- Its lack of any association with autoantibodies, e.g., anticentromere or antitopoisomerase-3 antibodies.
- Its absence of a paraproteinemia, which occurs commonly in scleromyxedema.
- Finally, dermatopathologists can also distinguish among NSF, scleroderma, and scleromyxedema by the absence of inflammatory cells in NSF (Table 11.2) (Cowper et al. 2001).

Myth: Rapid and fulminant NSF, which is associated with severe pain, limb immobility, and joint contractures, occurs in more than half of patients.

Reality: Only about 5% of patients present in a fulminant manner, with disease courses that advance rapidly over as little as 2 weeks (Cowper 2007, 2008). In such settings, NSF is marked by severe pain and accelerated loss of mobility with joint contractures, wheelchair dependence, and a bed-

bound state. This form of the disorder is highly morbid and associated with increased mortality due to complications such as hip fractures from falls and systemic involvement by the fibrosing process.

It is more common for NSF to develop subacutely. In most patients, NSF begins with symmetrical lower extremity edema that subsequently involves the upper extremities (Cowper 2008). The edema may be associated with erythema, blisters, and bullae. Upon resolution of the edema, the indurated skin is nonpitting and "unpinchable" (Fig. 11.1).

Resolution of the edema leads to the formation of firm plaques that progress to brawny induration and thickening of the dermis. Other dermal manifestations include superficial papules, nodules, and hyperpigmentation. Deeper skin involvement is manifested as cobblestoning, peau d'orange skin

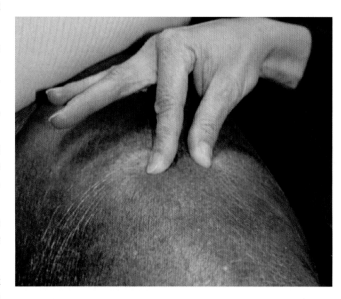

Fig. 11.1 NSF is characterized by edema that is nonpitting and unpinchable. Note the blanching of the fingertips of the person attempting to pinch the skin (From Girardi 2008. Reprinted with permission from Elsevier)

Table 11.2 Clinical and histopathological findings of fibrosing disorders considered in patients with nephrogenic systemic fibrosis (NSF) (Adapted from Cowper et al. 2001)

	NSF	Scleroderma, morphea, and eosinophilic fasciitis	Scleromyxedema
Distribution	Trunk and extremities (sparing of face)	Trunk, extremities, and face (particularly in scleroderma)	Trunk, extremities, and face
Paraproteinemia	Absent	Absent	Present
Systemic involvement	Sometimes (myocardium, pericardium, pleura, diaphragm)	Present (fibrosis of viscera, renal disease)	Present (internal mucin deposition)
Density of dermal fibroblasts	Increased numbers	Normal numbers or decreased	Increased numbers
Interstitial mucin	Present (early), but not in large collections	Present, large collections sometimes	Present, large collections sometimes
Inflammatory cells	Absent	Present, mixed infiltrates	Present, especially plasma cells

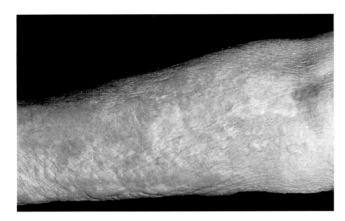

Fig. 11.2 Peau d'orange skin changes are noted in the arm of a patient with nephrogenic systemic fibrosis (With permission, Cowper 2001–2008)

changes (Fig. 11.2), and dermal tethering (Cowper 2008). These lesions are often extremely painful and may be associated with symptoms such as tightening, stiffness, burning, pruritus, paresthesias, and causalgia. Finally, flexion and extension contractures of large joints such as the hips, knees, elbows, hands, and feet develop in some patients, in processes that evolve over many months.

Pearl: Both clinical and histopathological findings are required to confirm the diagnosis of NSF.

Comment: NSF is a clinicopathological diagnosis (Cowper 2001). The diagnosis can be classified as certain, possible, or

excluded based on a combination clinical features and histopathological findings (Cowper 2008, personal communication). Other fibrosing disorders – e.g., systemic sclerosis (scleroderma), scleromyxedema, morphea, lipodermatosclerosis, and eosinophilic fasciitis – have clinical features that overlap substantially with NSF. These conditions may require laboratory testing or a skin biopsy for definitive diagnosis.

Myth: If dermal mucin deposits are absent, the diagnosis of NSF can be excluded.

Reality: Excess dermal mucin is a commonly encountered histopathological feature in cases of NSF (Fig. 11.3a). This observation led initially to comparisons of the disorder to scleromyxedema, which is also characterized by dermal mucinosis and fibrosis.

Although mucin deposition is characteristic of NSF, this finding is sometimes indistinct or even absent (Fig. 11.3b). The absence of mucin deposition within the skin should not exclude the diagnosis of NSF if the clinical and pathological findings otherwise favor it (Cowper et al. 2008).

Pearl: The diagnosis of NSF cannot be rendered accurately without clinical and histopathological correlation.

Comment: Neither the clinical nor the histopathological features of NSF are unique. The clinical features of NSF can be mimicked by scleromyxedema, scleroderma, morphea, lipodermatosclerosis, eosinophilic fasciitis, and other entities. The histopathological findings in NSF are virtually identical to those of scleromyxedema, but also overlap with other

Figs. 11.3 The cutaneous histopathological features of nephrogenic systemic fibrosis (NSF) may (**a**) or may not (**b**) reveal obvious mucin deposition. Mucin deposition is not required to make a histopathological diagnosis of NSF (Figure courtesy of Dr. Cowper)

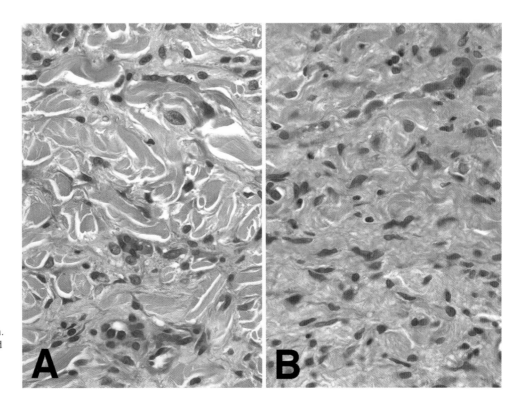

entities. The conclusions of published reports purported to describe NSF in the absence of histopathological evaluation should be viewed with skepticism, particularly if they diverge from the conclusions of studies that have employed rigorous clinicopathological correlation (Cowper et al. 2008).

Myth: NSF can develop in patients with any degree of kidney dysfunction.

Reality: Although NSF develops only in patients who suffer from kidney disease, it has not been described in patients with mild degrees of renal impairment. To be more specific, NSF has not been reported in any individual with an estimated glomerular filtration rate (eGFR) that exceeds 30 mL/min/1.73 m^2 (Grobner and Prischl 2008). A survey of the published literature (~264 cases) observed that NSF had been detected in patients with acute kidney injury, chronic kidney disease (stages IV and V), and end-stage renal disease on dialysis. Approximately 80% of patients with NSF have end-stage renal disease requiring dialysis. The other 20% suffers from either acute kidney injury (with or without dialysis) or stage IV or V chronic kidney disease (Grobner and Prischl 2008).

Myth: NSF can develop in any patient exposed to a gadolinium-based contrast agent.

Reality: In early 2006, Grobner published the observation that patients with end-stage renal disease on dialysis developed NSF within weeks to months of exposure to gadolinium-based contrast (Grobner 2006). Subsequently, numerous case series and case reports have verified the epidemiological association of gadolinium-based contrast exposure and NSF. Five case–control studies in patients with end-stage renal disease reported odds ratios between 22 and 46 for the development of NSF following exposure to gadolinium (Deo 2007; Collidge et al. 2007; Othersen et al. 2007; Marckmann et al. 2007; Broome et al. 2007).

As of 2008, all patients reported in the medical literature and the FDA MedWatch adverse events reporting system had underlying advanced kidney disease (eGFR <30 mL/min/1.73 m^2). No cases of NSF have been described in patients with normal kidney function or mild underlying renal disease.

Differences in the pharmacokinetics of gadolinium-based contrast in patients with advanced kidney disease probably explain much of the risk for NSF development. Most gadolinium-based contrast agents are cleared completely by glomerular filtration. Thus, as the GFR declines, the terminal half life ($T_{1/2}$) of gadolinium increases (Perazella and Rodby 2007). For example, the $T_{1/2}$ in the setting of normal kidney function is 1.3–1.9 h, with 95% excreted within 24 h. In contrast, the $T_{1/2}$ of gadolinium in the setting of kidney disease is approximately 5 h for stage III chronic kidney disease, approximately 9 h for stage IV, and approximately 27 h for stage V (Perazella and Rodby 2007). Among patients with

end-stage renal disease, hemodialysis reduces the $T_{1/2}$ to 2.1 h but requires up to four dialysis sessions to clear more than 95% of gadolinium from the plasma.

Peritoneal dialysis is less efficient than hemodialysis in clearing gadolinium. The $T_{1/2}$ of gadolinium-based contrast is approximately 53 h in a patient on peritoneal dialysis (Perazella and Rodby 2007).

Myth: All gadolinium-containing contrast agents are equally associated with NSF.

Reality: The majority of published cases of NSF originate in the United States, where six gadolinium-containing contrast agents are FDA-approved for MRI. In cases of NSF in which a gadolinium exposure could be identified with certainty, approximately 90% were exposed to gadodiamide (Omniscan®, GE Healthcare) and 10% to gadopentetate dimeglumine (Magnevist®, Bayer-Schering). Unpublished data and published case reports support this impression.

While marketing statistics are not readily available, it is generally accepted that, during this period, Magnevist® doses probably slightly exceeded Omniscan® doses in the US. This information suggests a higher propensity for Omniscan® to be associated with NSF, although recently European authorities have specifically banned the use of both agents in the renally impaired (MHRA 2007). A variety of lines of evidence suggest that GCCA with linear chelate molecules are more apt to induce NSF than those with macrocyclic chelates, and that "nonionic" formulations are more risky than "ionic" ones. These tendencies spring, in part, from the hypothesis that gadolinium dechelation is at the heart of NSF induction and, in part, from the observation of the relative reported frequencies of NSF to various GCCA (Cowper 2008).

Myth: Confirmation of a gadolinium exposure is required for the diagnosis of NSF.

Reality: NSF was defined by its clinical and pathological features several years before any association with gadolinium-containing contrast agents was made. Although the association between gadolinium exposure and NSF is strong, it is not clear that gadolinium is responsible for all cases of this syndrome. If a patient satisfies the clinicopathological criteria for NSF, then that diagnosis is appropriate, regardless of whether or not there is a known exposure to gadolinium. Detection of gadolinium within involved tissue is not required to make the diagnosis (Cowper et al. 2008).

Myth: Liver failure is an independent risk factor for NSF.

Reality: The admonition from the U.S. Food and Drug Administration that "patients with acute renal insufficiency of any severity due to the hepatorenal syndrome or in the perioperative liver transplantation period" should not receive gadolinium-containing contrast agents has led some practitioners to infer erroneously that liver disease is an independent risk

Table 11.3 Other postulated cofactors in the development of nephrogenic systemic fibrosis

Presence of an inflammatory disease state (infection, inflammation)
Presence of a thrombotic or hypercoagulable state
Recent surgical procedure (especially vascular procedures)
Metabolic disturbance (hyperphosphatemia, hypercalcemia)
Iron overload or recent intravenous iron therapy
High-dose erythropoietin exposure

factor for NSF (FDA 2007). Liver failure as an isolated finding has never been associated with NSF.

The FDA recommendations regarding the use of gadolinium-containing contrast agents are based on a risk assessment that includes calculation of the estimated glomerular filtration rate (eGFR) by the MDRD method. As the calculated value for eGFR is not validated for either acute kidney injury or the hepatorenal syndrome, the Food and Drug Administration highlighted these exceptions in their statements (Gonwa et al. 2004).

Pearl: Advanced kidney disease and exposure to gadolinium-based contrast appear necessary for the development of NSF, but other risk factors may also be required.

Comment: NSF develops predominantly in patients with advanced kidney disease (eGFR <30 mL/min/1.73 m²) who are exposed to a gadolinium-based contrast agent. The more severe the kidney dysfunction and the higher dose of gadolinium, the greater the risk of NSF. However, many patients who fulfill these risk criteria do not develop NSF, suggesting that other variables also impart risk (Perazella 2008). Other potential contributing factors, still unproven, are shown in Table 11.3.

Pearl: The best approach to prevent the development of NSF is to avoid exposure to gadolinium-based contrast agents in patients who are at high risk.

Comment: The strong epidemiological links between NSF and gadolinium exposure and the finding of significant amounts of Godolinium in NSF tissues (35–150 times higher than in non-NSF tissues) provide compelling evidence for gadolinium-based contrast agents as the causative agent in NSF (High et al. 2007). Further support is added by a rat model in which lesions that resemble NSF macroscopically and microscopically occur after gadolinium-based contrast agent exposure (Sieber et al. 2008). Because there remains no effective therapy for NSF, prevention is the best approach to this condition.

In high-risk patients, alternate imaging modalities must be considered if there is a reasonable hope that other approaches might address the clinical question. Certain MRI techniques that do not require gadolinium often provide sufficient information. As examples, three-dimensional time-of-flight MR

angiography, phase-contrast angiography, and arterial spin labeling MR techniques all provide excellent information about blood vessels and blood flow (Dawson and Punwani 2008). Ultrasound with various Doppler techniques or contrast-enhancement (intravenous microbubbles) is another option. Color, power, and spectral Doppler studies can visualize the direction and magnitude of blood flow through blood vessels, but these techniques are highly operator dependent (Dawson and Punwani 2008). Computed tomography without iodinated radiocontrast agents can provide all the information necessary in some settings. Radiocontrast agents pose significant risks of renal toxicity in patients with marginal renal function.

Pearl: NSF-like lesions can be induced in rats injected with gadolinium-containing contrast agents.

Comment: There have been published and unpublished reports indicating that cutaneous lesions clinically and histologically similar to NSF have been induced in rats subjected to high doses of certain gadolinium-containing contrast agents (Sieber et al. 2008). As these animals had intact renal function, doses of gadolinium were administered repeatedly to model the expected tissue levels of gadolinium-containing contrast agents in a human patient with renal dysfunction. In contrast to human disease, the animal model tended to manifest lesions on the dorsal trunk rather than on the extremities. In addition, the animal lesions tended to ulcerate or to be excoriated to the point of ulceration. Thus, although this rat model is not a perfect model of human NSF, this study lends further credibility to the hypothesis that NSF is caused by gadolinium-containing contrast agents' administration (Cowper 2008).

Pearl: Yellow scleral plaques are a useful diagnostic feature for NSF in patients younger than 45 years of age.

Comment: Yellow scleral plaques have been described in numerous case reports of NSF. In the experience of the Yale NSF Registry, scleral plaques are present in as many as 75% of cases. They commonly have surrounding vascular ectasia in their early stage (Fig. 11.4).

The yellow scleral plaques of NSF may be clinically indistinguishable from pinguecula in older patients. The younger the patient, the more specific scleral plaques are as an indicator of NSF (Cowper et al. 2008).

Pearl: NSF almost always presents on the extremities first. The lower extremities are involved before the upper extremities.

Comment: This distribution pattern nearly always holds true. In some cases, upper and lower extremity involvement develops simultaneously. The finding of both upper and lower extremity involvement is more specific for NSF than is lower extremity involvement alone. Isolated truncal involvement is

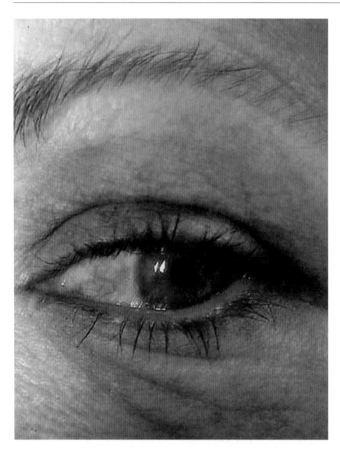

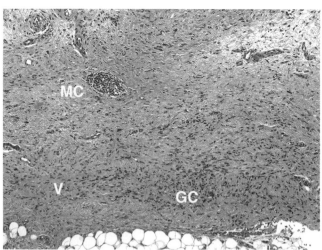

Fig. 11.5 A medium power image of the reticular dermal changes of nephrogenic systemic fibrosis. There is markedly increased cellularity, with increased fibroblast-like cells, occasional multinucleated giant cells (GC), and scant to absent mononuclear cells (MC). Vascularity (V) is increased, as is dermal collagen and mucin. This combination of features is highly suggestive of a dermal injury reaction (Figure courtesy of Dr. Cowper)

Fig. 11.4 Yellow scleral plaques: a distinctive feature of nephrogenic systemic fibrosis. In this relatively early phase of scleral plaque development, ectatic vessels are prominent (From Streams et al. 2003. Reprinted with kind permission from Elsevier)

uncharacteristic, and should prompt a search for an alternative explanation. In rare cases, NSF presents on the upper extremity, along the course of a peripherally inserted central catheter line (Cowper 2006a).

Pearl: The histopathological features of NSF strongly suggest a dermal tissue injury state.

Comment: NSF is characterized by a panoply of histopathologic components: fibrocyte-like cells, histiocytes, dermal dendritic cells, scar-like fibrosis, mucin, edema, calcification, and ossification (Fig. 11.5). All of these features are also encountered commonly in the setting of tissue repair. However, unlike tissue injury due to an infection or primary inflammatory condition, NSF lesions are devoid of significant numbers of lymphocytes, granulocytes, and plasma cells. This Pearl facilitates the histological diagnosis of NSF and is also consistent with the concept that NSF is a dermal reaction to injury (Cowper et al. 2003).

Myth: Several therapeutic agents are available to successfully stabilize and/or reverse the course of NSF.

Reality: Currently, no single therapeutic agent has been definitively proven to stabilize and reverse the course of NSF. In

general, the majority of cases of NSF follow a progressive course. Extracorporeal photopheresis has been associated with a slight improvement in skin thickening and joint mobility (Knopp and Cowper 2008; Linfert et al. 2008). Glucocorticoids, immunosuppressive agents, intravenous immune globulin, plasmapheresis, and thalidomide have all failed to improve the skin or joint manifestations of NSF. Anecdotal reports suggest that pentoxifylline, sodium thiosulfate, and imatinib mesylate might improve skin fibrosis (Linfert et al. 2008; Case Records of MGH 2008). The lack of efficacy for many agents used to treat NSF may relate to diagnosis of the process at a late stage, when the degree of fibrosis is advanced, and to repeated exposures of the patient to gadolinium-based contrast agents before recognition of the relationship between these agents and NSF. Early initiation of therapy and prevention of further gadolinium exposure might enhance treatment responses, but this hypothesis remains unproven.

Myth: Once NSF develops, reversal of the underlying fibrosing process is not possible.

Reality: In general, NSF is considered a fibrosing disorder that progresses relentlessly and is associated with permanent dermal and systemic end organ manifestations. However, the one circumstance in which NSF may stabilize or even improve (with softening of the skin and improved joint mobility) is recovery of the patient from acute kidney injury or the receipt of a renal allograft. Several patients with NSF associated with acute kidney injury were noted to develop spontaneous improvement in skin findings and joint mobility (Cowper et al. 2001; Mackay-Wiggan et al. 2003). Similarly, both published and anecdotal cases of improvements in NSF have been reported with kidney transplantation (Grobner 2006; Jan et al. 2003; Perazella 2007, personal observation). However, this is not a universal finding, perhaps depending on the chronicity of NSF at the time of renal transplantation and the level of kidney function achieved.

Pearl: Patients on peritoneal dialysis are at a substantially higher risk for the development of NSF compared with those who undergo hemodialysis.

Comment: Assuming that gadolinium dechelation is an important trigger for NSF, it is no surprise that peritoneal dialysis patients are at higher risk for this complication. Peritoneal dialysis is significantly less effective in removing gadolinium-containing contrast agents than is hemodialysis. A study from the Centers for Disease Control and Prevention provided the statistical evidence to substantiate this clinical impression (CDC 2007).

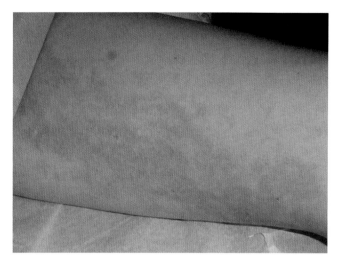

Fig. 11.6 Linear scleroderma. Linear scleroderma in an adult patient with left leg involvement. Notice the demarcation between normal and abnormal on the thigh (Figure courtesy of Dr. John Stone)

11.2 Localized Scleroderma

Pearl: Localized scleroderma is a distinct entity and should not be confused with limited cutaneous systemic sclerosis (limited SSc).

Comment: Localized scleroderma should not be confused with limited cutaneous systemic sclerosis. It is categorized as morphea (patches of thick skin) or linear scleroderma (an area of thickened skin demarcated clearly by a line) (Fig. 11.6). The latter includes scleroderma en coup de sabre, which affects the face or head (Fig. 11.7). Although restrictive lung disease has been reported in some pediatric patients with localized disease (Christen-Zaech et al. 2008), localized scleroderma is not usually associated with internal organ involvement.

Localized scleroderma is accompanied by a positive ANA in 30–50% of cases, but specific SSc-related autoantibodies such as anticentromere, antitopoisomerase I (Scl 70), and antiRNA polymerase III antibodies are absent (Takehara and Sato 2005). The absence of Raynaud phenomenon and sclerodactyly, along with the presence of typical lesions of morphea or of linear scleroderma, are additional clues that this is not systemic disease.

Pearl: Active morphea and linear SSc are warm to touch.

Comment: The examiner's hand can detect the activity of the lesion by feeling heat. Heat-sensitive Doppler equipment can be used to detect the activity of a lesion. As the lesion becomes inactive, the heat resolves. Skin affected by localized scleroderma is often pruritic, just as the cutaneous features of systemic sclerosis.

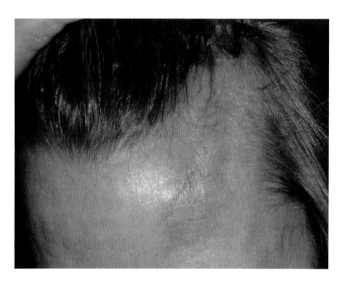

Fig. 11.7 En coup de sabre (Figure courtesy of Dr. John Stone)

11.3 Morphea

Myth: Morphea is caused by Lyme disease.

Reality: Uncontrolled studies have linked morphea with positive Lyme serologies or Borrelia burgdorferi DNA within skin lesions. However, the preponderance of data suggests that morphea is not associated with Lyme disease (Weide et al. 2000).

Pearl: Morphea often burns out in 2–5 years.

Comment: The Olmsted County study of morphea showed it was increasing in prevalence and that, for half the patients, there was resolution of the activity of the lesion by 3–4 years. Deeper lesions may take longer to resolve and are often accompanied by more disability (such as joint contractures) and damage depending on their location (Peterson et al. 1997).

Myth: Morphea is not an autoimmune disease.

Reality: Many patients with morphea have autoantibodies (ANA, RF), they have more relatives with autoimmune diseases, and there seems to be more autoimmune disease within morphea patients than would be expected such as diabetes, SLE, ITP, primary biliary cirrhosis, and vitiligo (Hawk and English 2001; Tuffanelli 1998).

Pearl: Morphea often has satellite lesions around the earlier lesions.

Comment: Many patients will have lesions active for a few years, but near to some of the original lesions, there may be more lesions that appear or even areas of pinkish discoloration and pigmentary changes slightly distant from the morphea plaque with seemingly normal skin in between.

Pearl: Antimalarials benefit many patients with morphea.

Comment: There are no systematic data about efficacy of antimalarials in morphea (Fig. 11.8), and it can be difficult to demonstrate meaningful improvement in this disease. However, anecdotal evidence suggests that when antimalarials are stopped in patients with morphea, they often develop new skin lesions.

Myth: Morphea is purely a skin disease.

Reality: About one third of patients with morphea have eosinophilic fasciitis, which has a clear systemic component. In addition, patients with morphea are more likely to have a second autoimmune disease (Peterson et al. 1995; Zulian et al. 2005).

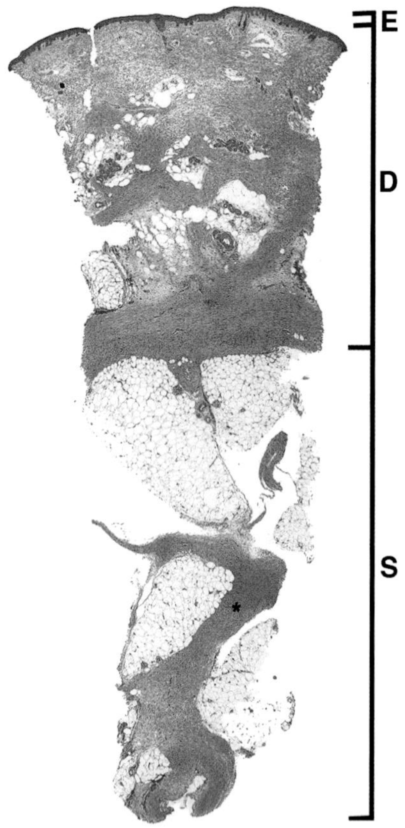

11.4 Scleromyxedema

Pearl: Scleromyxedema and NSF are often indistinguishable histologically but can be differentiated by their clinical features.

Comment: Two major features highlight the differences between NSF and scleromyxedema:

- *Pattern of skin involvement* – scleromyxedema tends to involve the head and neck rather than the extremities. In contrast, NSF involves the extremities first but virtually never involves the head and neck region.
- *Paraproteinemia* – the majority of patients with scleromyxedema have circulating paraproteins that are detectable by serum protein electrophoresis or immunoelectrophoresis. Patients with NSF almost never have such paraproteins unless their renal disease developed in the setting of multiple myeloma.

Subtle histopathological differences also exist in some cases. Scleromyxedema typically involves the dermis only, but NSF has a predilection for both the subcutis and dermis and sometimes the subcutis exclusively (Fig. 11.9). For this reason, a

Fig. 11.8 A deep biopsy of the skin in nephrogenic systemic fibrosis, revealing involvement of both the dermis (D) and subcutis (S). There is marked widening of subcutaneous septa (*asterisk*). The epidermis (E) is unaffected (Figure courtesy of Dr. Cowper)

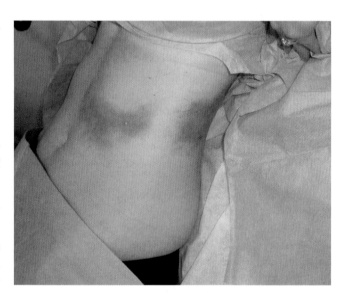

Fig. 11.9 Morphea (Figure courtesy of Dr. John Stone)

deep biopsy with a generous sampling of fat is the best diagnostic test for NSF (Cowper 2008). In this way, the approach to diagnosing NSF via skin biopsy is similar to those for diagnosing medium-vessel vasculitis, eosinophilic fasciitis, and other disorders with a predilection for the subcutaneous tissues.

Pearl: Patients with scleromyxedema should be evaluated for the presence of a paraprotein.

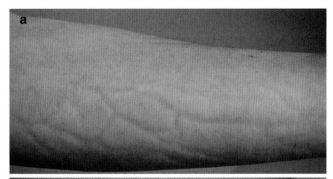

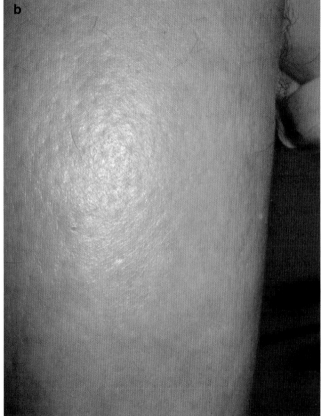

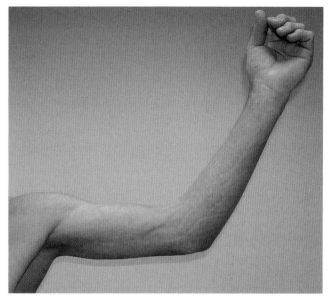

Fig. 11.11 Eosinophilic fasciitis. Note the enlargement of the arm distal to the elbow (Figure courtesy of Dr. John Stone)

skin of scleroderma and NSF, the overlying skin in eosinophilic fasciitis can be pinched. The easiest way for the examiner to do this is to place his or her thumbs on the patient's skin and then slide the thumbs together, pinching some skin gently between the opposing ends.

Eosinophilic fasciitis is associated with venous grooving (Fig. 11.10). This is observed most effectively on the skin of the medial upper arm as the patient externally rotates and abducts the arm.

Pearl: Eosinophilic fasciitis usually burns out.

Comment: Eosinophilic fasciitis often becomes inactive after several years. Early, aggressive treatment with glucocorticoids is important to minimize damage from this disorder. Limbs affected by eosinophilic fasciitis can have the appearance of pseudohypertrophied muscles (Fig. 11.11).

Fig. 11.10 Eosinophilic fasciitis. (a) Venous grooving in a patient with eosinophilic fasciitis. (b) Peaud' Orange skin on the back of the patient's calf (Figure courtesy of Dr. John Stone)

Comment: There is no Raynaud phenomenon, digital involvement, and dilated nailbed capillaries in scleromyxedema. However, the skin can look like SSc. If scleromyxedema is present, it can be associated with a monoclonal gammopathy of uncertain significance (MGUS) or myelodysplastic problems. Thus serum and urine protein electrophoresis evaluations should be performed.

11.5 Eosinophilic Fasciitis

Pearl: Eosinophilic fasciitis has "pinchable" skin.

Comment: The pathologic disturbance lies below the skin in eosinophilic fasciitis. Therefore, in contrast to the hidebound

References

Broome DR, Girguis MS, Baron PW, et al Gadodiamide-associated nephrogenic systemic fibrosis: why radiologists should be concerned. Am J Roentgenol. 2007;188:586–92

Case Records of MGH. Case 6-2008: A 46-year-old woman with renal failure and stiffness of the joints and skin. N Engl J Med. 2008;358:827–38

Centers for Disease Control (CDC). Nephrogenic fibrosing dermopathy associated with exposure to gadolinium-containing contrast agents– St. Louis, Missouri, 2002–2006. Morb Mortal Wkly Rep. 2007; 56(7):137–41

Christen-Zaech S, Hakim MD, Afsar FS, Paller AS. Pediatric morphea (localized scleroderma): Review of 136 patients. J Am Acad Dermatol. 2008;59(3):385–96

Collidge TA, Thompson PC, Mark PB, et al Gadolinium-enhanced MR imaging and nephrogenic systemic fibrosis: retrospective study of a renal replacement therapy cohort. Radiology 2007;245:168–75

Cowper SE. Gadolinium: is it to blame? J Cutan Pathol. 2008; 35(5):520–2

Cowper SE, Su L, Robin H, et al Nephrogenic fibrosing dermopathy. Am J Dermatopathol. 2001;23(5):383–93

Cowper SE, Bucala R. Nephrogenic fibrosing dermopathy: suspect identified, motive unclear [letter]. Am J Dermatopathol. 2003;25(4):35

Cowper SE, Boyer PJ. Nephrogenic systemic fibrosis: an update. Curr Rheumatol Rep. 2006a;8(2):151–7

Cowper SE, Bucala R, Leboit PE. Nephrogenic fibrosing dermopathy/ nephrogenic systemic fibrosis: Setting the record straight. Semin Arthritis Rheum. 2006b;35(4):208–10

Cowper SE, Rabach M, Girardi M. Clinical and histological findings in nephrogenic systemic fibrosis. Eur J Radiol. 2008;66(2):191–9

Cowper SE. Nephrogenic fibrosing dermopathy [NFD/NSF Website]. 2001–2008. 2007. http://www.icnfdr.org. Accessed 16 Apr 2008

Dawson P, Punwani S. Nephrogenic systemic fibrosis: non-gadolinium options for the imaging of CKD/ESRD patients. Sem Dial. 2008;51:160–5

Deo A, Fogel M, Cowper SE. Nephrogenic systemic fibrosis: a population study examining the relationship of disease development to gadolinium exposure. Clin J Am Soc Nephrol. 2007;2:264–7

FDA. Information for Healthcare Professionals Gadolinium-Based Contrast Agents for Magnetic Resonance Imaging (marketed as Magnevist, MultiHance, Omniscan, OptiMARK, ProHance). 2007. http://www.fda.gov/cder/drug/InfoSheets/HCP/gadolinium-containing contrast agents_200705.htm

Gonwa TA, Jennings L, Mai ML, et al Estimation of glomerular filtration rates before and after orthotopic liver transplantation: evaluation of current equations. Liver Transpl. 2004;10(2):301–9

Girardi M. Nephrogenic systemic fibrosis: a dermatologist's perspective. J Am Coll Radiol. 2008;5(1):40–4

Grobner T. GBC: a specific trigger for the development of nephrogenic fibrosing dermopathy and nephrogenic systemic fibrosis? Nephrol Dial Transplant. 2006;21:1104–8

Grobner T, Prischl FC. Patient characteristics and risk factors for nephrogenic systemic fibrosis following gadolinium exposure. Sem Dial. 2008;21:135–9

Hawk A, English JC III. Localized and systemic scleroderma. Semin Cutan Med Surg. 2001;20:27–37

High WA, Eng M, Ayers RA, Cowper SE. Gadolinium is quantifiable within the tissue of patients with nephrogenic systemic fibrosis. J Am Acad Dermatol. 2007;56:1–2

Jan F, Segal JM, Dyer J, et al Nephrogenic fibrosing dermopathy: two pediatric cases. J Pediatr. 2003;143:678–81

Knopp EA, Cowper SE. Nephrogenic systemic fibrosis: early recognition and treatment. Sem Dial. 2008;21:123–8

Linfert DR, Schell JO, Fine DM. Treatment of nephrogenic systemic fibrosis: limited options but hope for the future. Sem Dial. 2008;51:155–9

Mackay-Wiggan JM, Cohen DJ, Hardy MA, et al Nephrogenic fibrosing dermopathy (scleromyxedema-like illness of renal disease). J Am Acad Dermatol. 2003;48:55–60

Marckmann P, Skov L, Rossen K, et al Case-control study of gadodiamide-related nephrogenic systemic fibrosis. Nephrol Dial Transplant. 2007;22:3174–8

Medicines and Healthcare products Regulatory Agency (MHRA). Nephrogenic Systemic Fibrosis (NSF) and gadolinium-containing MRI contrast agents: Public Assessment Report. 2007. http://www.mhra.gov.uk/home/idcplg?IdcService=GET_FILE&dDocName=CON2030232&RevisionSelectionMethod=LatestReleased Accessed 15 Jul 2008

Othersen JB, Maize JC, Woolson RF, Budisavljevic MN. Nephrogenic systemic fibrosis after exposure to gadolinium in patients with renal failure. Nephrol Dial Transplant. 2007;22:3179–85

Perazella MA. Tissue deposition of gadolinium and development of NSF: a convergence of factors. Semin Dial. 2008;21:150–4

Perazella MA, Rodby RA. Gadolinium use in patients with kidney disease: a cause for concern. Semin Dial. 2007;20:179–85

Peterson LS, Nelson AM, Su WP. Classification of morphea (localized scleroderma). Mayo Clin Proc. 1995;70:1068–76

Peterson LS, Nelson AM, Su WP, Mason T, O'Fallon WM, Gabriel SE. The epidemiology of morphea (localized scleroderma) in Olmsted County 1960–1993. J Rheumatol. 1997;24(1):73–80

Sieber MA, Pietsch H, Walter J, et al A preclinical study to investigate the development of nephrogenic systemic fibrosis: a possible role for gadolinium-based contrast media. Invest Radiol. 2008;43(1):65–75

Streams BN, Liu V, Liegeois N, Moschella SM. Clinical and pathologic features of nephrogenic fibrosing dermopathy: a report of two cases. J Am Acad Dermatol. 2003;48:42–7

Swaminathan S, High WA, Ranville J, et al Cardiac and vascular metal deposition with high mortality in nephrogenic systemic fibrosis. Kidney Int 2008; 73(12):1413–18

Takehara K, Sato S. Localized scleroderma is an autoimmune disorder. Rheumatology (Oxford). 2005;44(3):274–9

Ting WW, Stone MS, Madison KC, Kurtz K. Nephrogenic fibrosing dermopathy with systemic involvement. Arch Dermatol. 2003;139: 903–6

Tuffanelli DL. Localized scleroderma. Semin Cutan Med Surg. 1998; 17:27–33

Weide B, Schittek B, Klyscz T, et al Morphoea is neither associated with features of Borrelia burgdorferi infection, nor is this agent detectable in lesional skin by polymerase chain reaction. Br J Dermatol. 2000;143(4):780–5

Zulian F, Vallongo C, Woo P, et al Localized scleroderma in childhood is not just a skin disease. Arthritis Rheum. 2005;52: 2873–81

Sjögren's Syndrome

12

Manuel Ramos-Casals, Troy E. Daniels, Robert I. Fox,
John P. Whitcher, George E. Fragoulis, Fotini N. Skopouli,
and Haralampos M. Moutsopoulos

12.1 Overview of Sjögren's Syndrome

> Primary Sjögren's syndrome (SjS) is a systemic auto-immune disease that is associated with early and gradually progressive lacrimal and salivary dysfunction.
> Secondary SjS occurs in association with other autoimmune disorders, the most common of which is rheumatoid arthritis.
> About 90% of patients with SjS are women.
> Minor salivary glands and lacrimal glands in SjS exhibit a particular pattern of periductal focal lymphocytic infiltration known as focal lymphocytic sialadenitis.
> Primary SjS has a community prevalence that ranges from 0.1 to 0.6%.
> The major eye problem in SjS is keratoconjunctivitis sicca, which leads to xerophthalmia. The principal oral manifestation of SjS is decreased salivary gland production, leading to xerostomia and a predilection for dental caries.
> Extraglandular manifestations of SjS include arthralgias, thyroiditis, renal involvement (leading to renal tubular acidosis (RTA)), peripheral neuropathy, cutaneous vasculitis, and lymphoma.
> The risk of lymphoma in SjS is approximately 5%.
> Most patients with SjS develop increased circulating polyclonal immunoglobulins and autoantibodies. These autoantibodies include two fairly specific antibodies directed against the Ro (SS-A) and La (SS-B) antigens.

12.2 Classification and Epidemiology

Myth: It doesn't matter which criteria are used for classifying or diagnosing patients with Sjögren's syndrome (SjS).

Reality: At least ten diagnostic/classification criteria for SjS have been published since the 1960s. The 2002 American–European Consensus Group classification criteria for SjS

(Vitali et al. 2002) were created to update the 1993/1996 European Community Criteria for Classifying SjS (Vitali et al. 1993, Vitali et al. 1996). These criteria sought to correct problems with earlier criteria sets by requiring that evidence of an autoimmune process characteristic of SjS be included. The 2002 Criteria stipulate that at least one criterion must be a positive anti-Ro/SSA or -La/SSB antibody assay or a positive labial salivary gland biopsy (Table 12.1) (Vitali et al. 2002).

The 2002 criteria have been criticized for excessive emphasis on glandular disease and failure to capture the full spectrum of other organ system involvement in SjS, particularly extraglandular disease features and the full spectrum of immunological abnormalities. Known prognostic factors in SjS, particularly the occurrence of hypocomplementemia, cryoglobulinemia, and vasculitis, are not captured in the 2002 criteria.

Pearl: Differences between primary SjS and secondary SjS have major clinical relevance.

Comment: Primary SjS and secondary SjS are related systemic autoimmune diseases, but important differences exist between these conditions (Pavlidis et al. 1982). Primary SjS is characterized by early and progressive salivary and lacrimal dysfunction. In addition, primary SjS also encompasses a host of extraglandular manifestations that can involve the thyroid gland, kidneys, liver, skin, peripheral nerves, lungs, and other organs. Patients with primary SjS rarely develop rheumatoid arthritis (RA), and secondary SjS often develops in the setting of RA. Approximately 30% of patients with RA develop secondary SjS, usually years after their RA diagnosis (Andonopoulos et al. 1987).

The three most common primary SjS symptoms are dry eyes, dry mouth, and musculoskeletal pain. Diagnosing primary SjS is more difficult than diagnosing secondary SjS because those with primary disease typically present with only one of these complaints to different specialists. All three complaints have their own differential diagnosis. Specialists who are addressing one complaint are often unfamiliar with the breadth of possibilities related to the others. A survey of more than 3,000 SjS patients in 2005 reported that the average time between occurrence of their first symptoms and diagnosis was more than 6 years (Sjögren's Syndrome Foundation 2006).

Table 12.1 American–European consensus group classification criteria for sjögren's syndrome

I. Ocular symptoms: a positive response to at least one of the following questions:
  1. Have you had daily, persistent, troublesome dry eyes for more than 3 months?
  2. Do you have a recurrent sensation of sand or gravel in the eyes?
  3. Do you use tear substitutes more than 3 times a day?

II. Oral symptoms: a positive response to at least one of the following questions:
  1. Have you had a daily feeling of dry mouth for more than 3 months?
  2. Have you had recurrently or persistently swollen salivary glands as an adult?
  3. Do you frequently drink liquids to aid in swallowing dry food?

III. Ocular signs: a positive result for at least one of the following two tests:
  1. Schirmer I test, performed without anesthesia (≤5 mm in 5 minutes)
  2. Rose Bengal[a] score or other ocular dye score (≥4 on the van Bijstervled scale)

IV. Histopathology: in minor salivary glands (obtained through normal-appearing mucosa) focal lymphocytic sialadenitis, evaluated by an expert histopathologist, with a focus score ≥1, defined as a number of lymphocytic foci (which are adjacent to normal-appearing mucous acini and contain more than 50 lymphocytes) per 4 mm^2 of glandular tissue.

V. Salivary gland involvement: a positive result for at least one of the following tests:
  1. Unstimulated whole salivary flow (≤1.5 mL in 15 minutes)
  2. Parotid sialography showing the presence of diffuse sialectasis (punctuate, cavitary, or destructive pattern), without evidence of major duct obstruction
  3. Saolivary scintigraphy showing delayed uptake, reduced concentration, and/or delayed excretion of tracer

VI. Autoantibodies: presence in the serum of the following:
  1. Antibodies to Ro(SS-A) or La(SS-B) antigens, or both

Rules for classification

For primary SS: in patients without any potentially associated disease
  a. Presence of any 4 four of the 6 six items indicates primary SjS as long as either item IV (histopathology) or VI (serology) is positive
  b. Presence of any 3 three of the 4 four objective criteria items (that is items III, IV, V, VI)
  c. The c lassification tree procedure (best used in clinical--epidemiological surveys)

For Secondary SjS: patients with a potentially associated disease (e.g., another well defined-connective tissue disease), the presence of item I or item II plus any 2 two from among items III, IV, and V.

Exclusion criteria: past head and neck radiation treatment; hepatitis C infection; acquired immunodeficiency disease (AIDS); pre-existing lymphoma; sarcoidosis; graft vs. host disease; use of anticholinergic drugs (since a time shorter than 4-fourfold the half life of the drug)

[a]Lissamine green has now replaced rose bengal for this test.
Adapted from (Vitali et al. 2002)

Myth: A patient is diagnosed with definite primary SjS if she or he fulfills at least four of the six American–European Classification Criteria.

Reality: The classification criteria have been derived to classify patients as primary SjS for the purpose of research studies, not clinical diagnosis (Vitali et al. 2002). For example, a patient who has recurrent bilateral parotid gland enlargement, autoantibodies to Ro/SSA and La/SSB, and a positive minor salivary gland biopsy has unequivocal primary SjS. However, some patients with objective measures of lacrimal or salivary gland dysfunction do not have clinical symptoms. In the absence of ocular or oral symptoms, antibodies to the Ro/SSA or La/SSB antigens, and a positive minor salivary gland biopsy, such patients do not fulfill classification criteria for SjS. Most of these patients take medications that explain their abnormal gland function.

Myth: SjS is an uncommon disease.

Reality: Epidemiological studies from Scandinavia and Greece have shown that primary SjS is less prevalent than RA (presuming a 1% prevalence for RA), but not by much (Jacobsson et al. 1989; Dafni et al. 1997). To a large extent,

the prevalence of SjS depends on the classification criteria applied. Studies based on the American–European criteria have reported a prevalence of primary SjS of 0.3% in the female population in Greece and up to 0.4% of females in the United Kingdom (Trontzas and Andrianakos 2005; Bowman et al. 2004).

Pearl: The expression of primary SjS in males is relatively muted when compared with its expression in females.

Comment: Various studies have described a less pronounced clinical phenotype among male SjS patients compared with female patients, regardless of whether one considers clinical, histological, sialographic, or immunologic criteria. In a series of 1,010 patients, the 73 male patients had a lower frequency of abnormal ocular tests and a lower prevalence of positive antinuclear antibodies, Raynaud's phenomenon, and thyroiditis (Ramos-Casals et al. 2008). These findings are consistent with the precept that most autoimmune diseases are more common in women. The relatively muted presentation in men can make the diagnosis more difficult.

Pearl: When SjS occurs in males, look for other clinical stigmata of Klinefelter syndrome.

Comment: In one study, up to 15% of the male SjS patients had symptoms of Klinefelter's syndrome (lack of reproductive capacity, low testosterone, and abnormal XXY karyotype) (Aoki, 1999). These findings are interesting in view of a finding in the BXSB mouse that involves the translocation of a portion of the X chromosome to the Y chromosome, because this is the only male mouse model to develop SjS- or SLE-like features (Krieg and Vollmer 2007).

12.3 Pathogenesis

Myth: The predominant cells comprising the focal lymphocytic infiltrates of labial minor salivary glands in primary SjS are T-lymphocytes.

Reality: The type of lymphocyte that predominates within minor salivary gland biopsies in primary SjS depends on the degree of glandular inflammation. In heavy lymphocytic infiltrates, B lymphocytes predominate and germinal centers are formed (Gerli et al. 1997). In mild to moderate degrees of lymphocytic infiltration, T cells predominate.

Pearl: SjS can be considered both a T cell and B cell disease.

Comment: The earliest lymphocytic infiltrates in salivary glands are composed of CD20 + B cells and T cells, mostly of the primed memory T helper phenotype. Later, other B cell phenotypes join the infiltrates (CD27 + memory and CD79a+). Clusters of plasma cells (CD38+) are present in both normal salivary glands and at the periphery of T cell and B cell infiltrates in SjS (Larsson et al. 2005). These infiltrates may exhibit lymphoid follicle formation in various stages of development as they enlarge. Their cellular portfolio comprises primarily CD20 + B cells and follicular dendritic cells, with a few helper T cells (Prochorec-Sobieszek et al. 2004).

The T cells have initiating roles in the pathogenesis of SjS and secrete many of the cytokines found within affected organs. The T-helper (Th) infiltrates in SjS include both proinflammatory Th1 cytokines such as interferon (IFN)-γ and interleukin (IL)-2, as well as antiinflammatory Th2 cytokines, such as IL-4, IL-5, and IL-13. Over time, these profiles shift; Th2 cytokines predominate early in SjS, but the balance shifts toward Th1 in more advanced disease (Mitsias et al. 2002).

The B cells not only lead to the circulating autoantibodies seen prominently in SjS, they also become the proliferating component. A B cell activating factor known as BAFF or BLyS (B cell activating factor/B lymphocyte stimulator), which is regulated by IFN-γ, promotes the survival and maturation of B cells. BAFF/BLyS is elevated in SjS serum. This factor is implicated in the polyclonal activation of B cells, correlates with the levels of circulating autoantibodies (Mariette et al. 2003), and may have a long-term role in the development of lymphoma. SjS-related lymphomas are almost always of B cell origin.

12.4 Sicca Features

12.4.1 Ocular Manifestations

Pearl: The predominant presenting complaints in patients with primary SjS are dry eyes and mouth.

Comment: More than ninety percent of patients with primary SjS complain of dry eyes and/or dry mouth (Skopouli et al. 2000). Patients with this disorder also sometimes present with recurrent or persistent parotid gland enlargement, Raynaud's phenomenon, bronchitis sicca, hypergammaglobulinemic purpura, peripheral neuropathy, or interstitial nephritis.

Myth: Concurrent symptoms of dry eyes and dry mouth (i.e., the "sicca complex") are all that one needs to diagnose SjS.

Reality: Dry mouth and dry eyes are both highly prevalent in SjS, but they do not occur in all patients. However, they occur in many other types of patients, as well, and can often be induced by medications (Tables 12.2 and 12.3). In a large cohort of participants in the NIH-sponsored International Sjögren's Syndrome registry, 91% of the patients complained of a dry mouth and 85% complained of dry eyes. However, the correlation between these symptoms and objective signs

Table 12.2 Dry mouth symptoms: differential diagnosis

Chronically administered systemic drugs with anticholinergic effects (e.g., antidepressants, parasympatholytics, neuroleptics)
Sjögren's syndrome[a]
Sarcoidosis, [a]tuberculosis
HIV[a] or hepatitis-C infection
Depression
Uncontrolled diabetes; amyloidosis
Therapeutic radiation to head and neck that includes major salivary glands in fields
Graft vs. host disease

[a]May also cause bilateral major salivary gland enlargement
(From Klippel et al. 2008. With kind permission from Springer Science + Business Media.)

Table 12.3 Dry eye symptoms: differential diagnosis

Sjögren's syndrome (keratoconjunctivitis sicca)
Chronically administered systemic drugs with anticholinergic effects
AIDS-associated keratoconjunctivitis sicca
Conjunctival cicatrization
Stevens–Johnson syndrome
Ocular cicatricial pemphigoid
Drug-induced pseudopemphigoid
Trachcoma
Graft vs. host disease
Trigeminal or facial nerve paralysis
Vitamin A deficiency ("xerophthalmia")

Adapted from (Whitcher et al. 1998)

of SjS was poor. In fact, neither symptom was associated with positivity for antibodies directed against the Ro/SSA or La/SSB antigents or focal lymphocytic sialadenitis in labial salivary gland biopsies (Daniels et al. 2007). Moreover, the symptom of dry eyes was only marginally associated with the presence of keratoconjunctivitis sicca (Daniels et al. 2007).

In short, symptoms of dry eyes and dry mouth are often caused by conditions other than SjS and are insufficient for the diagnosis of SjS.

Pearl: "Dry eyes" associated with SjS should be termed "keratoconjunctivitis sicca" rather than "xerophthalmia."

Comment: Xerophthalmia refers specifically to the dry eyes associated with hypovitaminosis A and should not be used in reference to SjS.

Pearl: Symptoms of keratoconjunctivitis sicca are more prevalent than xerostomia in patients who have SjS secondary to RA.

Comment: On close questioning, complaints consistent with keratoconjunctivitis sicca are elicited in nearly 40% of RA patients, but dry mouth is reported in only 6% (Andonopoulos et al. 1989). RA patients who have secondary SjS rarely mention sicca symptoms spontaneously and must be asked about them.

Patients with RA and secondary SjS rarely experience episodes of parotid gland swelling. In contrast, either intermittent or permanent parotid swelling is a hallmark of primary SjS, occurring in 34 of 65 patients (56%) in one study (Bloch et al. 1965).

Myth: The diagnosis of keratoconjunctivitis sicca is based on an abnormal Schirmer's test.

Reality: Both the sensitivity and specificity of the Schirmer's test are low for keratoconjunctivitis sicca (Paschides et al. 1989). The Schirmer's test measures lacrimal gland function, and many factors can interfere with the physiology of these glands: medications, older age, occupation, the time of day, the season of the year, and the patient's hydration status.

The test that provides unequivocal evidence of keratoconjunctivitis sicca is a slit lamp examination of the cornea and conjunctiva after rose Bengal or lissamine green staining (Fig. 12.1). In keratoconjunctivitis sicca, the stain collects within defects of the cornea caused by ocular drying and the consequent minor trauma to the eye.

Myth: The symptom of ocular foreign-body sensation is the best symptomatic indicator of keratoconjunctivitis sicca.

Reality: In comparing 449 patients referred to a SjS clinic, "ocular foreign body" sensation was the most prevalent of seven ocular symptoms. More than three fourths of the patients with keratoconjunctivitis sicca complained of an "ocular

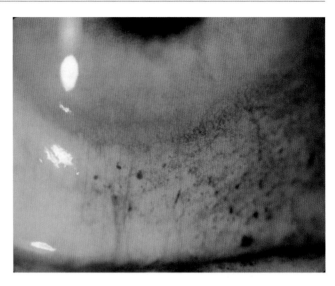

Fig. 12.1 Slit lamp examination of the cornea and conjunctiva after rose Bengal staining

foreign body" sensation. However, 61% of patients <u>without</u> keratoconjunctivitis sicca also offered that complaint, making its usefulness as a discriminator of true keratoconjunctivitis sicca rather limited.

Among the other seven ocular symptoms, "inability to tear," had the strongest association with keratoconjunctivitis sicca, but was experienced by a smaller proportion of patients with keratoconjunctivitis sicca (45%), compared with only 9% of those who did not have keratoconjunctivitis sicca ($p < 0.0001$) (Whitcher et al. 1998).

Pearl: Patients with keratoconjunctivitis sicca who need to use artificial tears chronically must use a product that is preservative-free.

Comment: Many commonly used artificial tears contain preservatives which, when used chronically, can elicit an inflammatory reaction in the cornea and conjunctiva that is painful. This preservative-induced effect is difficult to distinguish from those of true keratoconjunctivitis sicca. Prolonged use of preservative-containing artificial tears can result in conjunctival scarring that further complicates the clinical presentation.

SjS patients are particularly susceptible to ocular surface toxicity from these preservatives because of their aqueous tear deficiency. Preservative-free artificial tears should be used by all patients who instill them more than 4 times per day.

Myth: All patients diagnosed with keratoconjunctivitis sicca have SjS.

Reality: The term "keratoconjunctivitis sicca" was coined by Henrik Sjögren to describe a particular type of dry eye disease in 1933 . His description later came to define the ocular component of SjS. A few subsequent studies noted that not all patients with keratoconjunctivitis sicca exhibit evidence of the oral/salivary or serological components of SjS. One prospective study of 34 patients with keratoconjunctivitis sicca found that 44% had objective evidence of the salivary and serological components of SjS, but that 56% had no evidence of salivary gland dysfunction (Forstot et al. 1982). Some patients in the latter group were ANA positive, but none had antibodies to Ro/SSA or La/SSB.

A long-term study reexamined a group of 106 patients who had been diagnosed with keratoconjunctivitis sicca (Kruize et al. 1996). Repeat examinations up to 12 years after their initial diagnoses of keratoconjunctivitis sicca determined that 29% had primary SjS and 18% had secondary SjS, but 53% had isolated keratoconjunctivitis sicca.

Pearl: Ocular cosmetic procedures can exacerbate SjS.

Comment: Three specific types of cosmetic surgery are contraindicated in patients with SjS: blepharoplasty (eyelid "lift"), Lasik surgery, and Botox® injections.

Blepharoplasty may interrupt the basal tearing that occurs in the lower lid by the glands of Sherring. (These are the same glands that one stimulates by rubbing one's eyes). Stretching of the eyelid during blepharoplasty appears to disrupt the delicate neural interconnections within the network of glands. Blepharoplasty can also lead to increased zones of the cornea that are susceptible to exposure keratitis. Particularly when sleeping, the lower lid may not make adequate contact with the upper lid, leading to a zone of increased evaporative loss and resulting dessicative injury.

SjS is a contraindication to Lasik surgery because of the increased dryness that occurs after the procedure (Liang et al. 2008). This increased dryness presumably results from the "flap" cut by the microtome across the cornea, which severs the nerve bodies from afferent sensory nerves that innervate the cornea. The resulting "neuropathic" eye is more sensitive to abrasions as well as to the sensation of dryness (friction as the upper lid traverses the globe).

Finally, a standard model for induction of keratoconjunctivitis sicca is the injection of botulinum toxin (Lekhanont et al. 2007). The wisdom of avoiding this intervention in a patient with SjS is self-evident.

Pearl: SjS patients have unique ocular needs at the time of anesthesia and surgery.

Comment: Operating rooms and postoperative recovery rooms are notorious for their low humidity. SjS patients are at risk for exacerbations of their keratoconjunctivitis sicca or even for corneal abrasions in such environments. The risk is perhaps greatest in the recovery room, where the patient who is partially awake has fluttering eyelids and often receives unhumidified air directly to the face. These patients are unaware of ocular symptoms as they awaken from anesthesia. Ocular lubricants should be employed during surgery and during the recuperative period to prevent complications.

Anesthesiologists must limit the quantity of anticholinergic agents administered during intubation for patients with SjS. SjS patients may be unduly sensitive to these drugs and develop inspissated secretions that are not cleared easily. This can be particularly problematic after chest or abdominal surgery, when the expectoration of tenacious secretions is difficult even under better circumstances.

Finally, the use of oral saliva substitutes should be encouraged. It is expected that patients will be "NPO" prior to most surgeries. In the absence of normal saliva, patients with SjS experience unnecessary discomfort if they are not allowed to have their artificial saliva. This is particularly true when the patient's surgery is delated until later in the day.

Myth: Topical ophthalmological glucorticoids should not be used in SjS.

Reality: One randomized trial assigned SjS patients to either loteprednol 0.5% solution or placebo 4 times a day for 4 weeks (Pflugfelder et al. 2004). All patients had failed previous therapies with artificial tears. Patients in the topical glucocorticoid group demonstrated significant improvement and ability to return to traditional artificial tears after loteprednol. Thus, topical glucocorticoids may have a role in some patients, but they must be employed with caution in patients who have glaucoma or cataracts, especially if prolonged use is intended.

Pearl: The environment plays a key role in exacerbating patients' ocular symptoms.

Comment: Although SjS patients haves decreased rates of aqueous tear formation and increased rates of evaporative loss due to the inflammatory process, both of those processes are exacerbated by environmental factors. As examples, factors such as low humidity can be partially helped by humidifiers. The effect of dry winds are ameliorated by "wrap-around" sunglasses or side shields on glasses.

Additional factors such as the decreased "blink rate" associated with the use of computer monitors are underappreciated. The modern work place environment is typically an office with low humidity, where individuals spent large amounts of time staring at computer screens (Wolkoff et al. 2006). People concentrating on computer monitors have a 90% decrease in their baseline blink rate. Thus, concentration on "the screen" can override the normal corneal surface conditions that lead to blinking and spreading of the available tears.

12.4.2 Oral Manifestations

Myth: The most common cause of dry mouth symptoms is primary or secondary SjS.

Reality: The symptom of dry mouth (xerostomia) is highly prevalent in the general population. It is often associated with salivary hypofunction, but occurs in some patients with normal salivary flow rates. The most common cause of this symptom is the effect of one or more prescription drugs. Hundreds of drugs have the capacity to induce xerostomia. A list of these medications can be viewed at http://www.dry-mouth.info/practitioner/default.asp. In addition to SjS, other causes of dry mouth symptoms are listed in Table 12.2.

Pearl: One pattern of lymphocytic infiltration in salivary glands is diagnostic of the salivary component of SjS. Other patterns are not.

Comment: Diagnoses of the salivary component of SjS by the presence of a focal lymphocytic infiltrate in a labial salivary gland biopsy have been rendered since the 1960s (Daniels 1991). The ocular component of SjS (keratoconjunctivitis sicca) is significantly correlated with the presence of focal lymphocytic sialadenitis in labial salivary gland biopsies, but not with other patterns of chronic salivary inflammation commonly seen in those speicmens (Daniels and Whitcher 1994).

Diagnostic confusion among pathologists who review labial salivary gland biopsies is rife. In a prospective review of minor salivary gland biopsies from patients who had been referred to a SjS Clinic, 53% needed diagnostic revision. In 23% of the patients, the misclassification of the biopsy led to a diagnostic delay that ranged from a few months to more than 7 years (Vivino et al. 2002).

Myth: Minor labial salivary gland biopsy is a painful procedure often associated with unwanted side effects.

Reality: Minor labial salivary gland biopsy is a safe procedure that is associated with few adverse effects (Caporali et al. 2008). Hematoma, infection, and long-lasting numbness at the incision site occur rarely. The procedure provides valuable diagnostic confirmation of the salivary component of SjS and is often essential in parsing the differential diagnosis in patients who present with sicca symptoms (e.g., sarcoidosis, amyloidosis). Labial salivary gland biopsy also offers unusually easy access to an end-organ affected by autoimmune pathology, thus making it an important tool for research on disease pathophysiology.

Pearl: Several frequently forgotten causes of the sicca syndrome are type IV and V lipoproteinemias, amyloidosis, and sarcoidosis.

Comment: The patients with these conditions can present with dryness of the mouth and eyes. Patients with these disorders normally are negative on testing for antibodies to the Ro/SSA and La/SSB autoantigens. Labial minor salivary gland biopsy is of paramount diagnostic importance, because it can reveal fatty infiltrates in the lipoproteinemias; amorphous material within the blood vessel walls that stains positively for congo red in amyloidosis; and noncaseating granulomas in sarcoidosis (Fig. 12.2) (Reinertsen et al. 1980; Simon and Moutsopoulos 1979; Drosos et al. 1989).

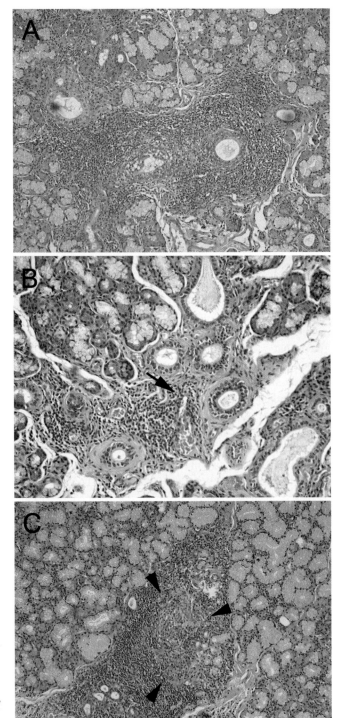

Fig. 12.2 (**a–c**) Contrasts between Sjögren's syndrome and sarcoidosis in the labial salivary glands. (**a**) Lymphocytic infiltrates within the labial minor salivary gland of a patient with primary Sjogren's syndrome. (**b**) Lymphocytic infi ltrates in within the minor salivary gland biopsy of a patient with SLE-SS overlap syndrome. The infiltrates are perivascular (*arrows*). (**c**) Granuloma formation within the minor salivary gland biopsy of a patient who also had erythema nodosum, arthritis, and bilateral hilar lymphadenopathy. Both the clinical picture and the histopathologic features depicted in (**c**) are compatible with sarcoidosis. [Figure courtesy of Dr. Haralampos M. Moutsopoulos]

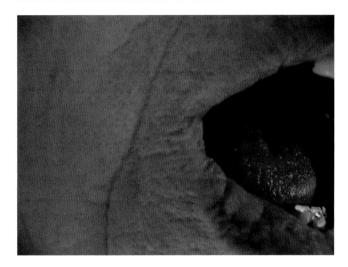

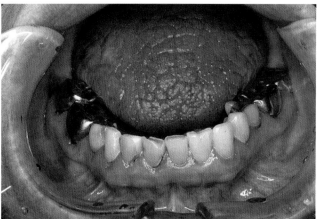

Fig. 12.3 Oral features of candidiasis, a common complication of Sjögren's syndrome. Angular cheilitis is present, along with a *red, beefy tongue* consistent with candidiasis [Figure courtesy of Dr. Haralampos M. Moutsopoulos]

Fig. 12.4 This patient with SjS exhibits signs of multiple dental caries and chronic erythematous candidiasis that are characteristic of chronic salivary dysfunction. Caries are seen next to the gingival margins in all of the teeth illustrated (including those with *gold crowns*) and three anterior teeth also have caries on their incisal edge. The diffuse atrophy of lingual filiform papillae is a clear sign of erythematous candidiasis [Figure courtesy of Dr. Troy Daniels]

Pearl: Angular cheilitis and a red tongue with atrophic papillae strongly suggest Candida overgrowth in the mouth.

Comment: Oral candidiasis is common in patients with primary SjS (Hernandez and Daniels 1989). This frequently presents as diffuse, painful erythema of the oral mucosa, particularly affecting the dorsal tongue and causing angular cheilitis (Fig. 12.3). A common symptom is intolerance to acidic or spicy foods. Several weeks of therapy with fluconazole are often required to cure this problem. In addition, patients with severe salivary hypofunction may require prolonged antifungal treatment with topical preparations that do not contain sugar (Daniels 2000). Recurrent candidiasis is common in some patients.

Myth: Periodontal disease is a very common problem among patients with primary SjS.

Reality: Periodontal disease is actually no more common in primary SjS patients as it is in healthy, age-matched controls (Boutsi et al. 2000). What is unique about the oral health of patients with SjS, however, is the patients' propensity to develop a characteristic pattern of dental caries (cavities) located along the gingival margins and cusp tips of multiple teeth (Fig. 12.4) (Daniels 2000). The treatment and prevention of these progressive lesions requires ongoing caries prevention activities and interaction with the patient's dentist.

Myth: Oral dryness in SjS results from the total destruction of the gland.

Reality: In fact, the glandular secretory elements are gradually replaced or "destroyed" by lymphocytic infiltration and proliferation. Even in patients with severe dryness, some normal-appearing ducts and acini remain but do not function well because of the inflammatory process that disrupts the ability of the residual secretory units to release or respond to neurotransmitters.

In a lip biopsy from an SjS patient with severe dryness, attention is usually focused on the dense lymphoid infiltrates (Fig. 12.5a). However, residual acinar units are still visible (arrows). Indeed, morphometric analysis has shown that only about 50% of the gland acinar or ductal tissue is replaced or destroyed (Fox 2002). This may seem surprising, because the kidneys and liver continue to function ably until their functional units are more than 90% destroyed.

Residual salivary gland tissue raises the possibility that substantial improvement is possible in SjS, presuming successful therapy against the glandular inflammation. The glandular tissue beyond the lymphoid infiltrate may retain its neural innervation. Studies in man and murine models have indicated the presence of receptors for acetylcholine and other critical neurotransmitters. The release of and response to neurotransmitters are strongly influenced by inflammatory cytokines, including Tumor necrosis factor (TNF) and IL-1. Unfortunately, broad-spectrum immunosuppressive approaches such as glucocorticoids and conventional immunosuppressive agents are not effective in treating the sicca symptoms of SjS. New treatment strategies are required.

Pearl: Salivary flow rates can be evaluated by minimally invasive methods.

Comment: Many individuals who do not have SjS complain of dry mouth. Moreover, patients' symptoms of dry mouth correlate very poorly with actual salivary flow rates. Thus, it is important to correlate patients' symptoms with objective signs of dryness. Technetium scans of salivary function are performed after coating the tongue with a lemon concentrate (Hakansson et al. 1994; Helman et al. 1987; Kohn et al. 1992). The uptake of contrast material by the gland and its rate of secretion into the mouth can be quantified reliably. Although the decreased flow rate is not specific to SjS, a Technetium scan can be useful

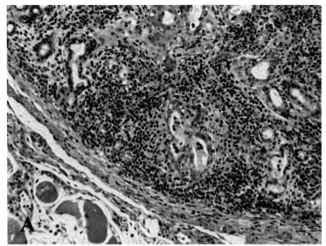

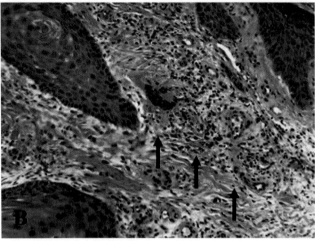

Figs. 12.5 (a, b) In a lip biopsy from a Sjögren's syndrome patient with severe dryness, attention is usually focused on the dense lymphoid infiltrates. In this biopsy of a labial minor salivary gland from a patient with primary SjS, follicular colonization of neoplastic B cell lymphocytes are evident (*arrowheads*). Remnants of follicular dentritic cells are also present (*arrows*) [Figure courtesy of Dr. H.M. Moutsopoulos]

in the evaluation of the patient who complains that "I don't feel any saliva in my mouth," yet has a normal salivary pool.

Pearl: The "sponge method" is more effective as a contraceptive than as a measure of salivary production.

Comment: A variety of methods of quantifying salivary production have been devised through the years. Most of these are as ineffective as they are cumbersome. As an example, in the Saxon test, saliva is collected on a preweighed sponge placed under the tongue (Kohler and Winter 1985). Substantial intra-patient variability is observed over the course of the same day. The Saxon test can be affected by factors such as the time since the last meal, teethbrushing, history of smoking, and medications (Stevens et al. 1990).

Pearl: Magnetic resonance imaging (MRI) sialography has virtually replaced invasive procedures for visualizing the ductal structure of major salivary glands.

Comment: Sialograms to assess the salivary status of SjS patients or to visualize the ductal structures for punctal sialadenitis are unnecessary. Sialograms have been largely replaced by gadolinium-enhanced MR studies with "fat suppression" views, which provide an excellent means of evaluating glandular tissues (Jungehulsing et al. 1999; Makula et al. 2000). This advance is fortunate, because few medical centers had sufficient experience with retrograde sialography to perform the procedure safely and well, anyway.

In any event, the role of ductal structure visualization in the assessment of the salivary component of SjS (by either injection sialography or MRI sialography) remains peripheral to other better established means such as minor gland biopsy or measuring unstimulated flow rate.

Pearl: A dry mouth is not necessarily a painful mouth.

Comment: The physician should look for signs of oral candidiasis such as angular cheilitis, atrophy or loss of filiform papillae on the dorsal tongue, or erythematous changes on the hard pallate, as well as lichen planus-like changes in buccal recess (see Fig. 12.3).

Many patients develop dry mouth as they age (Hershkovich et al. 2007; Nagler 2004). This is not a "normal part of the aging process," but rather a consequence of chronically administered prescription drugs. However, some event usually brings the patient to clinical attention. Frequently, a dry mouth is converted to a painful mouth by the occurrence of oral yeast infections, particularly in a patient who is on glucocorticoids or has recently been taking antibiotics (Abraham et al. 1998; Almstahl et al. 1999; Rhodus and Michalowicz 2005). Alterations in the oral microbial flora, as well as relative decreases in the salivary flow of naturally occurring antifungal agents such as transferrin or calprotectin, histatins, and other small molecules of the defensin family, further predispose the SjS patient to oral candidiasis.

Oral candidiasis can present as reddish petechiae in the mouth, generally found on the hard palate (see Fig. 12.3) (Daniels and Fox 1992; Daniels 2000). Denture removal may be required to observe the lesions.

Treatment of the oral candidiasis may require a rather prolonged treatment with topical antifungal drugs (Wu and Fox 1994), using mouth rinses similar to those employed by the radiation therapists and topical application of nystatins (Daniels 2000).

Pearl: Complaints of symptoms of "mouth burning" are common in clinical practice and often have explanations besides a systemic autoimmune condition such as SjS.

Comment: Other causes of burning mouth syndrome must also be considered, including: nutritional deficiencies, hormonal changes associated with menopause, local oral infections, denture-related lesions, hypersensitivity reactions, medications, and systemic diseases including diabetes mellitus

(Maltsman-Tseikhin et al. 2007; Patton et al. 2007). In many cases, no clear cause can be found, and the burning mouth is attributed to a local neuropathy or to a manifestation of depression.

In one study of 45 patients with the complaint of a burning mouth in whom no cause could be established (Patton et al. 2007), either a localized neuropathy or psychogenic etiology was suggested as the cause. A therapeutic trial of topical clonazapam and antioxidants (alpha-lipoic acid) was employed in some patients. Systemic agents such as gabapentin, pregabalin, or antidepressants with benefit in neuropathy (SjSRIs, SNSRIs, or NSRIs) have been employed in other patients. Agents with known anticholinergic side effects such as tricyclic antidepressants are not tolerated well.

Pearl: Decreased saliva volume can lead to complaints of dysphagia.

Comment: Subjective difficulty swallowing is one of the symptoms elicited in the diagnostic criteria for SjS. Some SjS patients have an underlying esophageal motility disorder that is part of their connective tissue disease syndrome. However, most patients with this complaint have adequate mechanical deglutition (Mandl et al. 2007a). The reported dysphagia results from the decreased volume and increased viscosity of saliva that are characteristic of SjS, which do not provide adequate "bulk" for swallowing (Belafsky and Postma 2003). This imbalance due to decreased saliva volume and content predisposes to dysfunction of the gastroesophageal sphincter, leading to gastroesophageal and laryngotracheal reflux. Laryngotracheal reflux should be suspected if the patient repeatedly clears her throat during conversation or has unexplained hoarseness.

Pearl: SjS patients have more difficulty swallowing certain types of tablets or capsules than other patients.

Comment: SjS patients have deglutition problems, as noted. As a result, they have difficulty with both swallowing and esophageal transit of many medications. When available, the use of smaller, "polished" tablets is preferred. An example is "branded" Plaquenil (hydroxychloroquine), which is a polished tablet, compared with some generic forms of the drug that are larger in size and contain a residue with bitter taste on the unpolished surface. Other unpolished capsules, e.g., those containing iron, can adhere to the dry esophageal mucosa, where they cause erosion. For these reasons, "polished" (coated) tablets are preferred to "sticky" capsules.

Myth: Symptoms and signs of chronic dry mouth are managed adequately by prescribing pilocarpine or cevimeline.

Reality: Sialogogues such as pilocarpine or cevimeline increase saliva production to some degree in all patients who have remaining salivary tissue. However, normal levels of secretion are not restored by these interventions. Although the drugs reduce oral symptoms in many patients, they do not have any effect on the prevention of dental caries, which are progressive in most patients with significant hyposalivation. They also seem to have no effect on reducing or preventing oral candidiasis.

Managing the oral manifestations of chronic hyposalivation varies with its severity, but in general requires: (1) that patients are supervised adequately in a program of dental caries prevention and treatment; (2) recognition and treatment of oral candidiasis (usually of the chronic erythematous type, which occurs in about one-third of SjS patients); and (3) reduction of their oral symptoms. Oral symptoms can be reduced by the prescription of a sialogogue, the use of a saliva substitute, and by the elimination of drugs with anticholinergic effects.

12.5 Parotid and Submandibular Involvement

Myth: Isolated submandibular gland enlargement is typical of SjS.

Reality: Patients with SjS have a range of major salivary gland involvement, but isolated submandibular gland enlargement is an atypical finding that should make one consider other

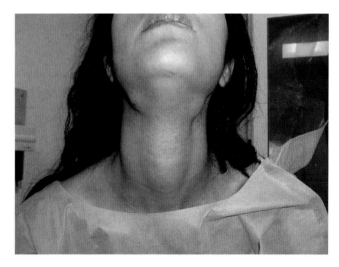

Fig. 12.6 Isolated submandibular gland enlargement. This finding is atypical of Sjögren's syndrome. This patient was sent for rheumatologic evaluation because of xerostomia and major salivary gland enlargement, but she had no parotid enlargement. A left submandibular adenectomy yielded the diagnosis of chronic sclerosing sialadenitis with intense IgG4-staining plasma cells within the gland. These findings were consistent with IgG4-associated systemic disease, a spectrum of conditions in which elevated levels of IgG4 are often found within serum and tissue infiltration of IgG4-producing plasma cells is found within the pancreas, biliary ducts, salivary glands, and other organs [Figure courtesy of Dr. John Stone]

disorders (Fig. 12.6). A variety of hematopoietic malignancies and carcinomas can cause submandibular gland enlargement, as can amyloidosis and certain chronic infections such as tuberculosis. A more recently recognized cause of submandibular gland enlargement is IgG4-associated systemic disease, a disorder in which IgG4-producing plasma cells infiltrate certain exocrine glands, e.g., the salivary glands, pancreas, and biliary tract (Kamisawa and Okamoto 2006).

In a classic paper on SjS, the clinical presentations of 62 SjS patients were reported (Bloch et al. 1965). Thirty-four of the patients (55%) had parotid gland enlargement and 10 (16%) had submandibular gland enlargement, but not a single patient had isolated submandibular gland disease (i.e., submandibular gland enlargement without parotid enlargement).

Myth: Parotid gland enlargement in patients with primary SjS often responds to a course of glucocorticoids.

Reality: Parotid gland enlargement does not respond to glucocorticoids. The recommended therapy is the local application of heat. If a superimposed infection is suspected, antibiotic therapy is mandatory.

Pearl: Salivary gland enlargement in SjS must be considered carefully.

Comment: Salivary gland enlargement is observed in approximately one-third of patients with primary SjS or secondary SjS. Enlarged salivary glands are usually bilateral, firm to palpation, either symmetrical or asymmetrical in size, and minimally symptomatic. Enlargement can be episodic, with gradual waxing and waning, or chronic, with gradual progression over months or years. The parotid glands, submandibular glands, or both may be affected. Reports from two well-documented cohorts found salivary gland enlargement on examination in 39 and 43% of primary SjS patients and 31 and 24% of secondary SjS patients, respectively (Bloch et al. 1965, Daniels et al. 1975). Other conditions that can cause bilateral salivary gland enlargement are listed in Table 12.4.

Table 12.4 Bilateral salivary gland enlargement – differential diagnosis

Sjögren's syndrome[a] (lymphoepithelial lesion)
Viral infections[b]
Chronic granulomatous diseases[a] (e.g., sarcoidosis)
Sialadenosis[c] (associated with: diabetes mellitus, acromegaly, gonadal hypofunction, hyperlipoproteinemia, hepatic cirrhosis, anorexia/bulimia, or pancreatitis)
Recurrent parotitis of childhood

[a]Associated with chronic salivary hypofunction
[b]Mumps is usually acute but CMV, HIV, and Coxsackie may cause prolonged enlargement
[c]Sialadenosis (idiopathic acinar hypertrophy) affects parotid glands only; always bilaterally symmetrical enlargement that is soft and nontender to palpation; not associated with symptoms or signs of salivary hypofunction; diagnosis by clinical presentation and disease association; biopsy of affected glands is unnecessary (From Klippel et al. 2008. With kind permission from Springer Science + Business Media.)

Gradually increasing swelling of parotid glands in SjS may be associated with an enlarging benign lymphoepithelial lesion or MALT lymphoma. An incisional biopsy is required to distinguish between these two entities. A rapid increase in the size of an enlarged gland associated with symptoms and signs of acute inflammation suggests a superimposed bacterial sialoadenitis and calls for systemic antibiotic treatment. However, rapid increase in glandular swelling without signs of acute inflammation often heralds transformation to a high-grade lymphoma or other malignant neoplasm. Tissue examination is obviously indicated in this setting.

Pearl: Glandular enlargement in SjS can wax and wane.

Comment: The course of glandular enlargement in SjS varies from patient to patient. Some develop parotid enlargement that persists largely unchanged for years. In others, the glandular involvement waxes and wanes over periods of several weeks or months. This is often asymmetric.

12.6 Extraglandular Involvement

Myth: Sicca symptoms are usually the first manifestation of SjS.

Reality: A chronic, asymmetric, purely sensory neuropathy can be the first manifestation of SjS. Sensory symptoms precede the development of other clinical features by several years in some patients (Mori et al. 2005; Denislic and Meh 1997). Sensory deficits may be accompanied by an autonomic neuropathy (Dyck 2005).

Pearl: Dysphagia in primary SjS patients can be caused by esophageal dysmotility.

Comment: Patterns of esophageal dysmotility observed in primary SjS include aperistalsis, triphasic tertiary contractions, frequent nonperistaltic contractions, and low contractions (Tsianos et al. 1985). These esophageal abnormalities do not correlate with the parotid flow rate, the degree of inflammatory infiltrate of the minor salivary glands, the extraglandular manifestations, or the presence of autoantibodies.

Myth: Cutaneous vasculitis in SjS is usually a lymphocytic vasculitis.

Reality: In fact, vasculitis of the skin in SjS is usually leukocytoclastic. The most common clinical feature of this is palpable purpura (Ramos-Casals et al. 2004a). Cryoglobulinemia is present in up to 30% of vasculitis cases associated with SjS. As discussed elsewhere in this chapter, this cryoglobulinemia is typically part and parcel of the SjS rather than a complication of a hepatitis C infection.

Other prominent features of skin vasculitis in SjS are:

- Urticarial lesions in approximately 25%.
- Medium-vessel disease that mimics polyarteritis nodosa (Fig. 12.7). Fortunately, this occurs in less than 5% of SjS patients with vasculitis.

Myth: Patients with primary SjS suffer from erosive symmetrical arthritis.

Reality: The arthritis of primary SjS is characterized by short-lived episodes of joint inflammation that remit spontaneously, usually within days. This arthropathy resembles a similar

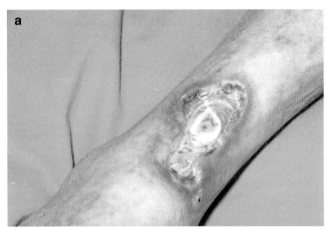

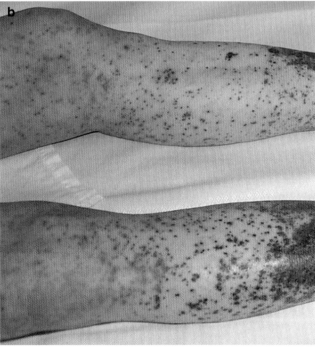

Figs. 12.7 (**a**, **b**) Medium-vessel vasculitis (**a**) that mimics polyarteritis nodosa is an unusual complication of Sjögren's syndrome (SjS), occurring in less than 5% of patients. The more common form of cutaneous vasculitis in SjS is palpable purpura (**b**), which is usually associated with a leukocytoclastic as opposed to lymphocytic vasculitis. [Figure 12.7a and b courtesy of Manuel Ramos-Casals and H.M. Moutsopoulos]

disease manifestation observed in patients with SLE. The recurrent arthritic episodes in primary SjS and SLE patients can lead to hand deformities called Jaccoud's arthropathy. In primary SjS, this arthritis is not one of an erosive, joint-destructive nature (Tsampoulas et al. 1986). In contrast, a patient who's SjS is secondary to rheumatoid arthritis typically develops joint erosions.

Pearl: The clinical course of Raynaud's phenomenon is milder in primary SjS than in other autoimmune diseases such as systemic sclerosis.

Comment: Raynaud's phenomenon is an early clinical feature of SjS in nearly 50% of patients and can appear before sicca symptomatology (Skopouli et al. 1990; Youinou et al. 1990; García-Carrasco et al. 2002b). The clinical course of Raynaud's phenomenon is milder in primary SjS than in other systemic autoimmune diseases such as systemic sclerosis, in which this complication is often associated with digital ulcers and ischemia. In primary SjS, Raynaud's phenomenon is rarely accompanied by vascular complications and only 40% of patients require pharmacological treatment.

Myth: Interstitial fibrosis is the predominant form of pulmonary involvement in primary SjS.

Reality: Various studies have recently analyzed pulmonary involvement in primary SjS (Papiris et al. 1999; Taouli et al. 2002; Franquet et al. 1999). Most investigators have reported a predominance of bronchial and bronchiolar involvement rather than interstitial disease. One study identified the ground-glass pattern as the predominant pattern observed on computed tomography, but this coexisted with bronchiectasis in some cases (Fig. 12.8) (Wright et al. 2003). The typical symptoms of patients with bronchial or bronchiolar disease are cough, dyspnea, and recurrent respiratory infections.

Pearl: SjS patients are more likely to develop mucus plugs.

Comment: SjS patients suffer not only from dryness of the eyes and mouth, but also from dryness of the skin, vagina, and bronchi. Bronchial dryness becomes especially important in two situations. First, in the presence of upper airway infection, there is a predilection to develop inspissated mucus plugs. This tendency can be exacerbated by over-the-counter cold preparations, which usually contain anticholinergic drugs. Second, mucus plugs may occur postoperatively as a result of both the anticholinergic drugs used during anesthesia and the dehydration sustained during surgery.

Pearl: Dry cough, a common manifestation of SjS, often indicates the presence of airway involvement and desiccation.

Comment: A chronic, nonproductive cough in a patient with primary SjS should alert the clinician to the possibility of bronchitis sicca. The most common symptom of laryngeal, tracheal, and bronchial involvement is a dry, persistent cough.

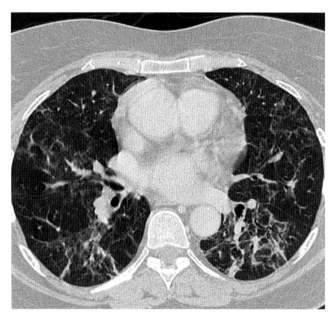

Fig. 12.8 Bronchiectasis and ground-glass pattern in a 62-year-old woman with primary Sjögren's syndrome and interstitial lung disease [Figure courtesy of Dr. Manuel Ramos-Casals]

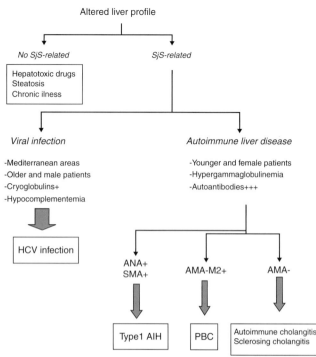

Fig. 12.9 Algorithm for the evaluation of abnormal liver function tests in Sjögren's syndrome. AIH = autoimmune hepatitis; PBC = primary biliary cirrhosis; ANA = antinuclear antibody; SMA = anti-smooth muscle antibody; AMA = antimitochondrial antibody [Figure courtesy of Dr. Manuel Ramos-Casals]

If the patient does not have other features of SjS, the diagnosis may be missed and the patient treated incorrectly for asthma or bronchitis. Despite the fact that upper airway symptoms afflict 50–70% of patients with SjS, only 20% have abnormalities that can be identified by rhinoscopy or indirect laryngoscopy (Freeman et al. 2005).

The underlying pathology in these patients consists of peribronchial infiltrates that lead to small airway disease (Papiris et al. 1999). The classic pulmonary function test manifestation of this disease complication is a decreased MEF25–75. Chest radiographs in these individuals are usually normal or show an ill-defined pattern of infiltrates that suggests interstitial lung disease. High-resolution computed tomography of the lungs reveals thickened bronchial walls. Lymphocytic interstitial pneumonitis evolves only rarely.

Bronchitis sicca does not respond well to bronchodilators. However, the oral administration of pilocarpine hydrochloride (20 mg/day) may be helpful.

Pearl: The development of pleurisy in a patient with SjS signals the presence of an additional autoimmune condition.

Comment: Pleurisy is an extremely rare manifestation of primary SjS. In contrast, in patients with secondary SjS, pleurisy occurs in up to 30% (Moutsopoulos et al. 1979b; Manoussakis et al. 2004).

Pearl: Hepatitis C virus (HCV) infection is an important cause of liver function test abnormalities in patients with SjS in some geographic areas.

Comment: Chronic HCV infection was the main cause of liver dysfunction in a large series of patients with SjS, with a

prevalence of 13% (Ramos-Casals et al. 2006b). HCV infections were nearly 3 times more common as a cause of liver disease than was autoimmune hepatitis. Of course, the prevalence of HCV infection varies widely in different regions of the world, but this finding (from Spain) underscores the importance of chronic HCV infection as a cause of liver disease in SjS patients from regions with a high HCV prevalence.

Myth: "Liver function tests" differentiate cleanly between autoimmune and viral hepatitis in patients with primary SjS.

Reality: The major forms of liver disease that are relevant to SjS are primary biliary cirrhosis, autoimmune liver disease, and HCV infection. The differential diagnosis of liver disease in patients with primary SjS is important, because the therapeutic approaches and prognoses of the various forms of hepatic dysfunction in this disease vary substantially (see Algorithm, Fig. 12.9). Unfortunately, routine laboratory tests are not helpful in distinguishing among the common forms of liver disease in SjS or in differentiating such hepatic complications from HCV infection. Serum concentrations of hepatic transaminases (aspartate and alanine aminotransferase), gamma glutaryl transferase, bilirubin, and alkaline phosphatase are all elevated to a similar degree in patients with primary biliary cirrhosis, autoimmune hepatitis, and HCV infection.

Immunological evaluations are also imperfect in differentiating among viral-associated and autoimmune causes of hepatic dysfunction (Ramos-Casals et al. 2006b). Patients with chronic HCV infection have a higher frequency of cryoglobulins and low complement levels, but patients with SjS can have these abnormalities, too. Patients with autoimmune liver disease have a higher frequency of autoantibodies such as antismooth muscle and antimitochondrial antibodies, but variability in the quality of autoantibody assays across different laboratories often makes these data less helpful than one would wish.

Pearl: Elevated liver enzymes (2–3 times) or antimitochondrial antibodies in the serum of a patient with primary SjS suggest that the patient has autoimmune cholangiitis.

Comment: Approximately 5% of patients with primary SjS have asymptomatic elevation of liver enzymes or antimitochondrial antibodies (Skopouli et al. 1994a). Liver biopsy in these patients shows lymphocytic infiltrates around bile ducts, reminiscent of early primary biliary cirrhosis (stage I-II). The progression of these lesions is very slow and usually does not lead to liver failure.

This clinical entity must be distinguished from the IgG4-associated systemic disease described above, which can mimic SjS through its involvement of submandibular glands and also affect the biliary tree (Kamisawa and Okamoto 2006).

Myth: An asymptomatic increase of serum amylase levels in a patient with primary SjS should alert the clinician to the possibility of pancreatic cancer development.

Reality: High serum amylase levels are detected in one-fourth of patients with primary SjS patients (Tsianos et al. 1984). In the majority of these individuals, the amylase arises from the inflamed salivary glands. In a small percentage of primary SjS patients, the amylase originates from the pancreas. The later group of individuals suffers from subclinical pancreatitis.

Myth: Pancreatitis is a common extraglandular feature of SjS.

Reality: Studies in the 1970s and 1980s found a high frequency of altered pancreatic function in primary SjS (>40%), although no data were presented on the clinical significance of these altered tests. These studies led to the consideration of pancreatic involvement as one of the typical extraglandular features of primary SjS. However, the frequency of clinical pancreatitis is very low in large series of patients with primary SjS (<2%) (Ramos-Casals et al. 2008). In patients with primary SjS, pancreatic involvement is usually asymptomatic and is demonstrated by altered pancreatic function tests. Clinically significant pancreatitis in primary SjS is rare.

Some of the early reports of "pancreatitis" occurring in association with "SjS" may actually represent cases of IgG4-related systemic disease, an emerging spectrum of illness that can affect multiple exocrine organs but which appears to be a different entity altogether compared with primary SjS

(Yamamoto et al. 2005). The concept of IgG4-related systemic disease is discussed elsewhere in this chapter.

Pearl: Glomerulonephritis is a rare complication of primary SjS.

Comment: Tubulointerstitial disease is regarded widely as the most common form of renal dysfunction in primary SjS. However, both tubular and glomerular diseases have important pathogenic, clinical, and prognostic implications in primary SjS. Among 27 SjS patients with documented renal biopsy reported in the literature (Bossini et al. 2001; Goules et al. 2000), 15 had tubulointerstitial nephritis, 11 had glomerulonephritis, and one had both tubulointerstitial disease and glomerulonephritis.

Among the patients with glomerulonephritis, the most common glomerular lesions were membranoproliferative (seven patients), mesangial proliferative (six patients), and membranous (two patients). Cryoglobulinemia was detected in half of the patients with glomerulonephritis. Only two patients ultimately developed end-stage renal disease.

Tubulointerstitial disease in SjS, which is usually found in younger patients, is characterized by an indolent course in which renal dysfunction is often subclinical. IgM and complement proteins comprise the primary deposits in the glomerulonephritis of SjS. This contrasts with the immunopathologic lesion of lupus nephritis, in which a "full house" of immunoreactant deposition (immunoglobulin and complement) is observed (Moutsopoulos et al. 1978). SjS glomerulonephritis usually responds to glucocorticoids at a starting dose of 0.5–1.0 mg/kg of body weight per day.

Pearl: Recurrent renal colic in a patient with primary SjS suggests that the patient has interstitial nephritis.

Comment: Interstitial nephritis can be an early manifestation of SjS (Goules et al. 2000). This condition is usually subclinical, and is manifested (if sought) by a low urine specific gravity (hyposthenuria) and an alkaline urine pH. An elevated serum creatinine seldom occurs as a complication of interstitial nephritis.

Nephrocalcinosis that presents with renal colic is a common clinical expression of distal renal tubular dysfunction in these patients. The classic renal manifestation of SjS is a distal RTA caused by interstitial nephritis. The distal RTA can lead to hypokalemia. Patients who develop distal RTAs may require spironolactone to control hypokalemia, but the use of loop diuretics should be discouraged as this may exacerbate hypokalemia. Proximal RTAs, which can lead to osteomalacia and the Fanconi syndrome, are rare in SjS (but reported) (Goules et al. 2000).

Pearl: A wide range of peripheral neuropathies can complicate SjS.

Comment: Early attention to peripheral neuropathies is extremely important. Sensory neuropathies and dorsal root ganglionopathies are the most common forms that afflict SjS patients (Mellgren et al. 2007). The pathological findings in cases of sensory ganglionopathy consist of loss of neuronal cell bodies and the infiltration of T cells.

Peripheral motor neuropathies can include mononeuritis multiplex (which stems from vasculitis) or CIDP (chronic idiopathic demyelinating polyneuropathy), the latter of which is linked in some cases to antimyelin associated glycoprotein. SjS patients can also suffer trigeminal and other cranial neuropathies, autonomic neuropathy, and mixed patterns of neuropathy.

Sural nerve biopsy may show vascular or perivascular inflammation of small epineurial vessels (both arterioles and venules) and in some cases necrotizing vasculitis. The loss of myelinated nerve fibers is common and loss of small-diameter nerve fibers occurs. Peripheral neuropathy in primary SjS often is refractory to treatment with currently available agents.

Pearl: Some patients with primary SjS present with a painful sensory neuropathy but normal nerve conduction studies.

Comment: Small-fiber neuropathy occurs in patients with primary SjS (Mori 2003; Gorson 2003). These patients often present with burning pain in the feet. Small-fiber neuropathy can develop either in isolation as the sole neurologic manifestation of disease, or in combination with larger sensory fiber involvement. The diagnosis often relies on quantitative sensory testing and sural nerve biopsy, but skin biopsy is an increasingly useful technique for demonstrating small-fiber neuropathy (Chai et al. 2005). The pathological finding on skin biopsy is a decrease in the density of epidermal nerve fibers (Gøransson et al. 2006). Patients with small-fiber neuropathy have normal nerve conduction studies, because the size of nerve fibers involved is below the resolution of conventional electrodiagnostic studies.

Pearl: Sensory neuropathy in primary SjS evolves in a chronic, insidious manner and usually demonstrates a poor response to glucocorticoids and immunosuppressive agents.

Comment: Sensory neuropathy becomes symptomatic before the underlying disorder is recognized in nearly half of primary SjS cases. The majority of patients with sensory neuropathies (>70%) have a long-term, insidious evolution of their symptoms (Font et al. 2003). The symptoms are generally refractory to treatment with glucocorticoids and immunosuppressive agents (Font et al. 2003). Recent reports have suggested a better therapeutic response to intravenous immunoglobulins and to rituximab (Gorson 2007).

Pearl: Patients who describe "light-headedness" should have their blood pressure and pulse checked when both supine and erect.

Comment: Autonomic neuropathy is common among SjS patients (Stojanovich et al. 2007; Mandl et al. 2007b).

Cardiovascular reflex tests are more likely to be abnormal in patients with SjS than among healthy controls.

Pearl: Trigeminal neuralgia is a common complication of primary SjS.

Comment: Peripheral neuropathy has been described in about 10–20% of patients with primary SjS. The major forms of neuropathy observed include sensory ataxic neuropathy, painful sensory neuropathy without sensory ataxia, trigeminal neuropathy, multiple mononeuropathy, multiple cranial neuropathy, autonomic neuropathy, and radiculoneuropathy. Trigeminal neuropathy is described in about 15% of patients with any kind of neuropathy. It is usually unilateral. The pain is distributed in the regions that are innervated by the branches of the trigeminal nerve.

Myth: Central nervous system vasculitis is among the most common extraglandular manifestations of primary SjS.

Reality: This association, described first in the late-1980s, is a matter of considerable controversy (Alexander et al. 1988). A wide variety of central nervous system (CNS) disease manifestations have been described in primary SjS patients. This pathology extends from cognitive dysfunction to dementia. Seizures, aseptic meningitis, multiple sclerosis-like lesions, and vasculitis have been also described. If the investigators of these studies had applied strict criteria for the classification of the disease, then the individuals with CNS involvement probably would have been categorized as suffering from overlap syndromes with features of both SjS and SLE (Ioannidis and Moutsopoulos 1999).

The frequency of true CNS disease among patients with "pure" primary SjS has probably been overestimated. In one study of more than 1,000 patients, symptomatic CNS involvement was observed in only 21 (<2%) (Ramos-Casals et al. 2008). Nevertheless, there is clearly a subset of patients who develop important neurological illnesses involving the brain and spinal cord. These comprise a subset of the patients who have antibodies directed against the Ro/SSA antigens. Some of these patients develop neurological features of a disease that are extremely difficult to distinguish from multiple sclerosis or from SLE associated with antiphospholipid antibodies (Delalande et al. 2004). The precise nature of this patient subset requires further study.

Pearl: SjS patients may develop myelopathy and optic neuritis, similar to "Devic's disease" in multiple sclerosis patients (MS).

Comment: The therapeutic issue for the rheumatologist is whether this represents central nervous system vasculitis that might require high-dose glucocorticoids or biologic agents, or whether the findings actually represent MS.

Initial studies on the correlation of MS and SjS were complicated by the "ascertainment" bias of patients with sicca symptoms that were referred to institutions specializing in MS. Other centers pointed out that MS patients often exhibit dryness in the absence of positive salivary gland biopsies, leading to the suggestion that their dryness is due to central nervous involvement involving the cholinergic outflow tracts.

Myth: An MS patient with a positive ANA has SjS.

Reality: A common clinical question is whether the finding of ANA in a patient with an abnormal brain MRI means that the patient has SjS with involvement of the central nervous system. Addressing this question has been challenging, because positive ANA results are found in normal individuals and in up to 20% of MS patients who lack any other evidence of a connective tissue disorder (Collard et al. 1997; Ferreira et al. 2005).

Pearl: More than 25% of patients with primary SjS have sensorineural hearing loss.

Comment: Sensorineural hearing loss was detected in 38 of 140 primary SjS patients (27%) whose results were pooled from four studies (Ramos-Casals et al. 2006a, b). Associations with immunologic parameters such as ANA, antiphospholipid antibodies, and anti-Ro/SSA or anti-La/SSB antibodies have been postulated but not proven. Sensorineural hearing loss in primary SjS preferentially affects high-frequency hearing, but deficits often remain subclinical (Boki et al. 2001). Retrocochlear disease and symptoms of vestibular dysfunction are not typical of SjS.

Pearl: Patients with primary SjS are at increased risk for lymphoma.

Comment: Primary SjS patients are at higher risk of lymphoma than are healthy individuals and patients with other autoimmune diseases (Kassan et al. 1978). Different studies have estimated the relative risk of lymphoma in patients with primary SjS when compared with the general population to range from 10- to 44-fold.

A meta-analysis of five studies in four different countries that included a combined total of 1,200 primary SjS patients confirmed the high risk of non-Hodgkin's lymphoma and calculated a standardized incidence rate (SIR) of 18.8 (Zintzaras et al. 2005). This SIR contrasts with those for SLE and RA of 7.4 and 3.9, respectively, from the same study.

Lymphoma tends to occur in a subgroup of SjS patients who express special risk factors early in their disease course. These risk factors include palpable purpura and C4 hypocomplementemia. This patient subgroup has increased mortality (Skopouli et al. 2000; Ioannidis et al. 2002). The long-term risk of lymphoma for patients with primary SjS is often estimated to be on the order of 5%.

Pearl: Persistently hard enlargement of the lacrimal or parotid glands in a patient with primary SjS should alert the clinician to the possibility of an extra-lymphoid lymphoma.

Comment: Lymphomas that develop in primary SjS patients are extranodal in 80% of cases. The most common site of extranodal lymphoma development is the salivary glands (Fig. 12.10). Ninety percent of primary SjS patients who develop lymphoma have histories of major salivary gland enlargement during their disease course (Fig. 12.11). Nearly 30% of such patients have persistent as opposed to intermittent glandular enlargement (Voulgarelis et al. 1999).

Myth: The incidence of fibromyalgia in SjS patients is the same as in the general population.

Reality: An increased prevalence of fibromyalgia is found in both SjS and SLE. In fact, the chronic fatigue and myalgias are such prevalent factors that they have made clinical drug development rather difficult, because fibromyalgia symptoms

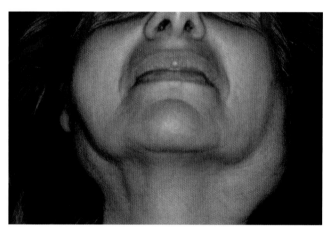

Fig. 12.10 The most common site of extranodal lymphoma development in Sjögren's syndrome is the salivary glands. This figure reveals parotid gland enlargement in a patient with primary SjS who has developed extranodal lymphoma during follow-up [Figure courtesy of Dr. Haralampos M. Moutsopoulos]

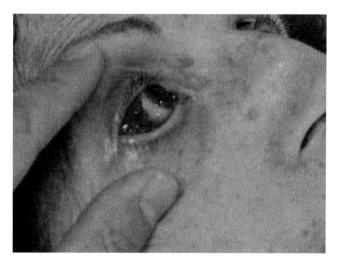

Fig. 12.11 Ocular B cell lymphoma in a patient with Sjögren's syndrome and chronic hepatitis C virus (HCV) infection [Figure courtesy of Dr. Manuel Ramos-Casals]

constitute a sizeable effect on patients' quality-of-life evaluations (Bowman et al. 2004; Pillemer et al. 2005).

Pearl: Thyroid disease is more frequent in SjS patients.

Comment: The most common thyroid disorder found in association with SjS is autoimmune thyroiditis (Jara et al. 2007). Subclinical hypothyroidism is common among patients with primary SjS. In one study, primary SjS was 10 times more frequent in patients with autoimmune thyroid disease, and autoimmune thyroiditis was 9 times more frequent in primary SjS.

One dissenting case-control study reported no significant differences in patients with primary SjS and a group of age- and sex-matched controls (Ramos-Casals et al. 2000). In that study, subclinical hypothyroidism affected 11% of the cases and 8% of the controls.

Pearl: Dyspareunia is a common premenopausal complaint of primary SjS.

Comment: Almost half of premenopausal women with primary SjS complain of dyspareunia (Skopouli et al. 1994b). Such symptoms are uncommon in age-matched control women and when present generally have an obvious etiology (trauma or inflammation). Despite dyspareunia, primary SjS patients appear to have similar frequency of sexual activity, fertility, and parity when compared with age-matched controls.

Pearl: Salivary gland toxicity may accompany the treatment of thyroiditis of 131-iodine.

Comment: Salivary gland toxicity is a potential adverse effect of high-dose radioiodine (131-I) (Hyer et al. 2007). One study of 20 patients revealed that 11 (15%) had symptoms of xerostomia within the first 48 h of receiving such therapy. These symptoms persisted for at least 12 months in seven patients. Medical or surgical interventions may be preferable to radioiodine administration in patients with SjS, whose salivary production is already compromised.

Pearl: Urinary tract symptoms and cystitis are underdiagnosed in primary SjS.

Comment: Two recent studies have investigated lower urinary tract symptoms in primary SjS. Severe urological symptoms (increased frequency, urgency, and nocturia) were reported in 61% of patients in one study (Walker et al. 2003). Biopsy-proven interstitial cystitis was found in some cases. Another study found that 5% of SjS patients fulfilled the criteria for interstitial cystitis (Leppilahti et al. 2003).

12.7 Laboratory Findings

Pearl: The height of the erythrocyte sedimentation rate (ESR) is SjS correlates with the level of immunoglobulins in the serum.

Comment: Elevated ESRs in SjS correlate directly with the degree of hypergammaglobulinemia (Ramos-Casals et al. 2002). Moreover, both these parameters are normally found in patients with primary SjS who are rheumatoid factor positive or who have autoantibodies directed against either the Ro/SSA or La/SSB antigens. Clinicians who observe high ESRs in patients with SjS should therefore not leap to conclusions about occult infections, subclinical malignancies, or the presence of systemic vasculitis; the abnormality may simply be the SjS itself. In such patients, the C-reactive protein is usually normal.

Pearl: Highly elevated serum C-reactive protein levels in a patient with primary SjS should raise the suspicion of an infection.

Comment: Patients with primary SjS typically do not mount an acute phase response related to their disease itself, at least not one associated with elevated C-reactive protein levels (Moutsopoulos et al. 1983a). The finding of a strikingly elevated serum C-reactive protein should trigger careful scrutiny for an infection. Systemic vasculitis occurring in the setting of primary SjS can also lead to an elevated C-reactive protein level.

Pearl: Patients with anti-Ro/SSA or anti-La/SSB antibodies often develop leukopenia or thrombocytopenia.

Comment: The relationship between anti-Ro/SSA antibodies and hematologic alterations was described in the early 1980s in a study of 75 patients (Alexander et al. 1983). This link was confirmed in a multivariate analysis of data on 400 primary SjS patients, which found that leukopenia was associated with anti-Ro/SSA antibodies and thrombocytopenia with anti-La/SSB antibodies (García-Carrasco et al. 2002a). In a series of 1,010 Spanish patients with primary SjS, the odds ratio of leukopenia associated with anti-Ro/SSA antibodies was 2.6. The odds ratio of thrombocytopenia associated with anti-La/SSB antibodies was 2.3 (Ramos-Casals et al. 2008).

Pearl: Neutropenia is a relevant hematologic finding in primary SjS.

Comment: The neutrophil count should be monitored in SjS patients, especially in those with recurrent infections. Nearly 30% of patients with primary SjS have autoimmune neutropenia (Brito-Zerón et al. 2008). The percentage of patients with SjS who develop this hematological complication is substantially higher than that of other cytopenias, e.g., leukopenia or thrombocytopenia. Neutropenia is associated with a higher rate of hospital admission due to infection.

The occurrence of agranulocytosis is rare in primary SjS (only about 2% of patients). Agranulocytosis is observed primarily in patients with a hematopoietic malignancy (mainly B cell lymphoma). The etiopathogenic role of antineutrophil antibodies in such patients, if any, is unclear. Two studies have found no correlation between autoantibodies to surface neutrophil antigens among SjS patients who had agranulocytosis (Coppo et al. 2003; Lamour et al. 1995).

12.8 Immunological Assays

Pearl: The most likely autoimmune disease to develop in a woman with Raynaud's phenomenon and autoantibodies to Ro/SSA and La/SSB is primary SjS.

Comment: Raynaud's phenomenon is a common manifestation of patients with primary SjS. This feature appears up to many years before the diagnosis of SjS in approximately one-third of patients (Skopouli et al. 1990; Youinou et al. 1990; García-Carrasco et al. 2002b).

Myth: Serum from patients with primary SjS who do not have autoantibodies to Ro/SSA and La/SSB should be examined every 6–12 months to detect the appearance of these autoantibodies.

Reality: Anti-Ro and anti-La antibodies are present in the sera of primary SjS patients at or before the time of diagnosis. The probability that a seronegative primary SjS patient will become seropositive during follow-up is low. Thus, continued monitoring of the sera of primary SjS patients for autoantibodies to these antigens makes little sense (Skopouli et al. 2000).

Pearl: The presence of low serum C4 or palpable purpura in a patient with SjS may predict the development of lymphoma in patients with primary SjS.

Comment: Lymphomas developing in SjS may occur in the salivary glands, gastrointestinal tract, or lungs. They often begin as B cell MALT lymphomas or, in lymph nodes, as marginal zone lymphomas. After years of slow progression, these indolent tumors can progress to rapidly growing, high-grade, large B cell lymphomas.

Various studies have identified risk factors for lymphoma development. These include cryoglobulinemia, hypocomplementemia, extremely low C4 levels, and palpable purpura (Ioannidis et al. 2002). Additional risk factors for lymphoma development include the onset of SjS at a young age and prolonged salivary gland enlargement.

Pearl: Antismooth muscle antibodies have no clinical significance in SjS.

Comment: ANA play a central role in the immunological expression of primary SjS, due to the fact that they are usually caused by antibodies directed against extractable nuclear antigens (ENAs). However, the clinical significance

of autoantibodies directed against nonnuclear antigens, such as antismooth muscle antibodies, has not been studied thoroughly. In a series of 335 patients, antismooth muscle antibodies were detected in 208 (62%) (Nardi et al. 2006). However, no particular associations with any clinical feature or laboratory abnormality are yet known.

Pearl: Clinical events associated with antiparietal cell antibodies and antiphospholipid antibodies are uncommon in primary SjS.

Reality: In a study of 335 SjS patients, 208 (27%) had antiparietal cell antibodies but only two had either pernicious anemia or atrophic gastritis (Nardi et al. 2006). A literature review revealed only four other reported cases of pernicious anemia in primary SjS. These data support the concept that the co-occurrence of SjS and pernicious anemia is uncommon, despite the fact that both are associated with autoimmunity. A similar study of 281 patients found that 36 (13%) had antiphospholipid antibodies, but only four fulfilled the classification criteria for the antiphospholipid syndrome (Ramos-Casals et al. 2006a).

Pearl: The finding of a positive ANA with an anticentromere pattern may have important clinical implications in primary SjS.

Comment: Anticentromere antibodies are detectable by the proper interpretation of an immunofluorescence assay for ANA. However, because of the time-intensive nature of immunofluorescence studies, these assays have been replaced in many laboratories by enzyme immunoassays. Thus, in some clinical settings, anticentromere antibodies must be assayed by specific enzyme immunoassays.

The finding of anticentromere antibodies in patients presumed to have primary SjS may be important, particularly if assays for antibodies to the Ro/SSA and La/SSB antigens are negative (Salliot et al. 2007). SjS patients who have anticentromere antibodies represent a specific clinical subset, which may be classified initially as having primary SjS but have a higher probability of developing limited systemic sclerosis. In one study, one-fourth of such patients developed limited scleroderma (Ramos-Casals et al. 2006a). Prominent Raynaud's phenomenon, sclerodactyly, and nailfold capillaroscopic changes are clues to the presence of this clinical phenotype (Figs. 12.12a and 12.12b).

The critical feature may be the presence or absence of antibodies to the Ro/SSA and La/SSB antigens. Patients who have such antibodies may be more likely to behave as SjS rather than as limited scleroderma.

Myth: ANCA positivity strongly suggests a coexisting systemic vasculitis in patients with primary SjS.

Reality: ANCA positivity in SjS patients is common when sera are tested by immunofluorescence. The preponderance of patients who are ANCA-positive have perinuclear

Figs. 12.12 (**a, b**) Sjögren's syndrome patients who have anticentromere antibodies often have a clinical phenotype that resembles limited scleroderma: Raynaud's phenomenon, sclerodactyly, and nailfold capillaroscopic changes. Some would term this combination of findings an "overlap" connective tissue disorder. [Figure courtesy of Dr. Manuel Ramos-Casals]

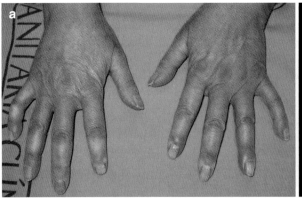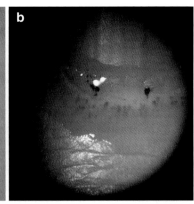

immunofluorescence pattern (Font et al. 1998). However, these ANCA are epiphenomena that appear irrelevant to disease pathogenesis or any particular clinical complication of the disease. When cutaneous or systemic vasculitis occurs in SjS, the usual underlying cause is cryoglobulinemia, not ANCA (Terrier et al. 2007).

Myth: A serum monoclonal gammopathy is associated with an underlying hematological neoplasm in most patients with primary SjS.

Reality: Circulating monoclonal immunoglobulins or/and free monoclonal light chains are detected in the serum of a considerable number of extraglandular SjS patients (Moutsopoulos et al. 1983b; Brito-Zerón et al. 2005). The monoclonal light chains are also detected in the urine of SjS patients (Moutsopoulos et al. 1985). The monoclonal spike in the serum usually consists of IgG, but other types of immunoglobulins have also been reported. Despite the high frequency of monoclonal immunoglobulins in SjS, only around 5% of SjS patients ultimately develop a B-lymphocyte malignancy.

Pearl: Serum monoclonal gammopathy often indicates the presence of an underlying type II mixed cryoglobulinemia.

Comment: In patients with primary SjS, detection of serum monoclonal immunoglobulins may indicate cryoglobulinemia. However, a significant percentage of patients with primary SjS and cryoglobulinemia have insufficient amounts of cryoprecipitate (<5%) for immunofixation testing (Brito-Zerón et al. 2005). The detection of an IgM kappa monoclonal spike on serum immunoelectrophoresis strongly suggests a type II mixed cryoglobulinemia. This consists most commonly of a monoclonal IgM kappa component and polyclonal IgG.

12.9 Differential Diagnosis

Pearl: SjS-associated with HCV has a distinct clinical and immunological profile but overlaps substantially with primary SjS.

Comment: The clinical expression of SjS-HCV is similar to primary SjS with respect to the prevalence of glandular features and the fulfillment of the 2002 criteria, but differs in having a higher prevalence of cryoglobulinemia, liver involvement, and neoplasia (mainly B cell lymphoma). The immunological expression of SjS-HCV includes a higher percentage of patients who are anti-Ro/SSA and anti-La/SSB antibody negative. Patients with SjS-HCV are also more likely to have cryoglobulins. This accounts for the higher prevalence of rheumatoid factor in their sera and hypocomplementemia (particularly C4 hypocomplementemia) (Ramos-Casals et al. 2005).

Pearl: The etiopathologic and clinical significance of HTLV-I infection in patients with SjS varies depending on the geographical area.

Comment: In Japan, where HTLV-I is endemic, nearly 25% of patients with primary SjS have HTLV-I infection (Nakamura et al. 2000). HTLV-I is now considered the viral counterpart in Asian countries to HCV in the Mediterranean region. Although genomic sequences of HTLV-I have been detected in European patients with primary SjS, in one study the prevalence of HTLV-I was similar between the SjS and control groups (Mariette et al. 2000).

Myth: Mikulicz disease is a specific clinical presentation of primary SjS.

Reality: In the late-1800s, Johann von Mikulicz reported a patient with painless, bilateral, symmetrical swelling of the lacrimal, parotid, and submandibular glands (Mikulicz, 1892). In 1953, Morgan and Castleman suggested that most cases classified as Mikulicz disease should actually be considered to be SjS, because the two conditions appear strikingly on routine histopathological staining (Morgan 1953).

More recent studies and the application of new techniques suggest that patients with Mikulicz disease have a distinct clinical, immunological, and histological profile. In contrast to primary SjS, patients with Mikulicz disease are predominantly male and have higher levels of serum IgG4 (Yamamoto et al. 2005). They also have lower titers of ANA and are negative for antibodies to the Ro/SSA and La/SSB antigens. The close association of Mikulicz disease with IgG4-related alterations suggests that its proper new classification is separate from SjS, part of a spectrum of "IgG4-related systemic disease."

The other components of this disease spectrum include many cases of "autoimmune pancreatitis," chronic sclerosing sialoadenitis (Küttner's tumor), Riedel's thyroiditis, some cases of cholangitis that mimic primary sclerosing cholangitis, some cases of retroperitoneal fibrosis, and some cases of tubulointerstitial nephritis (Takeda et al. 2004).

To date, most of the literature on this disease entity has derived from Japan, but increasingly the disorder is recognized worldwide. The principal importance of recognizing IgG4-related systemic disease relates to the fact that many cases of IgG4-related systemic disease respond briskly to glucocorticoids. In addition, many of the disease entities with which it can be confused do not (for example, adenocarcinoma of the pancreas, primary sclerosing cholangitis, and most features of SjS).

12.10 Prognosis and Outcome

Myth: The course of primary SjS involves an evolution from an organ-specific autoimmune disorder (autoimmune exocrinopathy) to a systemic inflammatory disease and concludes with a B cell malignancy.

Reality: Long-term follow-up of large primary SjS conhorts indicate that the majority of the patients – approximately 60% – maintain stable disease courses characterized by quantitative and qualitative changes in tear and saliva secretion, sicca symptoms, and circulating autoantibodies. These patients do not develop disease in other organ systems.

On the other hand, approximately 20% of patients demonstrated extraglandular involvement in addition to the exocrinopathy, early in their disease course. The extraglandular clinical manifestations in these patients include small airway disease, interstitial nephritis, and autoimmune cholangiitis. This patient subset has parenchymal disease that seldom compromises the function of the involved organs significantly. The mortality of these patients does not differ from that of healthy age- and sex-matched controls.

A third group of primary SjS patients express small-vessel vasculitis (palpable purpura) and low C4 levels early in their disease course. These patients are at high risk for systemic vasculitis and for the development of lymphoma when compared with other SjS patients, and have a higher mortality rate than healthy age- and sex-matched controls (Skopouli et al. 2000).

Pearl: The association between SjS and HCV infection may increase the risk of B cell lymphoma.

Comment: The sialotropism of HCV explains its close association with SjS and the sicca syndrome. Its lymphotropism, in turn, links the presence of HCV with the synthesis of cryoglobulins and lymphoma. This extrahepatic tropism suggests the possible development of both SjS and lymphoma in patients with chronic HCV infection. The following characteristics apply to patients with SjS who are infected with HCV (Ramos-Casals et al. 2007):

- Strongly positive rheumatoid factor serologies and type II mixed cryoglobulinemia
- A high frequency of parotid enlargement and vasculitis
- A high risk for the development of MALT lymphomas.

Among patients with SjS and HCV who do develop lymphomas, there is a high frequency of primary extranodal involvement in organs in which HCV replicates, e.g., the exocrine glands, liver, and stomach.

Myth: An abrupt decline in serum immunoglobulin levels and the loss of seropositivity for autoantibodies heralds the appearance of lymphoma in primary SjS.

Reality: Studies in the 1970s suggested that an abrupt decline in hypergammaglobulinemia precedes the development of lymphoma (Cummings et al. 1971). Other authors have described reductions in baseline serum IgM and IgM rheumatoid factor levels. This has not been confirmed by subsequent studies (Voulgarelis et al. 1999). More recent data suggest that the development of lymphoma is associated more closely with ongoing immunological abnormalities than with their disappearance (Pertovaara et al. 2001; Theander et al. 2004; Tzioufas et al. 1996; Brito-Zerón et al. 2007).

Pearl: Purpura, hypocomplementemia, and cryoglobulinemia are three key prognostic factors for adverse outcome in primary SjS.

Comment: Prospective studies of Spanish, Greek, and Swedish patients have identified cutaneous vasculitis, hypocomplementemia, and mixed cryoglobulinemia as factors associated with adverse outcomes (development of systemic vasculitis, B cell lymphoma, or death) (Brito-Zerón et al. 2007; Ioannidis et al. 2002; Theander et al. 2004). Serum complement levels and cryoglobulins are key immunological parameters for long-term monitoring.

Cryoglobulinemia in SjS is associated with an increased risk of both vasculitis and lymphoma. In one series, life-threatening vasculitis was related closely to cryoglobulinemia (Ramos-Casals et al. 2004a). Among the 52 patients with cutaneous vasculitis who were described, all six deaths occurred in patients with multisystemic cryoglobulinemic vasculitis. Cryoglobulins and vasculitis were independently associated with mortality in a multivariate analysis of data from 266 patients. Both these risk factors were associated with hazard ratios (relative risks) of more than 5.0 for mortality during the course of the study (Brito-Zerón et al. 2007).

Myth: Interstitial lung disease in SjS is associated with a poor prognosis and should be treated aggressively as in systemic sclerosis.

Reality: Interstitial lung disease can occur early in the course of SjS (Davidson et al. 2000). It tends to afflict patients who have anti-Ro/SSA antibodies, but rarely worsens over follow-up. Thus, a conservative approach that does NOT involve high-dose glucocorticoids and cyclophosphamide is advised.

12.11 Systemic Treatment

Pearl: Hydroxychloroquine is an excellent therapeutic option for treating general SjS symptomatology and musculoskeletal features.

Comment: Patients with primary SjS often present with constitutional symptoms, including fever, generalized pain, and fatigue. Antimalarial drugs have a beneficial effect in many such patients, similar to the effects they exert in SLE. Hydroxychloroquine (200 mg/day) has been reported to reduce markers of inflammation within saliva (Tishler et al. 1999). Hydroxychloroquine may mediate enhanced salivary secretion through the inhibition of glandular cholinesterase activity (Dawson et al. 2005).

One dissenting report came from a small double blind crossover trial of 400 mg/day that showed significant decrease in serum IgG and IgM in the treatment group. However, there was no beneficial clinical effect as expressed in preference for the active or placebo treatment with regard to symptoms and signs of primary SjS, nor was there any relevant change in tear gland activity or salivary gland scintigraphy (Kruize et al. 1993).

Myth: Hydroxychloroquine can alleviate sicca symptoms in patients with SjS.

Reality: Hydroxychloroquine is beneficial for the nonerosive arthritis and skin rashes that occur in primary SjS. Some experts suggest that this medication has a special role in hypergammaglobulinemic purpura because it fosters the lowering of immunoglobulin levels in serum (Kruize et al. 1993; Mavragani et al. 2006). However, as noted above, hydroxychloroquine is not likely to have any impact on a patient's sicca symptoms.

Pearl: TNF inhibition is of no value in the treatment of primary SjS.

Comment: TNF inhibition in primary SjS falls short of the expectations raised by its efficacy in other autoimmune conditions, including rheumatoid arthritis, the seronegative spondyloarthropathies, and inflammatory bowel disease. A randomized, double-blind, placebo-controlled trial of infliximab in primary SjS showed no evidence of efficacy (Mariette et al. 2004). Two small studies of etanercept came to similar conclusions (Zandbelt et al. 2004; Sankar et al. 2004).

Pearl: Aggressive diffuse B cell lymphomas in patients with primary SjS should be treated with chemotherapy (cyclophosphamide, doxorubicin, vincristine, and prednisone) in combination with rituximab, a B cell depleting agent.

Comment: Combination therapy of the diffuse large-cell lymphomas that sometimes complicate primary SjS has a dramatic impact on patient survival (Voulgarelis et al. 2006). This treatment strategy also appears to be effective in many cases of SjS complicated by palpable purpura or peripheral neuropathy. The combination chemotherapy regimen results in a decrease of circulating cryoglobulins, rheumatoid factor titers, and an increase in serum C4 levels.

Pearl: Ask patients about their use of Chinese or other herbal medications.

Comment: Many patients do not inform their physicians about herbal drugs, as they consider them "nutritional" supplements. However, the agents may have significant direct toxicities on the SjS patient. As an example, some supplements have been reported to cause profound hypokalemia in SjS patients with interstitial nephritis (Atalar et al. 2007).

In our experience, the "herbal" medicines come in the form of "Chinese" herbs or "Indian ayurvedic medicine." In addition to the adverse effect of the herb itself, the preparations may be contaminated with heavy metals (especially common in ayurvedic medications) or pesticides that were used at the time of crop harvesting. Because there is no regulation of the manufacture or sale of these "health supplements" by the Food and Drug Administration or any other regulatory body, patients use them at their own risk.

References

Abraham CM, al-Hashimi I, Haghighat N. Evaluation of the levels of oral Candida in patients with Sjögren's syndrome. Oral Surg Oral Med Oral Pathol Oral Radiol Endod. 1998;86:65–8

Alexander E, Arnett F, Provost T, Stevens MB. Sjögren's syndrome: association of anti-Ro(SS-A) antibodies with vasculitis, hematologic abnormalities, and serologic hyperactivity. Ann Intern Med. 1983;98:155–9

Alexander EL, Beall SjS, Gordon B, et al Magnetic resonance imaging of cerebral lesions in patients with the Sjögren syndrome. Ann Intern Med. 1988;108:815–23

Almstahl A, Kroneld U, Tarkowski A, Wikstrom M. Oral microbial flora in Sjögren's syndrome. J Rheumatol. 1999;26:110–4

Andonopoulos AP, Drosos AA, Skopouli FN, Acritidis NC, Moutsopoulos HM. Secondary Sjögren's syndrome in rheumatoid arthritis. J Rheumatol. 1987;14:1098–103

Andonopoulos AP, Drosos AA, Skopouli FN, Moutsopoulos HM. Sjögren's syndrome in rheumatoid arthritis and progressive systemic sclerosis. A comparative study. Clin Exp Rheumatol. 1989;7: 203–5

Aoki N. Klinefelter's syndrome, autoimmunity, and associated endocrinopathies. Intern Med. 1999;38:838–9

Atalar K, Afzali B, Lams B, et al Falls, hypokalaemia, and a dry mouth. Lancet. 2007;370(9582):192

Belafsky PC, Postma GN. The laryngeal and esophageal manifestations of Sjögren's syndrome. Curr Rheumatol Rep. 2003;5:297–303

Bloch KJ, Buchanan WW, Wohl MJ, Bunim JJ. Sjögren's syndrome. A clinical, pathological, and serological study of sixty-two cases. Medicine (Baltimore). 1965;44:187–231

Boki KA, Ioannidis JP, Segas JV, et al How significant is sensorineural hearing loss in primary Sjögren's syndrome? J Rheumatol. 2001;28: 798–801

Bossini N, Savoldi S, Franceschini F, et al Clinical and morphological features of kidney involvement in primary Sjögren's syndrome. Nephrol Dial Transplant. 2001;16:2328–36

Boutsi EA, Paikos S, Dafni UG, et al Dental and periodontal status of Sjögren's syndrome. J Clin Periodontol. 2000;27:231–5

Bowman SK, Ibrahim GH, Holmes G, et al Estimating the prevalence among Caucasian women of primary Sjögren's syndrome in two general practices in Birmingham, UK Scand J Rheumatol. 2004;33: 39–43

Brito-Zerón P, Ramos-Casals M, Bove A, et al Predicting adverse outcomes in primary Sjögren's syndrome: identification of prognostic factors. Rheumatology (Oxford). 2007;46(8):1359–62

Brito-Zerón P, Ramos-Casals M, Nardi N, et al Circulating monoclonal immunoglobulins in Sjögren syndrome: prevalence and clinical significance in 237 patients. Medicine (Baltimore). 2005;84(2): 90–7

Brito-Zerón P, Soria N, Muñoz S, et al Prevalence and clinical relevance of autoimmune neutropenia in patients with primary Sjögren's syndrome. Semin Arthritis Rheum. 2008;38(5):389–95

Caporali R, Bonacci E, Epis O, et al Safety and usefulness of minor salivary gland biopsy: retrospective analysis of 502 procedures performed at a single center. Arthritis Rheum. 2008;59:714–20

Chai J, Herrmann DN, Stanton M, et al Painful small-fiber neuropathy in Sjögren's syndrome. Neurology. 2005;65:925–7

Collard RC, Koehler RP, Mattson DH. Frequency and significance of antinuclear antibodies in multiple sclerosis. Neurology. 1997;49: 857–61

Coppo P, Sibilia J, Maloisel F, et al Primary Sjögren's syndrome associated agranulocytosis: a benign disorder? Ann Rheum Dis. 2003;62: 476–8

Cummings NA, Schall GL, Asofski R. Sjögren's syndrome. New aspects of research, diagnosis and therapy. Ann Intern Med. 1971;75: 937

Dafni UG, Tzioufas AG, Staikos P, et al Prevalence of Sjögren's syndrome in a closed rural community. Ann Rheum Dis. 1997;56: 521–5

Daniels T, Greenspan JS, Cox D, Criswell LA, DeSouza Y, Dong Y, et al Objective measures in Sjögren's syndrome are strongly associated with each other but not with sicca symptoms: analysis of 564 enrollees in the SICCA international registry and repository. Arthritis Rheum. 2007;56 Suppl:S446

Daniels T, Whitcher J. Association of patterns of labial salivary gland inflammation with keratoconjunctivitis sicca. Analysis of 618 patients with suspected Sjögren's syndrome. Arthritis Rheumatol. 1994;37:869–77

Daniels TE. Benign lymphoepithelial lesion and Sjögren's syndrome. Ch 6. In Ellis GL, Auclair PL, Gnepp DR, editors. Surgical pathology of the salivary glands. Philadelphia: W.B.Saunders; 1991. p. 83–106

Daniels TE, Fox PC. Salivary and oral components of Sjögren's syndrome. Rheum Dis Clin North Am. 1992;18(3):571–89

Daniels TE, Silverman S, Michalski JP, Greenspan JS, Sylvester RA, Talal N. The oral component of Sjögren's syndrome. Oral Surg Oral Med Oral Pathol. 1975;39:875–85

Daniels TE. Evaluation, differential diagnosis, and treatment of xerostomia. J Rheumatol. 2000;27(Suppl 61):6–10

Davidson BK, Kelly CA, Griffiths ID. Ten year follow up of pulmonary function in patients with primary Sjögren's syndrome. Ann Rheum Dis. 2000;59:709–12

Dawson LJ, Caulfield VL, Stanbury JB, et al Hydroxychloroquine therapy in patients with primary Sjögren's syndrome may improve salivary gland hypofunction by inhibition of glandular cholinesterase. Rheumatology (Oxford). 2005;44:449–55

Delalande S, de Seze J, Fauchais AL. Neurologic manifestations in primary Sjögren syndrome: a study of 82 patients. Medicine (Baltimore). 2004;83:280–91

Denislic M, Meh D. Early asymmetric neuropathy in primary Sjögren's syndrome. J Neurol. 1997;244(6):383–7

Drosos AA, Voulgari PV, Psychos DN, Tsifetaki N, Bai M. Sicca syndrome in patients with sarcoidosis. Rheumatol Int. 1999;18: 177–80

Dyck PJ. The clinical heterogeneity of immune sensory and autonomic neuropathies with (or without) sicca. Brain. 2005;128(Pt 11): 2480–2

Ferreira S, D'Cruz DP, Hughes GR. Multiple sclerosis, neuropsychiatric lupus and antiphospholipid syndrome: where do we stand? Rheumatology (Oxford). 2005;44:434–42

Font J, Ramos-Casals M, Cervera R, et al Antineutrophil cytoplasmic antibodies in primary Sjögren's syndrome: prevalence and clinical significance. Br J Rheumatol. 1998;37(12):1287–91

Font J, Ramos-Casals M, de la Red G, et al Pure sensory neuropathy in primary Sjögren's syndrome. Longterm prospective followup and review of the literature. J Rheumatol. 2003;30(7):1552–7

Forstot JZ, Forstot SL, Greer RO, Tan EM. The incidence of Sjögren's sicca complex in a population of patients with keratoconjunctivitis sicca. Arthritis Rheumat. 1982;25:156–60

Fox RI, Stern M. Sjögren's syndrome: mechanisms of pathogenesis involve interaction of immune and neurosecretory systems. Scand J Rheumatol Suppl 2002;(116):3-13

Franquet T, Diaz C, Domingo P, et al Air trapping in primary Sjögren syndrome: correlation of expiratory CT with pulmonary function tests. J Comput Assist Tomogr. 1999;23:169–73

Freeman SR, Sheehan PZ, Thorpe MA, Rutka JA. Ear, nose, and throat manifestations of Sjögren's syndrome: retrospective review of a multidisciplinary clinic. J Otolaryngol. 2005;34(1):20–4

García-Carrasco M, Ramos-Casals M, et al Primary Sjögren syndrome: clinical and immunologic disease patterns in a cohort of 400 patients. Medicine (Baltimore). 2002a;81(4):270–80

García-Carrasco M, Sisó A, Ramos-Casals M, et al Raynaud's phenomenon in primary Sjögren's syndrome. Prevalence and clinical characteristics in a series of 320 patients. J Rheumatol. 2002b;29: 726–30

Gerli R, Muscat C, Giansanti M, et al Quantitative assessment of salivary gland inflammatory infiltration in primary Sjögren's syndrome: its relationship to different demographic, clinical and serological features of the disorder. Br J Rheumatol. 1997;36:969–75

Gøransson LG, Herigstad A, Tjensvoll AB, et al Peripheral neuropathy in primary Sjögren syndrome: a population-based study. Arch Neurol. 2006;63:1612–5

Gorson KC, Ropper AH. Muscle Nerve 2003; 28(5):553–60. Positive salivary gland biopsy, Sjögren syndrome, and neuropathy: clinical implications

Gorson KC, Natarajan N, Ropper AH, Weinstein R. Rituximab treatment in patients with IVIg-dependent immune polyneuropathy: a prospective pilot trial. Muscle Nerve 2007; 35(1):66–9

Goules A, Masouridi S, Tzioufas AG, et al Clinically significant and biopsy-documented renal involvement in primary Sjögren's syndrome. Medicine (Baltimore). 2000;79:241–9

Hakansson U, Jacobsson L, Lilja B, et al Salivary gland scintigraphy in subjects with and without symptoms of dry mouth and/or eyes, and in patients with primary Sjögren's syndrome. Scand J Rheumatol. 1994;23:326–33

Helman J, Turner RJ, Fox PC, Baum BJ. 99mTc-pertechnetate uptake in parotid acinar cells by the Na + /K + /Cl- co- transport system. J Clin Invest. 1987;79:1310–3

Hernandez YL, Daniels TE. Oral candidiasis in Sjögren's syndrome: prevalence, clinical correlations, and treatment. Oral Surg Oral Med Oral Pathol. 1989;3:324–9

Hershkovich O, Shafat I, Nagler RM. Age-related changes in salivary antioxidant profile: possible implications for oral cancer. J Gerontol A Biol Sci Med Sci. 2007;62:361–6

Hyer S, Kong A, Pratt B, et al Salivary gland toxicity after radioiodine therapy for thyroid cancer. Clin Oncol (R Coll Radiol). 2007;19: 83–6

Ioannidis JP, Moutsopoulos HM. Sjögren's syndrome: too many associations, too limited evidence. The enigmatic example of CNS involvement. Semin Arthritis Rheum. 1999;29:1–3

Ioannidis JP, Vassiliou VA, Moutsopoulos HM. Long-term risk of mortality and lymphoproliferative disease and predictive classification of primary Sjögren's syndrome. Arthritis Rheum. 2002;46:741–7

Jacobsson LT, Axell TE, Hansen BU, et al Dry eyes or mouth: an epidemiological study in Swedish adults, with special reference to primary Sjögren's syndrome. J Autoimmun. 1989;2:521–7

Jara LJ, Navarro C, Brito-Zeron P, et al Thyroid disease in Sjögren's syndrome. Clin Rheumatol. 2007;26:1601–6

Jungehulsing M, Fischbach R, Schroder U, et al Magnetic resonance sialography. Otolaryngol Head Neck Surg. 1999;121:488–94

Kamisawa T, Okamoto A. Autoimmune pancreatitis: proposal of IgG4-related sclerosing disease. J Gastroenterol. 2006;41:613–25

Kassan SS, Thomas TL, Moutsopoulos HM, Hoover R, Kimberly RP, Budman DR, Costa J, Decker JL, Chused TM. Increased risk of lymphoma in sicca syndrome. Ann Intern Med. 1978;89:888–92

Kohler PF, Winter ME. A quantitative test for xerostomia. The Saxon test, an oral equivalent of the Schirmer test. Arthritis Rheum 1985; 28:1128–32

Kohn WG, Ship JA, Atkinson JC, et al Salivary gland 99mTc-scintigraphy: a grading scale and correlation with major salivary gland flow rates. J Oral Pathol Med. 1992;21:70–4

Krieg AM, Vollmer J. Toll-like receptors 7, 8, and 9: linking innate immunity to autoimmunity. Immunol Rev. 2007;220:251–69

Kruize AA, Hené RJ, Kallenberg CG, et al Hydroxychloroquine treatment for primary Sjögren's syndrome: a two year, double-blind crossover trial. Ann Rheum Dis. 1993;52:360–4

Kruize AA, Hene RJ, van der Heide A, Bodeutsch C, deWilde PCM, vanBijsterveld OP, et al Long-term followup of patients with Sjögren's syndrome. Arthritis Rheum. 1996;297–303

Lamour A, Le Corre R, Pennec YL, Cartron J, Youinou P. Heterogeneity of neutrophil antibodies in patients with primary Sjögren's syndrome. Blood. 1995;86:3553–9

Larsson X, Bredberg A, Henriksson G, Manthorpe R, Sallmyr A. Immunohistochemistry of the B cell component in lower lip salivary glands of Sjögren's syndrome and healthy subjects. Scand J Immunol. 2005;61:98–107

Lekhanont K, Leyngold IM, Suwan-Apichon O, et al Comparison of topical dry eye medications for the treatment of keratoconjunctivitis sicca in a botulinum toxin B-induced mouse model. Cornea. 2007;26: 84–9

Leppilahti M, Tammela TL, Huhtala H, et al Interstitial cystitis-like urinary symptoms among patients with Sjögren's syndrome: a population-based study in Finland. Am J Med. 2003;115:62–5

Liang L, Zhang M, Zou W, Liu Z. Aggravated dry eye after laser in situ keratomileusis in patients with Sjögren syndrome. Cornea. 2008;27: 120–3

Makula E, Pokorny G, Kiss M, et al The place of magnetic resonance and ultrasonographic examinations of the parotid gland in the diagnosis and follow-up of primary Sjögren's syndrome. Rheumatology (Oxford). 2000;39:97–104

Maltsman-Tseikhin A, Moricca P, Niv D. Burning mouth syndrome: will better understanding yield better management? Pain Pract. 2007; 7:151–62

Mandl T, Ekberg O, Wollmer P, et al Dysphagia and dysmotility of the pharynx and oesophagus in patients with primary Sjögren's syndrome. Scand J Rheumatol. 2007a;36:394–401

Mandl T, Wollmer P, Manthorpe R, Jacobsson LT. Autonomic and orthostatic dysfunction in primary Sjögren's syndrome. J Rheumatol. 2007b;34:1869–74

Manoussakis MN, Georgopoulou C, Zintzaras E, et al Sjögren's syndrome associated with systemic lupus erythematosus: clinical and laboratory profiles and comparison with primary Sjögren's syndrome. Arthritis Rheum. 2004;50:882–91

Mariette X, Agbalika F, Zucker-Franklin D, et al Detection of the tax gene of HTLV-I in labial salivary glands from patients with Sjögren's syndrome and other diseases of the oral cavity. Clin Exp Rheumatol. 2000;18:341–7

Mariette X, Ravaud P, Steinfeld S, et al Inefficacy of infliximab in primary Sjögren's syndrome: results of the randomized, controlled trial of remicade in primary Sjögren's syndrome (TRIPSjS). Arthritis Rheum. 2004;50:1270–6

Mariette X, Roux S, Zhang J, et al The level of BlyS (BAFF) correlates with the titer of autoantibodies in human Sjögren's syndrome. Ann Rheum Dis. 2003;62:168–71

Mavragani CP, Moutsopoulos NM, Moutsopoulos HM. The management of Sjögren's syndrome. Nat Clin Pract Rheumatol. 2006;2: 252–61

Mellgren SI, Goransson LG, Omdal R. Primary Sjögren's syndrome associated neuropathy. Can J Neurol Sci. 2007;34:280–7

Mikulicz J. Über eine eigenartige symmetrische Erkrankung der Tranen und Mundspeicheldrusen. Stuttgart: Beitr Chir Fortsch Gewidmet Theodor Billroth. 1892;610–30

Mitsias D, Tzioufas A, Veiopoulou C, et al The Th1/Th2 cytokine balance changes with the progress of the immunopathological lesion of Sjögren's syndrome. Clin Exp Immunol. 2002;128:562–8

Mori K, Iijima M, Sugiura M et al Sjögren's syndrome associated painful sensory neuropathy without sensory ataxia. J Neurol Neurosurg Psychiatry 2003; 74(9):1320–2

Mori K, Iijima M, Koike H, et al The wide spectrum of clinical manifestations in Sjögren's syndrome-associated neuropathy. Brain. 2005;128:2518–34

Moutsopoulos HM, Balow JE, Lawley TJ, et al Immune complex glomerulonephritis in sicca syndrome. Am J Med. 1978;64:955–60

Moutsopoulos HM, Elkon KB, Mavridis AK, et al Serum C-reactive protein in primary Sjögren's syndrome. Clin Exp Rheumatol. 1983a;1:57–8

Moutsopoulos HM, Webber BL, Vlagopoulos TP, et al Differences in the clinical manifestations of sicca syndrome in the presence and absence of rheumatoid arthritis. Am J Med. 1979;66:733–6

Moutsopoulos HM, Steinberg AD, Fauci AS, et al High incidence of free monoclonal lambda light chains in the sera of patients with Sjögren's syndrome. J Immunol. 1983b;130:2663–5

Moutsopoulos HM, Costello R, Drosos AA, et al Demonstration and identification of monoclonal proteins in the urine of patients with Sjögren's syndrome. Ann Rheum Dis. 1985;44:109–12

Nagler RM. Salivary glands and the aging process: mechanistic aspects, health-status and medicinal-efficacy monitoring. Biogerontology. 2004;5:223–33

Nakamura H, Kawakami A, Tominaga M, et al Relationship between Sjögren's syndrome and human T-lymphotropic virus type I infection: follow-up study of 83 patients. J Lab Clin Med. 2000;135: 139–44

Nardi N, Brito-Zerón P, Ramos-Casals M, et al Circulating auto-antibodies against nuclear and non-nuclear antigens in primary Sjögren's syndrome: prevalence and clinical significance in 335 patients. Clin Rheumatol. 2006;25(3):341–6

Papiris SA, Maniati M, Constantopoulos SH, et al Lung involvement in primary Sjögren's syndrome is mainly related to the small airway disease. Ann Rheum Dis. 1999;58:61–4

Paschides CA, Kitsios G, Karakostas KX, et al Evaluation of tear break-up time, Schirmer's-I test and rose bengal staining as confirmatory tests for keratoconjunctivitis sicca. Clin Exp Rheumatol. 1989;7:155–7

Patton LL, Siegel MA, Benoliel R, De Laat A. Management of burning mouth syndrome: systematic review and management recommendations. Oral Surg Oral Med Oral Pathol Oral Radiol Endod. 2007;103 Suppl:S39.e1–13

Pavlidis NA, Karsh J, Moutsopoulos HM. The clinical picture of primary Sjögren's syndrome: a retrospective study. J Rheumatol. 1982;9: 685–90

Pertovaara M, Pukkala E, Laippala P, et al A longitudinal cohort study of Finnish patients with primary Sjögren's syndrome: clinical, immunological, and epidemiological aspects. Ann Rheum Dis. 2001; 60:467–72

Pflugfelder SC, Maskin SL, Anderson B, et al A randomized, double-masked, placebo-controlled, multicenter comparison of loteprednol etabonate ophthalmic suspension, 0.5%, and placebo for treatment of keratoconjunctivitis sicca in patients with delayed tear clearance. Am J Ophthalmol. 2004;138:444–57

Pillemer SR, Smith J, Fox PC, Bowman SJ. Outcome measures for Sjögren's syndrome. J Rheumatol. 2005;32:143–9

Prochorec-Sobieszek M, Wagner T, Loukas M, Chwali ska-Sadowska H, Olesi ska M. Histopathological and immunohistochemical analysis of lymphoid follicles in labial salivary glands in primary and secondary Sjögren's syndrome. Med Sci Monit. 2004;10: BR115–21

Ramos-Casals M, Anaya JM, García-Carrasco M, et al Cutaneous vasculitis in primary Sjögren syndrome: classification and clinical significance of 52 patients. Medicine (Baltimore). 2004a;83(2): 96–106

Ramos-Casals M, Font J, Garcia-Carrasco M, et al Primary Sjögren syndrome: hematologic patterns of disease expression. Medicine (Baltimore). 2002;81(4):281–92

Ramos-Casals M, García-Carrasco M, Cervera R, et al Thyroid disease in primary Sjögren syndrome: study in a series of 160 patients. Medicine (Baltimore). 2000;79(2):103–8

Ramos-Casals M, la Civita L, De Vita S, et al For the SjS-HCV Study Group. Characterization of B cell lymphoma in patients with Sjögren's syndrome and hepatitis C virus infection. Arthritis Rheum. 2007;57(1):161–70

Ramos-Casals M, Loustaud-Ratti V, De Vita S, et al For the Sjögren syndrome associated with hepatitis C virus: a multicenter analysis of 137 cases. Medicine (Baltimore). 2005;84(2):81–9

Ramos-Casals M, Nardi N, Brito-Zerón P, et al Atypical autoantibodies in patients with primary Sjögren syndrome: clinical characteristics and follow-up of 82 cases. Semin Arthritis Rheum. 2006a; 35(5): 312–21

Ramos-Casals M, Sánchez-Tapias JM, Parés A, et al Characterization and differentiation of autoimmune versus viral liver involvement in patients with Sjögren's syndrome. J Rheumatol. 2006b;33(8): 1593–9

Ramos-Casals M, Solans R, Rosas J, et al Primary Sjögren syndrome in Spain: clinical and immunologic expression of 1010 patients. Medicine (Baltimore). 2008;87(4):210–9

Reinertsen JL, Schaefer EJ, Brewer HB, Moutsopoulos HM. Sicca-like syndrome in type V hyperlipoproteinemia. Arthritis Rheum. 1980;23: 114–8

Rhodus NL, Michalowicz BS. Periodontal status and sulcular Candida albicans colonization in patients with primary Sjögren's syndrome. Quintessence Int. 2005;36(3):228–33

Salliot C, Gottenberg JE, Bengoufa D, et al Anticentromere antibodies identify patients with Sjögren's syndrome and autoimmune overlap syndrome. J Rheumatol. 2007;34(11):2253–8

Sankar V, Brennan MT, Kok MR, et al Etanercept in Sjögren's syndrome: a twelve-week randomized, double-blind, placebo-controlled pilot clinical trial. Arthritis Rheum. 2004;50:2240–5

Simon BG, Moutsopoulos HM. Primary amyloidosis resembling sicca syndrome. Arthritis Rheum. 1979;22:932–4

Sjögren's Syndrome Foundation. And the survey says. The Moisture Seekers. 2006;24:1–3

Skopouli FN, Barbatis C, Moutsopoulos HM. Liver involvement in primary Sjögren's syndrome. Br J Rheumatol. 1994a;33:745–8

Skopouli FN, Dafni U, Ioannidis JP, Moutsopoulos HM. Clinical evolution, and morbidity and mortality of primary Sjögren's syndrome. Semin Arthritis Rheum. 2000;29:296–304

Skopouli FN, Papanikolaou S, Malamou-Mitsi V, et al Obstetric and gynaecological profile in patients with primary Sjögren's syndrome. Ann Rheum Dis. 1994b;53:569–73

Skopouli FN, Talal A, Galanopoulou V, et al Raynaud's phenomenon in primary Sjögren's syndrome. J Rheumatol. 1990;17:618–20

Stevens WJ, Swartele FE, Empsten FA, De Clerck LS. Use of the Saxon test as a measure of saliva production in a reference population of schoolchildren. Am J Dis Child. 1990;144:570–1

Stojanovich L, Milovanovich B, de Luka SR, et al Cardiovascular autonomic dysfunction in systemic lupus, rheumatoid arthritis, primary Sjögren syndrome and other autoimmune diseases. Lupus. 2007;16: 181–5

Takeda S, Haratake J, Kasai T, et al IgG4-associated idiopathic tubulointerstitial nephritis complicating autoimmune pancreatitis. Nephrol Dial Transplant. 2004;19:474–6

Taouli B, Brauner MW, Mourey I, et al Thin-section chest CT findings of primary Sjögren's syndrome: correlation with pulmonary function. Eur Radiol. 2002;12:1504–11

Terrier B, Lacroix C, Guillevin L, et al Diagnostic and prognostic relevance of neuromuscular biopsy in primary Sjögren's syndrome-related neuropathy. Arthritis Rheum. 2007;57(8):1520–9

Theander E, Manthorpe R, Jacobsson L. Mortality and causes of death in primary Sjögren's syndrome: a prospective cohort study. Arthritis Rheum. 2004;50:1262–9

Tishler M, Yaron I, Shirazi I, Yaron M. Hydroxychloroquine treatment for primary Sjögren's syndrome: its effect on salivary and serum inflammatory markers. Ann Rheum Dis. 1999;58:253–6

Trontzas PI, Andrianakos AA. Sjögren's syndrome: a population based study of prevalence in Greece. Ann Rheum Dis. 2005;64:1240–1

Tsampoulas CG, Skopouli FN, Sartoris DJ, et al Hand radiographic changes in patients with primary and secondary Sjögren's syndrome. Scand J Rheumatol. 1986;15:333–9

Tsianos EB, Chiras CD, Drosos AA, Moutsopoulos HM. Oesophageal dysfunction in patients with primary Sjögren's syndrome. Ann Rheum Dis. 1985;44:610–3

Tsianos EB, Tzioufas AG, Kita MD, et al Serum isoamylases in patients with autoimmune rheumatic diseases. Clin Exp Rheumatol. 1984;2: 235–8

Tzioufas AG, Boumba DS, Skopouli FN, Moutsopoulos HM. Mixed monoclonal cryoglobulinemia and monoclonal rheumatoid factor cross-reactive idiotypes as predictive factors for the development of lymphoma in primary Sjögren's syndrome. Arthritis Rheum. 1996;39:767–72

Vitali C, Bombardieri S, Moutsopoulos HM, Balestrieri G, Bencivelli W, Bernstein RM, et al Preliminary criteria for the classification of Sjögren's syndrome. Results of a prospective concerted action supported by the European Community. Arthritis Rheum. 1993;36: 340–7

Vitali C, Bombardieri S, Moutsopoulos HM, Coll J, Gerli R, Hatron Y, et al Assessment of the European classification criteria for Sjogren's syndrome in a series of clinically defined cases: results of a prospective multicentre study. Ann Rheum Dis. 1996;55:116–21

Vitali C, Bombardieri Jonsson R, Moutsopoulos HM, Alexander EL, Carsons SE, et al Classification criteria for Sjögren's syndrome: a revised version of the European criteria proposed by the American-European consensus group. Ann Rheum Dis. 2002;61:544–58

Vivino FB, Gala I, Hermann GA. Change in final diagnosis on second evaluation of labial minor salivary gland biopsies. J Rheumatol. 2002;29:938–44

Voulgarelis M, Dafni UG, Isenberg DA, Mousopoulos HM. Malignant lymphoma in primary Sjögren's syndrome. A multicenter, retrospective, clinical study by the European concerted action on Sjögren's syndrome. Arthritis Rheum. 1999;42:1765–72

Voulgarelis M, Giannouli S, Tzioufas AG, Moutsopoulos HM. Long term remission of Sjögren's syndrome associated aggressive B cell non-Hodgkin's lymphomas following combined B cell depletion therapy and CHOP (cyclophosphamide, doxorubicin, vincristine, prednisone). Ann Rheum Dis. 2006;65:1033–7

Walker J, Gordon T, Lester S, et al Increased severity of lower urinary tract symptoms and daytime somnolence in primary Sjögren's syndrome. J Rheumatol. 2003;30:2406–12

Whitcher J, Gritz D, Daniels T. The dry eye: a diagnostic dilemma. Int Ophthal Clin. 1998;38:23–37

Wolkoff P, Nojgaard JK, Franck C, Skov P. The modern office environment desiccates the eyes? Indoor Air. 2006;16:258–65

Wright SA, Convery RP, Liggett N. Pulmonary involvement in Sjögren's syndrome. Rheumatology (Oxford). 2003;42:697–8

Wu AJ, Fox PC. Sjögren's syndrome. Semin Dermatol. 1994;13:138–43

Yamamoto M, Takahashi H, Sugai S, Imai K. Clinical and pathological characteristics of Mikulicz's disease (IgG4-related plasmacytic exocrinopathy). Autoimmun Rev. 2005;4:195–200

Zandbelt MM, de Wilde P, van Damme P, et al Etanercept in the treatment of patients with primary Sjögren's syndrome: a pilot study. J Rheumatol. 2004;31:96–101

Zintzaras E, Voulgarelis M, Moutsopoulos H. The risk of lymphoma development in autoimmune diseases. Arch Intern Med. 2005; 165:2337–44

Klippel JH, Stone JS, Crofford L, White P. Primer on the Rheumatic Diseases. 13th Edition. 2008. Springer. London

Systemic Lupus Erythematosus

13

Michelle Petri, Rachel Abuav, Dimitrios Boumpas, Fiona Goldblatt, David Isenberg, Grant J. Anhalt, Victoria P. Werth, and R. John Looney

13.1 Overview of Systemic Lupus Erythematosus

> Systemic lupus erythematosus (SLE) is the prototypical autoimmune disease, associated with autoantibody production and evidence for immune complex deposition among the many aspects of its pathophysiology.
> SLE occurs most commonly in women during their reproductive years. The disease is approximately nine times more common among women than men.
> Virtually any organ can be affected by SLE. However, constitutional symptoms, mucocutaneous features, musculoskeletal involvement, and renal and central nervous system disease are the most common manifestations.
> Many aspects of SLE appear to be triggered by classic inflammatory mechanisms, accompanied by elevated acute phase reactants, and responsive to immunosuppressive therapies. Other aspects, such as those associated with antiphospholipid antibodies (aPL), are associated with hypercoagulability. Although inflammation contributes to these aspects as well, the approach to the treatment of aPL-mediated disease manifestations is usually centered on anticoagulation.
> Autoantibodies can occur in the absence of clinical features of SLE, but strong evidence implicates certain autoantibodies in the mediation of tissue damage in the kidney and other organs.
> Genetics plays a significant role in SLE, but the disease is clearly polygenic, with multiple genetic risk factors contributing incrementally to the overall genetic risk.
> Environmental risk factors are also critical. Established environmental risk factors for the disease include hormones, ultraviolet light, the exposure to certain medications, and possibly dietary exposures and infectious agents.

Issues related to pregnancy in patients with SLE are addressed in Chapter 17. The majority of Pearls and Myths related to the antiphospholipid syndrome are covered in Chapter 16.

13.2 Diagnosis

Myth: A patient must have at least 4 of the 11 American College of Rheumatology (ACR) classification criteria to be diagnosed with SLE.

Reality: The ACR classification criteria were devised to classify patients as having SLE for the purpose of research studies, not for clinical diagnosis (Table 13.1) (Hochberg 1997; Tan et al. 1982). These criteria are relatively easy to apply and help underscore the multisystem nature of SLE. Thus, it is understandable that they are frequently referred to and even used as "diagnostic" criteria.

However, because the criteria are historical and cumulative (i.e., a malar rash counts even if the patient had it last year but does not have it now), time is often required before a patient accrues four criteria. Some patients have only two criteria (e.g., a positive ANA and lupus nephritis demonstrated by renal biopsy), yet have unequivocal SLE. When it comes to making the diagnosis of SLE, clinical judgment trumps the ACR classification criteria.

Pearl: "ANA-negative lupus" still exists.

Comment: The sensitivity of ANA assays is suboptimal, particularly early in the disease course. Depending on which type of assay is used and the quality of the laboratory in which it is performed, the sensitivity of ANA testing can be less than 70% in patients who have SLE. This is particularly true in laboratories that employ ELISA or bead assays rather than immunofluorescence tests. Thus, a significant number of SLE cases will be missed if the diagnosis is discarded because the ANA assay is negative.

In patients who have features that are typical of lupus but no history of a positive ANA assay, the ANA must be repeated in an experienced laboratory that employs an indirect immunofluorescence assay, using Hep2 cells as the test substrate. In addition, assays for other autoantibodies such as those directed against Ro, La, Sm, RNP, and cardiolipin are important, and the measurement of complement levels (C3, C4, CH50) can also be informative. Biopsies of skin and kidney lesions are required in selected cases.

J. H. Stone (ed.), *A Clinician's Pearls and Myths in Rheumatology,*
DOI:10.1007/978-1-84800-934-9_13, © Springer Science + Business Media B.V. 2009

Table 13.1 The 1997 update of the 1982 American College of Rheumatology revised criteria for the classification of systemic lupus erythematosus[a]

Criterion	Definition
1. Malar Rash	Fixed erythema, flat or raised, over the malar eminences, tending to spare the nasolabial folds
2. Discoid rash	Erythematous raised patches with adherent keratotic scaling and follicular plugging; atrophic scarring may occur in older lesions
3. Photosensitivity	Skin rash as a result of unusual reaction to sunlight, by patient history or physician observation
4. Oral ulcers	Oral or nasopharyngeal ulceration, usually painless, observed by physician
5. Nonerosive Arthritis	Involving 2 or more peripheral joints, characterized by tenderness, swelling, or effusion
6. Pleuritis or Pericarditis	(a) Pleuritis – convincing history of pleuritic pain or rubbing heard by a physician or evidence of pleural effusion
	OR
	(b) Pericarditis – documented by electrocardigram or rub or evidence of pericardial effusion
7. Renal Disorder	(a) Persistent proteinuria > 0.5 g/day or > than 3+ if quantitation not performed
	OR
	(b) Cellular casts – may be red cell, hemoglobin, granular, tubular, or mixed
8. Neurologic Disorder	(a) Seizures – in the absence of offending drugs or known metabolic derangements; e.g., uremia, ketoacidosis, or electrolyte imbalance
	OR
	(b) Psychosis – in the absence of offending drugs or known metabolic derangements, e.g., uremia, ketoacidosis, or electrolyte imbalance
9. Hematologic Disorder	(a) Hemolytic anemia – with reticulocytosis
	OR
	(b) Leukopenia – < 4,000/mm^3 on ≥ 2 occasions
	OR
	(c) Lymphopenia – < 1,500/ mm^3 on ≥ 2 occasions
	OR
	(d) Thrombocytopenia – <100,000/ mm^3 in the absence of offending drugs
10. Immunologic Disorder	(a) AntiDNA: antibody to native DNA in abnormal titer
	OR
	(b) AntiSm: presence of antibody to Sm nuclear antigen
	OR
	(c) Positive finding of antiphospholipid antibodies on:
	an abnormal serum level of IgG or IgM anticardiolipin antibodies,
	a positive test result for lupus anticoagulant using a standard method, or
	a false-positive test result for at least 6 months confirmed by Treponema pallidum immobilization or fluorescent treponemal antibody absorption test
11. Positive Antinuclear Antibody	An abnormal titer of antinuclear antibody by immunofluorescence or an equivalent assay at any point in time and in the absence of drugs

[a]American College of Rheumatology webpage: http://www.rheumatology.org/publications/classification/SLE/1997UpdateOf1982RevisedCriteriaClassificationSLE.asp?aud=mem. Accessed May 26, 2009

Although the suboptimal sensitivity of ANA assays has come into clearer focus with the move of laboratories away from Hep2 cell-based immunofluorescence studies, the poor specificity for ANA assays has been known for a long time. As an example, a young woman with a positive ANA and arthralgias is more likely to have autoimmune thyroiditis than lupus.

Myth: The "lupus band test" is useful in diagnosis of problematic cases with possible SLE.

Reality: There was once a great deal of interest in using the so-called "lupus band test" to aid in the diagnosis of problematic cases with possible SLE. This test was based on the observation that some patients with SLE have deposition of immunoreactants in the basement membranes on normal-looking (nonlesional) skin. These lesions, when present, can be visualized by direct immunofluorescence studies of skin biopsies, and their detection was taken as presumptive evidence of SLE (Provost et al. 1980).

The term "positive lupus band test" has been applied inappropriately to the finding of immunoreactants in the basement membrane zone of lesional skin in SLE. The true concept of the lupus band test refers to findings in nonlesional skin.

Patients who have such deposits in nonlesional skin have a high frequency of antibodies against native DNA, depressed complement levels, nephritis, and poor survival rates (Gilliam et al. 1974). Thus, the lupus band test is really just a surrogate marker for patients who have circulating native DNA-containing immune complexes. Most SLE experts consider the lupus band test to be obsolete.

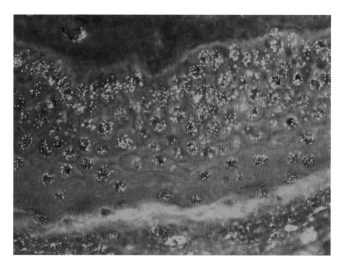

Fig. 13.1 An "in vivo ANA," demonstrated in a skin biopsy. This patient had a high-titer serum ANA associated with limited scleroderma. However, the finding of an in vivo ANA is an occasional artifact of performing direct immunofluorescence on a skin biopsy. An in vivo ANA does not always correlate with clinically relevant serum antibodies and a clinical diagnosis of rheumatic disease, but the phenomenon is more likely to occur if the serum ANA is strongly positive (Figure courtesy of Dr. Grant Anhalt)

Myth: The presence of an in vivo ANA on a skin biopsy is equivalent to finding a positive serum ANA.

Reality: Dermatopathologists sometimes report the finding of an "in vivo ANA" on skin biopsies submitted for direct immunofluorescence (Fig. 13.1). Is this finding equivalent to a positive serum assay for ANA? (Wells et al. 1979). Not necessarily. Here is why....

Tissue processed for immunofluorescence is not fixed. Thus, immunoglobulins are present within the interstitial spaces of the specimen. As the specimen is sectioned and incubated with antibody probes, ANA can diffuse into the open nuclei and bind to antigens within. This process is sometimes efficient enough that one observes a positive in vivo ANA even in the absence of a significant serum ANA titer. Thus, the finding of an incidental in vivo ANA on skin biopsy does not necessarily unmask an occult connective tissue disorder. As with any test, laboratory data must be correlated with the clinical context.

Pearl: Undifferentiated connective tissue diseases and "incomplete lupus" represent up to 10–20% of patients referred to rheumatologists.

Comment: The recognition that systemic rheumatic diseases have several common features has led to the concept of the undifferentiated connective tissue syndromes. These patients account for 10–20% of patients referred to tertiary care centers. Among patients presenting with symptoms suggestive of a connective tissue disease, only a small fraction (10–15%) fulfill classification criteria for SLE 5 years later. Factors

predictive of eventual evolution into SLE were young age, alopecia, serositis, discoid lupus, a positive Coombs test, and the presence of antiSm and antiDNA antibodies.

Latent or incomplete lupus describes patients who present with a constellation of symptoms suggestive of SLE, but do not qualify by clinical intuition or classification criteria as having classical SLE (Ganczarczyk et al. 1989; Graninger and Smolen 2001). These patients usually present with one or two of the ACR criteria and other features that are not included in the criteria. Most of these patients do *not* develop SLE ultimately or, if they do, their disease usually remains mild (Calvo-Alen et al. 1996).

Pearl: Not all lupus is diagnosed in patients before the age of 50.

Comment: This myth is perpetuated by clinicians who are reluctant to consider the diagnosis of SLE in older patients. SLE can present in older patients: up to 20% of patients with SLE develop their disease after the age of 50 (Font et al. 1991; Boddaert et al. 2004). The interval between symptom onset and diagnosis is often longer for older patients, because the clinical manifestations for patients in this subgroup can be insidious and atypical (Font et al. 1991).

The overwhelming female predominance that is typical of the peak incidence years is less evident among patients diagnosed later in life. In addition, older patients are less likely than are younger ones to have malar rashes, other cutaneous manifestations, clinically significant renal disease, and hypocomplementemia (Font et al. 1991; Domenech et al. 1992; Cervera et al. 1993). Serositis and sicca features are typical of late-onset SLE (Wilson et al. 1981; Costallat and Coimbra 1994; Ho et al. 1998; Formiga et al. 1999). The 5- and 10-year survival rates are lower in patients with late-onset disease, but mortality in the late-onset subgroup might reflect only the consequences of aging rather than disease-related differences (Boddaert et al. 2004).

13.3 Clinical Features

Myth: The major cause of death in SLE patients is: (a) active lupus; (b) complications of renal failure; or c) infection.

Reality: The correct answer: none of the above! In the 1970s, Urowitz and Gladman reported on the bimodal pattern of mortality in SLE. Whereas "early" deaths were caused predominantly by active SLE, "later" deaths were linked primarily to cardiovascular disease (Urowitz et al. 1976). Thus, although SLE patients certainly die of complications related directly to a, b, and c, the most common cause of death in many studies is accelerated atherosclerosis. This is even truer today than it was 3 decades ago.

The risk of myocardial infarction in SLE women aged 35–44 years is 50-fold higher when compared with age- and sex-matched controls (Manzi et al. 1997). This excess risk is not explained by traditional cardiovascular risk factors (Esdaile et al. 2001). Case-control studies have shown a two-fold increase in subclinical atherosclerosis, as measured by carotid duplex (Roman et al. 2003).

Myth: SLE causes pain.

Reality: The most frequent cause of a positive ANA and chronic pain is fibromyalgia! The failure to recognize that pain is NOT because of active SLE leads to much unnecessary glucocorticoid use and even the inappropriate use of narcotics. Unfortunately, SLE patients frequently have concomitant fibromyalgia (Akkasilpa et al. 2005; Middleton et al. 1994; Taylor et al. 2000). Estimates of the prevalence of fibromyalgia among patients with SLE range from 10 to 30%.

Arthralgias are the principal musculoskeletal feature of SLE, but synovitis also occurs. Patients describe their joint symptoms as "stiffness" and note an accentuation of the problem in the morning (the "gel phenomenon"). The PIPs, MCPs, wrists, and knees are involved in typical cases. SLE does not affect the neck, shoulder girdle, back, or trochanteric region. Pain in those areas in an SLE patient usually reflects fibromyalgia.

SLE patients also have pain from musculoskeletal damage (e.g., osteonecrosis) or from processes unrelated to SLE such as osteoarthritis, mechanical low back pain, bursitis, compression neuropathy, and a host of other conditions to which humans are prone. But beware the "lupus" patient who hurts all over: the correct diagnosis is probably fibromyalgia.

Myth: Fatigue is a sign of active SLE.

Reality: Fatigue is a major cause of the reduced quality of life reported by SLE patients and a significant contributor to disability. Acute fatigue often accompanies SLE flares, but this usually resolves along with the other features of active disease. However, for many patients with lupus, fatigue is a chronic symptom that is unresponsive to NSAIDs, glucocorticoids, and immunosuppressive medications. In these SLE patients, chronic fatigue is probably due to fibromyalgia. Thus, treating all chronic fatigue with glucocorticoids exposes many SLE patients to unnecessary toxicity.

Every SLE patient with chronic fatigue deserves an evaluation for comorbid processes, including anemia, hypothyroidism, adrenal insufficiency, sleep disorders, fibromyalgia, and depression. However, if no other cause is identified, then sensible advice is a brief daily nap. This nap should be sufficiently short that it does not interfere with the normal sleep–wake cycle. SLE patients with fatigue should also exercise daily (as should patients with fibromyalgia) (see Chapter 33, Fibromyalgia) (Iaboni et al. 2006; Omdal et al. 2002).

Myth: In a lupus patient, lymphadenopathy must be investigated aggressively to rule out lymphoma.

Reality: Lymphadenopathy occurs in approximately 40% of lupus patients. This finding is found typically at disease presentation and during disease flares. SLE patients with lymphadenopathy are more likely to have constitutional symptoms such as fever and malaise. Lymphadenopathy in SLE is characterized by soft, discrete, slightly tender lymph nodes. The involved lymph node chains are found usually in the cervical, axillary, and inguinal areas. Biopsies reveal areas of follicular hyperplasia and necrosis.

Features that suggest a pathological cause other than SLE include the absence of tenderness in the nodes; enlargement greater than three centimeters; induration; age older than 40, and a location above the clavicle (Vassilakopoulos and Pangalis 2000). Additional indicators of concern are splenomegaly and a monoclonal expansion of CD19+/CD22+ B lymphocytes in the peripheral blood (Table 13.2).

Lupus patients have a slightly increased risk for both Hodgkin's and non-Hodgkin's lymphoma. The standardized incidence ratios for these two disorders are 3.6 and 3.1, respectively, for patients with SLE. These risks persist even when the use of alkylating agents is taken into account.

Pearl: Up to one-third of lupus patients have one or more additional autoimmune diseases.

Comment: The association between SLE and other autoimmune diseases is well documented. Other autoimmune disorders often linked to SLE are Sjögren's syndrome, autoimmune thrombocytopenia, hypothyroidism, and polymyositis (Foote et al. 1982; Karpatkin 1985; Pyne and Isenberg 2002; Manoussakis et al. 2004). Approximately 30% of SLE patients manifest other autoimmune disorders; a smaller percentage develops more than one such condition (Table 13.3) (McDonagh and Isenberg 2000; Chambers et al. 2007).

Thus, the diagnosis of lupus should not be regarded as the end of the story. Vigilance is essential to detect the one-third of these patients who eventually develop additional autoimmune disease manifestations.

Myth: Autoimmune liver disease is common in SLE.

Reality: Autoimmune liver disease is relatively *uncom-*mon in SLE. It affects only about 2% of patients. Autoimmune

Table 13.2 When is lymphadenopathy in an SLE patient a cause for concern? lymphadenopathy out of proportion to SLE activity

Patient age > 40 years
Hardness of the affected nodes to palpation
An absence of tenderness but the presence of hardness
Enlargement of any node > 3 cm in diameter
Supraclavicular location
Splenomegaly
Monoclonal expansion of CD19+/CD22+ B lymphocytes in the peripheral blood
Modified from (Vassilakopoulos 2000)

Table 13.3 Prevalence of autoimmune diseases in patients with SLE compared to the UK population (From Chambers et al. 2007. Reprinted with permission from BMJ Publishing Group)

Autoimmune disease	Prevalence in UK (%)	Frequency in UCLH SLE cohort (total cohort n = 401), prevalence (%)
Sjögren's syndrome	3.3	45 (11.22)
Hashimoto's hypothyroidism	0.80	26 (6.48)
Antiphosholipid syndrome	No data	23 (5.7)
Myositis	0.002–0.01	14 (3.49)
Rheumatoid arthritis	0.44–1.16	14 (3.49)
ITP	No data	13 (3.24)
Graves disease/hyperthyroidism	0.65	8 (1.99)
Autoimmune hepatitis	0.014	5 (1.25)
AHA	No data	4 (0.99)
Fibrosing alveolitis	No data	3 (0.75)
Type 1 Diabetes Mellitus	0.34	3 (0.75)
Pernicious anaemia	0.13	3 (0.75)
Myasthenia gravis	0.015	3 (0.75)
Vitiligo	0.38	2 (0.50)
Coeliac disease	0.820	1 (0.25)

ITP Idiopathic thrombocytopaenia purpura; *AHA* Autoimmune haemolytic anaemia

Table 13.4 Autoimmune versus lupus-associated hepatitis

Feature	Autoimmune hepatitis	Lupus-associated hepatitis
Autoantibodies	Type I (classic): ANA, ASMA Type II: ALKM-1, ALC-1	ASMA, AMA only in 30% of the cases and usually in low titers; antiribosomal P
Serum chemistry (AST, ALT, LDH)	Variable elevations in serum liver biochemistry	Mild elevation (usually x3–4 normal)
Histology	Variable rates of periportal hepatitis with piece-meal necrosis	Rarely seen

* *ANA* antinuclear antibodies, *ASMA* antismooth muscle antibodies, *AMA* antimitochondrial antibodies, *ALKM-*1 antibodies to liver kidney microsomes, *ALC-*1 antibodies to liver cytosolic antigen

hepatitis, a separate disorder once known as "lupoid hepatitis" (Mackay et al. 1959), also has a predilection for young women. ALKM-1 (type 2) autoimmune hepatitis is generally a disease of girls and young women. This disorder is associated with antibodies to liver/kidney microsomes (ALKM-1) or to a liver cytosol antigen (ALC-1).

Autoantibodies help to distinguish between autoimmune hepatitis and liver disease associated with lupus (Irving et al. 2007). Positive ANA assays are the norm in both conditions. However, antismooth muscle and antimitochondrial antibodies occur in fewer than 30% of SLE patients and, when present, are usually found in low titers (Table 13.4). The absence of these antibodies suggests that any apparent liver inflammation might be due to SLE itself rather than the distinct condition of autoimmune hepatitis.

Elevations of the serum hepatic aminotransferases tend to be lower in lupus-associated hepatitis when compared with autoimmune liver disease. The alanine and aspartate aminotransferases are elevated generally to only three or four times the upper limit of normal in lupus-associated liver inflammation. Much higher elevations occur in autoimmune liver disease. When doubt persists about the cause of liver dysfunction in a patient with SLE or possible SLE, histopathology may resolve the question. Autoimmune hepatitis is associated with a characteristic periportal hepatitis and piecemeal necrosis.

Liver dysfunction can also exist in SLE as a result of issues that are not immunological in nature (Runyon et al. 1980). A wide variety of pathological lesions may be observed. Hepatic steatosis, a common finding, may occur as part of the disease process, as a complication of glucocorticoid use, or intercurrent factors such as alcohol use. Abnormalities of hepatic aminotransferases, lactate dehydrogenase, and alkaline phosphatase can also occur as a complication of NSAID or salicylate use.

Pearl: Primary biliary cirrhosis rarely occurs in SLE.

Comment: Primary biliary cirrhosis, an autoimmune disease of the liver that predominantly affects women over the age of 20, is unlikely to complicate SLE. In a female patient whose serum tests reflect a cholestatic pattern of liver injury, e.g., an unexplained elevation in alkaline phosphatase but normal bile ducts on ultrasound, a positive ANA, and a positive antimitochondrial antibody (AMA); Sjögren's syndrome and systemic sclerosis are both more likely concurrent disorders than is SLE.

Myth: The myositis of SLE resembles that of idiopathic inflammatory myopathies.

Reality: In lupus, generalized myalgia and muscle tenderness are common, especially during disease exacerbations. Inflammatory myositis involving the proximal muscles occurs in up to 10% of patients with SLE and may develop at any time during the course of the disease. However, this myositis is usually mild and responds well to moderate doses of glucocorticoids.

Electromyographic studies and elevations of the serum creatine phosphokinase (CK) or aldolase levels do not help differentiate idiopathic inflammatory myopathies from drug-induced conditions (both show myopathic patterns of tissue injury). Similarly, a low serum CK value even in the face of obvious muscle dysfunction can be found in patients with connective tissue disease, including SLE. Thus, a normal CK value in the presence of other symptoms and signs of myositis should not dissuade the clinician from pursuing that diagnosis through electrodiagnostic testing and muscle biopsy.

Myth: Autoimmune hemolytic anemia is the most common cause of anemia in lupus.

Reality: Autoimmune hemolytic anemia (AIHA) is found in approximately 10% of patients with SLE. AIHA is recognized by the finding of spherocytes on the peripheral blood smear, a sharp fall in hemoglobin (>3g/dL), an elevated reticulocyte count (>5%), a rise in the serum bilirubin level, and a positive Coombs test. In contrast to idiopathic AIHA, splenectomy is rarely indicated in SLE.

The most common causes of anemia in SLE are chronic disease and iron deficiency. In the absence of symptoms such as easy fatigability or dyspnea on exertion, the anemia of chronic inflammation does not require specific treatment. However, for lupus patients with stage 4 chronic kidney disease – which corresponds to a glomerular filtration rate of less than 30 mL/min – the Kidney Disease Outcomes Quality Initiative guidelines recommend maintaining a target hemoglobin of 11–12 mg/dL through the use of erythropoietin (http://www.kdoqi.org).

Myth: Erosive arthritis does not occur in patients with SLE.

Reality: Joint involvement is a common, early manifestation of SLE. Many clinicians believe that a critical discriminator between rheumatoid arthritis (RA) and SLE is the lack of erosive changes in lupus. As a general rule, this is true. However, up to 5% of patients with SLE develop an erosive arthropathy (Isenberg and Horsfall 1998).

Joint involvement in SLE can be categorized as follows:

- A non-deforming arthropathy
- A deforming but non-erosive arthropathy (Jaccoud's arthropathy) (Fig. 13.2)
- An erosive arthritis

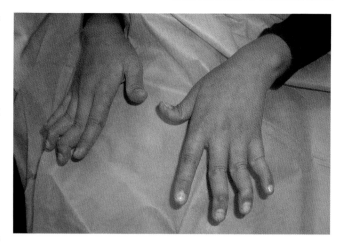

Fig. 13.2 Jaccoud's arthropathy. A deforming, non-erosive arthropathy in a patient with SLE. A hallmark of Jaccoud's arthropathy is the presence of marked but reducible flexion deformities (Figure courtesy of Dr. John Stone)

The erosive arthritis, sometimes termed "rhupus," comprises a clinical and serological overlap syndrome between RA and SLE.

In SLE patients with synovitis, antiCCP IgG antibodies are strongly associated with erosions (odds ratio 29; 95% confidence interval 5–174) (Chan et al. 2008). Furthermore, nearly all antiCCP antibody positive lupus patients fulfill criteria for both SLE and RA and thus have "rhupus" (Damian-Abrego et al. 2008). The HLA alleles associated with antiCCP antibodies in RA patients are also associated with antiCCP antibodies in SLE patients (Chan et al. 2008). Thus, from an immunological point of view, rhupus patients really appear to have both RA and SLE.

Lupus is associated with the production of type I interferon and a peripheral blood interferon "signature." The fact that type I and type II interferons are powerful inhibitors of osteoclasts is one likely explanation for the fact that only a small subset of lupus patients has bony erosions.

13.4 Cutaneous Lupus

Pearl: The malar rash of SLE is not transient.

Comment: A lupus rash should be substantiated by an experienced clinician. A "malar rash" that is transient may not be due to lupus at all: flushing, blushing, polymorphous light eruption, solar urticaria, glucocorticoid-induced acne, seborrheic keratosis, and rosacea can all lead to facial erythema.

Lupus rashes are inflammatory and therefore have texture: they are raised. Moreover, because inflammation takes time to resolve, lupus rashes do not resolve within hours. The malar rash of SLE spares areas shaded from ultraviolet light, such as the nasolabial folds and below the nares (Fig. 13.3a).

Pearl: The malar rash of lupus is often confused with other entities, even by dermatologists.

Comment: Dermatologists are often asked to evaluate patients who have a central facial eruption. The question is whether this represents rosacea, some other entity, or if it is indeed the butterfly rash of SLE.

In practice, the vast majority of such patients have rosacea, seborrheic dermatitis, or some other papulosquamous eruption. The classic butterfly eruption of SLE is observed typically only in patients with acute, fulminant SLE. Patients with chronic disease or those under treatment rarely develop malar rashes. When it does occur, it is a continuous lesion that goes from one cheek to the other and involves the nasal bridge. It is also scaly, red, and papular, and pustules are absent (Fig. 13.3b).

In contrast, the most commonly confused facial eruption is rosacea. Rosacea has discrete areas of involvement isolated to the cheeks, chin, and occasionally the central forehead. The nasal bridge is not involved in rosacea, but the bulb of the nose is often edematous and red. In active rosacea, one can see pustules on examination, although these may be quite small.

Seborrheic dermatitis usually involves the nasolabial folds, eyebrows, ears, and scalp. The scale often has a greasy appearance. Flaking of the scalp is common.

Finally, the cutaneous features of dermatomyositis can mimic SLE. Atypical skin rashes in dermatomyositis are sometimes confused with SLE (Fig. 13.4). Distinguishing features of dermatomyositis are the presence of violaceous, edematous plaques on the upper eyelids, forehead, and sides of the neck, with sparing of the underside of the chin. Dermatomyositis rashes often develop on a background of telangiectasia. Patients with dermatomyositis also often have scalp involvement that is highly pruritic (Fig. 13.5).

Pearl: Cutaneous LE is photosensitive.

Comment: The ACR definition of photosensitivity in the SLE classification criteria is paraphrased as follows: "A skin rash either observed by a physician or reported by the patient that occurs as a result of an unusual reaction to sunlight." Unfortunately, there are many photosensitive skin conditions that can fulfill this ACR criterion for SLE. Such conditions include polymorphous light eruption, photoallergic contact dermatitis, rosacea, dermatomyositis, and medication-induced photosensitivity.

The concept of photosensitivity in SLE also includes a phenomenon that does not manifest itself by a skin rash, yet still constitutes an abnormal reaction to sunlight. As an example, ultraviolet light can serve as the stimulus for flares of systemic signs and symptoms of SLE, not just those confined to the skin (Lin 2007).

Clinical evidence of photosensitivity is demonstrated most easily by the distribution of skin lesions. In the example

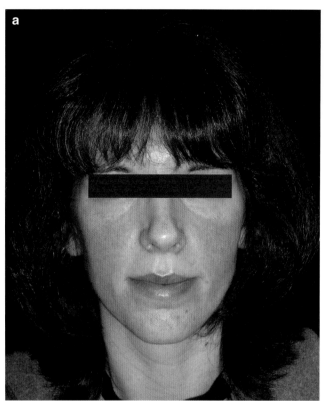

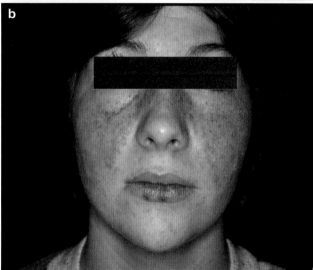

Figs. 13.3 (**a, b**) Malar Rashes. (**a**) One of the key features of a malar rash is that is spares the nasolabial folds, as illustrated in this figure. (**b**) The malar rash of SLE is a continuous plaque that extends over the bridge of the nose. There is distinct sparing of the nasolabial folds. There is substance to the plaque, which is not transient (Figure courtesy of Dr. Grant Anhalt)

demonstrated in Fig. 13.6, the underside of the chin, a sun-protected site, is spared. In contrast, widespread cutaneous lesions occur over areas of the head, neck, chest, and arms, all of which have greater sun exposure (Bijl and Kallenberg 2006).

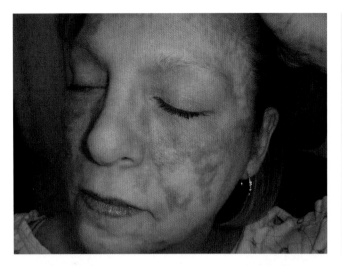

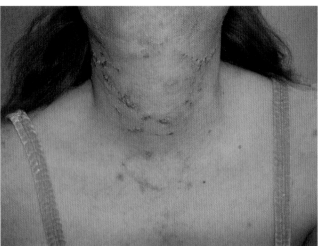

Fig. 13.4 Dermatomyositis masquerading as lupus. This patient was misdiagnosed as having systemic lupus erythematosus for years. Despite the atypical features of the facial eruption, clinical clues to the correct diagnosis of dermatomyositis are the heliotrope rash in the periocular area and the involvement of the scalp (Figure courtesy of Dr. Rachel Abuav)

Fig. 13.6 Photosensitivity. In this patient with systemic lupus erythematosus, there is a distinct sparing of the underside of the chin, a sun-protected area (Figure courtesy of Dr. Rachel Abuav)

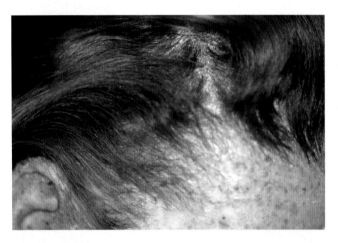

Fig. 13.5 Scalp involvement in dermatomyositis (Figure courtesy of Dr. John Stone)

Pearl: The clinical effects of UV light exposure can be delayed by months.

Comment: In the great majority of patients with SLE, UV light exposure results in an abnormally prolonged erythema of the skin. In many patients, this reaction ensues several weeks after the UV exposure. Furthermore, it appears that UV light can cause systemic disease flares up to 6 months after a prolonged UV light exposure (Lin 2007; Scheinfeld and Deleo 2004). In a photoprovocation study, UVB light triggered lesions in 33% of patients and UVA triggered lesions in 14%. In 53% of patients, however, both UVA and UVB were required to induce lesions of cutaneous LE.

Most types of cutaneous LE are photosensitive, but this relationship may not be appreciated by either the physician or the patient because of the delay in lesion formation that often follows UV light exposure (Tsokos 2004).

Myth: Patients with SLE who develop skin lesions most likely have a cutaneous manifestation of SLE.

Reality: Patients with SLE often develop non-lupus skin lesions that mimic cutaneous lupus. These can include scaly, erythematous macules or pustules on their skin or annular lesions with peripheral scale (Modi et al. 2008). It is important to consider the possibility of non-lupus diagnoses in such patients. As an example, tinea corporis is an excellent mimicker of both acute SLE and subacute cutaneous lupus erythematosus (SCLE).

The diagnosis of tinea can be made in SLE patients with scale or pustules by performing a potassium hydroxide (KOH) preparation of the scale or the contents of pustules to look for fungi. KOH digests the keratin, thereby facilitating the microscopic examination of the preparation for septated hyphae. Cutaneous scales can also be cultured in a microbiology laboratory. SLE patients who receive systemic immunosuppression for a cutaneous manifestation that is attributed to lupus but experience expansion of the cutaneous lesions should be evaluated carefully for a possible fungal infection of the skin (Fig. 13.7). Furthermore, treatment with topical glucocorticoids can alter the clinical appearance of tinea, rendering it "tinea incognito" (Fig. 13.8).

Other skin diseases, such as erythema annulare centrifugum, cutaneous T-cell lymphoma, and granuloma annulare are annular inflammatory skin diseases that can recur and have an appearance similar to SCLE. The possibility of these diagnoses underscores the importance of obtaining a skin biopsy on patients at the time they first develop skin disease.

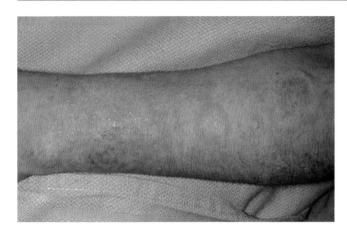

Fig. 13.7 Tinea in lupus. Extensive annular scaly plaques on the arm despite adequate control of systemic disease. Scraping and KOH examination revealed numerous hyphae. Fungal culture grew *Trichophyton rubrum*, the most common of pathogens that cause tinea corporis. The patient was treated successfully with a topical antifungal cream (Figure courtesy of Dr. Rachel Abuav)

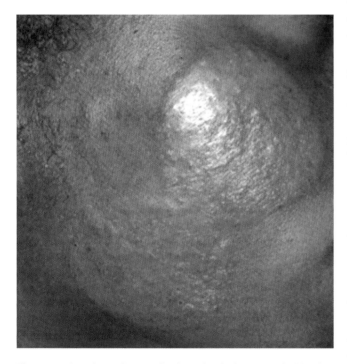

Fig. 13.8 Tinea incognito. Application of topical glucocorticoids often eliminates the surface scale associated with tinea faciei, making diagnosis tricky. A scraping and KOH examination of the plaque revealed hyphae. The patient's rash cleared with topical antifungal cream (Figure courtesy of Dr. Grant Anhalt)

Pearl: Bullous lupus erythematosus (LE) and epidermolysis bullosa acquisita are actually the same disease from the standpoint of the skin.

Comment: A small percentage of patients with acute SLE develop autoantibodies directed against type VII collagen in addition to the "usual" lupus autoantibodies against nuclear proteins and ribonuclear proteins. When this happens, such patients develop mucosal erosions in addition to large, tense blisters, usually on the head and neck or in the axillae and groin (Fig. 13.9a–c). This condition is known as bullous LE. Patients with bullous LE tend to have very aggressive disease courses and frequently have multiple other autoantibodies, e.g., those directed against double-stranded DNA and the Sm or RNP antigens. Hypocomplementemia, glomerulonephritis, arthritis, and serositis are other common disease complications in the setting of bullous LE.

When bullous LE lesions occur outside the context of SLE, the disorder is termed epidermolysis bullosa acquisita. In both conditions, patients with true bullous LE or epidermolysis bullosa acquisita have circulating autoantibodies that are directed against a dermal collagen protein called collagen type VII.

Patients with bullous LE and epidermolysis bullosa acquisita have tense blisters of the skin and mucosa that lead to scarring, because type VII collagen is present in the dermis below the basement membrane zone. Bullous LE and epidermolysis bullosa acquisita are both serious disorders that can involve the eyes, esophagus, or larynx. If left untreated, these disorders result in corneal blindness or laryngoesophageal stenosis.

The diagnosis of bullous LE depends on the demonstration of collagen type VII antibodies in skin or in the serum. Direct immunofluorescence of skin in perilesional tissue reveals thick, homogeneous deposition of IgG along the basement membrane zone (Fig. 13.10). Only skilled immunofluorescence laboratories will be able to distinguish bullous LE or EBA from other blistering disorders of the skin, such as bullous pemphigoid.

Pearl: All bullous lesions in SLE do not constitute bullous LE.

Comment: Bullous LE is a highly distinctive condition, with specific serologic markers. The medical literature is often confusing on this point. In cutaneous lupus, injury to the basal epithelial cells can cause what is called a "vacuolar degenerative change" at the interface of the dermis and epidermis. If this vacuolar interface change is severe enough, the epidermis separates from the underlying dermis at focal sites and a limited degree of blistering can ensue. However, this condition is separate from true bullous LE, which is associated with autoantibodies to type VII collagen (Schmidt et al. 2008).

Myth: Hair loss in SLE is usually due to systemic flares of the lupus.

Reality: Diffuse thinning of scalp hair can herald an exacerbation of SLE. However, there are many causes of diffuse, non-scarring alopecia in SLE. First, medications such as prednisone, methotrexate, mycophenolate mofetil, and hydroxychloroquine can be associated with significant hair

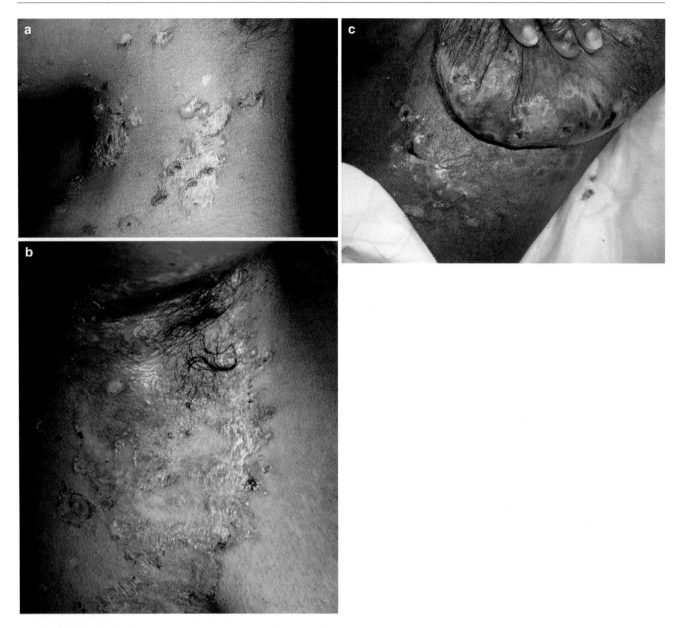

Fig. 13.9a–c Bullous lupus erythematosus. (**a**) Tense blisters on the neck of a young woman with acute SLE. Autoantibodies to type VII collagen were present (Figure courtesy of Dr. Grant Anhalt) (**b**) Extensive erosions and tense blisters in the axilla. This is a common site of involvement in bullous lupus erythematosus. Scarring is evident (Figure cour-

tesy of Dr. Grant Anhalt) (**c**) Extensive scarring of the inframammary region due to chronic blistering in this poorly compliant patient with bullous LE. The patient also had esophageal stenosis secondary to bullous LE. Note the complete and permanent destruction of the fingernail from scarring of the nail matrix (Figure courtesy of Dr. Rachel Abuav)

thinning. In addition, some patients who have lost hair because of a previous cause of diffuse loss, e.g., telogen effluvium associated with a lupus flare, do not regrow their hair to its pre-illness density because of pre-existing (genetically predetermined) androgenetic alopecia (Fig. 13.11). Eliciting a family history of androgenetic hair loss is helpful in identifying this phenomenon.

Patients with SLE are also at an increased risk of alopecia areata, another form of nonscarring hair loss that is mediated by the immune system. Some of these patients have large

areas of scalp involvement, although more typically there are circular areas of nonscarring hair loss (Werth et al. 1992).

Myth: Most nodules in patients with lupus are from lupus panniculitis.

Reality: Many cutaneous nodules in SLE patients are not due to lupus panniculitis. The incidence of erythema nodosum is increased in patients with lupus. Other possible causes of nodules in SLE are vasculitis, livedoid vasculopathy, panniculitic lymphoma, lipodermatosclerosis, and infections,

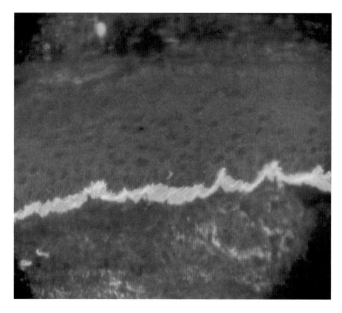

Fig. 13.10 Direct immunofluorescence of a skin biopsy that reveals a thick homogeneous band of IgG deposition along the basement membrane zone. The epidermis is above this band, and the dermis below. This finding is diagnostic of bullous lupus erythematosus or epidermolysis bullosa acquisita (Figure courtesy of Dr. Grant Anhalt)

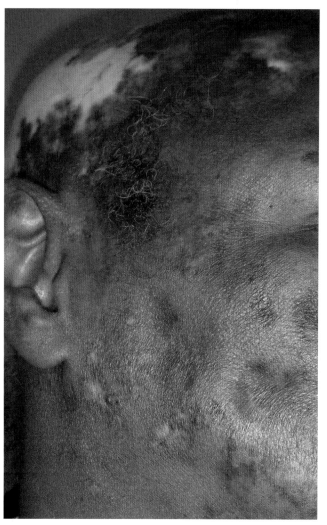

Fig. 13.12 Lupus panniculitis. Lupus panniculitis is manifest in this patient as depressions in the skin on her cheeks. Overlying skin changes are also prominent (Figure courtesy of Dr. Rachel Abuav)

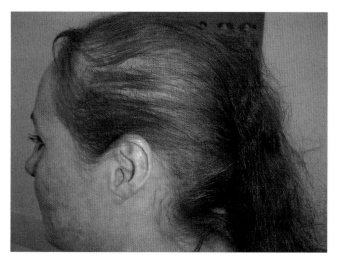

Fig. 13.11 Persistent alopecia in lupus. Despite prolonged remission following a severe lupus flare in which the patient developed alopecia, this patient's hair density has never returned to its pre-illness density. The lupus flare unmasked the presence of androgenetic alopecia (Figure courtesy of Dr. Rachel Abuav)

particularly bacterial, fungal, or atypical mycobacterial infections (Aguilera et al. 2007; Kroshinsky 2008). A skin biopsy that captures a sizeable amount of subcutaneous fat is critical to making the proper diagnosis in lupus patients with nodules.

Lupus panniculitis, a rare condition, has a characteristic morphology. Lupus panniculitis, which has a predilection for the malar region and the lateral deltoid fat pads, leads eventually to depressions in the skin (Fig. 13.12). Approxi-

mately half of all patients with lupus panniculitis have overlying skin changes that are evident such as scaling, erythema, and ulceration. Topical therapy is generally not an effective first-line therapy for lupus panniculitis. Intralesional glucocorticoids are employed on occasion (Callen 2006).

Pearl: The sudden onset of multiple nodules in SLE may be caused by eruptive dermatofibromas.

Comment: Dermatofibromas are common benign skin tumors of spindle cells. In general, they form on the arms and legs, but can be eruptive in SLE, leukemia, HIV infection, and other diseases of immune dysregulation. The sudden onset of numerous nodules in a patient with SLE may be caused by eruptive dermatofibromas (Fig. 13.13).

The patient shown in Fig. 13.13 developed numerous tender nodules at the time of a lupus flare. With prednisone, these lesions diminished in size but did not resolve completely.

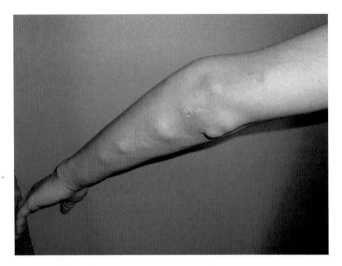

Fig. 13.13 Eruptive dermatofibromas in lupus. Numerous subcutaneous nodules appeared suddenly in the setting of an SLE flare. Skin biopsy of a nodule was consistent with a dermatofibroma. Prednisone diminished the size of the nodules but did not eliminate them completely (Figure courtesy of Dr. Rachel Abuav)

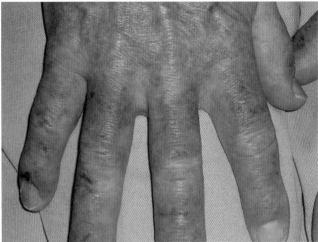

Fig. 13.14 Erythema over the phalanges in systemic lupus erythematosus. The location of erythema in lupus contrasts with the Gottron's papules typical of dermatomyositis (Figure courtesy of Dr. John Stone)

Treatment is not necessary but can include surgery, which is curative (Niiyama et al. 2002).

Pearl: Lupus can "Koebnerize."

Comment: Heinrich Koebner described the phenomenon that bears his name in 1876, when he observed new psoriatic lesions appearing in normal skin after a patient with psoriasis had been bitten by a horse. Since this description, the Koebner phenomenon has been witnessed in numerous other skin conditions, including SLE. Scratching induces discoid lesions in some patients. This has been confirmed by biopsying the lesions and finding histologic features that are characteristic of chronic cutaneous lupus. In addition, old scars can be a focus of new lesional lupus. These include burns, surgical scars, and vaccination sites. Oral lesions of lupus can be initiated by bite trauma (Ueki 2005).

Pearl: The location of erythema on the hands can distinguish SLE from dermatomyositis.

Comment: Although lupus may cause erythematous rashes that resemble those of dermatomyositis, involvement of the knuckles of the fingers (Gottron's papules) is atypical of SLE. SLE usually affects the areas between the small joints of the fingers and spares the knuckles (Fig. 13.14). Although there is significant overlap between SLE and dermatomyositis with regard to their cutaneous manifestations over the hands, this Pearl is a good "rule of thumb."

Myth: Oral ulcerations in SLE are due to necrotizing vasculitis.

Reality: One of the ACR criteria for the classification of SLE is oral ulceration. Oral ulcerations have been attributed to

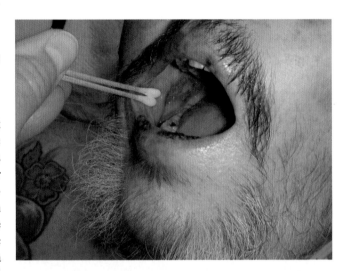

Fig. 13.15 Discoid lupus in the mouth. A discoid lupus erythematosus plaque on the buccal mucosa of a man with SLE (Figure courtesy of Dr. Rachel Abuav)

necrotizing vasculitis and alleged to predict severe systemic disease flares (Ropes 1976). This concept is cited widely today, despite subsequent studies that refute the notion. In one study of oral lesions in ten patients with SLE, biopsy of the ulcerations, erythema, and discoid lesions all showed interface mucositis (Jorizzo et al. 1992). None showed vasculitis.

Oral lesions occur in 20–25% of patients with cutaneous lupus and in 40% of patients with SLE. They range from erythematous patches to true discoid plaques (Fig. 13.15) to frank ulceration. The histopathological appearance of these lesions is one of interface mucositis with vacuolar degeneration of basal keratinocytes.

Myth: It is impossible to distinguish lip lesions of SLE from herpes simplex in an immunocompromised patient.

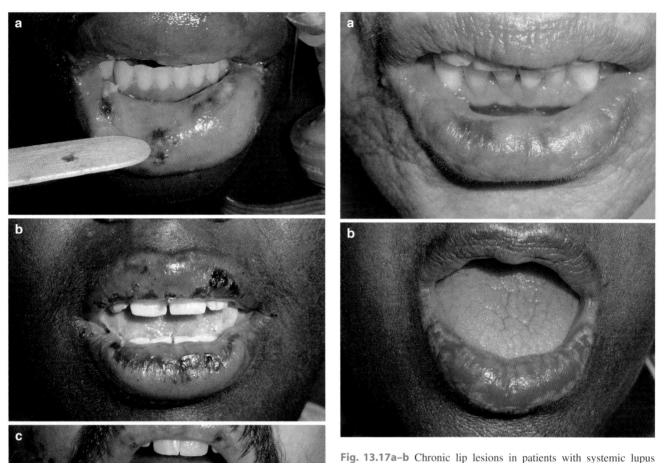

Fig. 13.16a–c Lesions of acute systemic lupus erythematosus (SLE) on the lips. Lip lesions in three patients with SLE flares. All lesions are centered on the "wet line" of the lip and extend onto the vermillion. There is hemorrhagic and serum crusting. The ulceration is shallow (Figure courtesy of Dr. Rachel Abuav)

Fig. 13.17a–b Chronic lip lesions in patients with systemic lupus erythematosus (SLE). These lesions are consistent with chronic cutaneous LE (discoid LE) and are centered on the "wet line" of the lip, extending onto the vermillion, but sparing the vermillion border (Figure courtesy of Dr. Rachel Abuav)

Reality: Lip lesions due to SLE are centered on the wet line of the lip and extend onto the vermillion border (Fig. 13.16a–c). In contrast, lip lesions due to the herpes simplex virus classically erupt on the vermillion border and extend onto the vermillion of the lip. Moreover, lip ulcers of SLE tend to be oval in shape and have ill-defined borders. SLE lesions tend to have an overlying hemorrhagic and serum crust. The edges are not heaped up; the center is typically rather shallow. Chronic SLE lesions have characteristic "discoid" borders with depigmentation and scar in the center (Figs. 13.17a and b).

Although lesions of orolabial HSV among immunocompromised patients can be atypical, these general principles often hold true:

- HSV on the lip erupts on the vermillion border with vesicles and crusting on an edematous base.
- In immunocompetent patients, intraoral lesions of HSV are restricted to mucosa affixed to bone: i.e., to the gingival and hard palate.
- Ulcerations due to HSV are typically punched out, edematous, and often grouped. In the lupus patient, ulcerations may occur more extensively and on areas not affixed to bone, but if one looks carefully, there will be lesions that are typical of orolabial HSV present. Along with viral cultures, these clinical clues make the diagnosis possible.

Of course, both lupus ulceration and reactivated HSV infections can occur concomitantly in patients with SLE. Because there can be morphologic overlap and reactivation of HSV within ulcerations caused by SLE, one should always obtain viral cultures of oral ulcerations in the lupus patient.

Pearl: Patients with a skin biopsy read as lupus actually may have dermatomyositis.

Comment: The skin biopsy findings in SLE, discoid lupus, subacute cutaneous lupus erythematosus, and dermatomyositis can be identical. Because cutaneous LE is more common than dermatomyositis, biopsies are frequently read as consistent with or diagnostic of lupus. Careful clinicopathologic correlation is required to determine a patient's true diagnosis. If a patient has a biopsy read as showing changes of lupus but has Gottron's papules, then that patient has dermatomyositis.

Pearl: Patients with subacute cutaneous lupus frequently have drug-induced disease.

Comment: Many medications are associated with the development of cutaneous lupus. Nearly all of these triggering medications are associated with a specific subset of lupus, namely subacute cutaneous lupus erythematosus, which is most often photosensitive (Fig. 13.18). If the patient is receiving a thiazide, calcium channel blocker, terbenifine, interferon, or an inhibitor of tumor necrosis factor, strong consideration should be given to stopping the drug. Many of these patients develop antiRo/SSA antibodies. Improvement may not be apparent for

months after stopping the culprit drug, but short-term treatment with prednisone and hydroxychloroquine leads to quick resolution. AntiRo/SSA antibodies can persist even after resolution of the skin disease (Sontheimer et al. 2008).

Pearl: Skin disease is uncommon in drug-induced lupus.

Comment: One must distinguish between drug-induced lupus and lupus-like drug eruptions. In patients with drug-induced lupus, the clinical manifestations are typically serositis and arthritis, but skin disease is rare (Tsokos 2004).

The most common forms of drug-induced lupus are due to drugs such as hydralazine, procainamide, and minocycline. These patients have a monomorphic serologic profile with antibodies directed only against histones, producing high titers of ANA that stain with a homogeneous pattern on immunofluorescence testing.

Pearl: The presence of discoid lupus lesions below the head and neck region is associated with an increased risk of developing systemic lupus.

Comment: Discoid lupus erythematosus (DLE) is the most common type of chronic cutaneous lupus erythematosus. It

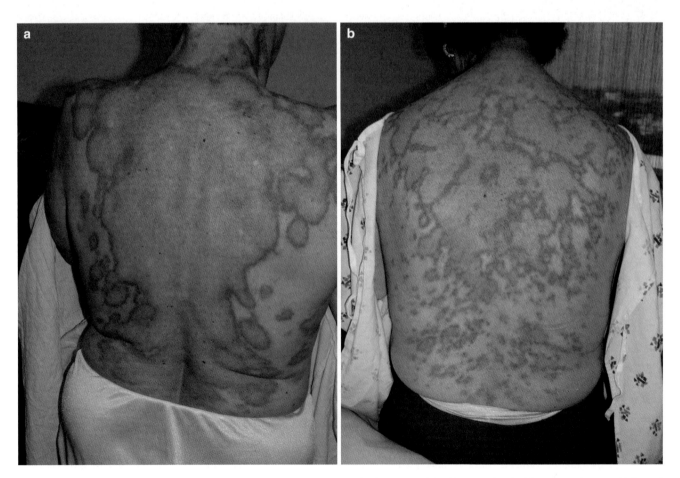

Fig. 13.18 (**a**, **b**) Subacute cutaneous lupus erythematosus. This annular, papulosquamous rash is often associated with extreme photosensitivity and antibodies directed against the Ro antigen (Fig. 13.18a courtesy of Dr. Victoria Werth, Fig. 13.18b courtesy of Dr. Rachel Abuav)

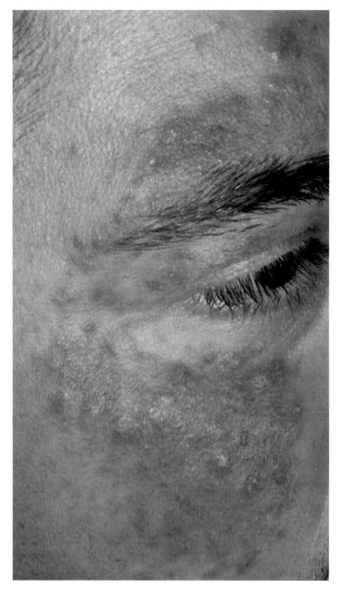

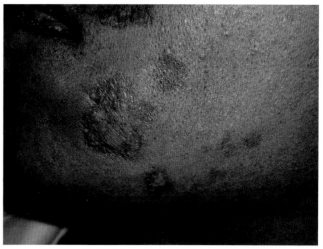

Fig. 13.20 Late discoid lupus erythematosus (DLE). In this patient, atrophy and pigmentary alteration denote scarring, which is irreversible. This is characteristic of established plaques of DLE (Figure courtesy of Dr. Rachel Abuav)

Among all patients with DLE, the risk of developing SLE is only about 5%. Among those with DLE lesions localized to the head and neck, the probability of a complete remission is on the order of 50% (Callen 2006).

Myth: Patients with cutaneous lupus should get some sun exposure to increase their vitamin D levels.

Reality: Vitamin D levels in cutaneous lupus patients are frequently low. This is probably related to sun avoidance and the use of sunscreens (Cusack et al. 2008). However, it is easy to provide oral supplementation of vitamin D to these patients, and the risks of vitamin D replacement are minimal relative to the potential for causing exacerbations of the underlying lupus through sun exposure.

Fig. 13.19 Early discoid lupus erythematosus (DLE). In this patient with early plaques of DLE, early treatment will avoid scarring (Figure courtesy of Dr. Grant Anhalt)

can be seen as an isolated finding; however, 15–20% of SLE patients have DLE lesions. Clinically, they are sharply demarcated, round (hence, "discoid") plaques that initially appear erythematous or violaceous (Fig. 13.19). With time, they become scaly and demonstrate follicular plugging. In the end stages, the rims are hyperpigmented and the centers are depigmented, scarred, and often atrophic (Fig. 13.20).

When DLE is found in isolation, the lesions are usually confined to the scalp, face, and neck, and demonstrate a photoaccentuated distribution. When lesions are extensive and present above and below the waist, the risk of developing SLE (if not already evident) appears high. Such patients usually have positive serologies and should be monitored closely for internal organ involvement.

13.5 Lupus Nephritis

Myth: Serum creatinine is a reliable indicator of renal function.

Reality: Measurement of the serum creatinine level is a practical but relatively insensitive indicator of abnormalities in the glomerular filtration rate. The serum creatinine level is affected by variables with little direct relationship to renal function, including sex, muscle mass, and age. Nevertheless, reproducible elevations in the serum creatinine level (e.g., ≥20–30% increase) are of concern, even if they fall within the normal range.

Pearl: In a pregnant lupus patient, substantial renal dysfunction can be present despite the finding of a normal serum creatinine level.

Comment: Normal pregnancies increase the glomerular filtration rate through expansion of the plasma volume. This leads to a decrease in serum creatinine levels in pregnancy. Thus, a "normal" serum creatinine level in a pregnant lupus patient might actually signal a substantial alteration of renal function (see Chapter 17).

Pearl: An experienced clinician recognizes the point of diminishing returns with the use of immunosuppression for glomerulonephritis.

Comment: It's not worth saving the kidneys if you've lost the patient. The efficacy of renal replacement therapy – both dialysis and transplantation – means that end-stage renal disease no longer marks the end of the line for a patient with SLE. Sometimes, it is prudent to let severely damaged kidneys go, rather than lose the patient to complications of immunosuppression.

As an example, end-stage renal disease at some point in the future is probably inevitable for a patient who has arrived at a serum creatinine of 4.0 mg/dL slowly. When in doubt, a renal biopsy showing Class VI (renal sclerosis) can provide sufficient evidence that the need for renal replacement therapy is unavoidable and that additional cyclophosphamide or mycophenolate mofetil is more likely to cause harm than good.

Pearl: Proteinuria can be diminished by 50% without prescribing a single milligram of prednisone.

Comment: Only a minority of patients with lupus nephritis achieve complete remission, even with modern treatment regimens. As an example, only 23% of patients treated with mycophenolate mofetil in one randomized trial achieved a complete remission (Ginzler et al. 2005). Our preoccupation with selecting and honing the proper regimen of immunosuppression can lead us to overlook other measures that play important roles in the long-term salvage of kidneys.

Renal-sparing protocols are underutilized in lupus nephritis. The reduction of proteinuria through ACE inhibition delays and prevents renal sclerosis, hyperlipidemia, hypercoagulability, and their concomitant complications. The use of ACE inhibitors and angiotensive receptor blockers can reduce proteinuria by up to 50%. Spironolactone also helps to reduce proteinuria (Chrysostomou and Becker 2001). (In men, eplerenone should be used, because of its lower risk of gynecomastia.)

Pearl: Proteinuria is a better indicator of lupus nephritis than is hematuria.

Comment: Hematuria is one of the renal manifestations of lupus listed on the SLE Disease Activity Index (SLEDAI) (Bombardier et al. 1992). However, sound clinical judgment is essential before ascribing hematuria to active lupus. SLE patients may have hematuria from a variety of causes, including menses, trauma, renal calculi, and thin basement membrane disease.

In the SELENA studies, the investigators amended the SLEDAI to require that hematuria only be used in the presence of proteinuria as a manifestation of lupus (Buyon et al. 2005; Petri et al. 2005).

Myth: The urinalysis is the poor man's renal biopsy.

Reality: If this were true, then he would be a poor man, indeed (and she a poor patient). Ample evidence suggests that the findings in a spun urine sample correlate poorly with the histopathologic features on biopsy (Christopher-Stine et al. 2007; Huong et al. 1999). Even in the setting of diffuse proliferative glomerulonephritis, minimal hematuria may be evident on urinalysis.

Yet the importance of a careful urinalysis in SLE should not be discounted. An abnormal urinalysis provides critical information. Urinalysis with microscopic examination of the urine sediment should be performed at every patient visit. However, in the setting of renal dysfunction of unclear etiology, the fundamental issue is tissue.

13.6 Central Nervous System Lupus

Myth: "Lupus headaches" are part and parcel of the disease.

Reality: Although "lupus headache" is one of the neurologic manifestations listed on the SLE Disease Activity Index (SLEDAI) (Bombardier et al. 1992), headaches are actually rare in lupus. Most women with SLE who have headaches have migraine physiology. Case-control studies have not shown any increase in headaches among SLE patients compared with controls (Fernandez-Nebro et al. 1999). Although headache is listed under the ACR neuropsychiatric case definitions, this symptom has poor specificity for SLE in population-based studies (ACR ad hoc committee on neuropsychiatric lupus 1999; Ainiala et al. 2001).

An SLE patient with a severe headache should have an evaluation designed to exclude brain hemorrhage or dural sinus thrombosis. Lumbar puncture is also appropriate to help exclude infection, malignancy, and pseudotumor cerebri. Lupus meningitis, manifested by a pleocytosis and elevated CSF protein, is a diagnosis of exclusion.

Pearl: When managing patients with neuropsychiatric lupus, improvement is likely to take several months. Patience is required.

Comment: A standardized nomenclature for neuropsychiatric lupus was developed by the American College of Rheumatology. This distinguishes three subsets of syndromes:

* Psychiatric, cognitive deficits, and acute confusional states
* Neurological syndromes of the central nervous system
* Neurological syndromes of the peripheral nervous system

In one single-center study, only 10 of 485 patients with SLE developed major neuropsychiatric disease manifestations (Pego-Reigosa and Isenberg 2008). In eight of these ten cases, the outcome was ultimately excellent but the time to recovery was long, often up to 12 months or longer for complete symptom resolution.

A critical feature in the management of some of these patients is to understand that improvement in the psychosis may require several months. Many patients attain significant and sustained resolution of symptoms following intensive immunosuppressive therapy, but in some the improvement does not occur quickly.

With regard to the treatment of lupus psychosis, there are no published controlled trials of any treatment strategy. Moreover, the long-term outcome of lupus psychosis is not well established. Several retrospective studies have reported the benefit using glucocorticoids and intravenous cyclophosphamide in patients with neuropsychiatric lupus in addition with antipsychotic, antidepressant, or anticonvulsant therapy (Boumpas et al. 1991; Neuwelt et al. 1995; Ramos et al. 1996; Baca et al. 1999; Takada et al. 2001).

Pearl: Practically speaking, it is often difficult to separate central nervous system disease manifestations that are due to inflammation from those that are caused by thrombosis.

Comment: Anticoagulation with warfarin is a cornerstone of treatment for lupus patients who present with neuropsychiatric events that are characteristic of the antiphospholipid syndrome (APS), e.g., stroke, intracerebral venous thrombosis, or chorea. However, the cause of a particular clinical syndrome is often not clearcut in lupus. When the relative contributions of "inflammatory" mechanisms as opposed to "thrombotic" pathways are unclear, the patient may require combination therapy with glucocorticoids, cytotoxic drugs, and warfarin.

Myth: Loss of vision in lupus is probably due to optic neuritis.

Reality: Significant ocular pain or reduction in vision requires urgent assessment by an ophthamologist (Sivaraj et al. 2007). Sight-threatening ocular disease in lupus may be due to a variety of processes at a number of ocular sites:

- Lens (cataract formation)
- Vitreous humor (hemorrhage)
- Retina (occlusion of retinal vein or artery, retinal detachment, toxic maculopathy from antimalarial agents or glucocorticoids)
- Choroid (choroidopathy, infarction, effusion)
- Neuro-ophthalmic tract (optic nerve, optic chiasm, or the occipital cortex).

Optic nerve disease occurs in fewer than 1% of patients with SLE and may be due to optic neuritis or ischemic optic neuropathy (anterior or posterior). Optic neuritis typically presents acutely with unilateral loss of vision and pain that is worse with eye movements. In contrast, optic neuropathy usually presents with acute unilateral vision loss that is painless, caused by occlusion of the small vessels to the optic nerve. Unilateral optic neuropathy appears to reflect a focal thrombotic event associated with the antiphospholipid syndrome.

In contrast to idiopathic optic neuritis or to that associated with multiple sclerosis, the visual prognosis in SLE is not always good, particularly in the setting of optic neuropathy. Recurrence is not unusual and further worsens the prognosis. In optic neuritis, glucocorticoids alone or in combination with immunosuppressive therapy are effective in almost 50% of the cases. In optic neuropathy, the outcome is worse. Some patients appear to respond to immunosuppressive therapy alone. For patients in whom antiphospholipid antibodies are identified, anticoagulation is appropriate.

Posterior reversible encephalopathy syndrome (PRES) is a rare neurologic condition associated with renal insufficiency, hypertension, acute intermittent porphyria, calcineurin inhibitors, and a variety of other conditions, including lupus. Patients present with headache, seizures, loss of vision from cortical blindness, and altered mental function. The pattern on magnetic resonance imaging studies is one of transient posterior cerebral hyperintensities on T2-weighted images (Fig. 13.21). Patients may respond to glucocorticoids and immunosuppressive therapy.

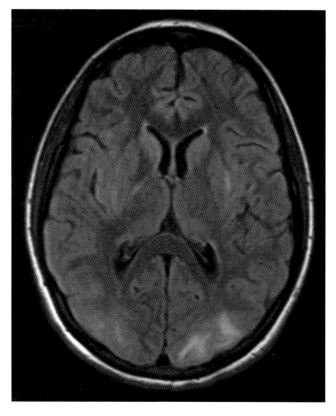

Fig. 13.21 Magnetic resonance imaging study in a lupus patient with the posterior reversible encephalopathy syndrome (PRES) (Figure courtesy of Dr. Arezou Khosroshahi)

13.7 General Management Points

Myth: A high erythrocyte sedimentation rate (ESR) indicates active clinical SLE.

Reality: Many SLE patients have dramatic elevations in their ESRs in the absence of apparent clinical disease activity. Similarly, hypocomplementemia and elevated titers of dsDNA antibodies also occur frequently in the absence of clinical disease. Such patients fall into the category of "serologically active but clinically quiescent" SLE (Walz LeBlanc et al. 1994). These patients should *not* be treated for active SLE, but rather be watched carefully: they are more likely to experience disease flares within the next year. Changes in serum complement levels and antidsDNA antibody titers do *not* predict disease flares over the following month (Ho et al. 2001a and b).

Serum levels of C-reactive protein (CRP) can also be elevated in SLE that is clinically quiescent. These patients also bear watching closely, but some data indicate that obesity, a problem in many patients with longstanding SLE, can lead to CRP elevations (Petri 2008).

Myth: In a febrile lupus patient, both C-reactive protein and procalcitonin levels are useful in excluding infection.

Reality: Infections account for approximately one-fourth of all deaths in lupus. These disease complications are attributable primarily to therapy, particularly glucocorticoids and cytotoxic drugs. When it comes to excluding infections in SLE, the stakes of being wrong are so high that one can never rely entirely on a single laboratory test. One study from the National Institutes of Health in the 1970s indicated that 60% of febrile episodes among SLE patients were due to active lupus, but 23% were caused by infections (Stahl et al. 1979).

The oft-quoted myth is that SLE flares do not increase either C-reactive protein or procalcitonin. This statement is wrong often enough to make it dangerous. In a study from the Netherlands, serum CRP levels were normal (less than 6 mg/L) in only 34% of patients with SLE flares (13 of 38 cases), and were also normal in 10% of those with a systemic infection (4 of 36 cases) (terBorg et al. 1990). Thus, even if the CRP level is normal, infections must be excluded rigorously in all SLE patients with fever. This is particularly true, of course, if the patient has a history of substantial immunosuppressive drug use (Roy and Tan 2001).

Two features of active lupus, namely arthritis and pleuropericarditis, are often associated with elevated CRP levels (Spronk et al. 1992; Hesselink et al. 2003). A 2-year prospective study reported that SLE flares associated with serositis were substantially more likely to be accompanied by an elevated CRP than were those without serositis (mean CRP level 76 mg/L versus 16 mg/L; P < 0.02).

Similar considerations apply to procalcitonin. Procalcitonin levels were alleged to remain low during SLE flares but

to increase in the setting of severe bacterial and fungal infections. Data on this point have been inconsistent. The test is currently not widely available, and is not recommended for general use.

Pearl: Lupus patients are immunosuppressed, even without our help.

Comment: Patients with SLE have an increased risk of certain viral, fungal, and bacterial infections even before their introduction to prednisone, glucocorticoid-sparing agents, and other treatments. SLE patients have difficulty with multiple viral infections, especially herpes zoster, cytomegalovirus, and papillomaviruses. They are also subject to fungal infections, especially oral candidiasis, but also onychomycosis. Perhaps because of splenic dysfunction, SLE patients have difficulty with encapsulated organisms such as the pneumococcus and meningococcus. Don't forget to vaccinate all SLE patients, especially the teenager with lupus who is going off to college (Petri 1998).

Pearl: Most infections in SLE are preventable.

Comment: Infection remains a leading cause of morbidity and mortality in patients with SLE (Zandman-Goddard and Shoenfeld 2003). This susceptibility is due to a combination of factors, including underlying immune dysregulation (manifested as defects in neutrophil chemotaxis), impaired clearance of opsonized bacteria, and functional hyposplenia (Iliopoulos and Tsokos 1996).

In addition, certain disease manifestations, principally renal involvement and treatment, also contribute to the occurrence, type, and severity of infections (Noel et al. 2001; Fessler 2002; Gladman et al. 2002). Serious but non-fatal infections are an independent risk factor for death 10 years after the diagnosis of SLE (Noel et al. 2001). Judicious use of glucocorticoids and the conscientious administration of immunizations decrease the frequency of infections (Gilland and Tsokos 2002).

Myth: Vaccines cause SLE flares.

Reality: Vaccines and lupus are a complicated story. There is no evidence that inactivated vaccines cause SLE flares. This has been studied rigorously for both the influenza vaccine and the pneumococcal vaccines, but the risk posed to lupus patients by the hepatitis B virus vaccination also appears negligible (Abu-Shakra et al. 2000; Klippel et al. 1979; Elkayam et al. 2002, 2005; Turner-Stokes et al. 1988). Because SLE patients may not mount vigorous vaccine responses, the pneumococcal vaccine should be administered every 5 years. The pneumococcal vaccine should never be omitted because SLE patients have particular problems with encapsulated organisms.

In short, clinicians should have no reticence about administering killed vaccines to patients with SLE. Common vaccine practice recommendations are shown in Table 13.5.

Table 13.5 Use of vaccinations in patients with systemic lupus erythematosus rated according to evidence (Adapted O'Neill 2006)

Vaccine	Type(s)	Evidence of efficacy in SLE[a]	Evidence of safety in SLE[a]	Concerns/comments
BCG	Live attenuated	No evidence available	No evidence available	CI if immunosuppressed
MMR	Live attenuated	No evidence available	Some evidence for use	CI if immunosuppressed
Varicella	Live attenuated	No evidence available	No evidence available	CI if immunosuppressed
Yellow Fever	Live attenuated	No evidence available	No evidence available	CI if immunosuppressed
Polio	Live attenuated (oral)	No evidence available	Some evidence for use	CI if immunosuppressed Available in some countries
	Inactivated (parenteral)	No evidence available	No evidence available	
Hepatitis B	Component (recombinant DNA)	Some evidence against	Some evidence for use	? Decreased efficacy
Hepatitis A	Inactivated	No evidence available	No evidence available	
Influenza	Inactivated component	Good evidence for use	Good evidence for use	
Meningococcus	Component polysaccharide	No evidence available	No evidence available	
	Conjugate	No evidence available	No evidence available	
Pertussis	Inactivated whole cell	No evidence available	No evidence available	
	Component	No evidence available	No evidence available	
Pneumococcus	Component polysaccharide	Good evidence for use	Strong evidence for use	Significant minority do not respond or response short lived
	Conjugate	No evidence available	No evidence available	
Haemophilus influenzae B	Conjugate	Good evidence for use	Good evidence for use	
Tetanus	Toxoid	Strong evidence for use	Strong evidence for use	
Diptheria	Toxoid	No evidence available	No evidence available	CI if immunosuppressed

MMR = Measles, mumps, rubella
[a]Represents overall impression from weighing up published series of the degree of evidence for or against the vaccines use in SLE. CI: Contraindicated

Pearl: The situation with live vaccines is more complex.

Comment: Although influenza and pneumococcal vaccines appear to be safe and effective in SLE, the story is not so clear-cut for live vaccines. Vaccines such as Varicella zoster and measles, mumps, and rubella (MMR) have been considered contraindicated in patients with SLE and any patient receiving more than 10 mg of prednisone a day or other immunosuppressive agents (O'Neill and Isenberg 2006). It has also been suggested that live vaccines should not be given for 3 months after cessation of immunosuppressive drugs. However, in June 2008, the Advisory Committee on Immunization Practices (ACIP) provided some new recommendations and raised several new questions.

The ACIP now recommends routine vaccination of all persons older than 60 years of age who have no contraindication (ACIP 2008). The recommendation includes individuals with chronic medical conditions. However, the panel felt that moderately or severely immunosuppressed (e.g., those on ≥ 20 mg/day prednisone for >2 weeks) or immunodeficient patients (e.g., AIDS or HIV with CD4+ T-lymphocyte values < 200 per mm^3 or <15% of total lymphocytes) should not receive the vaccine. Lower levels of immunosuppression, e.g.,

patients on <20 mg/day prednisone, methotrexate (<0.4 mg/kg/week), azathioprine (<3.0 mg/kg/day), or 6-mercaptopurine (<1.5 mg/kg/day) do not constitute contraindications to immunization against Varicella zoster. However, this is clearly an area where additional research is essential.

The panel did not comment on the additive effects of glucocorticoids plus immunosuppressive drugs. AntiTNF agents were felt to be too new to be sure of their impact on immunization against Varicella zoster. One reasonable approach is to discontinue TNF inhibitors for 1 month before administering the Varicella zoster vaccine and to wait 1 month before resuming TNF inhibition.

The situation in lupus is complex. Rheumatoid arthritis, psoriasis, polymyositis, sarcoidosis, and inflammatory bowel disease were all listed specifically as conditions in which vaccination might be allowed under appropriate circumstances. Lupus was not. Not only are lupus patients immunosuppressed by medications, they may also be significantly immunodeficient because of active lupus and to some degree because of the genetic defects associated with lupus.

Perhaps, for these reasons the ACIP did not make specific recommendations about Varicella zoster immunization in SLE patients. At this time, firm recommendations about

Varicella zoster immunization in SLE are not possible. Two points appear reasonable:

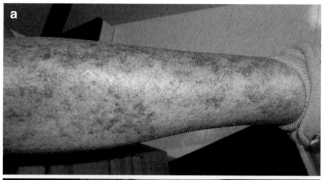

- Lupus patients whose disease is inactive and who are on stable doses of prednisone (<15 mg/day) with or without hydroxychloroquine may be appropriate candidates for Varicella zoster vaccination.
- Lupus patients with recently active disease should not receive this vaccination.

Additional studies to document the safety and efficacy of the zoster vaccine in SLE are needed.

Pearl: Pneumocystis carinii (jiroveci) prophylaxis should be employed in selected patients with SLE.

Comment: Patients with SLE are at increased risk for Pneumocystis carinii (jiroveci) pneumonia (PCP) (Porges et al. 1992). In a study of hospitalized patients, there were approximately 12 cases of PCP for every 10,000 SLE admissions, compared with only 2 cases of PCP for every 10,000 rheumatoid arthritis admissions (odds ratio = 2.5; 95% confidence interval 1.7–3.8) (Ward and Donald 1999).

SLE patients who develop PCP are usually (but not always) on high doses of glucocorticoids and immunosuppressive medications such as cyclophosphamide. (Godeau et al. 1994). Some patients who develop PCP are not on intensive immunosuppression at the time of their infection but have been on intensive immunosuppression in the preceding months (Suryaprasad 2008). PCP prophylaxis should be considered in an SLE patient on moderate to high doses of prednisone, particularly if another immunosuppressive drug is part of the treatment regimen or if the patient is severely lymphopenic.

Pearl: Lupus patients tolerate trimethoprim-sulfamethoxazole medications poorly.

Comment: Hypersensitivity to sulfonamides is more common among patients with SLE when compared with the general population. In addition, some investigations have indicated that sulfonamide use in SLE patients is associated with disease flares (Petri and Allbritton 1992). Maculopapular skin eruptions with or without fever are the most common adverse effect of sulfonamides in SLE (Fig. 13.22). Such reactions are probably type IV (cell-mediated) hypersensitivity responses (Pichler 2003). The rate of type I hypersensitivity (IgE-mediated) hypersensitivity responses does not appear to be markedly increased.

A high frequency of maculopapular rash and fever in response to sulfonamides has also been seen in patients infected with the human immunodeficiency virus (HIV). The pathophysiology for the increase in sulfonamide hypersensitivity has not been established. However, metabolism to reactive intermediates such as hydroxylamines and nitrososulfonamides, which leads to either direct cytotoxicity or to haptenization of host proteins, seems likely to play a role.

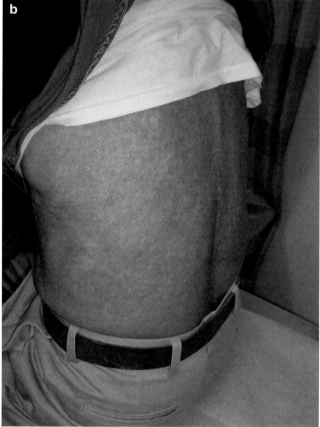

Fig. 13.22 (**a**, **b**) Eczema induced by trimethoprim/sulfamethoxazole (TMP/SMX). This lupus patient had been on TMP/SMX for approximately 2 months before he developed a diffuse cutaneous eruption (nonpalpable purpura on the lower extremities, blanching erythema on the back, abdomen, and trunk). The rash resolved following the discontinuation of TMP/SMX (Figure courtesy of Dr. John Stone)

These reactive intermediates are more likely to occur in slow acetylators and in the settings in which oxidative stress leads to low levels of glutathione, as seen in HIV and SLE (Perl et al. 2004).

Despite the increase in risk of hypersensitivity reactions in HIV, TMP-SMX is still used for the prophylaxis and treatment of PCP. Indeed, the potential benefit from TMP-SMX has led to the development of desensitization protocols for patients with a history of TMP-SMX hypersensitivity. These protocols are usually (but not always) successful. Of course, desensitization should not be attempted in patients with severe reactions such as Stevens–Johnson syndrome, toxic epidermal necrolysis, or serum sickness. Among patients with HIV, the gradual introduction of prophylactic TMP-SMX leads to fewer adverse reactions (Para et al. 2000).

Many similarities exist between patients with HIV and SLE with regard to sulfonamide hypersensitivity. One important difference, however, is the potential association of TMP-SMX use with disease exacerbation in SLE. Thus, the avoidance of sulfonamides for the treatment of routine bacterial infections in SLE patients seems a reasonable precaution. Whether to use TMP-SMX as opposed to dapsone, atovaquone, or aerosolized pentamidine for PCP prophylaxis in SLE remains a controversial issue. If the decision is made in favor of TMX-SMX, the medication should be introduced gradually over a 2-week period.

Pearl: The majority of patients with serologically active but clinically quiescent lupus are likely to flare at some point in the future, but the disease flare may not occur for many months or even several years.

Comment: A minority of patients with SLE enter a period in which their disease is serologically active but clinically quiescent. In the University College London Hospital Cohort, this state has been defined as an antidsDNA antibody titer greater than 50 units/mL on two occasions but a global BILAG score of less than 6 for at least 6 months.

In one cohort of patients with serologically active but clinically quiescent disease, 81% suffered a disease flare within 5 years (WalzLeBlanc et al. 1994; Ng et al. 2006). Approximately half of those patients had multiple flares during that time. The mean duration to first disease flare was 15 months (range: 2–46 months). Shorter times to disease flare correlated with high titers of antinucleosome antibodies and antidsDNA antibody titers that were five times above the normal limit (Ng et al. 2006).

Myth: Hormone replacement therapy (HRT) causes flares in patients with SLE.

Reality: The safety of exogenous estrogens in SLE patients remains a controversial topic. Estrogen use in SLE has special relevance because of the premature ovarian failure that these patients often experience as a result of treatment, the elevated risk of osteoporosis, and the rapid acceleration of atherosclerosis to which lupus patients are prone. Symptoms of estrogen deficiency are often particularly severe in younger women and frequently require long-term HRT.

Clinicians often avoid HRT in patients with SLE because the fear of inducing disease flares. The Safety of Estrogens in Lupus Erythematosus National Assessment (SELENA) trial found that patients who are prescribed HRT were more likely to experience mild to moderate disease flares more often

than those prescribed placebo (Buyon et al. 2005). However, severe flares were not more common in the HRT group.

Another study focused specifically on the influence of HRT on the occurrence of arterial and venous thrombotic events in post-menopausal women with SLE (Fernandez et al. 2007). That study reported no increase in vascular events among patients who were antiphospholipid antibody negative and had no history of such events. However, data from the Women's Health Study indicate that HRT increases the thrombotic risk in the general female population.

Decisions on the use of HRT in patients with SLE must be individualized according to each patient's risk profile. Data from the studies cited above cannot be extrapolated to patients with high titers of antiphospholipid antibodies or previous thrombotic events.

Myth: Statins should be used with caution in SLE patients because they heighten patients' risk of muscle injury.

Reality: Lupus patients have a substantially increased risk for accelerated atherosclerosis. Thus, cardiovascular risk factors, including dyslipidemia, should be sought and managed aggressively. Statins are both effective and generally safe in SLE. Severe myopathy affects only about 0.1% of all individuals who take statins. Thus, the issue with regard to statin use for many patients with SLE is not whether or not to use these drugs, but rather how to use them wisely.

Patients with significant renal insufficiency or hypothyroidism are at increased risk of skeletal muscle toxicity from statin use. Because SLE patients have a higher than normal likelihood of both renal and thyroid dysfunction, these factors should be considered before prescribing statins. Because some patients with connective tissue disease have low CK values, a normal serum CK in the presence of symptoms and signs of myositis does not exclude the possibility of muscle injury.

In the absence of clinical symptoms and weakness, a CK level more than three times the upper limit of normal that is attributed to statin use is an indication for discontinuing the medication. Patients should drink large quantities of fluids to facilitate the renal excretion of CK. After the CK has returned to baseline, patients may be tried on a statin less likely to cause muscle toxicity. Pravastatin and fluvastatin are both less likely to cause muscle injury than is lovastatin.

Pearl: Diffuse or focal myocarditis can mimic myocardial infarction.

Comment: The first order of business in a lupus patient with chest pain, regardless of the patient's age, is to exclude active coronary ischemia. Patients with SLE can and do develop coronary arteritis, leading to myocardial infarction.

However, in young patients with lupus who present with symptoms, signs, and laboratory findings consistent with acute coronary ischemia (e.g., angina, ST segment elevations on electrocardiography, and CK-MB or troponin concentration elevation), the clinician must bear in mind the possibility of myocarditis. Cardiac scintigraphy or magnetic resonance imaging can reveal diffuse or focal myocarditis in such patients.

Pearl: Fifty percent of SLE patients who have a lupus antico-agulant at diagnosis will suffer a thrombotic event.

Comment: This is true, and the lupus anticoagulant is a more powerful predictor of thrombotic risk than is anticardiolipin antibody (Somers et al. 2002; Wahl et al. 1997). However, the 50% risk of thrombosis associated with lupus anticoagulants is cumulative, occurring over 20 years. Thus, although empiric prophylactic therapy is worth considering, the choice of medication is determined by long-term safety concerns. The use of aspirin makes intuitive sense and has a better side-effect profile for most patients than does warfarin, but two clinical trials failed to demonstrate benefit of aspirin in the prevention of thrombotic events (Erkan et al. 2007; Ginsburg et al. 1992).

Despite the absence of evidence supporting its use, the absence of evidence is not evidence of absence: many clinicians use a daily baby aspirin to treat patients with antiphospholipid antibodies who have clinical manifestations of the antiphospholipid syndrome. Some data also indicate that hydroxychloroquine prevents antiphospholipid antibody-mediated thrombosis (Petri 1996; Pierangeli and Harris 1996).

The avoidance of medications that foster hypercoagulability is also important in managing patients at risk for thrombosis. Such medications include oral contraceptives, hormone replacement therapy, selective estrogen receptor modulators, thalidomide, and doses of erythropoietin that lead to overcorrection of anemia.

13.8 Treatment

Pearl: Immunosuppressive drug regimens in SLE are selected according to the pattern of organ involvement.

Comment: Clinicians who treat many patients with lupus tend to have "favorite" regimens that are prescribed according to the specific organs affected. Some generalizations are possible:

- Mycophenolate mofetil is the preferred medication for lupus nephritis because of its therapeutic equivalency with cyclophosphamide and its lower rate of adverse effects (Chan et al. 2000; Contreras et al. 2004; Ginzler et al. 2005).
- Azathioprine is probably equivalent to mycophenolate mofetil as a remission maintenance agent in lupus nephritis (Contreras et al. 2004).
- Methotrexate and leflunomide are the preferred agents for the treatment of arthritis in SLE (Sato 2001; Tam et al. 2004).

- Hydroxychloroquine is the drug of first choice for cutaneous SLE. For skin lupus refractory to hydroxychloroquine alone, the addition of quinacrine can be helpful.

Methotrexate and mycophenolate mofetil are useful second-line agents for cutaneous lupus. However, mycophenolate mofetil may require many months or even more than 1 year before its benefits in chronic cutaneous lupus are evident. Patients should be counseled about this.

- Thalidomide can be added for recalcitrant discoid lupus, but its toxicity profile (teratogenicity, neuropathy, premature gonadal failure, and thrombosis) makes its use unusual.

Pearl: Hydroxychloroquine should be put in the water supply.

Comment: At least in the water imbibed by lupus patients. Hydroxychloroquine has gained new respect as a preventive agent in SLE. Experienced lupus clinicians refer to this medication as "lupus health insurance". Hydroxychloroquine reduces the frequency of SLE flares and probably also reduces the "spread" of lupus to renal disease (Tsakonas et al. 1998; Fessler et al. 2005). Furthermore, it diminishes the likelihood of thrombosis caused by antiphospholipid antibodies (Petri 1996; Pierangeli and Harris 1996). Finally, the drug may have effects that are synergistic with those of other SLE medications. In one study of patients with lupus nephritis, patients who remained on hydroxychloroquine doubled their chance of responding to mycophenolate mofetil (Kasitanon et al. 2006).

Concern about hydroxychloroquine retinopathy is overblown. This retinal complication of this medication occurs quite rarely (on the order of 1 in 5,000 patients on long-term therapy), develops slowly, and is reversible if the medication is stopped promptly. A safe recommendation is to insist that patients treated with hydroxychloroquine have an annual ophthalmology examination.

The dose of hydroxychloroquine should be reduced in patients with significant renal dysfunction, in the elderly, and in patients with a low body mass index (e.g., children). The safety profile of chloroquine is less clear. Patients taking chloroquine should have more regular ophthalmic examinations (Marmor et al. 2002).

Pearl: Cigarette smoking is associated with an increased risk of cutaneous lupus and decreased responsiveness to antimalarial therapy.

Comment: Patients who smoke are more likely to have cutaneous lupus. In addition, there is good evidence that patients who are therapeutically resistant to the usual therapies, including antimalarials, immunosuppressive agents, and thalidomide are frequently smokers (Moghadam-Kia et al., in press; Jewell and McCauliffe 2000). Smoking cessation should be urged for a variety of reasons in SLE. Better control of skin disease is one of them (Miot et al. 2005).

Pearl: Quinacrine is a helpful adjunctive therapy when combined with hydroxychloroquine or chloroquine for the treatment of cutaneous lupus.

Comment: Quinacrine (100 mg/day) has an effect on cutaneous lupus that is synergistic with that of hydroxychloroquine (Feldman et al. 1994). The usual approach to cutaneous lupus is start hydroxychloroquine at a dose of <7.5 mg/kg/day. If there is insufficient improvement after 2 months, then quinacrine is added. Two additional months may be required for improvement to occur after the addition of quinacrine.

Recent studies suggest that hydroxychloroquine works by blocking Toll-like receptor (TLR) 9. Quinacrine appears to achieve its effects at least in part by the blockade of other TLRs, e.g., TLR7, and inhibition of dendritic cell migration (Kalia and Dutz 2007; Gorbache et al. 2007).

Quinacrine must be obtained in the United States now through compounding pharmacies. The main side effects of this medication are reversible discoloration of the skin and sclerae, occasional drug eruptions, and hyperpigmentation caused by the deposition of drug in the skin.

If patients do not respond to the combination of hydroxychloroquine and quinacrine, then hydroxychloroquine is frequently discontinued in favor of chloroquine. The higher likelihood of adverse effects with chloroquine (retinopathy, myopathy, and cardiomyopathy) compared with hydroxychloroquine is the major reason for reserving chloroquine for patients who have failed the combination of hydroxychloroquine and quinacrine.

Pearl: Patients who develop a drug exanthem to hydroxychloroquine frequently are able to tolerate chloroquine well.

Comment: Possible drug reactions to the antimalarial agents include exanthems, urticaria, hyperpigmentation, alopecia, and lichenoid drug eruptions. Patients who develop an exanthem with hydroxychloroquine should stop the medication. Once the eruption resolves, it is often possible to treat the patient with chloroquine without triggering a recurrence of the skin rash.

In contrast, patients who develop urticarial reactions to hydroxychloroquine frequently demonstrate cross-reactions with chloroquine treatment. Therefore, such patients should not be switched routinely from hydroxychloroquine to chloroquine. In addition, patients with cutaneous lupus or dermatomyositis can develop a lichenoid drug eruption when treated with antimalarials. Biopsy of this reaction can be difficult to distinguish from the underlying lupus or dermatomyositis, but eosinophils in the infiltrate of a skin biopsy point toward a lichenoid drug eruption rather than a rash related to the underlying disease (Geraminejad et al. 2004). An empiric trial of discontinuing a medication is often required to determine if a rash has been a result of the drug or the disease.

Myth: Ultrapotent topical glucocorticoids should never be used on the face for cutaneous lupus.

Reality: The truth is that dermatologists almost always use ultrapotent topical glucocorticoids for chronic cutaneous lupus, even on the face. Topical glucocorticoids generally work very well in early lesions. If this strategy is employed early enough, one can clear DLE lesions completely, leaving neither a scar nor a pigment abnormality. Patients should be monitored closely by a dermatologist to avoid adverse reactions.

Potential side effects of chronic application of topical glucocorticoids are classified into the categories of systemic and local. Systemic side effects include suppression of the hypothalamic–pituitary–adrenal axis, iatrogenic Cushing's syndrome, and growth retardation (infants and children). Side effects at the site of application include skin atrophy and striae, hypopigmentation, steroid-induced acne or rosacea, glaucoma, and cataracts.

Acne and slight hypopigmentation are the most common side effects of topical glucocorticoid therapy. Acne is generally managed easily with topical creams or a short course of systemic tetracycline antibiotics. Hypopigmentation is reversible on discontinuation of the topical glucocorticoid.

Pearl: The topical calcineurin inhibitors, tacrolimus and pimecrolimus, are effective in cutaneous lupus.

Comment: These topical agents are used for a variety of inflammatory dermatoses, including atopic dermatitis. They also appear to be efficacious in the treatment of cutaneous lupus. Tacrolimus and pimecrolimus are superior to cyclosporine for topical use because they are smaller molecules that have significantly greater cutaneous penetration.

In one clinical trial of 20 patients with cutaneous SLE that compared topical tacrolimus ointment (0.1%) to clobetasol proprionate ointment (0.05%), no significant difference in efficacy was observed between the two treatments (Tzung et al. 2007). However, 61% of the patients treated with clobetasol developed telangiectasia when compared with none in the tacrolimus group.

Pearl: Many SLE flares are due to noncompliance.

Comment: No one wants to have a chronic disease. Denial and medical non-compliance are greater problems with SLE than with chronic diseases that afflict middle-aged and elderly individuals, because SLE affects teenagers and young adults. One study showed that 51% of SLE patients prescribed hydroxychloroquine were not taking it (Koneru et al. 2007)! Noncompliance with prednisone might be even worse, because of the acne, moon facies, and weight associated with that medication.

Pearl: The development of end-stage renal disease in SLE is linked to poor medical compliance in many patients.

Table 13.6 Prognostic factors in lupus nephritis (Adapted from Faurschou 2006)

• Duration of glomerulonephritis signs for more than 6 months before biopsy
• Serum creatinine greater than XXXX mg/dL (140 μmol/L)
• Histopathological findings:
– Diffuse proliferative glomerulonephritis (WHO class IV)
– Tubular atrophy
• Treatment regimens
• Ethnicity

Comment: Up to 60% of patients with SLE in some centers develop renal involvement, and up to 20% eventually develop end-stage renal disease (Faurschou et al. 2006). The course of lupus nephritis is affected by multiple clinical, demographic, serological, and histopathological factors. Some major predictors of renal outcome in lupus nephritis are shown in Table 13.6.

When a patient does not respond as predicted, it is worth considering non-adherence to treatment. Treatment non-compliance is underrecognized as a negative prognostic factor in lupus nephritis. Convincing some patients with glomerulonephritis to take prednisone is difficult because the organ manifestation causes no symptoms that are obvious to the patient, yet the adverse effects of therapy are highly predictable (Bruce et al. 2000; Mok 2005; Adler et al. 2006; Petri et al 1991a). Between 30% and 50% of patients with lupus nephritis do not adhere to their prescribed treatment regimens (Bruce et al. 2000; Petri 1991a).

Pearl: Consider a short "burst" of glucocorticoids to manage mild to moderate SLE flares.

Comment: A common approach to the management of SLE patients is to maintain a low dose of glucocorticoids over extended periods of time. This is the "maintenance steroids" approach. In contrast, in other autoimmune diseases such as multiple sclerosis, which is also often characterized by a "relapsing-remitting" course, glucocorticoids are usually not maintained between flares (Barr et al. 1999). Because the average SLE patient has one flare per year, maintenance of the patient of prednisone during these interval periods may be unnecessary in some patients (Petri et al. 1991b).

The FLOAT study (*F*lares in *L*upus: *O*utcomes *A*ssessment *T*rial) evaluated the use of glucocorticoid "bursts" in the management of mild to moderate disease flares (Danowski et al. 2006). Patients were assigned randomly to receive either oral methylprednisolone dose packs or a single intramuscular injection of triamcinolone. Neither group received maintenance glucocorticoids between flares. The majority of patients in both arms achieved rapid resolution of their SLE activity.

Intramuscular triamcinolone ensures 100% compliance with the glucocorticoid regimen. However, intramuscular triamcinolone should be administered only in the buttocks because it can cause focal lipodystrophy.

Pearl: Don't be in too much of a hurry to stop the steroids altogether.

Comment: When lupus has gone into clinical remission, there is a tendency on the part of both the patient and the physician to want to stop the glucocorticoids. However, stopping the patient's prednisone too quickly often triggers a disease flare. One approach to preventing this is to continue glucorticoids at a stable low dose for at least 1 year. Prednisolone 5 mg/day is a reasonable lowest dose for remission maintenance. Once the decision is undertaken to taper glucocorticoids, the rate of decrease should not exceed 1 mg/day per month.

Pearl: If glucocorticoids are not working, consider potential pharmacologic issues.

Comment: Approximately 25% of all cases of glucocorticoid-resistant asthma are explained by either poor absorption or rapid clearance (Nimmagadda et al. 1996). Poor absorption is unusual and can sometimes be explained by interaction with other medications, e.g. antacids. Among patients with asthma, abnormal clearance of glucocorticoids is a more common explanation for low glucocorticoid levels in the blood. If no explanation for poor absorption is found, then switching from prednisone to methylprednisone or to liquid prednisone or liquid prednisolone can be helpful.

Glucocorticoid metabolism has not been evaluated extensively in SLE patients, perhaps because non-glucocorticoid immunosuppressive agents are usually effective in treating patients who do not respond to glucocorticoids alone. However, metabolic problems with glucocorticoids can be caused by some of the medications used commonly in SLE, particularly anticonvulsant agents and medications that upregulate hepatic p450 enzymes.

The effects of these drugs in SLE have not been studied, but flares or treatment failures have been found in other disorders such as asthma, giant cell arteritis, and renal transplantation (Brooks et al. 1972; Carrie et al. 1994; Wassner et al. 1976). The effect of drugs that induce p450 enzymes on glucocorticoid metabolism can be profound, with a reduction in area under the curve of blood levels by approximately 60%. Thus, the co-administration of such medications with glucocorticoids could require a doubling of the glucocorticoid dose in order to maintain effective blood levels.

Myth: Osteonecrosis is caused by doses of prednisone higher than 40–60 mg/day.

Reality: The threshold dose of prednisone for the risk of osteonecrosis is only 20 mg/day (Petri 1995). Other potential risk factors are ethnicity (African–Americans are at greater risk), vasculitis, Raynaud's phenomenon, and the presence of a hypercoagulable state such as the antiphospholipid syndrome.

Myth: In proliferative lupus nephritis, a "wait and see" approach can save the patient from the toxicity of immunosuppressive drugs.

Reality: Some clinicians, arguing that cyclophosphamide saves kidneys but not lives, delay the use of cytotoxic therapy in patients with proliferative lupus nephritis. Unfortunately, delay in cytotoxic therapy for such patients diminishes the likelihood of remission and increases the risk of subsesquent relapses and end-stage renal disease. Moreover, short-term induction courses (e.g., 6 months) without follow-up maintenance therapy increases the risk of relapse.

Serious lupus nephritis needs to be identified quickly and treated appropriately for a sufficient duration of time. For the majority of patients, this means either mycophenolate mofetil or intravenous cyclophosphamide.

Myth: Patients with lupus nephritis should receive the full NIH regimen of intravenous cyclophosphamide.

Reality: Few patients with lupus nephritis require the full duration of the NIH cyclophosphamide regimen, which called for treating patients for a minimum of 2 years (Austin et al. 1986). Patients with moderate lupus nephritis can be treated with glucocorticoids and mycophenolate mofetil (Appel et al., in press).

Pearl: A sizeable subset of patients with lupus nephritis can be treated with azathioprine.

Comment: Not all SLE patients with glomerulonephritis need cyclophosphamide (MacGowan et al. 2002; Grootscholten et al. 2006). Patients with mild renal disease can be treated with the combination of glucocorticoids and azathioprine (Glas-Vos et al. 1995; Nossent and Koldingsnes 2000).

Myth: With the introduction of mycophenolate mofetil, cyclophosphamide has become an "obsolete" therapy for SLE.

Reality: The LUNAR trial of rituximab for lupus nephritis showed no added benefit over mycophenolate mofetil.

In spite of earlier trials purporting to show that mycophenolate mofetil is superior to cyclophoshamide as induction therapy for proliferative lupus nephritis, this superiority has not been confirmed in subsequent studies. No long-term follow-up studies are available on patients treated with mycophenolate mofetil, and the efficacy of mycophenolate mofetil in patients with severe lupus nephritis (i.e., patients with crescents, fibrinoid necrosis, or substantial impairment of renal fuction) remains to be demonstrated.

Mycophenolate mofetil is a good alternative to pulse cyclophosphamide as induction therapy for patients with mild to moderate proliferative and/or membranous lupus nephritis. Failure to achieve complete remission within the first 4–6 months should evoke discussions about switching to the combination of pulse therapy of glucocorticoids with cyclophoshamide (Ioannidis et al. 2000; Boumpas et al. 2005).

Myth: Medications that cause drug-induced lupus cannot be used in idiopathic SLE.

Reality: The "big three" medications linked to drug-induced lupus are isoniazid, procainamide, and hydralazine. Contrary to popular opinion, these medications *can* be used in idiopathic SLE. There is no evidence that any of them exacerbates SLE.

TNF inhibitors have also been implicated in causing drug-induced lupus. The story of TNF inhibition and lupus remains to be told fully. Although TNF inhibitors can induce ANA, antidsDNA, and anticardiolipin antibodies, these medications may have a role in the treatment of some lupus patients (Aringer et al. 2004). Great caution is urged when using TNF inhibitors in patients with SLE, because the full implications of elevations in anticardiolipin and antidsDNA antibody titers remain unclear (Fusconi et al. 2007; Jonsdottir et al. 2004).

Myth: The management of lupus is empiric and varies widely among practicing physicians.

Reality: Although there are several areas in the management of lupus that require further investigation, reasonable recommendations exist based on a combination of evidence and expert opinion (Bertsias et al. 2008). The EULAR recommendations for the management of SLE cover general management as well as selected aspects of lupus such as the antiphospholipid syndrome, pregnancy, neuropsychiatric lupus, and nephritis. The recommendations provide a general framework for the management of lupus yet allow latitude for physician autonomy and patient preferences.

References

Abu-Shakra M, Zalmanson S, Neumann L, Flusser D, Sukenik S, Buskila D. Influenza virus vaccination of patients with systemic lupus erythematosus: Effects on disease activity. J Rheumatol 2000; 27(7):1681–1685

ACR ad hoc committee on neuropsychiatric lupus. The American College of Rheumatology nomenclature and case definitions for neuropsychiatric lupus syndrome. Arthritis Rheum 1999; 42:599–608

Adler M, Chambers S, Edwards C, Neild G, Isenberg D. An assessment of renal failure in an SLE cohort with special reference to ethnicity, over a 25-year period. Rheumatology 2006; 45:1144–1147

Advisory Committee on Immunization Practices (ACIP). Recommendations for the Prevention of Herpes Zoster Morbidity and Mortality Weekly Report Recommendations and Reports June 6, 2008/Vol. 57/ RR-5(www.cdc.gov/mmwr)

Aguilera P, Mascaró JM Jr, Martinez A, et al Cutaneous gamma/delta T-cell lymphoma: A histopathologic mimicker of lupus erythemato-susprofundus (lupus panniculitis). J Am AcadDermatol 2007; 56: 643–647

Ainiala H, Loukkola J, Peltola J, Korpela M, Hietaharju A. The prevalence of neuropsychiatric syndromes in systemic lupus erythematosus. Neurology 2001; 57(3):496–500

Akkasilpa S, Goldman D, Magder LS, Petri M. Number of fibromyalgia tender points is associated with health status in patients with systemic lupus erythematosus. J Rheumatol 2005; 32(1):48–50

Appel G, Contreras G, MA D, et al Mycophenolate Mofetil versus Cyclophosphamide as Lupus Nephritis Induction Treatment. J Am Soc Nephrol 2009; 20(5):1103–12

Aringer M, Graninger WB, Steiner G, Smolen JS. Safety and efficacy of tumor necrosis factor alpha blockade in systemic lupus erythematosus: An open-label study. Arthritis Rheum 2004; 50(10): 3161–3169

Austin H, Klippel J, Balow J, et al Therapy of lupus nephritis. Controlled trial of prednisone and cytotoxic drugs. NEJM 1986; 314:614–619

Baca V, Lavalle C, Garcia R, et al Favorable response to intravenous methylprednisolone and cyclophosphamide in children with severe neuropsychiatric lupus. J Rheumatol 1999; 26:432–439

Barr S, Zonana-Nacach A, Magder L, Petri M. Patterns of disease activity in systemic lupus erythematosus. Arthritis Rheum 1999; 42: 2682–2688

Bertsias G, Ioannidis JP, Boletis J, et al Task Force of the EULAR Standing Committee for International Clinical Studies Including Therapeutics. EULAR recommendations for the management of systemic lupus erythematosus. Report of a Task Force of the EULAR Standing Committee for International Clinical Studies Including Therapeutics. Ann Rheum Dis 2008; 67(2):195–205

Bijl M, Kallenberg CG. Ultraviolet light and cutaneous lupus. Lupus 2006; 15(11):724–727

Boddaert J, Huong D, Zahir A, Wechsler B, Godeau P, Piette J. Late-onset systemic lupus erythematosus: A personal series of 47 patients and pooled analysis of 714 cases in the literature. Medicine 2004; 83:348–359

Bombardier C, Gladman DD, Urowitz M, Caron D, Chang CH, the Committee on Prognosis Studies in SLE. Derivation of the SLEDAI: A disease activity index for lupus patients. Arthritis Rheum 1992; 35:630–640

Boumpas D, Yamada H, Patronas N, Scott D, Klippel J, Balow J. Pulse cyclophosphamide for severe neuropsychiatric lupus. Q J Med 1991; 81:975–984

Boumpas DT, Sidiropoulos P, Bertsias G. Optimum therapeutic approaches for lupus nephritis: what therapy and for whom? Nat Clin Pract Rheumatol 2005; 1(1):22–30

Brooks SM, Werk EE, Ackerman SJ, et al Adverse effects of phenobarbital on corticosteroid metabolism in patients with bronchial asthma. N Engl J Med 1972; 286:1125–1128

Bruce I, Gladmann D, Urowitz M. Factors associated with refractory renal disease in patients with systemic lupus erythematosus: The role of patient non-adherence. Arthritis Care Res 2000; 13:406–408

Buyon J, Petri MA, Kim MY, et al The effect of combined estrogen and progesterone hormone replacement therapy on disease activity in systemic lupus erythematosus: A randomized trial. Ann Intern Med 2005; 142:953–962

Callen JP. Cutaneous lupus erythematosus: A personal approach to management. Australas J Dermatol 2006; 47(1):13–27

Calvo-Alen J, Alarcon GS, Burgard SL, et al Systemic lupus erythematosus: Predictors of its occurrence among a cohort of patients with early undifferentiated connective tissue disease: Multivariate analyses and identification of risk factors. J Rheumatol 1996; 23:469–475

Carrie F, Roblot P, Bouquet S, et al: Rifampin-induced nonresponsiveness of giant cell arteritis to prednisone treatment. Arch Intern Med 1994; 154:1521–1524

Cervera R, Khamashta M, Font J, et al Systemic lupus erythematosus: Clinical and immunologic patterns of disease expression in a cohort of 1,000 patients. The European Working Party on Systemic Lupus Erythematosus. Medicine 1993; 72:113–124

Chambers S, Charman S, Rahman A, Isenberg D. Development of additional autoimmune diseases in a multiethnic cohort of patients with systemic lupus erythematosus with reference to damage and mortality. Ann Rheum Dis 2007; 66:1173–1177

Chan MT. Owen P. Dunphy J, et al Associations of erosive arthritis with anti-cyclic citrullinated peptide antibodies and MHC Class II alleles in systemic lupus erythematosus. J Rheumatol 2008; 35(1): 77–83

Chan TM, Li FK, Tang CS, et al Efficacy of mycophenolate mofetil in patients with diffuse proliferative lupus nephritis. Hong Kong-Guangzhou Nephrology Study Group. N Engl J Med 2000; 343 (16):1156–1162

Christopher-Stine L, Siedner M, Lin H, Haas M, Parekh H, Petri M, et al Renal biopsy in lupus patients with low levels of proteinuria. J Rheumatol 2007; 34: 332–335

Chrysostomou A, Becker G. Spironolactone in addition to ACE inhibition to reduce proteinuria in patients with chronic renal disease. N Engl J Med 2001; 345(12):925–926

Contreras G, Pardo V, Leclercq B, Lenz O, Tozman E, O'Nan P, et al Sequential therapies for proliferative lupus nephritis. N Engl J Med 2004; 350(10):971–980

Costallat L, Coimbra A. Systemic lupus erythematosus: Clinical and laboratory aspects related to age at disease onset. Clin Exp Rheumatol 1994; 12:603–607

Cusack C, Danby C, Fallon JC, et al Photo protective behaviour and sunscreen use: Impact on vitamin D levels in cutaneous lupus erythematosus. Photodermatol Photoimmunol Photomed 2008; 24: 260–267

Damian-Abrego G, Cabiedes J, Cabral A. Anti-citrullinated peptide antibodies in lupus patients with or without deforming arthropathy. Lupus 2008; 17:300–304

Danowski A, Magder L, Petri M. Flares in lupus: Outcome Assessment Trial (FLOAT), a comparison between oral methylprednisolone and intramuscular triamcinolone. J Rheumatol 2006; 33(1):57–60

Domenech I, Aydintug O, Cervera R, et al Systemic lupus erythematosus in 50 year olds. Postgrad med J 1992; 68:440–444

Elkayam O, Paran D, Caspi D, et al Immunogenicity and safety of pneumococcal vaccination in patients with rheumatoid arthritis or systemic lupus erythematosus. Clin Infect Dis 2002; 34:147–153

Elkayam O, Paran D, Burke M, et al Pneumococcal vaccination of patients with systemic lupus erythematosus: Effects on generation of autoantibodies. Autoimmunity 2005; 38:493–496

Erkan D, Harrison MJ, Levy R, Peterson M, Petri M, Sammaritano L, et al Aspirin for primary thrombosis prevention in the antiphospholipid syndrome: A randomized, double-blind, placebo-controlled trial in asymptomatic antiphospholipid antibody-positive individuals. Arthritis Rheum 2007; 56(7):2382–2391

Esdaile JM, Abrahamowicz M, Grodzicky T, Li Y, Panaritis C, du Berger R, et al Traditional Framingham risk factors fail to fully account for accelerated atherosclerosis in systemic lupus erythematosus. Arthritis Rheum 2001; 44(10):2331–2337

Faurschou M, Starklint H, Halberg P, Jacobsen S. Prognostic factors in lupus nephritis: Diagnostic and therapeutic delay increases the risk of terminal renal failure. J Rheumatol 2006; 33:1563–1569

Feldman R, Salmon D, Saurat JH. The association of the two antimalarialschloroquine and quinacrine for treatment-resistantchronic and subacutecutaneous lupus erythematosus. Dermatology 1994;186:425–427

Fernandez M, Calvo-Alen J, Bertoli A, et al Systemic lupus erythematosus in a multiethnic US cohort (LUMINA L II): Relationship between vascular events and the use of hormone replacement therapy in postmenopausal women. J Clin Rheumatol 2007; 13:261–265

Fernandez-Nebro A, Palacios-Munoz R, Gordillo J, Abarca-Costalago M, De Haro-Liger M, Rodriguez-Andreu J, et al Chronic or recurrent headache in patients with systemic lupus erythematosus: A case control study. Lupus 1999; 8(2):151–156

Fessler B. Infectious diseases in systemic lupus erythematosus:risk factors, management and prophylaxis. Best Pract Res Clin Rheumatol 2002; 16:281–291

Fessler BJ, Alarcon GS, McGwin G, Jr., Roseman J, Bastian HM, Friedman AW, et al Systemic lupus erythematosus in three ethnic groups: XVI. Association of hydroxychloroquine use with reduced risk of damage accrual. Arthritis Rheum 2005; 52(5):1473–1480

Font J, Pallares L, Cervera R, et al Systemic lupus erythematosus in the elderly: Clinical and immunological charracteristics. Ann Rheum Dis 1991; 50:702–705

Foote R, Kimbrough S, Stevens J. Lupus myositis. Muscle Nerve 1982; 5:65–68

Formiga F, Moga I, Pac M, Mitjavila F, Rivera A, Pujol R. Mild presentation of systemic lupus erythematosus in elderly patients assessed by SLEDAI. Lupus 1999; 8:462–465

Fusconi M, Vannini A, Dall'aglio AC, Pappas G, Bianchi FB, Zauli D. Etanercept and infliximab induce the same serological autoimmune modifications in patients with rheumatoid arthritis. Rheumatol Int 2007; 28(1):47–49

Ganczarczyk L, Urowitz MB, Gladman DD. Latent lupus. J Rheumatol 1989; 16:475–478

Geraminejad P, Stone MS, Sontheimer RD. Antimalarial lichenoid tissue reactions in patients with pre-existing lupus erythematosus. Lupus 2004; 13:473–477

Gilland WR, Tsokos GC. Prophylactic use of antibiotics and immunisations in patients with SLE. Ann Rheum Dis 2002 Mar; 61(3):191–192

Gilliam JN, Cheatum DE, Hurd ER, Stastny P Ziff M. Immunoglobulin in clinically uninvolved skin in systemic lupus erythematosus: Association with renal disease. J clin invest 1974; 53(5): 1434–1440

Ginsburg KS, Liang MH, Newcomer L, et al Anticardiolipin antibodies and the risk for ischemic stroke and venous thrombosis. Ann Intern Med 1992; 117:997–1002

Ginzler EM, Dooley MA, Aranow C, Kim MY, Buyon J, Merrill JT, et al Mycophenolate mofetil or intravenous cyclophosphamide for lupus nephritis. N Engl J Med 2005; 353(21):2219–2228

Gladman D, Hussain F, Ibanez D, Urowitz M. The nature and outcome of infection in systemic lupus erythematosus. Lupus 2002; 11:234–239

Glas-Vos Jd, Krediet R, Weening J, Arisz L. Treatment of proliferative lupus nephritis with methylprednisolone pulse therapy and oral azathioprine. Neth J Med 1995; 46:4–14

Godeau B, Coutant-Perronne V, Le Thi Huong D, et al Pneumocystis carinii pneumonia in the course of connective tissue disease: Report of 34 cases. J Rheumatol 1994; 21(2):246–251

Gorbache AV, Gasparian AV, Gurova KV, et al Quinacrine inhibits the epidermal dendritic cell migration initiating T cell-mediated skin inflammation. Eur J Immunol 2007; 37:2257–2267

Graninger, Smolen JS. Incomplete lupus erythematosus: Results of a multicentre study under the supervision of the EULAR Standing Committee on International Clinical Studies Including Therapeutic Trials (ESCISIT). Rheumatology (Oxford) 2001; 40:89–94

Grootscholten C, Ligtenberg G, Hagen E, et al Azathioprine/methylprednisolone versus cyclophosphamide in proliferative lupus nephritis. A randomized controlled trial. Kidney Int 2006; 70:732–742

Hesselink D, Aarden L, Swaak A. Profiles of the acute-phase reactants C-reactive protein and ferritin related to the disease course of patients with systemic lupus erythematosus. Scand J Rheumatol 2003; 32:151–155

Ho C, Mok C, Lau C, Wong R. Late onset systemic lupus erythematosus in southern Chinese. Ann Rheum Dis 1998; 57:437–444

Ho A, Magder L, Barr S, Petri M. Decreases in anti-double stranded DNA levels are associated with concurrent flares in patients with systemic lupus erythematosus. Arthritis Rheum 2001a; 44: 2342–2349

Ho A, Magder LS, Barr SG, Petri MA. A decrease in complement is associated with increased renal and hematologic flares in patients with systemic lupus erythematosus. Arthritis Rheum 2001b; 44: 2350–2357

Hochberg MC. Updating the American College of Rheumatology revised criteria for the classification of systemic lupus erythematosus [letter]. Arthritis Rheum 1997; 40:1725

Huong DL, Papo T, Beaufuls H, Wechsler B. Renal involvement in systemic lupus erythematosus: A study of 180 patients from a single center. Medicine (Baltimore) 1999; 78:148

Iaboni A, Ibanez D, Gladman DD, Urowitz MB, Moldofsky H. Fatigue in systemic lupus erythematosus: Contributions of disordered sleep, sleepiness, and depression. J Rheumatol 2006; 33(12):2453–2457

Iliopoulos A, Tsokos G. Immunopathogenesis and spectrum of infections in systemic lupus erythematosus. Semin Arthritis Rheum 1996; 25:318–336

Ioannidis JP, Boki KA, Katsorida ME, et al Remission, relapse, and re-remission of proliferative lupus nephritis treated with cyclophosphamide. Kidney Int 2000; 57(1):258–264

Irving KS, Sen D, Tahir H, et al A comparison of autoimmune liver disease in juvenile and adult populations with systemic lupus erythematosus-a retrospective review of cases. Rheumatology (Oxford) 2007; 46(7):1171–1173

Isenberg D, Horsfall A. Systemic lupus erythematosus-adult onset. In: Maddison P, Isenberg D, Woo P, Glass D (eds) Oxford textbook of rheumatology. Oxford, Oxford University Press, 1998, pp. 1145–1180

Jewell ML, McCauliffe DP. Patients with cutaneous lupus erythematosus who smoke are less responsive to antimalarial treatment. J Am AcadDermatol 2000; 42:983–987

Jonsdottir T, Forslid J, van Vollenhoven A, Harju A, Brannemark S, Klareskog L, et al Treatment with tumour necrosis factor alpha antagonists in patients with rheumatoid arthritis induces anticardiolipin antibodies. Ann Rheum Dis 2004; 63(9):1075–1078

Jorizzo JL, Salisbury PL, Rogers RS 3rd, Goldsmith SM, Shar GG, Callen JP, Wise CM, Semble EL White WL. Oral lesions in systemic lupus erythematosus. Do ulcerative lesions represent a necrotizing vasculitis?. J Am Acad Dermatolo 1992; 27(3):389–394

Kalia S, Dutz JP. New concepts in antimalarial use and mode of action in dermatology. DermatolTher 2007; 20:160–174

Karpatkin S. Autoimmune thrombocytopaenic purpura. Semin Haematol 1985; 22:260–288

Kasitanon N, Fine DM, Haas M, Magder LS, Petri M. Hydroxychloroquine use predicts complete renal remission within 12 months among patients treated with mycophenolate mofetil therapy for membranous lupus nephritis. Lupus 2006; 15(6):366–370

Klippel JH, Karsh J, Stahl NI, et al A controlled study of pneumococcal polysaccharide vaccine in systemic lupus erythematosus. Arthritis Rheum 1979; 22:1321–1325

Koneru S, Shishov M, Ware A, Farhey Y, Mongey AB, Graham TB, et al Effectively measuring adherence to medications for systemic lupus erythematosus in a clinical setting. Arthritis Rheum 2007; 57(6):1000–1006

Kroshinsky D, Stone JH, Bloch D, Stone JR. A 47-year-old woman with a nodular rash and numbness and pain in the legs. New England Journal of Medicine 2009; 360(7):711–20

Lee SS, Singh S, Magder LS, Petri M. Predictors of high sensitivity C-reactive protein levels in patients with systemic lupus erythematosus. Lupus 2008; 17:114–23

Lin A. Chapter 36: Topical calcineurin inhibitors. In: Wolverton SE (ed) Comprehensive dermatologic drug therapy (2nd edn). Philadelphia, PA, Saunders Elsevier, 2007, pp. 671–689

MacGowan J, Ellis S, Griffiths M, Isenberg D. Retrospective analysis of outcome in a cohort of patients with lupus nephritis treated between 1977 and 1999. Rheumatology 2002; 41:981–987

Mackay IR et al Lupoid hepatitis and the hepatic lesions of systemic lupus erythematosus. Lancet 1959; 1:65

Manoussakis M, Georgopoulou C, Zintzaras E, et al Sjogren's syndrome associated with systemic lupus erythematosus: Clinical and laboratory profiles and comparison with primary Sjogren's syndrome. Arthritis Rheum 2004; 50:882–891

Manzi S, Meilahn E, Rairie J, et al Age-specific incidence rates of myocardial infarction and angina in women with systemic lupus erythematosus: Comparison with the Framingham Study. Am J Epidemiol 1997; 145:408–415

Marmor MF, Carr RE, Easterbrook M, et al Recommendations on screening for chloroquine and hydroxychloroquine retinopathy. A report by the American Academy of Ophthalmology. Ophthalmology 2002; 109:1377–1382

McDonagh J, Isenberg D. Development of additional autoimmune disease in a population of patients with systemic lupus erythematosus. Ann Rheum Dis 2000; 59:230–232

Middleton GD, McFarlin JE, Lipsky PE. The prevalence and clinical impact of fibromyalgia in systemic lupus erythematosus. Arthritis Rheum 1994; 37(8):1181–1188

Miot HA, Bartoli MLD, Haddad GR. Association between discoid lupus erythematosus and cigarette smoking. Dermatology 2005; 211:118–122

Modi GM, Maender JL, Coleman N, et al. Tineacorporis masquerading as subacutecutaneous lupus erythematosus. Dermatol Online J 2008; 15; 14(4):8

Moghadam-Kia S, Chilek K, Gaines E, et al. Cross-sectional analysis of a collaborative web-based database for lupus erythematosus associated skin lesions: 114 prospectively enrolled patients. Arch Dermatol 2009; 145(3):255–60

Mok C. Prognostic factors in lupus nephritis. Lupus 2005; 14:39–44

Neuwelt C, Lacks S, Kaye B, Ellman J, Borenstein D. Role of intravenous cyclophosphamide in the treatment of severe neuropsychiatric systemic lupus erythematosus. Am J Med 1995; 98:32–41

Ng K, Manson J, Rahman A, Isenberg D. Association of antinucleosome antibodies with disease flare in serologically active clinically quiescent patients with systemic lupus erythematosus. Arthritis Care Res 2006; 55:900–904

Niiyama S, Katsuoka K, Happle R Hoffmann R. Multiple eruptive dermatofibromas: A review of the literature. Acta Derm Venereol 2002; 82(4):241–244

Nimmagadda SR, Spahn JD, Leung DY, Szefler SJ. Steroid-resistant asthma: Evaluation and management. [Review] [76 refs] [Journal Article. Research Support, Non-U.S. Gov't. Review] Ann Allergy Asthma Immunol 1996 Nov; 77(5):345–355; quiz 355–356

Noel V, Lortholary O, Casassus P, et al Risk factors and prognostic influence of infection in a single cohort of 87 adults with systemic lupus erythematosus. Ann Rheum Dis 2001; 60:1141–1144

Nossent H, Koldingsnes W. Long-term efficacy of azathioprine treatment for proliferative lupus nephritis. Rheumatology 2000; 39:969–974

Omdal R, Mellgren SI, Koldingsnes W, Jacobsen EA, Husby G. Fatigue in patients with systemic lupus erythematosus: Lack of associations to serum cytokines, antiphospholipid antibodies, or other disease characteristics. J Rheumatol 2002; 29(3):482–486

O'Neill S, Isenberg D. Immunizing patients with systemic lupus erythematosus: A review of effectiveness and safety. Lupus 2006; 15: 778–783

Para MF, Finkelstein D, Becker S, et al Reduced toxicity with gradual initiation of trimethoprim-sulfamethoxazole as primary prophylaxis for Pneumocystis carinii pneumonia: AIDS Clinical Trials Group 268. JAIDS 2000; 24(4):337–343

Pego-Reigosa JM, Isenberg DA. Psychosis due to systemic lupus erythematosus: Characteristics and long term outcome of this rare manifestation of the disease. Rheumatology 2008; 47:1498–1502

Perl A, Nagy G, Gergely P, et al Apoptosis and mitochondrial dysfunction in lymphocytes of patients with systemic lupus erythematosus. Methods Mol Med 2004; 102:87–114

Petri M. Musculoskeletal complications of systemic lupus erythematosus in the Hopkins Lupus Cohort: an update. Arthritis Care Res 1995; 8:137–145

Petri M. Thrombosis and systemic lupus erythematosus: The Hopkins Lupus Cohort perspective. Scand J Rheumatol 1996; 25:191–193

Petri M. Infection in systemic lupus erythematosus. Rheumatic Dis Clin N Am 1998; 24:423–456

Petri M, Allbritton J. Antibiotic allergy in systemic lupus erythematosus: A case-control study. J Rheumatol 1992; 19(2):265–269

Petri M, Perez-Gutthann S, Longenecker J, Hochberg M. Morbidity of systemic lupus erythematosus: Role of race and socioeconomic status. Am J Med 1991a; 91:345–353

Petri M, Genovese M, Engle E, Hochberg M. Definition, incidence and clinical description of flare in systemic lupus erythematosus: A prospective cohort study. Arthritis Rheum 1991b; 34:937–944

Petri M, Kim MY, Kalunian KC, et al Combined oral contraceptives in women with systemic lupus erythematosus. N Engl J Med 2005; 353:2550–2558

Pichler WJ. Delayed drug hypersensitivity reactions. Ann Intern Med 2003; 139(8):683–693

Pierangeli SS, Harris EN. In vivo models of thrombosis for the antiphospholipid syndrome. Lupus 1996; 5(5):451–455

Porges AJ, Beattie SL, Ritchlin C, et al Patients with systemic lupus erythematosus at risk for Pneumocystis carinii pneumonia. J Rheumatol 1992; 19(8):1191–1194

Provost TT, Andres G, Maddison PJ Reichlin M. Lupus band test in untreated SLE patients: Correlation of immunoglobulin deposition in the skin of the extensor forearm with clinical renal disease and serological abnormalities. J Invest Dermatol 1980; 74(6): 407–412

Pyne D, Isenberg D. Autoimmune thyroid diseases in systemic lupus erythematosus. Ann Rheum Dis 2002; 61:70–72

Ramos P, Mendez M, Ames P, Khamashta M, Hughes G. Pulse cyclophosphamide in the treatment of neuropsychiatric systemic lupus erythematosus. Clin Exp Rheumatol 1996; 14:295–299

Roman MJ, Shanker BA, Davis A, Lockshin MD, Sammaritano L, Simantov R, et al Prevalence and correlates of accelerated atherosclerosis in systemic lupus erythematosus. N Engl J Med 2003; 349(25):2399–2406

Ropes MW. Systemic lupus erythematosus. Cambridge, MA, Harvard University Press, 1976, p. 28

Roy S, Tan K. Pyrexia and normal C-reactive protein (CRP) in patients with systemic lupus erythematosus: Always consider the possibility of infection in febrile patients with systemic lupus erythematosus regardless of CRP levels. Rheumatology 2001; 40:349–350

Runyon BA, LaBrecque DR, Anuras S. The spectrum of liver disease in systemic lupus erythematosus. Report of 33 histologically-proved cases and review of the literature. Am J Med 1980; 69:187–194

Sato EI. Methotrexate therapy in systemic lupus erythematosus. Lupus 2001; 10(3):162–164

Scheinfeld N, Deleo VA. Photosensitivity in lupus erythematosus. Photodermatol Photoimmunol Photomed 2004; 20(5):272–279

Schmidt E, Brocker EB, Goebeler M. Rituximab in treatment-resistant autoimmune blistering skin disorders. Clin Rev Allergy Immunol 2008; 34(1):56–64

Sivaraj RR, Durrani OM, Denniston AK, et al Ocular manifestations of systemic lupus erythematosus. Rheumatology (Oxford) 2007; 46(12):1757–1762

Somers E, Magder LS, Petri M. Antiphospholipid antibodies and incidence of venous thrombosis in a cohort of patients with systemic lupus erythematosus. J Rheumatol 2002; 29(12):2531–2536

Sontheimer RD, Henderson CL, Grau RH. Drug-induced subacutecutaneous lupus erythematosus: A paradigm for bedside-to-bench patient-oriented translational clinical investigation Arch Dermatol Res 2009; 301(1):65–70

Spronk P, terBorg E, Kallenberg C. Patients with systemic lupus erythematosus and Jaccoud's arthropathy: A clinical subset with an increased C reactive protein response? Ann Rheum Dis 1992; 51:358–361

Stahl NI, Klippel JH, Decker JL. Fever in systemic lupus erythematosus. Am J Med 1979; 67:935–940

Suryaprasad A, Stone JH. When is it safe to stop Pneumocystis carinii (jiroveci) prophylaxis? Insights from cases complicating autoimmune diseases. Arthritis Care & Research 2008; 59(7):1034–9

Takada K, Illei G, Boumpas D. Cyclophosphamide for the treatment of systemic lupus erythematosus. Lupus 2001; 10:154–161

Tam LS, Li EK, Wong CK, Lam CW, Szeto CC. Double-blind, randomized, placebo-controlled pilot study of leflunomide in systemic lupus erythematosus. Lupus 2004; 13(8):601–604

Tan EM, Cohen AS, Fries JF, Masi AT, McShane DJ, Rothfeld NF, et al The 1982 revised criteria for the classification of systemic lupus erythematosus. Arthritis Rheum 1982; 25:1271–1277

Taylor J, Skan J, Erb N, Carruthers D. Lupus patients with fatigue: Is there a link with fibromyalgia syndrome? Rheumatology 2000; 39: 620–623

terBorg E, Horst G, Limburg P, vanRijswijk M, Kallenberg C. C-reactive protein levels during disease exacerbations and infections in systemic lupus erythematosus: A prospective longitudinal study. J Rheumatol 1990; 17:1642–1648

Tsakonas E, Joseph L, Esdaile JM, Choquette D, Senecal JL, Cividino A, et al A long-term study of hydroxychloroquine withdrawal on exacerbations in systemic lupus erythematosus. The Canadian Hydroxychloroquine Study Group. Lupus 1998; 7:80–85

Tsokos GC. Drugs, sun and T cells in lupus. Clin Exp Immunol 2004; 136(2):191–193

Turner-Stokes L, Cambridge G, Corcoran T, et al In vitro response to influenza immunisation by peripheral blood mononuclear cells from patients with systemic lupus erythematosus and other autoimmune disease. Ann Rheum Dis 1988; 47:532–535

Tzung TY, Liu YS Chang HW. Tacrolimus vs. clobetasol propionate in the treatment of facial cutaneous lupus erythematosus: A randomized, double-blind, bilateral comparison study. Br J Dermatol 2007; 156(1):191–192

Ueki H. Koebner phenomenon in lupus erythematosus with special consideration of clinical findings. Autoimmunity reviews 2005; 4(4): 219–223

Urowitz MB, Bookman AAM, Koehler BE, Gordon DA, Smythe HA, Ogryzlo MA. The bimodal mortality pattern of systemic lupus erythematosus. Am J Med 1976; 60:221–225

Vassilakopoulos TP, Pangalis GA. Application of a prediction rule to select which patients presenting with lymphadenopathy should undergo a lymph node biopsy. Medicine (Baltimore) 2000; 79(5): 338–347

Wahl DG, Guillemin F, de Maistre E, Perret C, Lecompte T, Thibaut G. Risk for venous thrombosis related to antiphospholipid antibodies in systemic lupus erythematosus: A meta-analysis. Lupus 1997;6: 467–473

Walz LeBlanc BAE, Gladman DD, Urowitz MB. Serologically active clinically quiescent systemic lupus erythematosus: Predictors of clinical flares. J Rheumatol 1994; 21:2239–2241

Ward MM, Donald F. Pneumocystis carinii pneumonia in patients with connective tissue diseases: The role of hospital experience in diagnosis and mortality. [Journal Article] Arthritis Rheum 1999 Apr; 42(4):780–789

Wassner SJ, Pennisi AJ, Malekzadeh MH, et al The adverse effect of anticonvulsant therapy on renal allograft survival. A preliminary report. J Pediatr 1976; 88:134–137

Wells JV, Webb J, Van Deventer M, et al In vivo anti-nuclear antibodies in epithelial biopsies in SLE and other connective tissue diseases. Clin Exp Immunol 1979; 38(3):424–435

Werth VP, Sanchez M, White W, et al Incidence of alopecia areata in lupus erythematosus. Arch Derm 1992; 128:368–371

Wilson H, Hamilton M, Spyker D, et al Age influences the clinical and serologic expression of systemic lupus erythematosus. Arthritis Rheum 1981; 24:1230–1235

Zandman-Goddard G, Shoenfeld Y. SLE and infections. Clin Rev Allergy Immunol 2003; 25:29–40

Pediatric Systemic Lupus Erythematosus

Earl D. Silverman

14

Pearl: A prolonged prothrombin time is likely the result of a prothrombin (factor II) deficiency as well as a lupus anticoagulant.

Comment: SLE is often associated with a prolonged partial thromboplastin time (PTT) because of the presence of a lupus anticoagulant (Chapter 16, Antiphospholipid Syndrome). However, in approximately 5% of lupus patients, there is also a prolonged prothrombin time (PT). The implications of a prolonged PT in lupus are altogether different. A prolonged PT in lupus is generally the result of an acquired deficiency of factor II or an acquired inhibitor to factor II. Patients with these defects generally present with hemorrhage rather than thrombosis, the hematological event normally linked with lupus anticoagulants.

The treatment approach to an acquired factor II deficiency or inhibitor is immunosuppression. Prednisone is the only medication required in most circumstances, and high doses of this medication (e.g., 1–2 mg/kg/day) usually lead to a rapid normalization of the PT (Eberhard et al. 1992; Hudson et al. 1997; Massengill et al. 1997; Taddio et al. 2007).

Pearl: Headaches in lupus can be caused by cerebral vein thrombosis.

Comment: Cerebral vein thrombosis is generally seen in the presence of a lupus anticoagulant. Venograms performed noninvasively by either computed tomography or magnetic resonance imaging are usually adequate to make the diagnosis, and the therapy (obviously) is anticoagulation with coumadin or low molecular weight heparin. Pediatric patients may be at higher risk of cerebral vein thrombosis than are adults (Brik et al. 1995; Carhuapoma et al. 1997).

As with many cases of pathological thrombosis, more than one defect in the coagulation cascade may be present and a thorough search for all known clotting lesions is important. Factor V Leiden mutation in combination with a lupus anticoagulant has been reported on one patient with cerebral vein thrombosis (Uthman et al. 2004).

Pearl: New-onset chorea is more likely to be associated with antiphospholipid antibodies than with rheumatic fever.

Comment: At least, this is true in developed nations. The significant decline in the incidence of rheumatic fever in developed countries has meant that cases of Sydenham's chorea are increasingly rare. Cases of new-onset chorea in Western countries are now more likely to be caused by antiphospholipid antibodies. However, there has been no formal study of the relative incidence of the two disorders in Western countries (or anywhere else).

Distinguishing between Sydenham's chorea and the antiphospholipid syndrome can be challenging, as patients with rheumatic fever can have anticardiolipin antibodies (Figueroa et al. 1992). The additional finding of a lupus anticoagulant favors the antiphospholipid syndrome (Avcin et al. 2008). Among pediatric patients, chorea is almost always associated with SLE rather than the primary antiphospholipid syndrome (Sanna et al. 2003; Olfat et al. 2004). In SLE, the APS (and, for that matter, acute rheumatic fever) chorea is more common in children than in adults and may be either unilateral or bilateral (Cervera et al. 1997). Other movement disorders associated with aPL are hemidystonia, hemiballismus, myoclonus, and Parkinsonism (Martino et al. 2006).

Pearl: Children and adolescents require higher doses of glucocorticoids than adults with SLE.

Comment: The current treatment standard for severe SLE in the pediatric age group is 2 mg/kg/day prednisone as an initial dose. Most pediatric rheumatologists do not use more than a total of 60 mg of prednisone per day, but starting doses of 80 mg/day are sometimes employed for short periods. This approach results in a standard dose of 2 mg/kg in patients who weigh 30 kg or less, but somewhat less than 2 mg/kg in patients who weigh more.

The requirement for these relatively higher doses of prednisone in smaller children probably results from increased metabolism and a larger volume of distribution of the drug in smaller children. Younger children do not appear to have worse glucocorticoid side-effects, despite the higher dose per kg when compared with adolescents and adults. This is not to say that adverse effects of glucocorticoids do not occur in young children: they do.

J. H. Stone (ed.), *A Clinician's Pearls and Myths in Rheumatology,*
DOI:10.1007/978-1-84800-934-9_14, © Springer Science + Business Media B.V. 2009

Table 14.1 Manifestations of neonatal lupus[a] (Frequency data derived from Cimaz et al. 2003 and Boros et al. 2007)

Clinical feature	Frequency among consecutive 124 pregnancies in women with anti-Ro/SSA or –La/SSB antibodies (%)
Complete congenital heart block	1.6
Rash	16
Hepatitis	26
Hematologic abnormalities (usually neutropenia)	27
Neurologic abnormalities/ macrocephaly[*]	8
Chondrodysplasia punctata	0

[a]Data from 87 consecutive pregnancies

Myth: Children with congenital heart block frequently do have mothers with known SLE (or Sjögren's syndrome).

Reality: Neonatal lupus erythematosus (NLE) is associated with the transplacental passage of maternal anti-Ro/SSA and anti-La/SSB antibodies. Large, prospective studies of mothers with SLE and anti-Ro/SSA or anti-La/SSB antibodies indicate that the incidence of congenital heart block is between 1% and 2%. Many mothers who deliver children with congenital heart block (CHB) are well or have subclinical features more consistent with Sjögren's syndrome than with SLE. Because Sjögren's syndrome (SjS) tends to develop or become clinically manifest later in life than does SLE, many women with SjS and anti-Ro/SSA or -La/SSB antibodies are asymptomatic at the time of delivery of a child with CHB.

For most babies, unfortunately, the fact of these maternal autoantibodies is identified first as a consequence of the evaluation for congenital heart block rather than from routine fetal echocardiographic screening of pregnancies in women whose anti-Ro/SSA or –La/SSB antibodies are known (Waltuck and Buyon 1994; Press et al. 1996; Julkunen et al. 1998; Lawrence et al. 2000; Brucato et al. 2001; Jaeggi et al. 2002; Costedoat-Chalumeau 2004).

All pregnant women with anti-Ro/SSA antibodies should be screened with serial fetal echocardiograms beginning at gestational week 18. Currently, it is recommended that at the time of diagnosis of autoantibody-associated CHB, the mother of the fetus should be treated with dexamethasone (a steroid that crosses the placenta) to try to minimize the damage to the developing fetal heart. This therapy appears to decrease the incidence of intrauterine and neonatal death but does not permanently reverse the heart block.

Among women who have had one child with congenital heart block, the likelihood of recurrence in a second pregnancy is on the order of 15–20% (Gladman et al. 2002).

Myth: Congenital heart block is the most common manifestation of neonatal lupus.

Reality: One in 14,000 live births is complicated by complete congenital heart block. Approximately 90% of these cases are secondary to neonatal lupus erythematosus. The most *serious* complication of neonatal lupus erythematosus is complete congenital heart block or complete atrioventricular block. However, conduction defects are not the most common manifestation of this disorder. The clinical manifestations of neonatal lupus are shown in Table 14.1.

Only about one-third of babies born to women with the relevant antibodies have no clinical or laboratory abnormalities (Cimaz et al. 2003). The rash can be subtle and difficult to diagnose if it is in a non-sun exposed area. The rash may be present at birth but is most commonly seen at age 6–7 weeks and usually resolves without treatment by age 4 months. Both liver test abnormalities and hematologic abnormalities are almost always asymptomatic and will usually resolve with 4–6 months without sequelae (Cimaz et al. 2003). Fulminant liver failure is a rare complication of neonatal lupus (Lee et al. 2002).

Pearl: Neonatal lupus erythematosus can be caused by anti-RNP antibodies in the absence of anti-Ro/SSA or anti-La/SSB antibodies.

Comment: In 5% of the cases of cutaneous neonatal lupus erythematosus, serum from both the mother and baby are negative for anti-Ro/SSA and–La/SSB antibodies but positive for antibodies to ribonucleoprotein (anti-RNP antibodies) (Provost et al. 1987; Sheth et al. 1995; Su et al. 2001). Thus, the finding of a cutaneous rash or other findings consistent with neonatal lupus should trigger screening for anti-RNP antibodies in addition to anti-Ro/SSA and–La/SSB antibodies.

Pearl: Cutaneous neonatal lupus may be associated with long-term sequelae.

Comment: Cutaneous neonatal lupus presents with a characteristic annular rash that often appears around the eyes in a so-called "raccoon distribution." The rash also occurs commonly on the trunk and back. Although the rash of neonatal lupus is often photosensitive, it can be present at birth and in areas not exposed to the sun.

Ninety percent of cases resolve without scarring within several months, after the maternal antibodies have disappeared from the infant's serum (Neiman et al. 2000). Systemic or topical therapy is seldom required. However, in approximately 10% of patients, the rash heals with puckering or telangiectasiae (Thornton et al. 1995; High and Costner 2003). These telangiectasiae are classically in the area of the temples, and may develop in that area even if the active rash did not affect that region clinically (Fig. 14.1). The telangiectasiae usually heal slowly with time but may be removed by laser surgery if they persist.

Pearl: Hydrocephalus should be excluded in all children born to mothers with anti-Ro/SSA and anti-La/SSB autoantibodies.

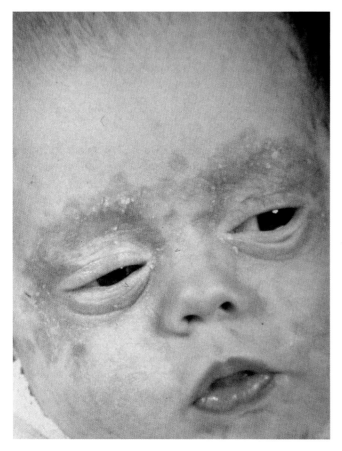

Fig. 14.1 Cutaneous neonatal lupus

Comment: Neurologic abnormalities have been described in patients with neonatal lupus (Cabanas et al. 1996; Inoue et al. 2002; Prendiville et al. 2003; Boros et al. 2007). The most important neurological manifestation is macrocephaly, which can occur with or without hydrocephalus (Nakayama-Furukawa et al. 1994; Boros et al. 2007). The head circumference of infants born to mothers with anti-Ro/SSA antibodies is larger on average than that of infants whose mothers do not have these antibodies. These large heads tend to return to normal as the child by age two. However, in rare cases, hydrocephalus develops and can require surgical intervention.

Pearl: Patients with culture-negative sepsis should be considered to have the macrophage activation syndrome.

Comment: Patients with systemic juvenile idiopathic arthritis are at risk for the macrophage activation syndrome (MAS). Patients with SLE are also at risk for this condition. Early recognition of the MAS is the key to its successful management. Patients with MAS are acutely ill, toxic-appearing, and hypotensive. They appear to have overwhelming sepsis, but all cultures are negative.

One of the keys to the diagnosis of MAS is the relative preservation of urine output in the face of hypotension. However, patients with MAS can have azotemia and

significant urinalysis abnormalities. Laboratory features include a pancytopenia with elevation of the serum hepatic aminotransferases, lactate dehydrogenase, ferritin, triglyceride, and C-reactive protein levels. Elevated levels of d-dimers are typical of the MAS, but serum fibrinogen levels tend to be low relative to the degree of inflammation.

MAS is not restricted to pediatric patients but is well described in adults with rheumatic conditions and in particular SLE (Lambotte et al. 2006; Ruperto et al. 2006; Pringe et al. 2007; Qian and Yang 2007).

Pearl: Herpes virus infections can cause significant leukopenia and lymphopenia.

Comment: SLE is characterized by a leukopenia that may include both a lymphopenia and a neutropenia. (Many clinicians focus on the tendency to lymphopenia, because this is one of the American College of Rheumatology criteria for the classification of SLE.)

Among SLE patients who are leukopenic, however, the total white blood cell count usually remains above 3,000/dL. When counts are decreased to a level significantly below this figure, systemic herpes virus infections must be considered. These include cytomegalovirus, varicella-zoster virus, and Epstein–Barr virus (EBV) infections.

Herpes virus infections can be present at the diagnosis of SLE or, more likely, develop over the course of the illness. The potential for the reactivation of EBV is particularly a problem in patients who are immunosuppressed (Chung and Fas 1998; Dror et al. 1998; Rappaport and Tang 2000; Nakahara et al. 2001; Sekigawa et al. 2002; Verdolini et al. 2002; Hirose et al. 2006; Kasapcopur et al. 2006; Pluchinotta et al. 2007; Takei et al. 2007).

Myth: The arthritis of SLE is painful.

Reality: It can be, but is not always. The arthritis of SLE is regarded generally as a painful, symmetrical polyarthritis. Arthritis in lupus usually does not cause erosive disease unless the patient also has a positive serum rheumatoid factor. In such cases, the overall clinical designation of "rhupus" is often used to indicate the clinical and radiologic overlap between rheumatoid arthritis and lupus.

Although the arthritis of lupus is not associated typically with joint erosions (except in rhupus), tendon and ligament abnormalities can occur secondary to SLE and lead to joint deformities. More commonly in patients with pediatric SLE, as many as 50% of patients have an arthritis that is relatively painful although there may be some mild discomfort and morning stiffness and does not usually lead to permanent joint damage. This is not to be confused with the less commonly seen painless arthritis, which may lead to joint deformities that resemble Jaccoud's arthropathy. These forms of arthritis may cause few symptoms but must be considered as an additional activity measure in SLE.

Myth: African–American patients with proliferative lupus nephritis require cyclophosphamide.

Reality: African–American patients with proliferative lupus nephritis have poor disease outcomes when compared with many other SLE subsets. Many investigators have suggested, consequently, that African–American patients should be treated with pulse cyclophosphamide. However, large series of pediatric and adult African–American patients with proliferative nephritis have reported poor outcomes despite the use of pulse cyclophosphamide (or perhaps, in the case of some patients, because of it) (Dooley et al. 1997; Vyas et al. 2002; Flower et al. 2006).

One trial that compared intravenous pulse cyclophosphamide to mycophenolate mofetil for the treatment of lupus nephritis reported that African–Americans had a poorer outcome than predicted by the NIH studies in the cyclophosphamide arm. One of the major differences was that the majority of patients in the NIH study were white (Contreras et al. 2004).

The proper conclusion from this experience may be that African–American patients with proliferative lupus nephritis have a poorer outcome than other patients with other racial/ethnic backgrounds and therefore should not be exposed to more toxic therapy, which does not appear to improve long-term outcome.

Myth: Magnetic resonance imaging studies are useful in the evaluation of SLE patients with diffuse central nervous system involvement.

Reality: Sorting out the cause of diffuse central nervous system (CNS) dysfunction, i.e., acute confusional states, mood disorders, headaches, psychosis, or cognitive impairment is challenging. Laboratory investigations in many such patients indicate that the usual parameters measured in the hope of gleaning insight on disease activity – serum complement levels, anti-dsDNA antibody levels, and acute phase reactants – are normal or unchanged from the patients' baseline.

Much hope has been placed in MRI investigations of these patients, particularly in the potential specificity of FLAIR and diffusion imaging in delineating active neuropsychiatric SLE from other conditions. Unfortunately, studies of this imaging modality indicate that many patients with diffuse CNS disease have only non-specific changes or even normal examinations on MRI (Sabbadini et al. 1999; Jennings et al. 2004; Sundgren et al. 2005; Castellino et al. 2008). One of the most common findings in this setting, volume loss, can be secondary to acute SLE but also to prior glucocorticoid treatment (Jennings et al. 2004). This helps neither the clinician nor the patient in most cases.

Many of these imaging tests distinguish normal controls from SLE patients, but no one needs a $1,500 test to do that.

MRI is not sufficiently specific to distinguish SLE patients with diffuse CNS dysfunction but not CNS involvement nor specific CNS syndromes from patients with SLE without CNS involvement. However, currently the diagnosis of CNS involvement remains a clinical diagnosis.

Pearl: Patients with chronic ITP should be monitored for the development of lupus.

Comment: Idiopathic thrombocytopenic purpura (ITP) is a common disorder, even among individuals who do not have SLE. When this illness becomes chronic and/or resistant to therapy, screening of these patients with an ANA is indicated. In many patients, repeat screening is required; the ANA may become positive only months to years after the diagnosis of ITP.

Between 10% and 25% of patients with chronic ITP and a positive ANA develop overt SLE over time. This percentage is even higher if a Coombs'-positive hemolytic anemia is present in addition to the thrombocytopenia (the so-called "Evans' syndrome").

Pearl: Some patients with Evans' don't have classic lupus, but rather a defect in the Fas–Fas ligand pathway known as "ALPS": the autoimmune lymphproliferative syndrome.

Comment: ALPS is a heritable disorder of the Fas (CD95)-Fas ligand pathway that leads to a defect in lymphocyte apoptosis. The disorder usually presents between the ages of 1 and 18 with a median age of presentation of 2 years. ALPS is associated with mutations in the following genes: TNFRSF6, Fas ligand (TNFSF6), caspase 8, and 10, but these known mutations do not account for all recognized cases. ALPS is categorized into three recognized subtypes: (1) Type 1a due to mutations in TNFRSF6; (2) Type 1b due to mutations in TNFSF6 and (3) Types IIa and IIb due to defects in caspase-10 and caspase-8 respectively; and (4) Type III without a known mutation. The diagnostic laboratory features are the presence of T lymphocytes, which express the alpha/beta T-cell receptor but lack expression of either CD4 or CD8 (alpha/beta double negative T cell) and defective in vitro Fas-mediated apoptosis.

As may be expected by the name, this syndrome is clinically characterized by lymphoproliferation, which includes "massive" lymphadenopathy, hepatomegaly, splenomegaly, and hypersplenism. Less common clinic findings include urticaria, uveitis, vasculitis, arthritis, oral ulcers, panniculitis, and occasionally glomerulonephritis. Many of these features may be seen in patients with SLE. Other autoimmune features include autoimmune hemolytic anemia, autoimmune thrombocytopenia, and autoimmune neutropenia. Many patients are ANA positive and may have specific autoantibodies.

The diagnosis of ALPS can be confirmed by either genetic studies, the persistence of elevated levels of double negative alpha/beta T-cells, or the characteristic defect in Fas-mediated apoptosis. Lymph node biopsies show marked expansion of paracortical T cells, the majority of which are double negative alpha/beta T cells. These cells show active expansion but very little apoptosis. Probably, as a result of abnormal survival of lymphocytes and the potential role of Fas as a tumor suppressor gene, these patients are at an increased risk for the development of malignancy and approximately 10% of patients will develop a malignancy. These patients are at particular risk for hematologic malignancies with very high relative risks for lymphomas but thyroid cancer, hepatocellular carcinoma, colon cancer, and skin cancers have also been described. The major clinical problems seen in patients with ALPS are related to the persistent cytopenias, which may be life-threatening. They generally respond well to corticosteroid therapy but frequently these patients become steroid-dependent and may require immunosuppressive agents. Recently, there have been reports of good responses to mycophenolate mofetil.

Pearl: Discoid lesions in children and adolescents are likely secondary to SLE, not to isolated discoid Lupus Erythematosus.

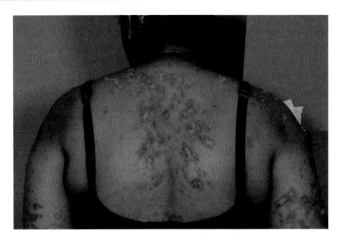

Fig. 14.3 Discoid lupus erythematosus lesion. When this cutaneous finding is present in a child, the patient usually evolves features of systemic lupus erythematosus over time. In contrast, in adults, discoid lupus lesions are associated with a low likelihood of the development of systemic lupus erythematosus (Courtesy of Dr. Rachel Abuav)

Comment: Discoid lupus lesions comprise a scarring dermopathy that is characterized by lesions involving the skin of the head and neck (classically the ears, face, or scalp) (Fig. 14.2). Many adults with discoid lesions have no features of systemic involvement and are believed to have a low likelihood of evolution to SLE. In contrast, discoid lesions are rarely observed in children. When discoid lesions are present in children, however, they indicate a high likelihood that SLE will develop eventually, albeit many months or years may elapse before the onset of systemic disease (Fig. 14.3).

References

Avcin T, Benseler SM, et al A followup study of antiphospholipid antibodies and associated neuropsychiatric manifestations in 137 children with systemic lupus erythematosus. Arthritis Rheum 2008; 59(2):206–213

Boros CA, Spence D, et al Hydrocephalus and macrocephaly: New manifestations of neonatal lupus erythematosus. Arthritis Rheum 2007; 57(2):261–266

Brik R, Padeh S, et al Systemic lupus erythematosus in children in Israel. Harefuah 1995; 129(7–8):233–235, 296, 295

Brucato A, Frassi M, et al Risk of congenital complete heart block in newborns of mothers with anti-Ro/SSA antibodies detected by counterimmunoelectrophoresis: A prospective study of 100 women. Arthritis Rheum 2001; 44(8):1832–5

Cabanas F, Pellicer A, et al Central nervous system vasculopathy in neonatal lupus erythematosus. Pediatr Neurol 1996; 15(2):124–126

Carhuapoma JR, Mitsias P, et al Cerebral venous thrombosis and anticardiolipin antibodies. Stroke 1997; 28(12):2363–2369

Castellino G, Padovan M, et al Single photon emission computed tomography and magnetic resonance imaging evaluation in SLE patients with and without neuropsychiatric involvement. Rheumatology (Oxford) 2008; 47(3):319–323

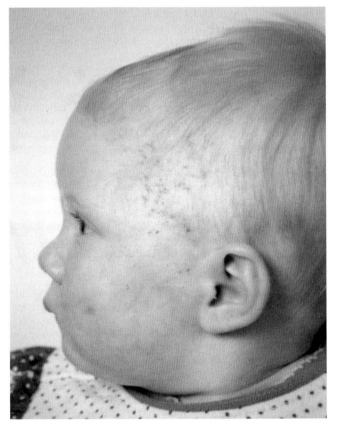

Fig. 14.2 Telangiectasias occurring over the temple region in a child with a history of neonatal lupus

Cervera R, Asherson RA, et al Chorea in the antiphospholipid syndrome. Clinical, radiologic, and immunologic characteristics of 50 patients from our clinics and the recent literature. Medicine (Baltimore) 1997; (3):203–212

Chung AB Fas N. Successful acyclovir treatment of herpes simplex type 2 hepatitis in a patient with systemic lupus erythematosus: A case report and meta analysis. Am J Med Sci 1998; 316(6):404–407

Cimaz R, Spence DL, et al Incidence and spectrum of neonatal lupus erythematosus: A prospective study of infants born to mothers with anti-Ro autoantibodies. J Pediatr 2003; 142(6):678–683

Contreras G, Pardo V, Baudouin L, Lenz O, Tozman E, O'Nan P, Roth D. Sequential therapies for proliferative lupus nephritis. N Engl J Med 2004; 350(10):971–980

Costedoat-Chalumeau N, Amoura Z, et al Outcome of pregnancies in patients with anti-SSA/Ro antibodies: a study of 165 pregnancies, with special focus on electrocardiographic variations in the children and comparison with a control group. Arthritis Rheum 2004; 50(10):3187–3194

Dooley MA, Hogan S, et al Cyclophosphamide therapy for lupus nephritis: Poor renal survival in black Americans. Glomerular Disease Collaborative Network. Kidney Int 1997; 51(4):1188–1195

Dror Y, Blachar Y, et al Systemic lupus erythematosus associated with acute Epstein-Barr virus infection. Am J Kidney Dis 1998; 32(5):825–828

Eberhard A, Couper R, et al Exocrine pancreatic function in children with systemic lupus erythematosus. J Rheumatol 1992; 19(6):964–967

Figueroa F, Berrios X, et al Anticardiolipin antibodies in acute rheumatic fever. J Rheumatol 1992; 19(8):1175–1180

Flower C, Hennis A, et al Lupus nephritis in an Afro-Caribbean population: Renal indices and clinical outcomes. Lupus 2006; 15(10):689–694

Gladman G, Silverman ED, et al Fetal echocardiographic screening of pregnancies of mothers with anti-Ro and/or anti-La antibodies. Am J Perinatol 2002; 19(2):73–80

High WA Costner MI. Persistent scarring, atrophy, and dyspigmentation in a preteen girl with neonatal lupus erythematosus. J Am Acad Dermatol 2003; 48(4):626–628

Hirose I, Ymamaguchi H, et al Fatal varicella infection in a girl with systemic lupus erythematosus after oral acyclovir prophylaxis. Eur J Pediatr 2006; 165(4):280–281

Hudson N, Duffy CM, et al Catastrophic haemorrhage in a case of paediatric primary antiphospholipid syndrome and factor II deficiency. Lupus 1997; 6(1):68–71

Inoue K, Fukushige J, et al Central nervous system vasculopathy associated with neonatal lupus. Pediatr Neurol 2002; 26(1):68–70

Jaeggi ET, Hamilton RM, et al Outcome of children with fetal, neonatal or childhood diagnosis of isolated congenital atrioventricular block. A single institution's experience of 30 years. J Am Coll Cardiol 2002; 39(1):130–137

Jennings JE, Sundgren PC, et al Value of MRI of the brain in patients with systemic lupus erythematosus and neurologic disturbance. Neuroradiology 2004; 46(1):15–21

Julkunen H, Kaaja R, et al Immune-mediated congenital heart block (CHB): Identifying and counseling patients at risk for having children with CHB. Semin Arthritis Rheum 1998; 28(2):97–106

Kasapcopur O, Ergul Y, et al Systemic lupus erythematosus due to Epstein-Barr virus or Epstein-Barr virus infection provocating acute exacerbation of systemic lupus erythematosus? Rheumatol Int 2006; 26(8):765–767

Lambotte O, Khellaf M, et al Characteristics and long-term outcome of 15 episodes of systemic lupus erythematosus-associated hemophagocytic syndrome. Medicine (Baltimore) 2006; 85(3):169–182

Lawrence S, Luy L, et al The health of mothers of children with cutaneous neonatal lupus erythematosus differs from that of mothers of children with congenital heart block. Am J Med 2000; 108(9):705–709

Lee LA, Sokol RJ, et al Hepatobiliary disease in neonatal lupus: prevalence and clinical characteristics in cases enrolled in a national registry. Pediatrics 2002; 109(1):E11

Martino D, Chew NK, et al Atypical movement disorders in antiphospholipid syndrome. Mov Disord 2006; 21(7):944–949

Massengill SF, Hedrick C, et al Antiphospholipid antibodies in pediatric lupus nephritis. Am J Kidney Dis 1997; 29(3):355–361

Nakahara C, Hayashi D, et al Delayed onset of systemic lupus erythematosus in a child with endothelial tubuloreticular inclusion. Clin Nephrol 2001; 56(4):332–335

Nakayama-Furukawa F, Takigawa M, et al Hydrocephalus in two female siblings with neonatal lupus erythematosus. Arch Dermatol 1994; 130(9):1210–1212

Neiman AR, Lee LA, et al Cutaneous manifestations of neonatal lupus without heart block: Characteristics of mothers and children enrolled in a national registry. J Pediatr 2000; 137(5):674–680

Olfat MO, Al-Mayouf SM, et al Pattern of neuropsychiatric manifestations and outcome in juvenile systemic lupus erythematosus. Clin Rheumatol 2004; 23(5):395–399

Pluchinotta FR, Schiavo B, et al Distinctive clinical features of pediatric systemic lupus erythematosus in three different age classes. Lupus 2007; 16(8):550–555

Prendiville JS, Cabral DA, et al Central nervous system involvement in neonatal lupus erythematosus. Pediatr Dermatol 2003; 20(1):60–67

Press J, Palayew K, et al Antiribosomal P antibodies in pediatric patients with systemic lupus erythematosus and psychosis. Arthritis Rheum 1996; 39(4):671–676

Pringe A, Trail L, et al Macrophage activation syndrome in juvenile systemic lupus erythematosus: An under-recognized complication? Lupus 2007; 16(8):587–592

Provost TT, Watson R, et al The neonatal lupus syndrome associated with U1RNP (nRNP) antibodies. N Engl J Med 1987; 316(18):1135–1138

Qian J, Yang CD. Hemophagocytic syndrome as one of main manifestations in untreated systemic lupus erythematosus: Two case reports and literature review. Clin Rheumatol 2007; 26(5):807–810

Rappaport KD, Tang WM. Herpes simplex virus type 2 acute retinal necrosis in a patient with systemic lupus erythematosus. Retina 2000; 20(5):545–546

Ruperto N, Ravelli A, et al The pediatric rheumatology international trials organization/American College of Rheumatology provisional criteria for the evaluation of response to therapy in juvenile systemic lupus erythematosus: prospective validation of the definition of improvement. Arthritis Rheum 2006; 55(3):355–363

Sabbadini MG, Manfredi AA, et al Central nervous system involvement in systemic lupus erythematosus patients without overt neuropsychiatric manifestations. Lupus 1999; 8(1):11–19

Sanna G, Bertolaccini ML, et al Neuropsychiatric manifestations in systemic lupus erythematosus: Prevalence and association with antiphospholipid antibodies. J Rheumatol 2003; 30(5):985–992

Sekigawa I, Nawata M, et al Cytomegalovirus infection in patients with systemic lupus erythematosus. Clin Exp Rheumatol 2002; 20(4):559–564

Sheth AP, Esterly NB, et al U1RNP positive neonatal lupus erythematosus: Association with anti-La antibodies? Br J Dermatol 1995; 132(4):520–526

Su CT, Huang CB, et al Neonatal lupus erythematosus in association with anti-RNP antibody: A case report. Am J Perinatol 2001; 18(8):421–426

Sundgren PC, Jennings J, et al MRI and 2D-CSI MR spectroscopy of the brain in the evaluation of patients with acute onset of neuropsychiatric systemic lupus erythematosus. Neuroradiology 2005; 47(8):576–585

Taddio A, Brescia AC, et al Steady improvement of prothrombin levels after cyclophosphamide therapy in pediatric lupus anticoagulant hypoprothrombinemia syndrome (LAHPS). Clin Rheumatol 2007; (12):2167–2169

Takei M, Yamakami K, et al A case of systemic lupus erythematosus complicated by alveolar hemorrhage and cytomegalovirus colitis. Clin Rheumatol 2007; 26(2):274–277

Thornton CM, Eichenfield LF, et al Cutaneous telangiectases in neonatal lupus erythematosus. J Am Acad Dermatol 1995; 33(1):19–25

Uthman I, Khalil I, et al Lupus anticoagulant, factor V Leiden, and methylenetetrahydrofolate reductase gene mutation in a lupus patient with cerebral venous thrombosis. Clin Rheumatol 2004; 23(4):362–363

Verdolini R, Bugatti L, et al Systemic lupus erythematosus induced by Epstein-Barr virus infection. Br J Dermatol 2002; 146(5):877–881

Vyas S, Hidalgo G, et al Outcome in African-American children of neuropsychiatric lupus and lupus nephritis. Pediatr Nephrol 2002; 17(1):45–49

Waltuck J, Buyon JP. Autoantibody-associated congenital heart block: Outcome in mothers and children. Ann Intern Med 1994; 120(7): 544–551

Mixed Connective Tissue Disease

15

Robert W. Hoffman

Overview of Mixed Connective Tissue Disease

> Mixed connective tissue disease (MCTD) is often viewed as a "cousin" of systemic lupus erythematosus (SLE), with which it shares many disease features.

> Some experts regard MCTD as a variant of SLE because of the considerable overlap in clinical and serological manifestations. Others consider it to be a unique disorder because of the frequency with which certain phenotypic features occur in patients classified as MCTD.

> Patients with MCTD by definition have antibodies directed against ribonuceoprotein, i.e., anti-RNP antibodies.

> Common clinical manifestations of MCTD are arthritis, Raynaud's phenomenon, digital ischemia progressing to fingertip ulceration, pulmonary hypertension, interstitial lung disease, and gastrointestinal hypomotility.

> Some patients with MCTD evolve with time to a clinical phenotype that is more easily classified as SLE. Others, perhaps a majority, evolve over time to clinical syndromes most compatible with systemic sclerosis.

> MCTD must be distinguished from "undifferentiated" connective tissue diseases (in which a clear-cut rheumatological process may or may not emerge with time) and also from "overlap" connective tissue diseases, in which the disease features of two or more well-defined connective tissues diseases are present in the same patient. As example of an overlap connective tissue disease is the occurrence of SLE and polymyositis in the same patient. Such a patient would not be regarded as a "mixed" connective tissue disease (MCTD), but rather as the co-occurrence of two diseases in the same patient.

Myth: Mixed Connective Tissue Disease (MCTD) is rare.

Reality: No definitive epidemiologic studies related to MCTD have been published, but clinical studies from the United States, Mexico, and Japan indicate that MCTD is less common than lupus but more common than scleroderma or dermatomyositis (Kotajima et al. 1999). Although "rare" is relative when it comes to rheumatic diseases, MCTD is actually more common than some other connective tissue diseases that have a higher profile among both medical practitioners and the general public.

Myth: MCTD, undifferentiated connective tissue disease (UCTD), and "overlap syndrome" are all synonymous terms.

Reality: These three terms are frequently confused and often used interchangeably, particularly by non-rheumatologists. The term "UCTD" was coined to describe patients who fail to meet classification criteria for certain distinct rheumatic disorders, particularly scleroderma, SLE, or Sjögren's syndrome.

UCTD patients typically have disease of recent onset. Over time, their clinical features often evolve to resemble a "clear cut" rheumatic disease (or perhaps more than one) more closely. Many such rheumatic conditions are "difficult to pigeonhole" early in their course, but in many such cases, the patients ultimately develop features that are recognizable as a disease sanctioned by ACR classification criteria. As an example, the importance of making the diagnosis of SLE in some patients with fewer than four ACR criteria for the classification of that disorder is discussed elsewhere (*see Systemic Lupus Erythematosus, chapter 13*).

All that said, within 5 years of the onset of symptoms, long-term follow-up studies have demonstrated that nearly all patients with possible MCTD can be classified confidently as having MCTD or another distinct rheumatic disease within 5 years of their symptom onset (Burdt et al. 1999). A subset of patients fails to meet classification criteria for MCTD or any other rheumatic disease at that time. These patients should be considered truly "undifferentiated," i.e., UTCD. Long-term follow-up studies of these true UCTD patients suggest a generally good outcome (Mosca et al. 1999).

Finally, an *overlap* CTD is one in which there are unequivocal features of two autoimmune diseases recognized in textbooks as being separate. One classic example of an overlap

J. H. Stone (ed.), *A Clinician's Pearls and Myths in Rheumatology*,
DOI:10.1007/978-1-84800-934-9_15, © Springer Science + Business Media B.V. 2009

CTD is the occurrence of symptoms of polymyositis and systemic sclerosis in the same patient. In such cases, there is nothing "undifferentiated" about the manifestations of either disease: a muscle biopsy confirms the histopathologic features of polymyositis, and the patient has skin thickening and other disease manifestations of scleroderma. This overlap of polymyositis and systemic sclerosis actually has a unique autoantibody: PM/Scl autoantibodies. These antibodies are directed against a nuclear antigen complex that consists of 11–16 proteins, the precise cellular function of which remains unknown (Treadwell et al. 1984).

Pearl: Sicca symptoms are common in MCTD.

Comment: Keratoconjunctivitis sicca and xerostomia are detected often whenever MCTD patients are asked in a systematic manner about these symptoms. Symptoms and signs of Sjögren's syndrome have been identified in more than half of all MTCD patients in some studies. These findings, considered to represent secondary Sjögren's syndrome rather than an overlap CTD (see above), are often accompanied by the development of anti-SSA/Ro autoantibodies.

Pearl: MCTD can present as a unilateral or bilateral trigeminal neuropathy.

Comment: A well-recognized complication of MCTD, early in the disease course, is a fifth cranial nerve palsy. A similar or identical finding (of equally obscure pathogenesis) has been reported in systemic sclerosis (Farrell and Medsger 1982). The common link between the occurrence of this neurological lesion and these two rheumatic diseases might be the presence of anti-RNP antibodies.

The development of trigeminal nerve dysfunction in MCTD or systemic sclerosis is bilateral as often as it is unilateral. The clinical features of this problem consist of the sudden onset of either unilateral or bilateral facial numbness, with or without pain or paresthesias. In one series of 442 consecutive scleroderma patients from the University of Pittsburgh, 6 of the 16 patients (38%) with trigeminal neuropathies were strongly positive for antibodies to RNP. In contrast, only 8% of those who did not have trigeminal neuropathy had antibodies to RNP.

Myth: MCTD is simply a subset of either lupus or scleroderma.

Reality: The etiology and pathogenesis of all three of these conditions remain unknown. Consequently, any classification scheme for such diseases is potentially flawed and subject to refinement in the light of future scientific advances. In a follow-up study of the original group studied by Sharp et al. and in longitudinal long-term outcome studies, investigators found that with treatment there was a reduction over time in the inflammatory features of the disease, including arthralgias/arthritis, esophageal dysmotility, Raynaud's phenomenon, serositis, and skin rash (Nimelstein et al. 1980; Burdt et al. 1999). However, both persistent and new clinical features, including sclerodactyly, pulmonary hypertension, and peripheral neuropathy, became the dominant features of the illness later in the course of the disease. After some years of disease, some patients meet the ACR classification criteria for scleroderma.

Despite its challenges with regard to disease classification, the concept of MCTD has been recognized widely since its formulation in the early 1970s (Sharp et al. 1972). MCTD has been identified in a variety of different populations across the world. Although some iconoclasts continue to grouse about "defining a disease by the presence of an autoantibody" (a practice that no true MCTD expert endorses), the notion of a distinct MCTD phenotype rings true with experienced clinicians, and most consider it a valid entity.

Myth: MCTD is no longer a clinically relevant term.

Reality: The primary disease-related cause of death in MCTD is pulmonary hypertension. This feature marks a striking divergence of this disease from SLE, a disorder in which clinically significant pulmonary hypertension rarely becomes an issue. Advances in our ability to diagnose and treat pulmonary hypertension effectively in recent years strengthen the argument for early recognition of the MCTD clinical phenotype.

Pearl: Periodic screening of patients using with pulmonary function tests (PFTs) and two-dimensional echocardiography helps identify incipient pulmonary hypertension.

Comment: Annual PFTs with DLco measurement as well as two-dimensional echocardiograms are recommended for patients with MCTD. Substantial pulmonary hypertension can exist in MCTD even in the setting of mild clinical symptomatology and a normal chest radiograph. A declining DLco or elevated right-sided cardiac pressures should lead to further evaluations, including a high-resolution chest CT or right heart catheterization.

Pearl: The emergence of anti-RNP antibodies is linked closely to the onset of clinical manifestations of disease.

Comment: The development of anti-RNP autoantibodies bears a close temporal relationship to the onset of clinical signs and symptoms in MCTD. A retrospective analysis of serum samples in patients subsequently diagnosed with a rheumatic disease found that most patients develop clinical signs and symptoms within 6 months of the appearance of anti-RNP antibodies (Arbuckle et al. 2003). Moreover, the presence of anti-RNP antibodies is rare among individuals who are asymptomatic at testing.

Myth: Mixed connective tissue disease (MCTD) can be diagnosed by the presence of anti-RNP antibodies.

Reality: Although anti-RNP antibodies are not diagnostic of MCTD in and of themselves, the diagnosis should be viewed with great skepticism if these antibodies are absent. Anti-RNP reactivity is extremely rare in the absence of an autoimmune disease but does occur with some frequency in overlap connective tissue disorders, systemic lupus erythematosus (SLE), and scleroderma. Thus, anti-RNP antibodies are *necessary but not sufficient* for the diagnosis of MCTD.

Anti-RNP antibodies are required for the *classification* of an individual as having MCTD (Sharp et al. 1972; Burdt et al. 1999). However, there are no validated *diagnostic* criteria for MCTD. (The same is true for many, if not most, other rheumatic diseases.) Classification criteria developed for the purpose of research cannot be applied reliably to the diagnosis of individual patients, even though clinicians are often tempted to do so.

Pearl: Diffuse swelling of the fingers that extends to the dorsum of the hand may be a persistent feature in MCTD. This can lead to the misdiagnosis of rheumatoid arthritis.

Comment: Diffuse swelling of the fingers is a hallmark of MCTD. This is sometimes related to synovitis, but more often corresponds to a soft tissue swelling not arthritis. Non-arthritic soft tissue swelling can extend to the dorsum of the hands, persist for years, and progress to sclerodactyly in some patients. It also resolves with treatment in other patients. In addition to diffuse swelling, tapering of the fingers is also characteristic (but not pathognomonic) of MCTD in many patients (Fig. 15.1).

Arthralgias or arthritis can also be a primary MCTD feature. Rheumatoid factor is detectable in the sera of 50–75% of MCTD patients. Antibodies to cyclic citrullinated peptide have also been reported in MCTD. The presence of the major histocompatibility gene encoding HLA-DR4 appears to be a risk factor for this disease (Hoffman et al. 1990).

Pearl: Gastroesophageal reflux responds well to proton-pump inhibitors but less well to older classes of agents for this problem.

Comment: Proton pump inhibitors offer an effective form of therapy for what was once one of the more refractory features of MCTD, reflux esophagitis. MCTD patients bear a striking resemblance to patients with systemic sclerosis in their tendency to develop gastroesophageal reflux, as well as in the frequency with which Raynaud's phenomenon, digital ulceration (Fig. 15.2), and pulmonary hypertension complicate the disease.

Myth: Myositis is common in MCTD.

Reality: Although an inflammatory myopathy was included as part of the initial disease description (Sharp et al. 1972), myositis actually tends to be quite mild in most patients with MCTD. Myositis remains clinically silent in many patients unless sought specifically. Often a mild serum creatine kinase (CK) elevation provides the only clue to muscle inflammation. The typical MCTD patient with muscle involvement has a serum CK level elevated not higher than two or three times the

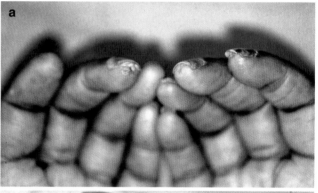
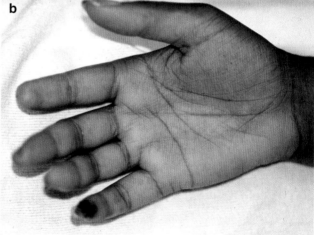

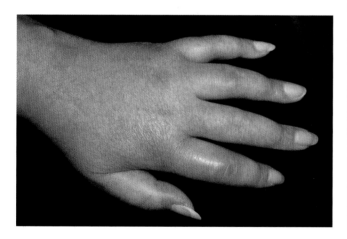

Fig. 15.1 Sclerodactyly often leads to pronounced finger tapering in patients with mixed connective tissue disease. This feature is not pathognomonic of mixed connective tissue disease but is a marker for a variety of disorders in the "connective tissue disease" spectrum (Figure courtesy of John H. Stone)

Fig. 15.2 Sclerodactyly and digital ischemia in patients with mixed connective tissue disease. (**a**) shows digital pitting, a long-term consequence of digital ischemia. (**b**) shows gangrenous changes in the distal part of one finger (Figures courtesy of John H. Stone)

upper limit of normal. Even more important than low serum CK levels, however, is the fact that few MCTD patients develop clinical muscle weakness. The inflammatory myopathy may be so mild that it does not affect treatment considerations.

Pearl: Raynaud's phenomenon is nearly universal among patients with MCTD.

Comment: Pointed questioning unearths this symptom in almost every case of MCTD. This finding heightens the suspicion that an autoimmune disorder might be present in a patient with otherwise nondescript symptoms.

Myth: MCTD is more severe in children than in adults.

Reality: Initial studies on MCTD from the Los Angeles County Children's Hospital suggested that the disease was more severe on average in children than in adults (Singsen et al. 1977). As the recognition of MCTD has grown more widespread, it has become apparent that a range of manifestations exists among pediatric patients and the long-term outcomes in this population are variable. Studies from Missouri, Minnesota, Germany, and Japan have demonstrated that the course and prognosis of MCTD in children is similar to that in adults (Hoffman 1993; Burdt et al. 1999; Michels 1997).

Pearl: MCTD can cause a nasal septal perforation.

Comment: The etiology is not clear, but MCTD joins Wegener's granulomatosis, relapsing polychondritis, sarcoidosis, and a smattering of other conditions that sometimes lead to a nasal septal perforation.

References

Arbuckle MR, McClain MT, Rubertone MV, et al Development of autoantibodies before the clinical onset of systemic lupus erythematosus. N Engl J Med 2003; 349:1526–1533

Burdt MA, Hoffman RW, Deutscher SL, et al Long-term outcome in mixed connective tissue disease: Longitudinal clinical and serologic findings. Arthritis Rheum 1999; 42:899–909

Farrell DA, Medsger TA Jr. Trigeminal neuropathy in progressive systemic sclerosis. Am J Med 1982; 73:57–62

Kotajima L, Aotsuka S, Sumiya M, et al Clinical features of patients with juvenile onset mixed connective tissue disease: Analysis of data collected in a nationwide collaborative study in Japan. J Rheumatol 1999; 23:1088–1094

Michels H. Course of mixed connective tissue disease in children. Ann Med 1997; 29:359–364

Mosca M, Neri R, Bombardieri S. Undifferentiated connective tissue diseases (UCTD): A review of the literature and a proposal for preliminary classification criteria. Clin Exp Rheumatol 1999; 17: 615–620

Nimelstein SH, Brody S, McShane D, Holman HR. Mixed connective tissue disease: A subsequent evaluation of the original 25 patients. Medicine 1980; 59:239–248

Sharp GC, Irvin WS, Tan EM, et al Mixed connective tissue disease: An apparently distinct rheumatic disease syndrome associated with a specific antibody to extractable nuclear antigen (ENA). Am J Med 1972; 52:148–159

Singsen BH, Kornreich HK, Koster-King K, et al Mixed connective tissue disease in children. Arthritis Rheum 1977; 20(2 Suppl): 355–360

Treadwell EL, Alspaugh MA, Wolfe JF, Sharp GC. Clinical relevance of PM-1 antibody and physiochemical characterization of PM-1 antigen. J Rheumatol 1984; 11(5):658–662

The Antiphospholipid Syndrome

16

David P. D'Cruz and Munther Khamashta

16.1 Overview of the Antiphospholipid Syndrome

> The antiphospholipid syndrome (APS) is a multi-system autoimmune disorder characterized by recurrent arterial and venous thromboses and pregnancy morbidity (Hughes 1983).

> The most common clinical manifestations of the APS are shown in Table 16.1.

> Cutaneous manifestations of the APS include livedo reticularis (livedo racemosa), leg ulcers, skin necrosis, superficial thrombophlebitis, splinter hemorrhages, digital ischemia, and gangrene. Many of these features must be distinguished from vasculitis, which can also be associated with these findings.

> The APS is linked to multiple central nervous system manifestations. These are listed in Table 16.2.

> The APS can occur in a primary form which is not associated with another underlying condition. In addition, it can develop concurrently with disorders such as systemic lupus erythematosus (SLE).

> Antiphospholipid antibodies (aPL) are a heterogeneous group of immunoglobulins directed at phospholipid binding proteins. Three antibodies are central to the diagnosis of APS: the lupus anticoagulant (LA), anticardiolipin antibodies (aCL), and β-2-glycoprotein 1.

> aCL and β-2-glycoprotein 1 are detected by enzyme-linked immunosorbent assays. The LA is commonly detected by the dilute Russell viper venom time, but other assays are also available (Brandt et al. 1995).

> aPL are found in less than 1% of healthy populations of all ages. However, the figure is substantially higher among healthy older populations – as high as 5%. The prevalence in SLE is substantially higher, on the order of 24% for IgG aCL, 13% for IgM aCL, and 15% for LA (Cervera et al. 1993).

> APS has a significant impact on morbidity and mortality (Shah et al. 1998; Jouhikainen et al. 1993; Schulman et al. 1998; Ruiz-Irastorza et al. 2004). In one longitu-

dinal study of SLE patients, aPL-related thromboses accounted for 27% of all deaths in the cohort (Cervera et al. 1993).

> The term "catastrophic APS" refers to a rare but potentially lethal disorder characterized by accelerated thrombosis, multiple organ involvement that includes renal thrombotic microangiopathy and death in a high percentage of patients (Bucciarelli et al. 2006).

> The combination of anticoagulation, glucocorticoids, and plasma exchange is a useful treatment approach to the catastrophic APS (Bucciarelli et al. 2006). Immunosuppression, particularly with cyclophosphamide, should be avoided.

> Arterial and venous events associated with the APS are treated initially with unfractionated or low molecular weight heparins, followed by oral anticoagulation with warfarin.

> Women with APS are at high risk of complications during pregnancy and in the postpartum period. In the postnatal period, women with Thrombotic APS should be given thromboprophylaxis with subcutaneous heparin followed by the resumption of oral anticoagulation as soon as possible. Controversies in the management of patients during pregnancy are discussed.

Myth: The lupus anticoagulant indicates that the patient has systemic lupus erythematosus.

Reality: This is a common misconception among patients (and some physicians). The term "lupus anticoagulant" is among the more confusing terms in medicine, for several reasons. The lupus anticoagulant (LA) is in fact a pro-thrombotic autoantibody directed against phospholipid-binding proteins. (This is true for all antiphospholipid antibodies.) In addition, despite the fact that the updated classification criteria for systemic *lupus* erythematosus include the presence of a *lupus* anticoagulant, many patients with *lupus* anticoagulants do not have and will not develop lupus (Hochberg 1997).

J. H. Stone (ed.), *A Clinician's Pearls and Myths in Rheumatology,*
DOI:10.1007/978-1-84800-934-9_16, © Springer Science + Business Media B.V. 2009

Table 16.1 Most common cumulative clinical manifestations of the antiphospholipid syndrome in 1,000 patients followed prospectively (Adapted from Cervera et al. 2002)

Deep vein thrombosis (38.9%)
Pulmonary embolism (14.1%)
Cutaneous manifestations, especially livedo reticularis/racemosa (24.1%)
Neurological manifestations including migraine (20.2%) (see Table 16.2)
Stroke (19.8%)
  Transient ischemic attacks (11.1%)
  Epilepsy (7.0%)
  Cardiac valve disease (11.6%) (Fig. 16.5)
Myocardial infarction (5.5%)
Hematological manifestations
  Thrombocytopenia (29.6%)
  Hemolytic anemia (9.7%)
Obsteric complications
  Early and late fetal loss (52.5%)
  Pre-eclampsia (9.5%)
  Premature delivery (10.6%)
Renal disease (2.7%)

Table 16.2 Central nervous system manifestations of the antiphospholipid syndrome (Adapted from Sanna et al. 2006)

Classic cerebrovascular disease complications:
• Ischemic strokes
• Transient ischemic attacks
• Acute ischemic encephalopathy
• Cerebral venous sinus thrombosis
Other well-recognized (but often unproven) associations:
• Headaches, including migraine
• Cognitive dysfunction, including dementia
• Seizures, abnormal electroencephalography
• Chorea
• Transverse myelopathy
• Demyelinating syndromes
• Idiopathic intracranial hypertension
• Sensorineural hearing loss
• Guillain–Barre syndrome
• Transient global amnesia
• Ocular ischemic syndromes
• Dystonia–Parkinsonism
• Progressive supranuclear palsy

Pearl: Multiple different autoantibodies can cause the lupus anticoagulant phenomenon.

Comment: A broad spectrum of autoantibodies that are directed against phospholipid-binding proteins can be associated with LA activity. Such autoantibodies include those directed against prothrombin, phosphatidylserine, phosphatidylethanolamine, and β2-glycoprotein 1. However, clinical testing for such other specific antibodies seldom adds much to the standard laboratory aPL assays for aCL antibodies and LA.

Myth: A normal activated partial thromboplastin time (aPTT) excludes an LA.

Reality: A prolonged aPTT suggests the possibility of an LA, but only about half of all patients with documented LAs have an abnormal aPTT. The dilute Russell viper venom time (dRVVT) test is more sensitive and specific for the detection of an LA than is prolongation of the aPTT.

Myth: The LA affects the aPTT, not the prothrombin time (PT).

Reality: On the contrary, an LA does affect the PT in some cases. A prolonged PT might indicate an extremely high level of LA. Two tests that are not commonly affected by LA are the chromogenic factor X and the prothrombin–proconvertin time. However, these assays are not available routinely in most laboratories (Moll and Ortel 1997).

Pearl: Many medications may be associated with the production of aPL.

Comment: Many conditions other than the primary APS and SLE can be associated with the finding of aPL in serum. However, in many other such instances, the finding of aPL does not indicate an individual at heightened risk for thrombosis or other APS complications. As examples, aPL occur frequently in infections such as HIV and syphilis, as well as in association with some types of malignancy or following exposure to certain drugs. However, unless these antibodies are directed against β-2-glycoprotein-1, the likelihood that they are clinically significant is very low.

Pearl: Many clinical features widely acknowledged to be associated with the APS are not included in classification criteria for definite cases of this condition.

Comment: Classification criteria for definite APS have been validated (Table 16.3) (Wilson et al. 1999; Lockshin et al. 2000) and updated (Miyakis et al. 2006). These classification criteria were developed for use in research studies rather than as diagnostic criteria, which as yet do not exist. Many clinical manifestations generally considered to be present in some patients with the APS, e.g., thrombocytopenia, hemolytic anemia, transient ischemic attacks, seizures transverse myelitis (Fig. 16.1), livedo reticularis, valvular heart disease, demyelinating syndromes (Fig. 16.2), chorea, and migraine were not included in the final criteria established for "definite" APS (Miyakis et al. 2006). The exclusion of such criteria from the classification criteria results in higher specificity but lower sensitivity.

In clinical practice, sound judgment often dictates that a clinician consider a patient with such clinical features in the context of persistently positive aPL to have the APS and treat the patient accordingly.

Myth: A patient with thrombosis and/or pregnancy morbidity can only be diagnosed with APS with moderate to high titers

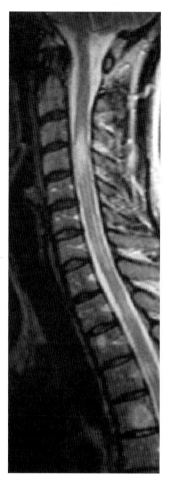

Fig. 16.1 Transverse myelitis in a patient with SLE and aPL. A large high signal lesion is seen in the upper cervical cord with cord edema (D'Cruz et al. 2004)

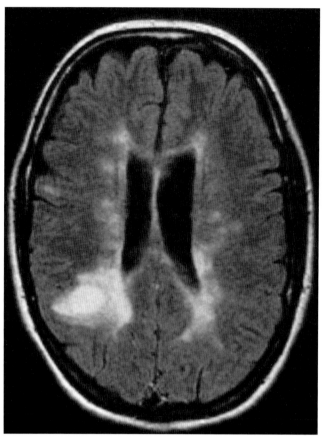

Fig. 16.2 White matter hyper-intense lesions on MRI in a patient with aPL resembling demyelination

of aCL antibodies and/or a positive LA and/or anti-β-2-gly-coprotein 1 antibodies tested at least 12 weeks apart.

Reality: This myth gets at another common point of confusion between classification and diagnostic criteria. There are no diagnostic criteria for the APS. The current classification criteria were designed to be highly specific so as to avoid bias and to foster homogeneity within research study populations. High specificity inevitably comes at a cost of lower sensitivity and means that many patients whose clinical diagnosis is the APS do not meet classification criteria.

A 35-year-old woman with extensive livedo reticularis and a previous pregnancy resulting in intrauterine death of the fetus who presents with a pulmonary embolism in the context of persistent low-titer aCL antibodies would be considered by most experts to have APS. However, the patient would not meet the APS classification criteria.

Once anticoagulation with warfarin has begun, it is often difficult to interpret LA assays. This fact complicates the point within the classification criteria that requires retesting a minimum of 12 weeks later. Strict classification of the patient then becomes difficult, particularly if antibodies to aCL and β2-glycoprotein 1 are negative and the patient's sole aPL antibody has been the LA.

Pearl: The only types of aCL that are associated with an increased risk of thrombosis are those that are dependent on β2-glycoprotein 1.

Comment: This point was mentioned above but is worth re-emphasizing. Patients with positive aCL tests but negative assays for anti-β2glycoprotein 1 are not at increased risk for clotting or other APS manifestations. These β2glycoprotein 1 independent antibodies are commonly found in infections such as HIV, hepatitis C, leprosy, syphilis, and other infections, as well as in association with certain drugs.

16.2 Risk Factors for Thrombosis in APS

Pearl: Previous thrombosis is the strongest predictor of future events.

Comment: History of a clinical event compatible with the APS in the context of persistent moderate to high aCL levels or LA is the most powerful predictor of a future APS event (Akimoto et al. 2005). The importance of previous thrombosis was highlighted by the recurrence rate in a retrospective

Table 16.3 Classification criteria for the antiphospholipid syndrome (From Miyakis et al. 2006. Reprinted from J Thromb Haemost, with kind permission from Wiley Interscience)

Antiphospholipid antibody syndrome (APS) is present if at least one of the clinical criteria and one of the laboratory criteria that follow are met

Clinical criteria

1. Vascular thrombosis

One or more clinical episodes of arterial, venous, or small vessel thrombosis, in any tissue or organ. Thrombosis must be confirmed by objective validated criteria (i.e. unequivocal findings of appropriate imaging studies or histopathology). For histopathologic confirmation, thrombosis should be present without significant evidence of inflammation in the vessel wall

2. Pregnancy morbidity

  (a) One or more unexplained deaths of a morphologically normal fetus at or beyond the 10th week of gestation, with normal fetal morphology documented by ultrasound or by direct examination of the fetus, or

  (b) One or more premature births of a morphologically normal neonate before the 34th week of gestation because of:
(i) eclampsia or severe preeclampsia defined according to standard definitions, or (ii) recognized features of placental insufficiency, or

  (c) Three or more unexplained consecutive spontaneous abortions before the 10th week of gestation, with maternal anatomic or hormonal abnormalities and paternal and maternal chromosomal causes excluded

In studies of populations of patients who have more than one type of pregnancy morbidity, investigators are strongly encouraged to stratify groups of subjects according to a, b, or c above.

Laboratory criteria

1. Lupus anticoagulant (LA) present in plasma, on two or more occasions at least 12 weeks apart, detected according to the guidelines of the International Society on Thrombosis and Haemostasis (Scientific Subcommittee on LAs/phospholipid-dependent antibodies)

2. Anticardiolipin (delete extra 'c') (aCL) antibody of IgG and/or IgM isotype in serum or plasma, present in medium or high titer (i.e. >40 GPL or MPL, or >the 99th percentile), on two or more occasions, at least 12 weeks apart, measured by a standardized ELISA

3. Anti-beta2 glycoprotein-I antibody of IgG and/or IgM isotype in serum or plasma (in titer > the 99th percentile), present on two or more occasions, at least 12 weeks apart, measured by a standardized ELISA, according to recommended procedures

study in which patients with the APS and previous thrombosis had a recurrence rate of 20% per patient-year of follow-up (Khamashta et al. 1995).

Other risk factors also contribute to the development of a first thrombotic event in the presence of aPL. For example, at the time of the initial thrombosis, 50% of aPL-positive patients have coincident risk factors (Giron-Gonzalez et al. 2004). These include recent surgery and prolonged immobilization (associated with venous thrombosis), and hypercholesterolemia and arterial hypertension (linked to arterial thrombosis). SLE itself is a risk factor for thrombosis, regardless of the patient's aPL status. Finally, multivariate models in studies of APS patients have demonstrated independent associations of smoking, older age, disease activity over

time, mean dose of glucocorticoids, and shorter disease duration (Calvo-Alen et al. 2005).

Pearl: aPL are found in approximately 30–40% of patients with "idiopathic" immune thrombocytopenia (ITP).

Comment: The recognition of aPL in ITP is important because conventional thinking associates ITP with an increased risk of bleeding. In contrast, patients with aPL may suffer thromboses even in the setting of thrombocytopenia (Diz-Küçükkaya et al. 2001).

Pearl: Livedo reticularis is strongly associated with the occurrence of arterial ischemic events in the APS.

Comment: Livedo reticularis is strongly associated with arterial lesions in APS. In one study that involved 200 consecutively evaluated patients, livedo reticularis was associated with cerebral or ocular ischemic events with an odds ratio of 10.8 (95% CI 5.2 – 22.5) (Francès et al. 2005). In contrast, livedo reticularis was observed with decreased frequency in patients who only experienced venous thromboses (odds ratio 0.2; 9% CI 0.1 – 0.5).

Myth: Livedo reticularis is the most common cutaneous manifestation of APS.

Reality: The literature is remarkably muddy here. This issue is whether the proper term for the lacy discoloration of the skin in this condition is livedo reticularis as opposed to livedo racemosa. Since the earliest descriptions of the APS, the term "livedo reticularis" has been used rather indiscriminately. Clinicians have used livedo reticularis in the context of the APS when, in many instances, livedo racemosa would have been the more accurate term. Livedo racemosa, a term coined by Ehrmann in 1907 (Ehrmann 1907), is a much more striking cutaneous finding than is livedo reticularis, and livedo racemosa is far more likely to indicate a serious medical condition, be it the APS, polyarteritis nodosa, or something else.

Livedo racemosa is the most common dermatologic manifestation of APS and is frequently associated with cerebrovascular events, arterial thrombosis, and pregnancy morbidity. The racemosa pattern may be distinguished by the broken pattern, widespread extent (especially on the trunk), and its minimal alteration during cool temperatures (Fig. 16.3). In contrast to livedo racemosa, livedo reticularis often occurs in physiologic settings such as cold weather and is not always associated with an underlying disease.

Livedo racemosa versus livedo reticularis is also discussed in the chapter on polyarteritis nodosa (Chapter 26).

Pearl: APS nephropathy may complicate lupus nephritis and should be considered in all patients with SLE, renal disease, and positive assays for aPL.

Comment: APS nephropathy is a distinct entity with characteristic clinical and histological features (Tektonidou 2004).

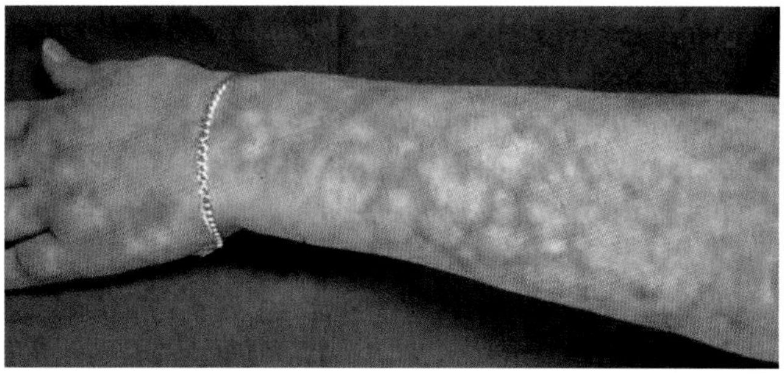

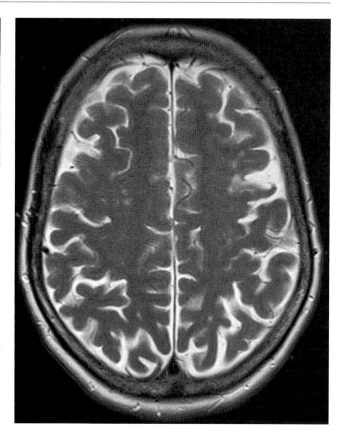

Fig. 16.3 Livedo racemosa. The extensive "broken" pattern indicates pathologic rather than physiological livedo reticularis

All renal vessels may be affected by the thrombotic microangiopathy, but glomerular lesions comprised of basement membrane wrinkling and reduplications appear to be pathognomonic. As acute lesions heal, focal areas of fibrosis and atrophy may develop. Renal impairment may ensue, depending on the extent and severity of these processes.

Recent studies have also confirmed the importance of livedo reticularis (racemosa) as a clinical marker of this syndrome in association with hypertension. In addition, asymptomatic renal artery stenosis may be more common than suggested by early case reports (Sangle 2003). Clinicians should thus assess aPL positive patients very carefully for the development of renal disease and patients with lupus nephritis who develop an additional APS nephropathy should be considered for long-term anticoagulation as well as immunosuppression (D'Cruz 2005).

Anticoagulation is the mainstay of treatment for APS nephropathy, but this strategy remains imperfect. Close attention to other risk factors, especially hypertension and the traditional Framingham risk factors, may reduce the risk of end-stage renal failure in these patients.

Myth: High signal lesions on brain MRI indicate cerebral vasculitis.

Reality: This problem arises especially in patients with SLE in whom the radiologist reports high signal lesions as being consistent with "cerebral vasculitis." In fact, true cerebral vasculitis is extremely rare in SLE. Moreover, vasculitis is not part of the APS. High signal white matter lesions correlate with older age, but also with aPL (Fig. 16.4) (Sanna et al. 2003).

Myth: APS is a bland disorder characterized by thrombosis in the absence of signs of systemic inflammation.

Reality: "Straightforward" APS is usually not associated with signs of systemic inflammation. However, inflammation, particularly complement activation, does appear to play a central role in the pathophysiology of this condition (Girardi et al. 2006).

There is one important exception to the "bland inflammation" rule in the APS. This occurs in the setting of the

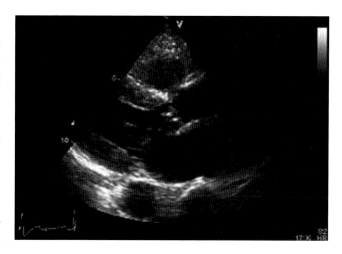

Fig. 16.4 High signal lesions on MRI compatible with small vessel ischemia in a patient with APS

Fig. 16.5 Aortic valve vegetation in a patient with APS presenting with a stroke

catastrophic APS, which is often accompanied by the systemic inflammatory response syndrome (SIRS). The catastrophic APS is difficult to distinguish it from thrombotic thrombocytopenic purpura/hemolytic uremic syndrome (Asherson et al. 2007).

Pearl: Patients with the APS should not receive estrogen-containing medications.

Comment: No discussion here. Both the combined oral contraceptive pill and hormone replacement therapy are absolutely contraindicated in APS patients because of their association with thromboembolic disease.

Myth: A baby aspirin a day is useful in primary prophylaxis for patients who have aPL but no history of clinical events compatible with the APS.

Reality: Many clinicians recommend low-dose aspirin for primary prevention in patients without previous thrombosis, particularly if titers of aPL are high. However, there is little in the way of solid data to support this. Indeed, one placebo-controlled trial did not show any protective benefit against thrombosis, albeit follow-up in that trial was limited (Erkan et al. 2007). Although not treating asymptomatic aPL-positive individuals with aspirin remains a reasonable option (Lim et al. 2006), many expert clinicians give aspirin anyway in the interest of doing something that might help and is unlikely to cause harm.

For SLE patients, some evidence supports the use of hydroxychloroquine in this setting. In the LUMINA study, hydroxychloroquine was protective against thrombosis in univariate analysis but not in multivariate analysis (Ho et al. 2005). A recent systematic review endorsed antimalarial therapy for both its disease-modifying (i.e., "anti-inflammatory") effects as well as its protective effects against thrombosis (Ruiz-Irastorza et al. 2008).

Pearl: Patients with aPL who undertake long airplane flights are increased risk of venous thrombosis.

Comment: Prolonged journeys in which passengers are seated in cramped conditions for lengthy periods of time may be associated with "traveller's thrombosis" (Hughes et al. 2003). No studies have addressed the possible relevance of aPL in this syndrome. In the absence of evidence, it seems reasonable to recommend simple measures such as support stockings, hydration, exercises, and, for patients on treatment, ensuring therapeutic levels of anticoagulation for APS patients who undertake long journeys by any mode of transportation.

In high-risk aPL-positive individuals who have not suffered thromboses but who are deemed to be at high risk for thrombosis for one reason or another (e.g., high aPL titers or the presence of both aCL and an LA), some clinicians recommend a single injection of low molecular weight heparin prior to commencing the journey, provided that the patient's renal function is normal. Other high-risk periods for patients with aPL include the post-operative period, especially after abdominal, gynecological, and orthopedic surgery, and the post-partum period.

Pearl: Anticoagulation in a patient with the APS should be lifelong.

Comment: Several studies support this consensus view (Lim et al. 2006). However, lifelong anticoagulation is not without

hazard. Major bleeds occur in up to 40% of patients in some long-term studies of non-APS patients (Fihn et al. 1993). Data on APS patients from both retrospective cohort reviews and randomized controlled trials suggest that the risk of recurrent thrombotic events exceeds the risk of bleeding, which is relatively low (Finazzi 2005; Crowther et al. 2003; Cervera et al. 2008).

The intensity of anticoagulation has been debated. Randomized controlled trials have suggested that INR levels between 2.0 and 3.0 are sufficient in uncomplicated APS patients with only venous thrombotic events (Finazzi et al. 2005; Crowther et al. 2003). However, in patients with arterial events or with recurrent thrombotic events, an INR between 3.0 and 4.0 may be required (Ruiz-Irastorza et al. 2007).

Once patients are established on warfarin, aspirin does not confer any added advantage and can be discontinued.

Myth: A young woman who has suffered a stroke and has strongly positive aPL assays can be managed safely with aspirin alone and secondary prevention measures.

Reality: Among patients with the APS, strokes tend to occur a mean of 2 decades earlier when compared with the general population (Verro et al. 1998; Brey 2004). Indeed, one systematic review suggested that aPL were an independent risk factor for incidental ischemic stroke, although data on their role in recurrent ischemic stroke was less clear (Verro et al. 1998). Nonetheless, once ischemic stroke occurs, secondary prevention becomes a major issue.

Stroke management in APS patients has been extremely controversial. Older retrospective studies have shown that recurrent thrombotic events are significantly less likely on warfarin therapy with a target INR > 3.0 with or without low-dose aspirin (Khamashta et al. 1995; Rosove and Brewer 1992). One retrospective case series that examined the outcomes of 66 APS patients with previous thrombosis reported an alarming rate of recurrent thrombosis: 9.1 cases per 100 patients-years (95% CI, 3.3 – 19.6) (Ruiz-Irastorza et al. 2002). Most recurrent events developed at INRs between 2.1 and 2.6, a level of anticoagulation assumed by many clinicians to be therapeutic.

Results and the recommendations stemming from the Antiphospholipid Antibodies and Stroke Study (APASS) proved to be very controversial. In that study, 1770 aPL-positive patients with ischemic stroke were allocated randomly to receive either aspirin (325 mg/day) or warfarin (target INR: 1.4–2.8) (The APASS Investigators 2004). Over a 2-year follow-up period, the presence of aPL among patients with ischemic strokes did not predict subsequent thromboembolic events. Recurrent thrombotic events developed in 24% of patients with or without aPL.

The main study conclusions of the APASS were: (a) LA or aCL testing was not important for prognosis or treatment of unselected patients with recent ischemic stroke; (b) in patients with stroke who tested positive for aPL, warfarin therapy with a target INR of 1.4–2.8 was not associated with fewer recurrent events than aspirin. The small group of 120 patients who tested positive for both aCL and LA had a higher risk of thromboembolic events or death regardless of the type of treatment. Unfortunately, several important study flaws hamper generalization of the results to the APS population (Ruiz-Irastorza et al. 2007).

Pearl: Anticoagulation with warfarin may be continued in patients with mild stable thrombocytopenia.

Comment: Thrombocytopenia is common among APS patients. Paradoxically, however, such patients remain at risk for thrombosis despite their thrombocytopenia. Warfarin should be continued at therapeutic levels unless the degree of thrombocytopenia is severe.

In patients with severe thrombocytopenia, glucocorticoids and intravenous immunoglobulins are usually effective. Other agents such as danazol, dapsone, and even aspirin have been tried. There is some debate as to the effectiveness of splenectomy in APS patients, but some studies suggest that splenectomy contributes to more effective control of thrombocytopenia over the long term (Hakim et al. 1998; Galindo et al. 1999).

Pearl: Women with menorrhagia may be managed with hormonal intrauterine devices.

Comment: A frequent problem in the management of female patients is menorrhagia, particularly when INRs are maintained at high levels. In this situation, the "Mirena" coil, an intrauterine coil with a silastic capsule containing levonorgestrel, is helpful in decreasing the volume of menstrual flow (Pisoni et al. 2006).

Pearl: Data on the optimal management of women with the APS during pregnancy are conflicting.

Comment: The current choices are aspirin, heparin, or both (Petri and Qazi 2006). This area remains controversial, especially since a randomized controlled trial demonstrated that good pregnancy success rates were achievable with low-dose aspirin alone and there appeared to be no advantage to adding low molecular weight heparin (Farquharson et al. 2002). These data contrasted with previous controlled trials that showed a significant benefit of heparin with aspirin over aspirin alone (Rai et al. 1997; Kutteh 1996).

Heparin does not cross the placenta and is not known to cause any adverse fetal effects (Baglin et al. 2006). In contrast, warfarin exposure between 6 and 12 weeks of gestation can be associated with an embryopathy characterized by stippled epiphyses and nasal hypoplasia. Thus, if heparin is selected, the change from warfarin to heparin should be achieved prior to 6 weeks gestation.

The risk of osteoporosis in the mother from long-term heparin has probably been overestimated. A controlled study showed that bone loss is a feature of normal pregnancy and that low molecular weight heparin does not exacerbate this loss (Carlin et al. 2004).

Pearl: Women with aPL and previous pregnancy morbidity are at increased of future thrombosis.

Comment: Many women with recurrent fetal losses as the sole manifestation of APS attend recurrent miscarriage clinics. However, once these women deliver successfully, they are often discharged from these clinics without counseling to reduce the risk of a future thrombotic event. There is a consensus that these women should be considered to be at increased risk of a future thrombotic event and management should aim to reduce potential risk factors. However, there is no consensus on the best primary prevention strategy. Many experts prescribe low-dose aspirin therapy, but there are no robust data to support this practice.

References

Akimoto T, Kobayashi S, Tamura N, et al Risk factors for recurrent thrombosis: Prospective study of a cohort of Japanese systemic lupus erythematosus. Angiology 2005; 56:601–609

Asherson RA, Pierangeli SS, Cervera R. Is there a microangiopathic antiphospholipid syndrome? Ann Rheum Dis 2007; 66:429–342

Baglin T, Barrowcliffe TW, Cohen A, et al Guidelines on the use and monitoring of heparin. Br J Haematol 2006; 133:19–34

Brandt JT, Triplett DA, Alving B, et al Criteria for the diagnosis of lupus anticoagulants: An update. On behalf of the Subcommittee on Lupus Anticoagulant/Antiphospholipid Antibody of the Scientific and Standardisation Committee of the ISTH. Thromb Haemost 1995; 74:1185–1190

Brey RL. Management of the neurological manifestations of APS – what do the trials tell us? Thromb Research 2004; 114:489–499

Bucciarelli S, Espinosa G, Cervera R, et al Mortality in the catastrophic antiphospholipid syndrome: Causes of death and prognostic factors in a series of 250 patients. Arthritis Rheum 2006; 54:2568–2576

Calvo-Alén J, Toloza SM, Fernández M, et al Systemic lupus erythematosus in a multiethnic US cohort (LUMINA). XXV. Smoking, older age, disease activity, lupus anticoagulant, and glucocorticoid dose as risk factors for the occurrence of venous thrombosis in lupus patients. Arthritis Rheum 2005; 52:2060–2068

Carlin AJ, Farquharson RG, Quenby SM, et al Prospective observational study of bone mineral density during pregnancy: Low molecular weight heparin versus control. Hum Reprod 2004; 19:1211–1214

Cervera R, Khamashta MA, Font J, et al Systemic lupus erythematosus: Clinical and immunologic patterns of disease expression in a cohort of 1,000 patients. The European Working Party on Systemic Lupus Erythematosus. Medicine (Baltimore) 1993; 72:113–124

Cervera R, Piette JC, Font J, et al Antiphospholipid syndrome: Clinical and immunologic manifestations and patterns of disease expression in a cohort of 1,000 patients. Arthritis Rheum 2002; 46:1019–1027

Cervera R, Khamashta MA, Shoenfeld Y, et al Morbidity and mortality in the antiphospholipid syndrome during a 5-year period: A multicenter prospective study of 1,000 patients. Ann Rheum Dis 2008 Sep 18 [Epub ahead of print]

Crowther MA, Ginsberg JS, Julian J, et al A comparison of two intensities of warfarin for the prevention of recurrent thrombosis in patients with the antiphospholipid antibody syndrome. N Engl J Med 2003; 349:1133–1138

D'Cruz DP. Renal manifestations of the antiphospholipid syndrome. Lupus 2005; 14:45–48

Diz-Küçükkaya R, Hacihanefioğlu A, Yenerel M, et al Antiphospholipid antibodies and antiphospholipid syndrome in patients presenting with immune thrombocytopenic purpura: A prospective cohort study. Blood 2001; 98:1760–1764

Ehrmann S. Ein Gefaessprozess Bei Lues. Wien Med Wochenschr. 1907;57:777

Erkan D, Harrison MJ, Levy R, et al Aspirin for primary thrombosis prevention in the antiphospholipid syndrome: A randomized, double-blind, placebo-controlled trial in asymptomatic antiphospholipid antibody-positive individuals. Arthritis Rheum 2007; 56: 2382–2391

Farquharson RG, Quenby S, Greaves M. Antiphospholipid syndrome in pregnancy: A randomized, controlled trial of treatment. Obstet Gynecol 2002; 100:408–413

Fihn SD, McDonell M, Martin D, et al Risk factors for complications of chronic anticoagulation. A multicenter study. Warfarin Optimized Outpatient Follow-up Study Group. Ann Intern Med 1993; 118: 511–520

Finazzi G, Marchioli R, Brancaccio V, et al A randomized clinical trial of high-intensity warfarin vs. conventional antithrombotic therapy for the prevention of recurrent thrombosis in patients with the antiphospholipid syndrome (WAPS). J Thromb Haemost 2005; 3:848–853

Francès C, Niang S, Laffitte E, et al Dermatologic manifestations of the antiphospholipid syndrome: Two hundred consecutive cases. Arthritis Rheum 2005; 52:1785–1793

Galindo M, Khamashta MA, Hughes GR. Splenectomy for refractory thrombocytopenia in the antiphospholipid syndrome. Rheumatology (Oxford) 1999; 38:848–853

Girardi G, Yarilin D, Thurman JM, et al Complement activation induces dysregulation of angiogenic factors and causes fetal rejection and growth restriction. J Exp Med 2006; 203:2165–2175

Giron-Gonzalez JA, Garcia del Rio E, Rodriguez C, et al Antiphospholipid syndrome and asymptomatic carriers of antiphospholipid antibody: Prospective analysis of 404 individuals. J Rheumatol 2004; 31: 1560–1567

Hakim AJ, Machin SJ, Isenberg DA. Autoimmune thrombocytopenia in primary antiphospholipid syndrome and systemic lupus erythematosus: The response to splenectomy. Semin Arthritis Rheum 1998; 28:20–25

Ho KT, Ahn CW, Alarcon GS, et al Systemic lupus erythematosus in a multiethnic cohort (LUMINA): XXVIII. Factors predictive of thrombotic events. Rheumatology (Oxford) 2005; 44:1303–1307

Hochberg MC. Updating the American College of Rheumatology revised criteria for the classification of systemic lupus erythematosus. Arthritis Rheum 1997; 40:1725

Hughes GRV. Thrombosis, abortion, cerebral disease, and the lupus anticoagulant. Br Med J 1983; 287:1088–1089

Hughes RJ, Hopkins RJ, Hill S, et al Frequency of venous thromboembolism in low to moderate risk long distance air travellers: The New Zealand Air Traveller's Thrombosis (NZATT) study. Lancet 2003; 362:2039–2044

Jouhikainen T, Stephansson E, Leirisalo-Repo M. Lupus anticoagulant as a prognostic marker in systemic lupus erythematosus. Br J Rheumatol 1993; 32:568–573

Khamashta MA, Cuadrado MJ, Mujic F, et al The management of thrombosis in the antiphospholipid antibody syndrome. N Engl J Med 1995; 332:993–997

Kutteh WH. Antiphospholipid antibody-associated recurrent pregnancy loss: Treatment with heparin and low-dose aspirin is superior to low-dose aspirin alone. Am J Obstet Gynecol 1996; 174:1584–1589

Lampropoulos CE, Koutroumanidis M, Reynolds PP, et al Electroencephalography in the assessment of neuropsychiatric manifestations in antiphospholipid syndrome and systemic lupus erythematosus. Arthritis Rheum 2005; 52:841–846

Lim W, Crowther MA, Eikelboom JW. Management of antiphospholipid antibody syndrome: A systematic review. JAMA 2006; 295:1050–1057

Lockshin MD, Sammaritano LR, Schwartzman S. Validation of the Sapporo criteria for antiphospholipid syndrome. Arthritis Rheum 2000; 43:440–443

Miyakis S, Lockshin MD, Atsumi T, et al International consensus statement on an update of the classification criteria for definite antiphospholipid syndrome (APS). J Thromb Haemost 2006; 4:295–306

Moll S, Ortel TL. Monitoring warfarin therapy in patients with lupus anticoagulants. Ann Intern Med 1997; 127:177–185

Petri M, Qazi U. Management of antiphospholipid syndrome in pregnancy. Rheum Dis Clin North Am 2006; 32:591–607

Pisoni CN, Cuadrado MJ, Khamashta MA, Hunt BJ. Treatment of menorrhagia associated with oral anticoagulation: Efficacy and safety of the levonorgestrel releasing intrauterine device (Mirena coil). Lupus 2006; 15:877–880

Rai R, Cohen H, Dave M, Regan L. Randomised controlled trial of aspirin and aspirin plus heparin in pregnant women with recurrent miscarriage associated with phospholipid antibodies (or antiphospholipid antibodies). BMJ 1997; 314:253–257

Rosove MH, Brewer PM. Antiphospholipid thrombosis: clinical course after the first thrombotic event in 70 patients. Ann Intern Med 1992; 117:303–308

Ruiz-Irastorza G, Khamashta MA, Hunt BJ, et al Bleeding and recurrent thrombosis in definite antiphospholipid syndrome. Arch Intern Med 2002; 162:1164–1169

Ruiz-Irastorza G, Egurbide MV, Ugalde J, Aguirre C. High impact of antiphospholipid syndrome on irreversible organ damage and survival of patients with systemic lupus erythematosus. Arch Intern Med 2004; 164:77–82

Ruiz-Irastorza G, Hunt BJ, Khamashta MA. A systematic review of secondary thromboprophylaxis in patients with antiphospholipid antibodies. Arthritis Rheum (Arthritis Care Res) 2007; 57:1487–1495

Ruiz-Irastorza G, Ramos-Casals M, Brito-Zeron P, Khamashta MA. Clinical efficacy and side effects of antimalarials in systemic lupus erythematosus: A systematic review. Ann Rheum Dis 2008 Dec 22 [Epub ahead of print]

Sangle SR, Jan W, Lau IS, et al Coeliac artery stenosis and antiphospholipid (Hughes) syndrome/antiphospholipid antibodies. Clin Exp Rheumatol 2006; 24:349

Sanna G, Bertolaccini ML, Cuadrado MJ, et al Neuropsychiatric manifestations in systemic lupus erythematosus: Prevalence and association with antiphospholipid antibodies. J Rheumatol 2003; 30:985–992

Sanna G, D'Cruz D, Cuadrado MJ. Cerebral manifestations in the antiphospholipid (Hughes) syndrome. Rheum Dis Clin North Am 2006; 32:465–490

Schulman S, Svenungsson E, Granqvist S, The Duration of Anticoagulation Study Group. Anticardiolipin antibodies predict early recurrence of thromboembolism and death among patients with venous thromboembolism following anticoagulant therapy. Am J Med 1998; 104:332–338

Shah NM, Khamashta MA, Atsumi T, Hughes GRV. Outcome of patients with anticardiolipin anti-bodies: A 10 year follow up of 52 patients. Lupus 1998; 7:3–6

Tektonidou MG, Sotsiou F, Nakopoulou L, et al Antiphospholipid syndrome nephropathy in patients with systemic lupus erythematosus and antiphospholipid antibodies: Prevalence, clinical associations, and long-term outcome. Arthritis Rheum 2004; 50: 2569–2579

The APASS Investigators. Antiphospholipid antibodies and subsequent thrombo-occlusive events in patients with ischemic stroke. JAMA 2004; 291:576–584

Verro P, Levine SR, Tietjen GE. Cerebrovascular ischemic events with high positive anticardiolipin antibodies. Stroke 1998; 29:2245–2253

Wilson W, Gharavi A, Koike T, et al International consensus statement on preliminary classification for definite antiphospholipid syndrome. Report of an International Workshop. Arthritis Rheum 1999; 42:1309–1311

Pregnancy in the Rheumatic Diseases

17

Megan E.B. Clowse and Rosalind Ramsey-Goldman

17.1 Overview of Pregnancy in the Rheumatic Diseases

> Few conditions in rheumatology are fraught with greater concern and more unknowns than those of fertility and pregnancy.

> Patients with rheumatologic disease are not at higher risk for infertility than the general population, unless they have received cyclophosphamide.

> In general, the inflammation from active rheumatologic disease is more dangerous to a pregnancy than immunosuppressant medications.

> Medications to continue if needed to control disease: hydroxychloroquine, azathioprine, sulfasalazine, and prednisone.

> Medications to discontinue prior to pregnancy: methotrexate, leflunamide, mycophenolate mofetil, cyclophosphamide.

> Normal pregnancy can alter laboratory findings. In particular, the creatinine should fall and proteinuria may increase mildly. The sedimentation rate and complement may increase.

> Flares in lupus during pregnancy tend to be mild. Patients at highest risk for a severe flare have active lupus at the time of conception.

> Even treated with low molecular weight heparin and aspirin 81mg a day, up to 25% of pregnancies in women with antiphospholipid syndrome will result in a pregnancy loss.

> Maternal SSA/Ro and SSB/La antibodies put a baby at risk for neonatal lupus. Up to 50% of these mothers do not fit criteria for a rheumatologic disease.

> Rheumatoid arthritis will improve in many women during pregnancy, but often flares post-partum. Medications may be tapered during pregnancy but should be restarted following delivery to avoid a severe flare.

17.2 Introduction

Few conditions in rheumatology are fraught with greater concern and more unknowns than those of patients' fertility and pregnancy. Women with rheumatic disease pose special problems during the periconception period and puerperium due to the effects of pregnancy on their underlying disease, the impact of their underlying disease on pregnancy, and the influence of medications on both. In this chapter, we begin with General Considerations, then discuss the use of specific medications in pregnancy, and conclude with Pearls and Myths related to individual rheumatic disorders and their interactions with pregnancy.

17.3 General Considerations

Myth: Women with rheumatic diseases cannot become pregnant because of infertility.

Reality: Infertility is not more common among women with rheumatologic diseases in general. Women with systemic lupus erythematosus (SLE) have rates of pregnancy similar to those of sisters and friends, but lupus pregnancies are more likely to result in gestational loss (Petri and Allbritton 1993). In addition, fertility may be impaired in individual patients by anovulation during episodes of active disease or chronic renal failure, or administration of high dose of glucocorticoids and cyclophosphamide. Patients requiring cyclophosphamide may be protected from infertility by the use of godanotrophins releasing analogs (Somers et al. 2005; Raptopoulou et al. 2004).

There is a debate about whether antinuclear antibodies (ANAs) and antiphospholipid antibodies (aPL) impair implantation, leading to infertility (Kikuchi et al. 2003). Positive ANAs and aPL are more common among women evaluated in infertility clinics. Treatment directed at the underlying rheumatic disease, e.g., with anticoagulation or low-dose glucocorticoids, may improve pregnancy rates in patients suffering from infertility.

Women with rheumatoid arthritis (RA) have (on average) smaller families than do women without RA, but this is more likely the result of personal choice and difficulty with intercourse than of intrinsic infertility (Katz 2006).

Myth: Ovarian stimulation can induce or exacerbate SLE.

Reality: In theory, ovulation stimulation as a fertility treatment could induce SLE, but studies have not confirmed this potential side effect. On the other hand, patients with SLE or primary APS, who are undergoing infertility treatment, could be at risk of flare or thrombosis. When carefully monitored in selected patients, assisted reproductive technologies do not appear to exacerbate SLE in patients whose disease is inactive.

Stable autoimmune diseases that are not associated with major organ damage probably do not affect the outcomes of pregnancies conceived through assisted reproductive technologies (Lockshin 2004). The children born from pregnancies conceived through assisted reproductive technologies are apparently normal at birth, whether or not the genetic or birth mother has autoimmune disease. Few long-term follow-up data are available on the children from these pregnancies.

For patients with antiphospholipid syndrome (or, in selected cases with antiphospholipid antibodies without clinical events), most experts recommend prophylaxis to prevent thrombosis during the conception period. The combination of unfractionated or low molecular weight heparin and aspirin is the regimen employed most often. Anticoagulation should be suspended 24 h before oocyte retrieval and reinstituted 24 h after to reduce the risk of hemorrhage (Costa and Colia 2008). Anticoagulation is extended if pregnancy results.

Myth: There is no way to decrease the risk of preeclampsia.

Reality: Preeclampsia, the combination of hypertension and proteinuria induced by pregnancy, typically develops in the third trimester but can start as early as the 20th week of gestation. Eclampsia, a more severe form of preeclampsia, includes grand mal seizures. Up to a quarter of women with SLE develop significant hypertension or preeclampsia during pregnancy (Clowse et al. 2008). Preeclampsia places both mother and child at increased risk for death. The best treatment for preeclampsia is delivery. The mother's symptoms usually resolve completely within a few days of delivery.

Daily low-dose aspirin taken throughout pregnancy decreases the risk of preeclampsia by about 20% among patients who do not have SLE (Duley et al. 2007). This intervention has not been tested in women with rheumatologic disease, but daily treatment with low-dose aspirin may decrease the risk of preeclampsia in this high-risk population.

Myth: An elevated erythrocyte sedimentation rate (ESR) during pregnancy is a bad prognostic sign.

Reality: The ESR is an unreliable marker of inflammation in pregnancy. Pregnancy itself commonly causes an elevation of the ESR, to greater than 100 mm/h in some cases. Thus, measurements of the ESR should be avoided in pregnant women; it rarely provides useful information but may cause undue concern. The C-reactive protein (CRP) might be a better measure of inflammation in pregnancy, but this has not been confirmed in prospective investigations.

Myth: Dyspnea during pregnancy means that the woman has pleurisy or a pulmonary embolism.

Reality: Dyspnea is a common finding during pregnancy in healthy women. In the first trimester, increased levels of progesterone lead to an increased respiratory rate, but this is rarely associated with the sensation of shortness of breath. In the third trimester, the increasing size of the uterus leads to compression of the lungs, which can promote dyspnea. This dyspnea may be accompanied by pain in the lower chest or abdomen from the baby, but this pain should be distinguishable from pleurisy.

Pregnancy is a hypercoagulable state, probably because the body has evolved to prevent bleeding from the highly vascular placenta. For this reason, healthy women are at a threefold increased risk for deep venous thrombosis (DVT) or pulmonary embolism (PE) during pregnancy and the puerperium. Women with SLE or the antiphospholipid syndrome (APS) are at higher risk for these complications when not pregnant, and the risk is even greater during pregnancy (Clowse et al. 2008). Low-dose aspirin may attenuate this risk to some extent, but this intervention is not an evidence-based therapy. Vigilant evaluation of symptoms, such as unequal swelling of the legs or new dyspnea, is important.

Pearl: A creatinine value of 1.0 mg/dL is likely to be abnormal in a woman who is pregnant.

Comment: During pregnancy, a woman's blood volume increases by 50%, leading to increased renal perfusion and a physiologic lowering of the serum creatinine level. One should anticipate a decline in the creatinine level for all women during pregnancy, with a normal creatinine considered to be between 0.4 and 0.7 mg/dL. A serum creatinine of 1.0 mg/dL is therefore often a cause for concern.

Pearl: An increase in proteinuria during pregnancy does not necessarily indicate a flare of renal lupus.

Comment: In normal pregnancies, the maternal blood volume increases by 50%. This leads to an increase in renal blood flow that causes, in turn, an increase in proteinuria from previously damaged kidneys. A 24-h urine protein measurement of up to 300 mg is considered within the normal range for a healthy pregnant woman. For women with a history of lupus nephritis who have some proteinuria at baseline, the amount of proteinuria can double simply as a function of the increase in renal perfusion. For this reason, an assessment of baseline proteinuria early in pregnancy helps enormously in the interpretation of subsequent questions of renal problems suggested by rising proteinuria.

17.4 Medications

Pearl: Some rheumatic disease medications should be continued during pregnancy.

Comment: A healthy mother is the best environment for the fetus. Thus, medications should be used before and during pregnancy if they promote maternal health. Balancing the risks and benefits of rheumatologic medications to the mother and fetus is essential to the decision to continue or discontinue medications during pregnancy. A comprehensive review of the safety of rheumatic disease medications during pregnancy was published in 2006 and updated in 2008 (Østensen et al. 2006, 2008).

For SLE, active disease (particularly renal disease) within 6 months of conception and the discontinuation of SLE medications are both associated with active disease during pregnancy and poor pregnancy outcomes (Clowse et al. 2005, 2006b ; Clowse 2007(a,b); Ramsey-Goldman et al. 1993).

Approximately 50% of women with SLE have some measurable disease activity during pregnancy. Most SLE activity in these situations represents mild to moderate disease, but treatment is often necessary to minimize the potential effects of active disease on the mother and fetus. Up to 30% of women with SLE have pregnancies that are complicated by the occurrence of very active disease. Under these circumstances, increases in the doses of the patient's SLE medications or the addition of new treatments may be required.

The opposite course can be anticipated in RA, which tends to improve during pregnancy. Some women with RA are able to taper their medications altogether during pregnancy. Unfortunately, the risk of a postpartum flare is high among women with RA. Most RA patients are compelled to resume their prepregnancy medication regimen shortly after delivery (Barrett et al. 1999). This is discussed in greater detail below.

Myth: Clinicians should wait until pregnancy is an established fact before making any changes in a patient's medical regimen.

Reality: Preconception counseling is important to discuss medication options, to adjust medications according to published recommendations, and to monitor the mother for approximately 6 months before attempting conception (Clowse et al., 2005; Clowse 2007). Plans must be in place to switch patients with the antiphospholipid syndrome from warfarin low molecular weight heparin. "Adjunct" medications must be reviewed carefully along with medications use to treat SLE directly. As examples, both angiotensin converting enzyme inhibitors and statins are associated with congenital malformations with exposure during the first trimester (Taguchi et al. 2008).

Similar strategies are also utilized when adjusting medications prior to conception in women with RA. For example, methotrexate should be stopped 3–6 months prior to pregnancy. Leflunomide levels in serum should be assessed and cholestyramine administered if appropriate for women with a history of leflunomide use. However, NSAIDs, sulfasalazine, azathioprine, hydroxychloroquine, and glucocorticoids can be continued during pregnancy.

Pearl: A steroid is not a steroid during pregnancy.

Comment: Prednisone is metabolized by placental 11-hydroxygenase before it reaches the fetal circulation. Thus, the fetus is exposed to only 10% of the maternal dose. In contrast, fluorinated glucocorticoids such as betamethasone and dexamethasone are not metabolized by placental 11-hydroxygenase. Much larger doses of those medications reach the fetal circulation. (This is why betamethasone or dexamethasone is administered to foster lung maturity in fetuses at risk for preterm delivery and to fetuses that appear to have early congenital heart block.) Short-acting preparations, including hydrocortisone, prednisone, prednisolone, and methylprednisolone are recommended for maternal disease indications.

All glucocorticoid preparations, regardless of their fluorination state, have the potential for causing the maternal complications of hypertension, osteopenia, osteonecrosis, diabetes, increased susceptibility to infection, cataracts, weight gain, acne, and proximal muscle weakness in both the nonpregnant and pregnant state. The lowest dose needed to treat either maternal or fetal indications is recommended (Ramsey-Goldman and Schilling 1996; Lin et al. 2007).

Pearl: Men may have an even higher risk of infertility following cyclophosphamide therapy than do women.

Comment: Most of the data on fertility risk in men exposed to cyclophosphamide comes from the oncology literature, where it is emphasized that just one exposure can compromise fertility, even in younger men. This contrasts with the data on women exposed to cyclophosphamide, whose older age and cumulative dose are important risk factors for premature menopause.

One study of male patients with SLE indicated that the testes are highly susceptible to the toxic effects of cyclophosphamide (Soares et al. 2007). Persistent damage from this drug is reflected in the primordial sperm cells, leading to significant sperm alterations. Abnormal testicular function, noted even 5 years after drug exposure, was associated with elevated FSH levels and lower testicular volumes (Soares et al. 2007).

Thus, the story with regard to cyclophosphamide and infertility may be at least as glum for men as it is for women. Sperm cyroprecipitation should be discussed early in the disease course, especially if the use of cyclophosphamide is anticipated. It is usually wise for a male patient to bank at least six samples, because a higher number of samples available provides greater options for conception. Samples can be collected every other day.

Myth: All fetuses exposed to methotrexate or leflunomide will be born with birth defects.

Reality: The congenital anomalies described in animals and humans exposed to methotrexate in utero during the first trimester usually involve the central nervous system, skeletal system, and palate (Wilson et al. 1979; Milunsky et al. 1968). Intrauterine growth restriction has also been observed. Methotrexate is used as an abortifacient for women with tubal pregnancies. When used for this purpose, the methotrexate dose is approximately three times higher than that used normally to treat arthritis. A recent study of 38 pregnancies exposed to methotrexate reported 21 live births (55%), eight elective abortions (21%), seven spontaneous abortions (18%), and three babies with congenital anomalies (14% of live births) (Chakravarty et al. 2003).

Leflunomide causes skeletal and central nervous system malformations in rats and rabbits exposed in utero to this drug. Premature birth, blindness, and cerebral palsy were reported in one human child exposed to leflunomide during the first 16 weeks of pregnancy (Neville and McNally 2007). However, preliminary results from a study of 63 pregnancies exposed to leflunomide during the first trimester showed no increased risk of miscarriage or malformation (Østensen et al. 2008).

Based on the data currently available, we do not recommend routine pregnancy termination for fetuses exposed to methotrexate or leflunomide. Instead, careful obstetrical care and evaluation should be implemented to identify abnormalities as early as possible.

Pearl: Leflunomide must be discontinued long in advance of any planned pregnancy.

Comment: The active metabolite of leflunomide is detectable in plasma up to 3 years after discontinuation of the drug. Thus, cholestyramine or active charcoal should be given to enhance elimination from the body when conception is desired. Conception should only be attempted after the plasma level is undetectable (Østensen et al. 2006, 2008).

Pearl: Mycophenolate mofetil (MMF) and azathioprine are used in comparable clinical scenarios, but considerations in the pregnant patient differ substantially for these two medications.

Comment: Both MMF and azathioprine are categorized as class D medications by the U.S. Food and Drug Administration, indicative of positive evidence of risk to a human fetus (FDA 2007). However, the practical implications for use in pregnant patients are quite different. MMF is associated with an increased risk of spontaneous abortion and congenital malformations (FDA 2007). The reported malformations include bilateral microtia or anotia (malrotation of the ears), abnormalities of the external auditory canals, oral clefts, anomalies of the limbs, heart, esophagus, and kidney (Østensen et al. 2008). Data from the U.S. National Transplantation Pregnancy Registry indicated that among 33 MMF-exposed pregnancies in 24 transplant patients, 15 (45%) resulted in spontaneous abortions. In addition, 4 of the 18 live born infants (22%) had congenital malformations.

Azathioprine is also a category D drug in pregnancy. However, this medication is used routinely in pregnant women who have received organ transplants as well as in those with immune-mediated conditions such as inflammatory bowel disease and SLE who need the drug to control their underlying disease. No recurrent patterns of malformations have been identified among infants exposed to azathioprine, despite isolated reports of malformations, intrauterine growth restriction, and transient chromosomal anomalies in clinically normal infants, severe immune deficiency, cytomegalovirus infections, temporary neonatal lymphopenia, and depressed hematopoesis (Østensen et al. 2006).

The upshot: even though azathioprine bears a category D label, this medication is recommended when indicated for control of inflammatory disease in the mother. Azathioprine should be used in place of MMF during pregnancy.

Pearl: Stopping hydroxychloroquine before or after conception leads to an increased risk of a lupus flare during pregnancy.

Comment: Early reports of in utero chloroquine toxicity led to reluctance to use this medication during pregnancy (Paufique and Magnard 1969). However, these concerns have been diminished by more recent reports on pregnancies in mothers with connective tissue disorders who were exposed to daily hydroxychloroquine or chloroquine during the first trimester (Levy et al. 1991; Parke and West 1996; Costedoat-Chalumeau et al. 2003; Clowse et al. 2006b). No increases in congenital malformations or cardiac conduction disturbances were detected in these studies. A consensus workshop concluded that antimalarials are recommended to manage disease activity in SLE during pregnancy and its use did not increase the risk of fetal malformations (Østensen et al. 2006). Women who continue hydroxychloroquine require lower doses of prednisone during pregnancy when compared to women who do not take this medication (Clowse et al. 2006b).

Myth: Biologic agents are generally regarded as safe during pregnancy.

Reality: Experience with TNF-inhibitors (infliximab, etanercept, adalimumab) and other biologic agents, remains too limited to claim safety during pregnancy. There are also insufficient data to infer anything about the potential effects of these medications on spermatogenesis. Experts recommend stopping rituximab prior to pregnancy (Østensen et al. 2008).

Pearl: Breastfeeding does not increase the risk of developing a rheumatologic illness.

Comment: If there is a relationship between breastfeeding and the rheumatic diseases, it may be a protective one. In four cohort studies, breastfeeding for 13–24 months appeared to reduce the likelihood that the mother would develop RA by approximately 50% (Brun 1995; Merlino et al. 2003; Karlson et al. 2004; Pikwer et al. 2008). Two cohort studies that utilized data from the Nurses' Health Study found no increase in the risk of incident SLE among mothers who breastfed their infants (Costenbader et al. 2007; Simaard et al. 2008).

Pearl: Ibuprofen is the NSAID of choice for women who are breastfeeding.

Comment: NSAIDs, prednisone, antimalarial agents, and sulfasalazine can be used safely by lactating mothers. Ibuprofen is the NSAID of choice for women who breastfeed because of its extremely low levels in breast milk and its short half-life. In addition, the therapeutic dose for an infant is significantly higher than that found in breast milk.

Peak levels of prednisone in breast milk are found about 2 h after the mother takes a dose, but levels decline rapidly thereafter. Breastfeeding women may attempt to time their feedings accordingly. Several studies have confirmed the absence of adverse effects in infants exposed to prednisone through breast milk.

Drug levels of hydroxychloroquine also peak in the breast milk 2 h after a dose and decline over the next 9 h. In a study of 19 children treated with daily exposure to hydroxychloroquine through breast milk for periods of up to 30 months, no retinal, motor, or growth abnormalities were observed during a 12-month follow-up period.

Sulfasalazine is compatible with breastfeeding in healthy, full-term infants, but caution is indicated in preterm infants or in babies with hyperbilirubinemia. Sulfasalazine metabolites may contribute to neonatal jaundice.

17.5 Systemic Lupus Erythematosus

Myth: Women with SLE should never get pregnant.

Reality: The majority of women with SLE have safe pregnancies and deliver healthy, full-term babies. Pregnancy involves assuming a significant risk of a disease flare, but most flares that occur can be managed effectively. Furthermore, some can be avoided through the timing of conception to coincide with a period of relative disease quiescence. We recommend that women avoid pregnancy for at least 6 months after an SLE flare.

Up to one-fourth of women with SLE have significant hypertension or preeclampsia (Clowse et al. 2008). These complications normally resolve following delivery. The incidence of end-stage renal disease following pregnancy is low, with only a few cases reported in the literature. Women at greatest risk for these complications are those with active SLE, particularly lupus nephritis, at the time of conception.

Some circumstances related to SLE do elevate pregnancy-associated risks to a level above that acceptable to most women. For example, women with a history of stroke secondary to the antiphospholipid syndrome are at high risk for a recurrent stroke or other arterial thrombosis during pregnancy. Women whose disease has recently required cyclophosphamide or MMF for SLE control may not tolerate 9 months without these drugs. Women with a prior myocardial infarction, significant pulmonary hypertension, or interstitial lung disease may not tolerate the added cardiopulmonary strain of pregnancy poorly. These patients usually are served best by physicians who discourage them from considering pregnancy.

Pearl: Oral contraceptives are not inappropriate for all women with SLE.

Comment: For most SLE patients, the avoidance of oral contraceptives that contain estrogen appears prudent. However, the dogma that oral contraceptives are contraindicated in all patients with SLE was challenged by the SELENA study, which showed that oral contraceptives do not increase the rate of SLE flares in women with mild SLE (Petri et al. 2005). The SELENA study did not include women with moderate to severely active SLE, so no statements about the appropriateness of oral contraceptive use in that setting are possible. For patients known to have risk factors for hypercoagulability, the avoidance of estrogen-containing contraceptives is prudent.

Reliable alternatives to estrogen-based contraceptives are available to women with SLE. Progestin-only contraceptives, either in the form of an injection every 3 months or progesterone-only pills that are taken daily, do not increase SLE activity or the risk for thrombosis. The depot form is particularly effective in preventing pregnancy. An intrauterine device, also an excellent long-term contraceptive option, is not contraindicated in women with rheumatologic disease.

In the event that a woman has unprotected intercourse, the over-the-counter emergency contraceptive pill ("Plan B") contains only progestin. Thus, it is safe for women with SLE.

Table 17.1 Clinical features helpful in distinguishing a lupus flare from preeclampsia

Flare of systemic lupus erythematosus	Preeclampsia/eclampsia
• Can develop at any time during the pregnancy	• Never develops before the 20th week of gestation
• Rash	• Pathologically brisk reflexes
• Arthritis	• Clonus
• Serositis	• Elevated serum levels of hepatic transaminases
• Increase in uric acid level less common than in preeclampsia/eclampsia	• Increased serum uric acid level
• Fever	• Decreased urine calcium concentration
• Active urine sediment	

Pearl: In some patients, it is impossible to distinguish preeclampsia from lupus nephritis.

Comment: Preeclampsia presents with hypertension (or a rising blood pressure when compared with the patient's pregnancy baseline) and new-onset proteinuria. Preeclampsia never occurs before 20 weeks of gestation and usually not before the third trimester. Thus, the timing of proteinuria onset helps distinguish preeclampsia from active SLE.

Unfortunately, in the third trimester, preeclampsia can mimic a lupus flare closely. Clinical features that help distinguish a lupus flare from preeclampsia are shown in Table 17.1. Several laboratory tests are helpful in identifying preeclampsia, including an elevated serum uric acid and a decreased urine calcium concentration (Meads et al. 2008). In some situations, treatment for both conditions may be required: delivery for the preeclampsia and immunosuppression for the lupus.

Pearl: Lupus can complicate a pregnancy, even if the disease remains quiescent during the pregnancy itself.

Comment: Quiet lupus promotes a healthy pregnancy. However, the lingering effects of previously active SLE (i.e., damage) can still impact a pregnancy's outcome, even if no flare occurs during gestation. Up to 30% of pregnancies in women who's SLE remains quiescent are delivered preterm. Damage to the kidney incurred before pregnancy promotes hypertension and preeclampsia. In addition, the elevated thrombotic risk shared by many patients with SLE is enhanced several times over by pregnancy. Many SLE experts prescribe low-dose aspirin throughout pregnancy in the hope of obviating thrombotic complications (Duley et al. 2007).

Myth: Normal complement levels during pregnancy make the likelihood of a disease flare low.

Reality: Complement levels increase between 10 and 50% during normal pregnancies. Thus, complement level measurements during lupus pregnancies are unpredictable and have poor prognostic value for either SLE flares or pregnancy outcomes. In the Johns Hopkins Lupus Cohort, 50% of women had a low level of complement at some point during pregnancy. Those with low complement had a slightly higher risk of preterm birth. Complement levels were most helpful when evaluating clinically evident lupus activity: women with moderately active lupus and low complement had far worse pregnancy outcomes than women with similarly active lupus but normal complement (Clowse et al. 2004).

Although the trend of the complement levels is more helpful than any single measurement, complement levels seldom provide definitive direction for clinical decision-making lupus pregnancies. Information about serial complement measurements must be correlated with the clinical picture. There remains a large margin for good clinical judgment.

Pearl: Thrombocytopenia during pregnancy is not always due to active lupus.

Comment: Up to 8% of healthy women develop moderate thrombocytopenia during pregnancy, with platelet counts in the 80–120,000/mm^3 range. This moderate drop in platelets is not pathologic and recovers following delivery. Thrombocytopenia may also be a sign of the HELLP syndrome (Hemolysis, Elevated Liver tests, and Low Platelets), a severe form of preeclampsia that is typically seen in the third trimester.

Myth: Pregnancy is contraindicated in patients with renal allografts.

Reality: More than 14,000 pregnancies in women with renal allografts have been documented over the past 50 years. The majority of these pregnancies resulted in a live baby and a functional renal transplant in the mother. An estimated 75% of such pregnancies result in live births, half of which are preterm (Armenti et al. 2004). Fewer than 5% of women experience an episode of allograft rejection during pregnancy.

On the other hand, approximately 10% of patients lose kidney function within 2 years of delivery, a rate that is higher than expected (Armenti et al. 2004). Thus, pregnancy does pose some risk the health of renal allografts. It is generally recommended that women wait at least 1 year after undergoing renal transplantation before attempting to conceive and that the patient's blood pressure and allograft function be stable before conception (McKay et al. 2005). Vaginal deliveries are possible in half of patients with renal allografts, despite the pelvic location of the transplanted kidney (Armenti et al. 2004a).

Myth: The great majority of women with lupus suffer disease flares during or after pregnancy.

Reality: The estrogen-driven theory of SLE does not extend to many women in pregnancy. Estrogen levels in the third trimester increase to levels 100-fold higher than prepregnancy levels, yet the majority of women remain relatively symptom-free. More than 85% of women whose SLE was quiescent during the 6 months prior to conception have no more than mild SLE activity during pregnancy (Clowse et al. 2005).

The majority of SLE flares in pregnancy involve the skin and joints. These flares can occur at any time during pregnancy or in the months following delivery. Flares during pregnancy are best prevented by continuing SLE medications, particularly hydroxychloroquine, during the gestational period (Clowse et al. 2006b).

17.6 Antiphospholipid Syndrome (APS)

Pearl: Pregnancy losses occur despite low-molecular weight heparin and aspirin treatment in 25% of women with the APS.

Comment: This is true. Although a 25% loss rate is far from optimal, it is better than the estimated 90% loss rate without any treatment and 40% loss rate with aspirin alone (Empson et al. 2005). For a woman who suffers a pregnancy loss despite treatment, a standard approach is to attempt pregnancy again with low molecular-weight heparin and aspirin. For patients with repeat pregnancy losses, intravenous immune globulin is endorsed by some reproductive immunologists. However, evidence-based support for this approach is lacking.

Pearl: Heparin and aspirin should be continued for 6 weeks after delivery in women with the APS.

Comment: Mothers are at increased risk for thrombosis during and immediately after pregnancy. Low-molecular weight heparin and aspirin should be continued for 6 weeks following delivery to prevent venous thrombotic events during this period of relative immobility (Empson et al. 2005).

17.7 Neonatal Lupus Syndromes

Myth: Congenital heart block in neonatal lupus always leads to fetal demise.

Reality: Neonatal lupus is an example of acquired autoimmunity. This syndrome is caused by the passage across the placenta of maternal autoantibodies following the 16th week of gestation (Izmirly et al. 2007). Organ involvement in this disorder includes cardiac, cutaneous, hepatic, hematologic, and other manifestations. Organ involvement in neonatal lupus is associated with antibodies in both the maternal and fetal serum directed against the Ro or La antigens (or, in a minority of cases, against RNP).

Most of the organ manifestations of neonatal lupus are self-limited and benign. However, congenital heart block can result in significant morbidity and even fetal death. Approximately 50% of newborns with complete heart block require cardiac pacing early in life. Such babies require lifelong cardiac pacing. One-year mortality among infants with congenital heart block ranges from 12 to 41%. Most deaths occur in utero or within the first 3 months of life. The risk of death continues through age 4, with mortality figures on the order of 3–4% after the first year of life (Gordon 2007).

In rare cases, death attributed to congenital heart block has occurred in adulthood (Moak et al. 2001). The main cause of early and late death in those affected with congenital heart block is cardiac failure due to dilated cardiomyopathy. Predictors of early mortality include a fetal heart rate less than 55/min, delivery before 34 weeks of gestation, and hydrops fetalis.

Pearl: Many mothers who deliver babies with neonatal lupus have no established connective tissue disorder at the time of their child's birth.

Comment: Most mothers who give birth to a baby with the neonatal lupus syndrome have a connective tissue disorder but do not know it. Up to 66% of mothers who deliver a baby with neonatal lupus have no recognized symptoms of a connective tissue disorder at the birth of the affected child. SLE, Sjögren's syndrome, and undifferentiated connective tissue disorders can all be associated with the birth of babies with neonatal lupus.

In a study of 229 mothers of babies with neonatal lupus who were followed for a mean of 6 years, approximately half of the mothers who were initialy asymptomatic developed some symptoms of a rheumatic disorder (Gordon 2007; Izmirly 2007). However, progression to a recognized connective tissue disorder occurred in less than 15% of patients. The underlying diagnoses in 321 mothers of babies with the neonatal lupus syndrome are shown in Table 17.2.

Table 17.2 Diagnoses of connective tissue disease in 321 mothers of babies with the neonatal lupus syndrome (Adapted from Izmirly et al. 2007)

23% asymptomatic (no connective tissue disorder diagnosis)
24% undifferentiated connective tissue disorder
15% systemic lupus erythematosus
22% had Sjögren's syndrome
17% systemic lupus erythematosus with secondary Sjögren's syndrome

Myth: Babies with the neonatal lupus syndrome are at high risk of developing rheumatic disorders as adults.

Reality: Limited data are available on the long-term outcomes of infants with the neonatal lupus syndrome. One study investigated 55 mothers of babies with neonatal lupus, including 49 affected babies and 45 unaffected siblings (Martin et al. 2002). Six children (12%) who had had neonatal lupus as babies developed definite autoimmune conditions between the ages of 2 and 13. Their diagnoses included juvenile rheumatoid arthritis (n = 2), Hashimoto's thyroiditis (1), psoriasis and iritis (1), diabetes mellitus and psoriasis (1), and congenital hypothyroidism and nephrotic syndrome (1). None of the unaffected siblings developed rheumatologic disease. These data suggest that most children's risk of autoimmune disease expression disappears along with the maternally derived autoantibodies at approximately 6 months of life. During adolescence and young adulthood, neither individuals with neonatal lupus nor their unaffected siblings appear to have increased risks of developing autoimmune conditions (Martin et al. 2002).

17.8 Rheumatoid Arthritis

Pearl: Women with rheumatoid arthritis generally improve during pregnancy but flare in the postpartum phase.

Comment: Up to 75% of women with RA have significant improvement in their arthritis during pregnancy. Some women enjoy complete remissions during this time. The improvement is more modest in others, but still sufficient to permit a decrease in RA medications during pregnancy.

Approximately 20% of women with RA actually experience a worsening of their inflammatory arthritis during pregnancy (Barrett and Brennan 1999). Moreover, within 1 month of delivery, 66% of women note exacerbations of their RA. Within 6 months, 77% of patients have flared.

Myth: If a pregnant woman has swollen joints, it means that her rheumatoid arthritis is getting worse.

Reality: This is a pretty good rule if the joint swelling is accompanied by pain. However, pregnant women often develop swollen joints independent of rheumatoid arthritis. This is sometimes secondary to the generalized swelling caused by changes in sodium excretion from the kidney in the third trimester. In these cases, the swelling includes the soft tissues of the hands and feet as well as the joints. Some women also develop bland knee effusions during pregnancy.

17.9 Scleroderma

1. Women with scleroderma should never get pregnant.

In the older literature, patients with scleroderma were thought to be at high risk for poor fetal and maternal outcome. However, in several more recent retrospective case-control studies, fewer adverse pregnancy outcomes were observed. Careful planning, close monitoring and appropriate therapy allows many of these patients to have a successful pregnancy. Retrospective case-control studies clearly show an increased frequency of pre-term births and small full-term infants but the frequency of miscarriage and neonatal survival rate did not differ from healthy controls. (Steen, Conte et al. 1989; Miniati, Guiducci et al. 2008)

Women with scleroderma usually do not have a worsening of their disease during pregnancy provided that the disease is stable at conception. However, new onset scleroderma has been reported during pregnancy and postpartum. The later stages of pregnancy are associated with an increase in cardiac output, and, as a consequence symptoms related to Raynauds phenomenon improve or even abate completely. Skin changes may improve during pregnancy and may then worsen postpartum. Gastroesophageal reflux and dyspnea are common in both healthy pregnant women and those women with scleroderma. The development of hypertension during pregnancy in a woman with scleroderma must be evaluated for pre-eclampsia, hemolytic anemia, elevated liver enzymes and low platelets (HELLP) syndrome, and scleroderma renal crisis. Daily increases in serum creatinine and the absence of proteinuria characterize scleroderma renal crisis from pre-eclampsia or HELLP. Recurrent renal crisis is more likely to occur within 5 years of the initial event, therefore women are advised to wait 3-5 years after an episode of renal crisis before considering a pregnancy. (Steen 1999)

Since ACE inhibitors are life saving in scleroderma renal crisis, they may need to be continued during pregnancy despite their teratogenic potential in the first trimester and renal effects in the third trimester if nifedipine or other calcium channel blockers fail to control blood pressure. (Barr 1994; Cooper, Hernandez-Diaz et al. 2006) Appropriate counseling is necessary to discuss the disease course and medications in women with scleroderma.

2. Pulmonary hypertension is an absolute contraindication to pregnancy.

One of the most lethal complications of scleroderma is pulmonary hypertension. The prevalence of pulmonary hypertension in scleroderma is estimated to occur in 10-20% of individuals with this disorder. (Note to the editor: could refer to the scleroderma section for more details on this topic). Women with scleroderma or primary pulmonary hypertension (without systemic sclerosis) have significantly increased rates of maternal complications including hypertensive disorders, pre-eclampsia and longer hospital stays. (Chakravarty, Khanna et al. 2008) Even though there is a case report of a successful pregnancy in a woman with both systemic sclerosis and pulmonary hypertension, pregnancy in the setting of systemic sclerosis and pulmonary hypertension is not recommended. (Baethge and Wolf 1989) Furthermore, we would agree with the recommendation to perform an evaluate for pulmonary hypertension as part of the pre-conception counseling workup in women with scleroderma, and if it is detected, would recommend not conceiving due to the high mortality rate associated with this disease manifestation. (Gayed and Gordon 2007)

(Cooper, Hernandez-Diaz et al. 2006; Schwarz and Manzi 2008)

References

Armenti VT, Radomski JS, et al Report from the National Transplantation Pregnancy Registry (NTPR): outcomes of pregnancy after transplantation. Clin Transpl 2004;103–114

Baethge, B. A. and R. E. Wolf (1989). "Successful pregnancy with scleroderma renal disease and pulmonary hypertension in a patient using angiotensin converting enzyme inhibitors." Ann Rheum Dis 48(9): 776–8

Barr, M., Jr. (1994). "Teratogen update: angiotensin-converting enzyme inhibitors." Teratology 50(6): 399–409

Barrett JH, Brennan P, et al Does rheumatoid arthritis remit during pregnancy and relapse postpartum? Results from a nationwide study in the United Kingdom performed prospectively from late pregnancy. Arthritis Rheum 1999; 42:1219–1227

Brun JG, Nilssen S, Kvale G. Breast feeding, other reproductive factors and rheumatoid arthritis: A prospective study. Br J Rheumatol 1995; 34:542–546

Chakravarty EF, Sanchez-Yamamoto D, Bush TM. The use of disease modifying antirheumatic drugs in women with rheumatoid arthritis of childbearing age: A survey of practice patterns and pregnancy outcomes. J Rheumatol 2003; 30:241–246

Chakravarty, E. F., D. Khanna, et al (2008). "Pregnancy outcomes in systemic sclerosis, primary pulmonary hypertension, and sickle cell disease." Obstet Gynecol 111(4): 927–34

Cooper, W. O., S. Hernandez-Diaz, et al (2006). "Major congenital malformations after first-trimester exposure to ACE inhibitors." N Engl J Med 354(23): 2443–51

Clowse M. Lupus activity in pregnancy. Rheum Dis Clin N Amer 2007; 33:237–252

Clowse MEB, Witter F, et al Complement and anti-double stranded DNA antibodies predict pregnancy outcomes in lupus patients. Arthritis Rheum 2004; 50(suppl):S689

Clowse ME, Magder LS, et al The impact of increased lupus activity on obstetric outcomes. Arthritis Rheum 2005; 52:514–521

Clowse ME, Magder L, et al Hydroxychloroquine in lupus pregnancy. Arthritis Rheum 2006a; 54:3640–3647

Clowse ME, Magder LS, et al Early risk factors for pregnancy loss in lupus. Obstet Gynecol 2006b; 107(2 Pt 1):293–299

Clowse ME, Jamison M, et al A national study of the complications of lupus in pregnancy. Am J Obstet Gynecol 2008; 199:127.e1–e6

Costa M, Colia D. Treating infertility in autoimmune patients. Rheumatology (Oxford) 2008; 47(Suppl 3):38–41

Costedoat-Chalumeau N, Amoura Z, Duhaut P, et al Safety of dyroxychloroquine in pregnant patients with connective tissue diseases: A study of one hundred thirty-three cases compared with a control group. Arthritis Rheum 2003; 48:3207–3211

Costenbader KH, Feskanich D, Stampfer MJ, Karlson EW. Reproductive and menopausal factors and risk of systemic lupus erythematosus in women. Arthritis Rheum 2007; 56:1251–1262

Duley L, Henderson-Smart DJ, et al Antiplatelet agents for preventing pre-eclampsia and its complications. Cochrane Database Syst Rev 2007; (2):CD004659

Empson M, Lassere M, et al Prevention of recurrent miscarriage for women with antiphospholipid antibody or lupus anticoagulant. Cochrane Database Syst Rev 2005; (2):CD002859

FDA, 2007.www.fda.gov/cder/drug/InfoSheets/HCP/mychephelolate-HCP.htm

Gayed, M. and C. Gordon (2007). "Pregnancy and rheumatic diseases." Rheumatology (Oxford) 46(11): 1634–40

Gordon PA. Congenital heart block: Clinical features and therapeutic options. Lupus 2007; 16:642–646

Izmirly PM, Rivera TL, Buyon JP. Neonatal lupus syndromes. Rheum Dis Clin N Amer 2007; 33:267–285

Karlson EW, Mandl LA, Hankinson SE, Grodstein F. Do breast-feeding and other reproductive factors influence future risk of rheumatoid arthritis. Arthritis Rheum 2004; 50:3458–3467

Katz PP. Childbearing decisions and family size among women with rheumatoid arthritis. Arthritis Rheum 2006; 55:217–223

Kikuchi K, Shibahara H, et al Antinuclear antibody reduces the pregnancy rate in the first IVF-ET treatment cycle but not the cumulative pregnancy rate without specific medication. Am J Reprod Immunol 2003; 50:363–367

Levy M, Buskila D, Gladman DD, Urowitz MB, Koren G. Prengnancy outcome following first trimester exposure to chloroquine. Am J Perinatol 1991; 8:174–178

Lin P, Bonaminio P, Ramsey-Goldman R. Pregnancy & rheumatic diseases. In: Imboden J, Hellmann D, Stone J (eds) Current diagnosis & treatment. Rheumatology (2nd edn). New York, McGraw-Hill, 2007, pp. 146–159

Lockshin MD. Autoimmunity, infertility and assisted reproductive technologies. Lupus 2004; 13(9):669–672

Martin V, Lee LA, Askanase AD, Katholi M, Buyon JP. Long-term followup of children with neonatal lupus and their unaffected siblings. Arthritis Rheum 2002; 46:2377–2383

McKay DB, Josephson MA, et al Reproduction and transplantation: Report on the AST Consensus Conference on reproductive issues and transplantation. Am J Transplant 2005; 5:1592–1599

Meads CA, Cnossen, et al Methods of prediction and prevention of pre-eclampsia: Systematic reviews of accuracy and effectiveness literature with economic modelling. Health Technol Assess 2008; 12(6):iii–iv, 1–270

Merlino LA, Cerhan JR, Criswell LA, Mikuls TR, Saag KG. Estrogen and other female reproductive risk factors are not strongly associated with the development of rheumatoid arthritis in elderly women. Semin Arthritis Rheum 2003; 33:72–82

Milunsky A, Graef JW, Gaynor MF. Methotrexate-induced congenital malformations. Med J Aust 1968; 2:1076–1077

Miniati, I., S. Guiducci, et al (2008). "Pregnancy in systemic sclerosis." Rheumatology (Oxford) 47 Suppl 3: iii16–8

Moak JP, Barron KS, Hougen TJ, et al Congenital heart block: Development of late-onset cardiomyopathy, a previously underappreciated sequela. J Am Coll Cardiol 2001; 37:238–242

Neville CE, McNally J. Maternal exposure to leflunomide associated with blindness and cerebral palsy (letter). Rheumatol 2007; 46:1506

Østensen M, Khmashta M, Lockshin M, et al. Anti-inflammatory and immunosuppressive drugs in reproduction. Arthritis Res Ther 2006; 8:1–19

Østensen M, Lockshin M, Doria A, et al Update on safety during pregnancy of biological agents and some immunosuppressive antirheumatic drugs. Rheumatol 2008; 47:iii28–iii31

Parke AL, West B. Hydroxychloroquine in pregnant patients with systemic lupus erythematosus. J Rheumatol 1996; 23:1715–1718

Paufique L, Magnard P. Retinal degeneration in 2 children following preventive anitmalarail treatment of the mother during pregnancy. Bull Soc Ophtalmol Fr 1969; 69:466–467

Petri M, Allbritton J. Fetal outcome of lupus pregnancy: A retrospective case-control study of the Hopkins Lupus Cohort. J Rheumatol 1993; 20:650–656

Petri M, Kim MY, et al Combined oral contraceptives in women with systemic lupus erythematosus. N Engl J Med 2005; 353(24): 2550–2558

Pikwer M, Bergströom U, Nilsson J-Å, Jacobsson L, Berglund G, Turesson C. Breast feeding, but not use of oral contraceptives, is associated with a reduced risk of rheumatoid arthritis. Ann Rheum Dis online May 14, 2008 as 10.1136/aard.2007.084707

Ramsey-Goldman R, Schilling E. Optimum use of disease-modifying and immunosuppressive antirheumatic agents during pregnancy and lactation. Clin Immunother 1996; 5:40–58

Ramsey-Goldman R, Mientus JM, Kutzer JE, Mulvihill JJ, Medsger TA Jr. Pregnancy outcome in women with systemic lupus erythematosus (SLE) treated with immunosuppressive drugs (ISD). J Rheumatol 1993; 20:1152–1157

Raptopoulou A, Sidiropoulos P, Boumpas D. Ovarian failure and strategies for fertility preservation in patients with systemic lupus erythematosus. Lupus 2004; 13(12):887–890

Schwarz, E. B. and S. Manzi (2008). "Risk of unintended pregnancy among women with systemic lupus erythematosus." Arthritis Rheum 59(6): 863–6

Simaard JF, Karlson EW, Costenbader KH, Hernán MA, Stampfer MJ, Liang MH, Mittlemen MA. Perinatal factors and adult-onset lupus. Arthritis Rheum (Arthritis Care Res) 2008; 59: 1155–1161

Soares PMF, Borba EF, Bonfa E, Hallak J, Corrêa AL, Silva CAA. Gondal evalution in male systemic lupus erythematosus. Arthritis Rheum 2007; 56:2352–2361

Somers EC, Marder W, Christman GM, et al Use of a gonadotropin-releasing hormone analog for protection against premature ovarian failure failure during cyclophosphamide therapy in women with severe lupus. Arthritis Rheum 2005; 52(9): 2761–2767

Steen, V. D. (1999). "Pregnancy in women with systemic sclerosis." Obstet Gynecol 94(1): 15–20

Steen, V. D., C. Conte, et al (1989). "Pregnancy in women with systemic sclerosis." Arthritis Rheum 32(2): 151–7

Taguchi N, Rubin ET, Hosokawa A, et al Prenatal exposure to HMG-CoA reductase inhibitors: Effects on fetal and neonatal outcomes. Reproductive Toxicology 2008 [Epub]

Wilson JG, Scott WJ, Ritter EJ, Fradkin R. Comparative distribution and embryo toxicity of methotrexate in pregnant rats and rhesus monkeys. Teratology 1979; 19:71–98

Inflammatory Myopathies

18

Ira N. Targoff, Chester V. Oddis, Paul H. Plotz, Frederick W. Miller, and Mark Gourley

18.1 Overview of the Inflammatory Myopathies

> The idiopathic inflammatory myopathies (IIM) are a heterogeneous group of disorders characterized by varied patterns of inflammation within striated muscle.

> The major disease categories among the IIM are dermatomyositis (DM), polymyositis (PM), inclusion body myositis (IBM), myositis associated with connective tissue diseases, and myositis associated with malignancy.

> The skin, joints, lungs, heart, and gastrointestinal tract are also involved in different forms of these disorders.

> Muscle weakness that is proximal, symmetrical, and painless is a hallmark feature of the inflammatory myopathies. Patients with IBM are also prone to distal, asymmetric muscle involvement.

> Measurement of serum concentrations of muscle enzymes, skin and muscle biopsy, electromyography, and magnetic resonance imaging can assist in the diagnosis.

> Testing for serum autoantibodies is helpful both in diagnosis and in predicting the clinical phenotype and response to therapy.

> A minority of patients with DM and PM have myositis that is associated with an underlying malignancy. The risk is greatest for middle-aged to elderly patients with DM. Approximately 15% of DM patients have malignancy-associated disease.

> Most malignancies present within 1 year before or after the diagnosis of inflammatory myopathy.

18.2 Dermatomyositis Versus Polymyositis

Myth: Dermatomyositis is polymyositis with a rash.

Reality: Although dermatomyositis (DM) and polymyositis (PM) share the term "myositis," these disease entities should not be considered the same for many reasons. Pathologic differences suggest that DM is a humorally mediated vasculopathy. In contrast, PM results from T cell-directed injury to the myocyte. Histologic examination of inflamed muscle in DM reveals more B cells, complement deposition, and CD4-positive T cells in perivascular regions. In contrast, PM is characterized by a predominantly CD8+ T cell infiltrate, with fewer B cells. Although the same autoantibodies can be found in DM and PM, some are associated with specific IIM subsets such as antisignal recognition particle (SRP) in PM and anti-Mi-2 in DM. Other differences include a substantially greater interferon-α/β-induced gene expression in DM when compared to PM.

Response to therapy also differentiates the myopathies. DM typically responds readily to glucocorticoids, but PM responds more slowly and often requires the addition of a second-line immunosuppressive agent.

18.3 Skin Disease

Pearl: Biopsy of any of the skin lesions in DM shows the same histology.

Comment: This is almost entirely correct! With the exception of the uncommon subcutaneous cystic lesions, biopsy of any skin lesion in DM will show focal epidermal atrophy, liquefaction, and degeneration of the basal cell layer

J. H. Stone (ed.), *A Clinician's Pearls and Myths in Rheumatology,*
DOI:10.1007/978-1-84800-934-9_18, © Springer Science + Business Media B.V. 2009

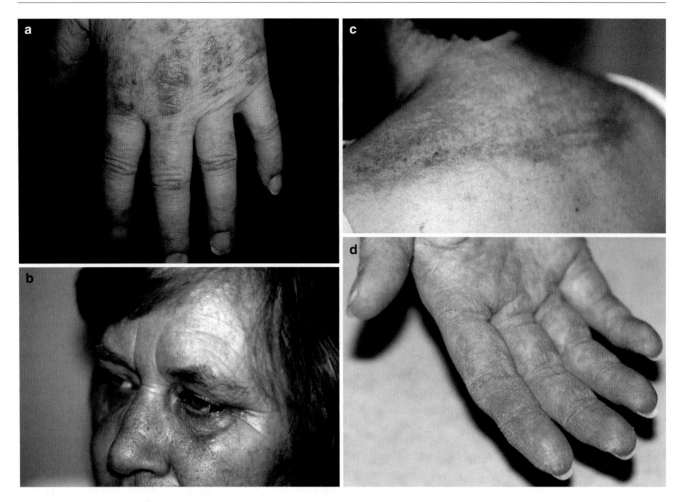

Fig. 18.1 Cutaneous findings of dermatomyositis. Skin biopsy of any of these lesions shows the same histopathologic features (see Fig. 18.2) (**a**) Gottron's papules (**b**) Heliotrope erythema (**c**) Shawl sign (**d**) Mechanic's hands (Figures Courtesy of Dr. John Stone)

and a perivascular or upper dermal mononuclear or lymphocytic infiltrate. Immunofluorescence studies confirm the presence of an interface dermatitis, with positive staining for immunoglobulin or complement at the dermal–epidermal junction. Biopsies of Gottron's papules (Fig. 18.1a), heliotrope erythema (Fig. 18.1b), the shawl sign (Fig. 18.1c), and mechanic's hands (Fig. 18.1d) all reveal the same histopathological features. The dermatopathology of these lesions is depicted in Fig. 18.2.

Myth: Patients must have muscle disease to make a diagnosis of DM.

Reality: The original Bohan and Peter criteria required that patients have muscle disease in order to receive a diagnosis of DM (Bohan and Peter 1975). However, the pathognomonic skin findings in patients with DM permit the diagnosis of "amyopathic" DM in the absence of muscle findings. The hallmark skin findings of DM include Gottron's papules and erythema over the extensor surfaces of joints, particularly the

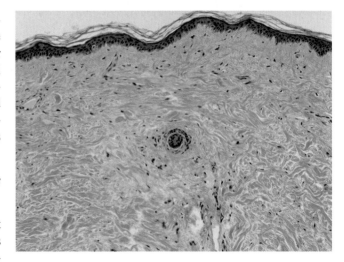

Fig. 18.2 Histopathology of the skin in dermatomyositis. A hematoxylin and eosin stain of a skin biopsy (× 100 magnification) reveals an atrophic epidermis, extensive dermal mucin deposition (pink-colored material), and only a mild dermal inflammatory infiltrate are seen (Figure courtesy of Dr. Mai Hoang, Massachusetts General Hospital)

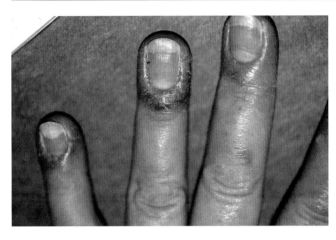

Fig. 18.3 Periungual erythema in a patient with dermatomyositis (Figure courtesy of Dr. John Stone)

metacarpophalangeal and interphalangeal joints, the elbow, the malleoli, and the knee along with a heliotrope rash. Other characteristic but not pathognomonic findings include periungual erythema (Fig. 18.3) or capillary changes, dystrophic cuticles, and a violaceous erythema found in a photodistribution.

Patients with amyopathic DM have undiminished muscle strength, no muscle pain, and normal muscle enzymes (Gerami et al. 2006). Approximately one-third of DM patients who present to dermatologists have amyopathic DM. Another third has minimal muscle symptoms, with only subclinical evidence of myositis on laboratory and electrophysiologic evaluation and radiographic imaging (Quain et al. 2007).

Myth: Patients with amyopathic DM do not have the same risk of lung disease as those with DM who have muscle inflammation as well as skin disease.

Reality: Patients with amyopathic DM can have interstitial lung disease in the absence of muscle inflammation. In fact, one study reported that 25% of patients with amyopathic DM had interstitial lung disease (Quain et al. 2007). As a result, patients with amyopathic DM must be screened with pulmonary function tests (PFTs) that include measurement of diffusion capacity. Further evaluation of the lungs is required if this screen detects any abnormalities. Annual PFTs are appropriate assessments in patients with DM and PM.

Some patients with interstitial lung disease have erythema and/or roughness of the palmar surface and sides of the fingers and palm, otherwise known as "mechanic's hands." This skin finding is associated with the antisynthetase syndrome (Quain et al. 2007).

Pearl: Patients with amyopathic DM should be screened for underlying malignancies.

Comment: Patients with DM have a higher risk of malignancy than do patients with PM (Buchbinder et al. 2001).

Patients with amyopathic DM are also at an increased risk for cancer and the frequency of malignancy is likely similar in both classic DM and amyopathic DM (Gerami et al. 2006); thus, patients should be screened accordingly (Callen 2001). The cancers that are particularly increased in DM include lung, ovary, pancreas, stomach, colon, and rectum, as well as non-Hodgkin's lymphoma (Hill et al. 2001).

18.4 Muscle Enzymes

Myth: All patients with active myositis have an elevated creatine kinase concentration.

Reality: Serum creatine kinase (CK) activity levels do not correlate perfectly with muscle inflammation or weakness in myositis as muscle inflammation and weakness can be present without CK elevation. This is most often seen in DM, in both the adult and juvenile subsets (see below). The mechanism by which this occurs is not understood completely. Some patients may have an inhibitor of enzyme function that leads to an underestimation of the CK activity (Kagen and Aram 1987). The serum CK activity level may correlate better with the degree of muscle inflammation early in the course of the disease as opposed to later when muscle atrophy is more likely.

In patients with a normal CK, one or more of the other muscle enzymes (e.g., aldolase, lactic dehydrogenase (LDH), aspartate aminotransferase (AST), alanine aminotransferase (ALT)), or another muscle factor (e.g., myoglobin) may be elevated. However, as discussed below, serum enzyme concentrations should not exclusively guide treatment.

Even if the serum CK activity level remains within the range of normal, changes in activity levels within this range may be significant as elevations of the CK above the patient's baseline activity level may be important. Magnetic resonance imaging of the muscle is helpful in the assessment of disease activity when muscle weakness is present in the absence of muscle enzyme elevations.

Pearl: Muscle inflammation in the setting of a normal serum CK activity level is more likely in DM than in PM.

Comment: Active myositis with a normal CK is more common in DM than in PM, but must be distinguished from amyopathic DM (in which there is no clinical or laboratory evidence of muscle involvement). Even if cases of amyopathic DM are excluded, serum CK activity levels correlate less well with the severity of muscle involvement in DM than they do in PM.

PM is unlikely in the setting of a normal CK and is more difficult to diagnose than DM when the CK is not elevated. In fact, "definite" PM cannot be diagnosed according to the

Bohan and Peter criteria without an elevation of serum muscle enzymes (Bohan and Peter 1975). Some reports indicate that normal CK activity levels in the setting of active myositis are likely to occur in patients with malignancy-associated myositis or inflammatory myopathy associated with a connective tissue disease, but reports of series of such patients are too small to permit definitive conclusions on this point.

Myth: The most important parameter in assessing disease activity in myositis patients is the concentration of muscle enzymes.

Reality: The main clinical manifestation of myositis is muscle weakness that translates into functional impairment and disability. Since the principal objective of treatment is the recovery and maintenance of normal strength through the suppression of muscle inflammation, the most important parameter to monitor is muscle strength, not serum enzyme concentrations.

This concept was incorporated into the consensus definition of improvement for myositis established by a panel of experts (Rider et al. 2004). Muscle strength is most often assessed by manual muscle testing, but function can be ascertained by other approaches, including patient questionnaires. The serum CK and other muscle enzymes are indirect measures of muscle inflammation and can be misleading so the notion that myositis treatment should focus on CK normalization is a Myth.

However, despite the shortcomings of serum muscle enzyme measurements as a biomarker of disease activity, these determinations still play a role in the assessment of most myositis patients. Indeed, CK activity levels correlate well with other measures of disease activity in many patients and an increase in the serum CK in an otherwise stable patient serves as a potential warning of a disease exacerbation, assuming there is no intercurrent process such as muscle injury, hypothyroidism, or medication use to explain the abnormality.

Myth: Serum concentrations of ALT do not rise during periods of active inflammatory muscle disease because this enzyme is specific to the liver, not skeletal muscle.

Reality: Elevations in the serum ALT concentration can occur in muscle injury as well as with liver damage. Although there is more aspartate aminotransferase (AST) than ALT in muscle, serum ALT can rise when injury to skeletal muscle is significant.

The fact that ALT elevation can occur in muscle disease complicates the clinician's ability to detect medication-induced liver toxicity. The failure of the AST and ALT concentrations to fall in conjunction with the CK activity level as muscle strength improves may unmask the presence of drug-induced hepatotoxicity.

Myth: An elevated CK-MB activity level is a sign of cardiac damage in patients with myositis.

Reality: The CK-MB activity level and its proportional activity level when compared to that of the total CK can increase in myositis even in the absence of detectable cardiac muscle inflammation or injury. This is usually attributed to an increased proportion of CK-MB production by myoblasts in regenerating muscle. Cardiac muscle inflammation does occur in myositis and is sometimes clinically significant, but the more frequent occurrence of CK-MB elevation from noncardiac sources in patients with myositis makes it difficult to use CK-MB as a sign of cardiac damage.

Serum troponin-T levels have also been proposed as specific markers of myocardial disease, but they too have been associated with myositis disease activity unrelated to cardiac involvement (unpublished observations and Erlacher et al. 2001). On the other hand, serum concentrations of cardiac troponin-I are usually normal in patients with PM or DM who do not have cardiac involvement (Erlacher et al. 2001). Consequently, elevations of cardiac troponin-I support an inflammatory process in the myocardium.

Myth: Aldolase is a muscle-specific enzyme.

Reality: Elevations of the serum CK are usually derived from muscle, particularly when the isotype is CK-MM. Skeletal muscle injury also results in the elevation of the serum aldolase activity, because skeletal muscle is rich in aldolase A. The CK activity level is generally a more sensitive and specific marker of muscle injury than is aldolase. The aldolase may be elevated in hemolytic states, with liver damage and in CNS disorders as aldolase B is found in the liver and other tissues. However, in some myositis patients, the serum CK may not correlate with disease activity and the serum aldolase is more useful in such unusual and rarely reported cases.

18.5 Myositis-Specific Autoantibodies

Myth: The "myositis-specific autoantibodies" are specific for myositis, as patients with one of these antibodies always have myositis.

Reality: The term "myositis-specific autoantibodies" (MSA) was first used to identify a group of autoantibodies that is associated primarily with myositis. MSAs have been distinguished from "myositis-associated autoantibodies" (MAAs), which may occur in myositis as well as other connective tissue diseases (CTD). The MSAs originally included the following:

- Antisynthetase antibodies (anti-Jo1 antibodies being the most common, but now also including at least seven other antibodies directed against aminoacyl-tRNA synthetases)
- Anti-SRP antibodies
- Anti-Mi-2 antibodies

These antibodies, when assessed by immunoprecipitation methods, generally have a specificity for myositis on the order of 90% or more, but previous studies have reported antisynthetase antibody-positive patients with ILD who do not have any clinical evidence of muscle inflammation (Friedman et al. 1996; Tillie-Leblond et al. 2008), or late onset myositis in the course of other CTDs (Tillie-Leblond et al. 2008; Schmidt et al. 2000). Anti-SRP autoantibodies may also not be as specific for myositis as originally reported (Kao et al. 2004), and although anti-Mi-2 autoantibodies are relatively specific for myositis by immunoprecipitation assays, antibodies to Mi-2 peptides may be seen in other conditions when measured by ELISA or immunoblotting (Hengstman et al. 2005).

The greatest utility of the MSAs occurs when the diagnosis is unclear, such as in the setting of possible myositis or another immunologic disorder where autoimmunity is presumed, such as in patients with ILD of unclear etiology (see below).

Pearl: Not all of the autoantibodies relevant to the IIMs have been identified.

Comment: The list grows longer every year. In addition to the antisynthetase, anti-SRP, and anti-Mi2 autoantibodies, several additional autoantibodies appear to have a primary association with PM or DM. These include the anti-hPMS-1 antibody, the anti-p155/140 antibody, an antibody against small ubiquitin-like modifier activating enzyme (anti-SAE antibody), the anti-caDM140 antibody, and others. The specificities of these autoantibodies have not been studied as extensively as those of traditional MSAs, but they appear to have diagnostic utility. These tests are not yet commercially available.

Myth: Patients with antisynthetase antibodies always have myositis.

Reality: The antisynthetase antibodies are more specific for an underlying connective tissue disease or an autoimmune syndrome rather than for myositis itself. For each of the antisynthetase antibodies, patients have been reported who have the antibody but do not have myositis. However, these patients have had other features of the antisynthetase syndrome such as interstitial lung disease or an inflammatory arthropathy. Antisynthetase antibody testing should be considered in patients whose interstitial lung disease may have an autoimmune basis, even in the absence of evidence of myositis (Tillie-Leblond et al. 2008). This is particularly true

if clinical features such as arthritis, Raynaud's phenomenon, mechanic's hands, or fevers are present.

Pearl: Patients with antisynthetase antibodies often present with features other than myositis but may develop myositis later.

Comment: Patients with antisynthetase antibodies do not always develop myositis, but in those who do, myositis may neither be the presenting or the symptom that brings the patient to medical attention (Schmidt et al. 2000). Such patients may present with interstitial lung disease, a syndrome that resembles rheumatoid arthritis, fever or even the rash of dermatomyositis.

Pearl: Certain antisynthetase antibodies are associated with a higher frequency of myositis than are others.

Comment: Although anti-Jo1 antibodies are detected in some patients with interstitial lung disease who do not have myositis (see above), this clinical picture is more common in patients with the non-Jo-1 antisynthetase autoantibodies. The frequency of myositis is lower in patients who are anti-PL-12 (anti-alanyl-tRNA synthetase), anti-OJ (anti-isoleucyl-tRNA synthetase), or anti-KS (anti-asparaginyl-tRNA synthetase) antibody positive (Targoff and Arnett 1990; Targoff et al. 1993; Sato et al. 2007; Hirakata et al. 2007). The frequency of myositis associated with particular antisynthetases may vary with the ethnic population under study (Hirakata et al. 2007).

Myth: Patients who have MSAs should be antinuclear antibody (ANA) positive if an indirect immunofluorescent assay is used.

Reality: Antisynthetases are directed at aminoacyl-tRNA synthetases, which are cytoplasmic in location. Thus, these autoantibodies usually cause cytoplasmic (not nuclear) patterns of fluorescence on indirect immunofluorescent ANA testing. Cytoplasmic staining may or may not be reported by commercial laboratories; thus, patients with myositis and antisynthetase antibodies are often ANA negative. In patients with antisynthetase antibodies who are ANA positive, coexistent autoantibodies may be present in the serum. Patients with anti-SRP autoantibodies also usually demonstrate cytoplasmic staining upon immunofluorescence testing for similar reasons as patients with an antisynthetases antibody.

Conversely, patients with anti-Mi-2 and anti-PM-Scl autoantibodies should have a positive ANA test. The anti-Mi-2 antibody yields a nuclear speckled pattern, and anti-PM-Scl antibodies cause a combined nuclear and nucleolar pattern. Anti-p155/140 antibodies usually cause a nuclear speckled pattern, but is less consistent and usually lower in titer.

Pearl: The finding of diffuse cytoplasmic immunofluorescence on ANA testing can be a clue to the presence of antisynthetase or anti-SRP autoantibodies.

Comment: In a patient who has clinical manifestations of an inflammatory myopathy, the finding of a cytoplasmic pattern by indirect immunofluorescence is an indication for obtaining a more thorough analysis for potential MSAs and MAAs. Antiribosomal P antibodies can also give this pattern.

Pearl: Many patients with myositis do not have a myositis-specific autoantibody (MSA).

Comment: Only about 30–40% of patients with DM or PM have antisynthetase, anti-SRP, or anti-Mi2 autoantibodies. By testing for more recently described antibody specificities (see Table 18.1), the frequency of autoantibody identification in these patients increases to greater than 50%. Although a percentage of myositis patients have MAAs, some patients with myositis have no currently identifiable autoantibodies (MSA or MAA) by either commercial or investigational testing.

One study that employed multiple assay techniques in a group of 100 patients detected MSAs or MAAs in 80% of the cohort (Koenig et al. 2007). Although numerous antibodies and combinations of antibodies were found, the study did not include detection of recently described antibodies known to be associated with myositis so the 80% figure may be somewhat low.

Myth: Mechanic's hands are specific for the antisynthetase syndrome.

Reality: Mechanic's hands, the cracking and/or fissuring of the lateral and palmar aspects of the fingers, are associated with the antisynthetase syndrome (see Fig. 18.1d). However, mechanic's hands can occur with other autoantibodies, e.g., anti-PM-Scl antibodies (Oddis et al. 1992).

Not all roughened hands are mechanic's hands. This finding must be distinguished from psoriasis, dyshydrotic eczema, and simple calluses.

Myth: All patients with anti-SRP antibodies have a severe myopathy and a disease course characterized by treatment refractoriness.

Reality: Most studies note that anti-SRP patients have more severe weakness than myositis patients without this antibody (Kao et al. 2004; Miller et al. 2002) and some have a rapidly progressive and relatively treatment-resistant course (Love et al. 1991). However, some anti-SRP antibody positive patients are more treatment-responsive and do well with glucocorticoids and other immunosuppressive agents (Hengstman et al. 2006; Kao et al. 2004).

Pearl: Patients with anti-SRP autoantibody frequently have less lymphocytic inflammation and relatively greater myofiber necrosis on their muscle biopsy.

Comment: The muscle biopsy in patients whose myositis is associated with antibodies to SRP often demonstrates a necrotizing myopathy with little or no inflammation (Dimitri et al. 2007; Hengstman et al. 2006; Kao et al. 2004; Miller et al. 2002). The lack of the classic inflammatory changes of myositis may lead to difficulty with diagnosis. The presence of a necrotizing myopathy and severe muscle weakness should suggest the diagnosis of SRP-associated PM, particularly in the presence of a cytoplasmic pattern on ANA testing (see above). Patients with anti-SRP antibodies rarely have the cutaneous findings of DM.

Pearl: Patients with antisynthetase or anti-PM-Scl autoantibodies can have a significant arthropathy.

Table 18.1 Myositis-specific autoantibodies

1. Antibodies to aminoacyl-tRNA synthetases ("anti-synthetase antibodies"):
• Anti-Jo1 antibodies, directed against histidyl-tRNA synthetase
Other antisynthetase antibodies are directed against other specific synthetases:
• The OJ, EJ, PL-7, PL-12, KS, and Zo antigens
– The antisynthetase antibodies are associated with interstitial lung disease, Raynaud's phenomenon, inflammatory arthritis, and mechanic's hands
2. Antibodies to signal recognition particle (anti-SRP antibodies)
• Associated with necrotizing myopathy and treatment-refractory disease
3. Antibodies to Mi-2
• Associated with dermatomyositis
4. Other:
• Antibodies to hPMS-1
• Antibodies to a 155-kiloDalton antigen
• Anti-Ku and anti-PM-Scl antibodies
– associated with overlapping features of polymyositis and scleroderma
• Anti-CADM-140 antibodies
– associated with amyopathic dermatomyositis
• Anti-155/140 antibody
– Distinct from the anti-155 and anti-CADM-140 antibodies. Associated with flagellate erythema and malignancies.

Comment: Arthritis is found in up to 90% of patients with the antisynthetase syndrome (Love et al. 1991) and is the presenting feature in some patients, leading to a diagnosis of rheumatoid arthritis before other features of the syndrome become evident (see above). The arthritis is not usually erosive, but it can be deforming (Oddis et al. 1990). Patients with anti-PM-Scl can also have arthritis as part of an overlap syndrome that may also demonstrate features of myositis (either PM or DM) and/or scleroderma.

Pearl: The myositis associated with anti-PM-Scl and anti-U1RNP tends to be milder and easier to treat than the myositis associated with antisynthetase and anti-SRP autoantibody subsets.

Comment: The myositis associated with anti-PM-Scl antibodies often occurs in overlap with scleroderma. These patients have milder and more responsive myositis than other autoantibody subsets (Jablonska and Blaszczyk 1999) and respond to lower doses of glucocorticoids than are usually used in myositis. Similarly, patients with myositis and the U1RNP autoantibody generally respond well to lower doses of glucocorticoids and have less long-term morbidity related to their myopathy when compared to the generally poor outcomes seen in myositis patients with antisynthetase and anti-SRP autoantibodies.

Pearl: The presence of anti-p155/140 antibodies and the absence of other MSAs or MAAs are associated with an increased risk of malignancy in adult DM.

Comment: Three studies have found an increased frequency of cancer in adult DM patients who have an autoantibody that immunoprecipitates 155 and 140 kD proteins (Chinoy et al. 2007; Kaji et al. 2007; Targoff et al. 2006). The group with cancer-associated myositis also has a low frequency of other MSAs and MAAs. When used together, these features are helpful in assessing the likelihood of cancer in patients with DM (Chinoy et al. 2007). Unfortunately, testing for this "doublet" is not commercially available and can only be done in research laboratories specializing in the testing of MSAs and MAAs.

18.6 Imaging

Pearl: Magnetic resonance imaging (MRI) findings may distinguish PM from IBM.

Comment: MRI of the thighs with T1 and short tau inversion recovery (STIR) sequences can be helpful in distinguishing PM from sporadic IBM (sIBM) (Fig. 18.4). PM is characterized by

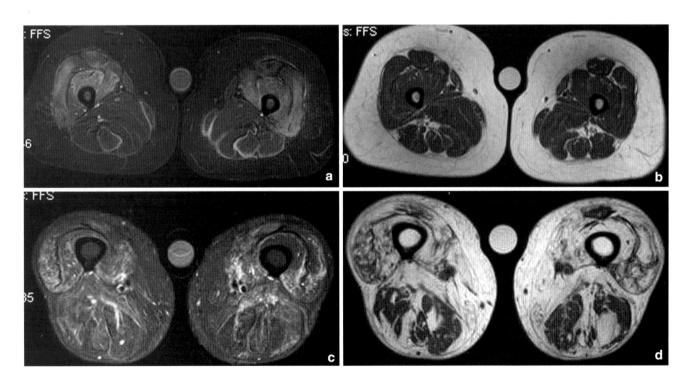

Fig. 18.4 Axial STIR and T1-weighted MRI images through the mid-section of the thighs of two patients – one with polymyositis (**a**) (top left and (**b**) *top right*), the other with inclusion body myositis (**c**) bottom left and (Fig. 18.4d bottom right). Note the widespread inflammation and atrophy in all musculature in inclusion body myositis, particularly intense in the anterior muscle group. Polymyositis tends to show inflammation and atrophy in a fascial distribution (Figure courtesy of Dr. Mark Gourley)

isolated inflammation that is symmetrical and generally favors the posterior muscle group. IBM is more likely to be asymmetric with fatty replacement and to involve muscles of the anterior thigh and more distal musculature (Dion et al. 2002).

18.7 Inclusion Body Myositis

Myth: The presence of rimmed vacuoles on muscle biopsy is diagnostic of IBM.

Reality: Although rimmed vacuoles are a characteristic pathological feature in IBM, they may also occur in other neuromuscular disorders, such as distal myopathies, oculopharyngeal myopathy, PM, rigid spine syndrome, congenital myopathies, limb girdle muscular dystrophies, and various neurogenic diseases. The patient's clinical features, the full pathologic picture, the response to therapy, and the overall disease course are all critical components in establishing the diagnosis of IBM. Similarly, the classic finding of rimmed vacuoles in the muscle biopsy of patients with IBM may require repeated biopsies over time.

Myth: Dysphagia is less common in patients with IBM than DM and PM.

Reality: When dysphagia is found in a patient with an inflammatory myopathy, IBM is the most likely diagnosis. In a study of 62 patients with IIM-associated dysphagia, 42% had IBM, 29% had DM, 15% had PM, and 15% had overlap syndromes (Oh et al. 2007). The dysphagia of IBM is reported by the patient as feeling like a "blocking sensation" with swallowing. It is often associated with the findings of cricopharyngeal spasm or achalasia on cinesophagram studies.

Pearl: The presence of a foot drop in a patient with "refractory PM" is IBM until proven otherwise.

Comment: Although distal weakness may occur in the IIMs, this is often in the setting of severe and/or chronic PM or DM. However, IBM is associated with both distal and asymmetric muscle weakness as well as muscle atrophy. The finding of a foot drop (which may be subtle), manifested by weakness of the ankle dorsiflexors should lead the clinician to consider IBM. This may be unilateral but may be bilateral and variable in severity between both lower extremities.

18.8 Treatment

Myth: Many cases of PM are refractory to immunosuppressive therapy.

Reality: This statement is true in cases associated with anti-SRP autoantibodies. However, many "steroid-refractory" PM cases are in fact mimickers of PM. Common mimickers of PM are IBM, muscular dystrophies, mitochondrial or metabolic myopathies, and drug-induced syndromes, the prime example of which is a statin myopathy.

Myth: Exercise is contraindicated in patients with inflammatory myopathy during the initial phase of treatment.

Reality: A supervised exercise program is a necessary prescription when treating patients with an inflammatory myopathy. The long-held belief that exercise harms patients who have active myositis has been disproved by studies demonstrating benefits in strength, improvements in quality of life, and the absence of muscle disease exacerbations when an appropriately structured exercise program is initiated (Alexanderson et al. 2007). The program should be supervised and instituted in a graded manner so as not to cause muscle pain or worsening weakness.

Pearl: Combination therapy with methotrexate and azathioprine may be effective in the treatment of refractory myositis when either agent alone is ineffective.

Comment: Although methotrexate or azathioprine in conjunction with glucocorticoids is often at least partially effective in the treatment of myositis, some patients are refractory to either methotrexate or azathioprine alone. The combination of oral methotrexate and azathioprine has evidence-based support for its use in refractory myositis, showing benefit in some patients who previously demonstrated an inadequate response to either methotrexate or azathioprine alone (Villalba et al. 1998). Clinicians should consider combination therapy in myositis in a fashion similar to that utilized in other connective tissue diseases.

Pearl: Clinical improvement in muscle weakness lags behind the response in the serum CK and an increase of the serum CK often predates a flare of myositis.

Comment: Although the serum CK should not be used as the only determinant of treatment in patients with myositis (see above), it can provide useful clues in the management of myositis. Many times patients will continue to complain of some degree of muscle weakness even though their CK has normalized. They should be reassured that the clinical response to therapy lags behind the biochemical response and that with continued glucocorticoid tapering (and the maintenance of other immunosuppressive therapy, as appropriate), their muscle strength will likely improve. Similarly, patients who are clinically stable but demonstrate a rising CK from the normal range to elevated values may be headed for a disease flare. Although the clinician would not want to simply increase immunosuppressive therapy in such instances, he/she should carefully monitor such patients for an impending disease flare.

Myth: The presence or absence of peripheral eosinophilia helps distinguish methotrexate lung from other causes of interstitial lung disease.

Reality: The initial cases reported of methotrexate lung described peripheral eosinophilia (Whitcomb et al. 1972). More comprehensive studies performed subsequently, however, reveal that eosinophilia is a nonspecific finding found in only about one-third of the cases of methotrexate lung.

References

Alexanderson H, Dastalmachi M, Esbjornsson-Liljedahl M, et al Benefits of intensive resistance training in patients with chronic polymyositis or dermatomyositis. Arthritis Care Res 2007; 57:768.

Bohan A, Peter JB. Polymyositis and dermatomyositis. Parts 1 and 2 N. Engl J Med 1975; 292:344–3447,403–407

Buchbinder R, Forbes A, Hall S, Dennett X, Giles G. Incidence of malignant disease in biopsy-proven inflammatory myopathy. A population-based cohort study. Ann Intern Med 2001; 134:1087–1095.

Callen JP. Relation between dermatomyositis and polymyositis and cancer. Lancet 2001; 357:85–86

Chinoy H, Fertig N, Oddis CV, et al The diagnostic utility of myositis autoantibody testing for predicting the risk of cancer-associated myositis. Ann Rheum Dis 2007; 66:1345–1349

Dimitri D, Andre C, Roucoules J, et al Myopathy associated with anti-signal recognition peptide antibodies: Alinical heterogeneity contrasts with stereotyped histopathology Muscle Nerve 2007; 35:389–395

Dion E, Cherin P, Payan C, et al Magnetic resonance imaging criteria for distinguishing between inclusion body myositis and polymyositis. J Rheumatol. 2002; 29:1897

Erlacher P, Lercher A, Falkensammer J, et al Cardiac troponin and beta-type myosin heavy chain concentrations in patients with polymyositis or dermatomyositis. Clin Chim Acta 2001; 306:27–33

Friedman AW, Targoff IN, Arnett FC. Interstitial lung disease with autoantibodies against aminoacyl- tRNA synthetases in the absence of clinically apparent myositis. Semin Arthritis Rheum 1996; 26:459–467

Gerami P, Schope JM, McDonald L, et al A systematic review of adult-onset clinically amyopathic dermatomyositis (dermatomyositis sine myositis): A missing link within the spectrum of the idiopathic inflammatory myopathies. J Am Acad Dermatol 2006; 54:597–613

Hengstman GJ, van Brenk L, Vree Egberts WT, et al High specificity of myositis specific autoantibodies for myositis compared with other neuromuscular disorders. J Neurol 2005; 252:534–537

Hengstman GJ, ter Laak HJ, Vree Egberts WT, et al Anti-signal recognition particle autoantibodies: Marker of a necrotising myopathy. Ann Rheum Dis 2006; 65:1635–1638

Hill CL, Zhang Y, Sigurgeirsson B, Pukkala E, Mellemkjaer L, Airio A, Evans SR, Felson DT. Frequency of specific cancer types in dermatomyositis and polymyositis: a population-based study. Lancet 2001; 357:96–100

Hirakata M, Suwa A, Takada T, et al Clinical and immunogenetic features of patients with autoantibodies to asparaginyl-transfer RNA synthetase. Arthritis Rheum 2007; 56:1295–1303

Jablonska S, Blaszczyk M. Scleroderma overlap syndromes. Adv Exp Med Biol 1999; 455:85–92

Kagen LJ, Aram S. Creatine kinase activity inhibitor in sera from patients with muscle disease. Arthritis Rheum 1987; 30: 213–217

Kaji K, Fujimoto M, Hasegawa M, et al Identification of a novel autoantibody reactive with 155 and 140kDa nuclear proteins in patients with dermatomyositis: An association with malignancy. Rheumatology 2007; 46:25–28

Kao AH, Lacomis D, Lucas M, et al Anti-signal recognition particle autoantibody in patients with and patients without idiopathic inflammatory myopathy. Arthritis Rheum 2004; 50:209–215

Koenig M, Fritzler MJ, Targoff IN, et al Heterogeneity of autoantibodies in 100 patients with autoimmune myositis: Insights into clinical features and outcomes. Arthritis Res Therapy 2007; 9:R78

Love LA, Leff RL, Fraser DD, et al A new approach to the classification of idiopathic inflammatory myopathy: Myositis-specific autoantibodies define useful homogeneous patient groups. Medicine 1991; 70:360–374

Miller T, Al Lozi MT, Lopate G, et al Myopathy with antibodies to the signal recognition particle: Clinical and pathological features. J Neurol Neurosurg Psychiatry 2002; 73:420–428

Oddis CV, Medsger TA Jr., Cooperstein LA. A subluxing arthropathy associated with the anti-Jo-1 antibody in polymyositis/dermatomyositis. Arthritis Rheum 1990; 33:1640–1645

Oddis CV, Okano Y, Rudert WA, et al Serum autoantibody to the nucleolar antigen PM-Scl: clinical and immunogenetic associations. Arthritis Rheum 1992; 35:1211–1217

Oh TH, Brumfield KA, Hoskin TL, et al Dysphagia in inflammatory myopathy: Clinical characteristics, treatment strategies, and outcome in 62 patients. Mayo Clin Proc 2007; 82:441–447

Quain RD, Teal V, Taylor L, et al Number, characteristics, & classification of dermatomyositis patients seen by dermatology & rheumatology at a tertiary medical center. J Am Acad Dermatol 2007; 57:937–943

Rider LG, Giannini EH, Brunner HI, et al International consensus on preliminary definitions of improvement in adult and juvenile myositis. Arthritis Rheum 2004; 50:2281–2290

Sato S, Kuwana M, Hirakata M. Clinical characteristics of Japanese patients with anti-OJ (anti-isoleucyl-tRNA synthetase) autoantibodies. Rheumatology 2007; 46:842–845

Schmidt WA, Wetzel W, Friedlander R, et al Clinical and serological aspects of patients with anti-Jo-1 antibodies–an evolving spectrum of disease manifestations. Clin Rheumatol 2000; 19:371–377

Targoff IN, Arnett FC. Clinical manifestations in patients with antibody to PL-12 antigen (alanyl-tRNA synthetase). Am J Med 1990; 88: 241–251

Targoff IN, Trieu EP, Miller FW. Reaction of anti-OJ autoantibodies with components of the multi-enzyme complex of aminoacyl-tRNA synthetases in addition to isoleucyl-tRNA synthetase. J Clin Invest 1993; 91:2556–2564

Targoff IN, Mamyrova G, Trieu EP, et al A novel autoantibody to a 155-kd protein is associated with dermatomyositis Arthritis Rheum 2006; 54:3682–3689

Tillie-Leblond I, Wislez M, Valeyre D, et al Interstitial lung disease and anti-Jo-1 antibodies: Difference between acute and gradual onset. Thorax 2008; 63:53–59

Villalba L, Hicks J, Adams E, et al Treatment of refractory myositis: A randomized crossover study of two new cytoxic regimens. Arthritis Rheum 1998; 41:392–399

Whitcomb ME, Schwarz MI, Tormey DC. Methotrexate pneumonitis: Case report and review of the literature. Thorax 1972; 27(5):636–639

Juvenile Dermatomyositis

19

Ann M. Reed, Clarissa A. Pilkington, Brian M. Feldman,
Lauren M. Pachman, and Lisa G. Rider

19.1 Overview of Juvenile Myositis

> Children with inflammatory myopathies have clinical
> and laboratory features, as well as risk factors and out-
> comes that overlap with their adult counterparts.
> However, a number of important differences exist
> between pediatric and adult disease.
> Juvenile dermatomyositis (JDM), the most common of
> this group of illnesses in children, has an incidence of
> approximately 3.2 cases/million children/year.
> JDM has a gender ratio of 2 girls:1 boy.
> JDM has a mean age of 6.7 years at disease onset.
> The duration of active disease before the time of diag-
> nosis alters the patients' features at presentation as
> well as their clinical outcomes.
> Environmental and genetic factors affect the child's
> susceptibility to these conditions and also alter the
> inflammatory response, adding heterogeneity to disease
> pathophysiology.

*Pearl: JDM is not just a muscle condition, but rather a sys-
temic disease.*

Comment: The pathological basis of JDM is systemic vasculopathy, which affects the smallest blood vessels. Consequently,
a variety of organ systems can be affected (Table 19.1).
Interstitial lung disease, dyspnea on exertion, dysphonia, dysphagia, vasculopathy (vasculitis) of the gastrointestinal tract,
and bowel dysmotility are relatively common in JDM.
Cerebral, ocular, and cardiac manifestations are rare in JDM,
but can be life threatening.

Myth: The diagnosis of JDM requires a muscle biopsy.

Reality: The classical criteria for inflammatory myopathies
(Bohan and Peter 1975 a,b) require the presence of characteristic rashes, including the heliotrope rash (Fig. 19.1) or

Gottron's papules (Fig. 19.2), for the classification of a
patient as having JDM. In addition, a patient must have at
least two of the following clinical or laboratory criteria:

- Symmetric, proximal muscle weakness
- Elevation of one or more "muscle" enzyme in the blood
  (CK, aldolase, alanine aminotransferase (ALT), AST, or
  LDH)
- Abnormal electromyogram, with polyphasic small motor
  unit potentials, high-frequency discharges, spontaneous
  fibrillations, positive sharp waves, or increased insertional
  irritability
- An abnormal muscle biopsy

In the absence of characteristic rashes, a diagnosis of juvenile polymyositis would require at least three of the clinical
or laboratory features.

Muscle biopsies are extremely helpful in supporting the
diagnosis of myositis, in confirming the specific type if the
clinical differentiation is unclear, and in excluding a number of
inflammatory myopathy mimickers (Table 19.2). Typical biopsy
findings in JDM include perifascicular atrophy, perivascular
inflammatory infiltrate, degenerating and regenerating myofi-
bers, and centralization of nuclei. However, many patients with
JDM fulfill three clinical and laboratory features, including the
presence of weakness, characteristic rashes, and elevation of
serum muscle enzyme levels. Therefore, a muscle biopsy is
not necessary in every case of JDM.

Fewer than 40% of the surveyed pediatric rheumatologists
in North America and Europe rely on a muscle biopsy for
diagnosis. Most rely upon magnetic resonance imaging (MRI)
findings (Fig. 19.3) to confirm the diagnosis (Brown et al.
2006). However, muscle histopathologic features provide
important prognostic information in many cases (Wedderburn
et al. 2007b; Miles et al. 2007; Lopez de Padilla et al. 2007).

A muscle biopsy should be performed in patients who do
not have a rash characteristic of JDM (i.e., heliotrope erythema or Gottron's papules). A muscle biopsy is also indicated if atypical features are present.

*Myth: Muscle weakness and inflammation in a child always
indicates a diagnosis of idiopathic juvenile myositis.*

Table 19.1 Clinical features typically seen in patients with juvenile dermatomyositis (From Feldman et al. 2008. Reprinted with permission from Elsevier)

Constitutional
- Fever: 16–65%
- Adenopathy: 20%
- Lethargy: 10%

Pulmonary
- Dyspnoea: 7–43%

Gastrointestinal
- Dysphonia or dysphagia: 18–44%
- Gastrointestinal symptoms: 22–37%

Musculoskeletal
- Weakness: 95%
- Myalgia or arthralgia: 25–73%
- Arthritis: 23–58%
- Contractures: 26–27%
- Raynaud's disease: 9–14%

Cutaneous
- Gottron's papules: 57–100%
- Heliotrope rash: 66–100%
- Nailfold capillary changes: 91%
- Malar or facial rash: 42–73%
- Mouth ulcers: 35%
- Skin ulcers: 23–30%
- Limb oedema: 11–32%
- Calcinosis: 6–30%
- Lipodystrophy: 10–14%

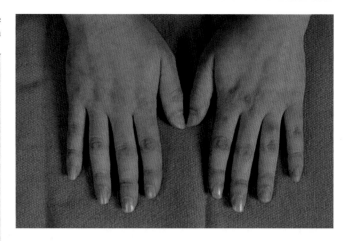

Fig. 19.2 Gottron's papules. Raised erythematous patches overlying the knuckles, which are characteristic lesions of dermatomyositis

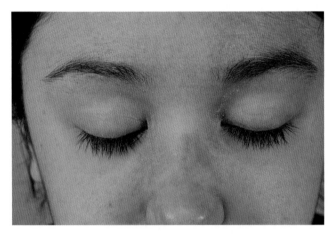

Fig. 19.1 Heliotrope discoloration of the eyelids and malar/facial erythema

Reality: Muscle weakness or fatigue may result from primary muscle tissue abnormalities or from factors that affect muscle tissue only indirectly. Chronic muscle inflammation may result from infection, medications, local trauma, or be idiopathic, as in juvenile dermatomyositis (JDM). However, many other myopathies other than juvenile myositis can lead to muscle weakness or fatigue, and some may have associated muscle inflammation (see Table 19.2).

Patients with myositis have certain clinical and laboratory clues, which suggest the diagnosis of myositis and distinguishing myositis from other causes of muscle dysfunction (Miller 2005). Patients with myositis often have features of systemic rheumatic diseases, including fever, photosensitive rashes, periungual capillary changes, and arthritis. Approximately 70% of children with myositis have a positive anti-nuclear antibody. They may also have a family history of other forms of autoimmune disease.

Patients with myositis have a characteristic pattern of weakness that is symmetric and involves primarily proximal and axial muscles. In other forms of muscle dysfunction in children, the weakness can involve both proximal and distal muscles; affect the facial, ocular, or scapular muscles; be asymmetric; or be worsened by fasting or exercise. The level of creatine kinase (CK) elevation can rise to several thousand units per liter (U/L) (a normal value is in the order of 250 U/L). However, a significant percentage of patients with JDM have normal CK levels. Finally, in contrast to patients with other pediatric muscle disorders, patients with myositis usually respond well to glucocorticoids and other immunosuppressive therapy.

Myth: The serum CK level is a good indicator of disease activity in childhood myositis.

Reality: The serum concentration of enzymes derived from muscle has been used traditionally as an indicator of JDM disease activity and to discriminate active disease (Guzman et al. 1994). However, serum levels of CK and other muscle-derived enzymes often correlate poorly with measures of muscle strength in JDM; CK concentrations may improve without a corresponding improvement in muscle strength. Serum CK levels sometimes return to normal even when the illness remains active (Rider 2002). The longer the delay in the diagnosis of JDM, the greater the likelihood that serum levels of CK and other muscle enzymes will be normal upon measurement (Pachman et al. 2006). The points apply equally

Table 19.2 Differential diagnosis of childhood idiopathic inflammatory myopathies. In many of these conditions, a diagnosis is facilitated by muscle biopsy; muscle biopsy should be strongly considered in the absence of typical rashes of juvenile dermatomyositis, including heliotrope or Gottron's papules. For further information, see http://www.neuro.wustl.edu/neuromuscular/index.html (From Feldman et al. 2008. Reprinted with permission from Elsevier)

Group	Condition
Weakness alone	
Muscular Dystrophies (MD)	Limb-girdle dystrophies
	Dystrophinopathies
	Fascioscapulohumeral dystrophy
	Other dystrophies
Metabolic myopathies	Muscle glycogenocses (glycogen storage diseases)
	Lipid storage disorders
	Mitochondrial myopathies
Endocrine myopathies	Hypothyroidism
	Hyperthyroidism
	Cushing syndrome/exogenous steroid myopathy
	Diabetes Mellitus
Drug-induced myopathy	Consider in patients taking any of the following drugs or biologic therapies: statins, interferon α, glucocorticoids, hydroxychloroquine, diuretics, amphotericin b, "caine" anesthetics, growth hormone, cimetidine, and vincristine.
Neuromuscular transmission disorders	Myasthenia gravis
Spinal muscular atrophy	
Infectious myopathy	
Viral	Enterovirus, influenza, coxsackievirus, echovirus, parvovirus, poliovirus, hepatitis B, HTLVI
Bacterial and parasitic organisms	Staphylococcus, streptococcus, toxoplasmosis, trichinosis, Lyme borreliosis
Other rheumatic conditions	Systemic lupus erythematosus (SLE), scleroderma, juvenile idiopathic arthritis, mixed connective tissue disease, idiopathic vasculitis
Other inflammatory conditions	Inflammatory bowel disease, celiac disease
Rash without weakness	Psoriasis, eczema, allergy

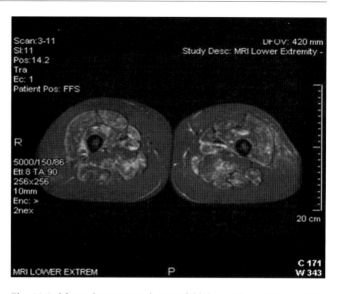

Fig. 19.3 Magnetic resonance image of thigh muscles, axial view. This short tau inversion recovery image demonstrates muscle edema, seen in active myositis

well to aldolase, lactate dehydrogenase (LDH), and aspartate aminotransferase (AST) as to CK.

Current data suggest that serum LDH may be the most clinically useful serum muscle-derived enzyme, as it best predicts the global disease activity in JDM patients with longstanding disease (Rider 2002). The combination of LDH in combination with AST may be best in predicting flares of JDM activity (Guzman et al. 1994).

Other proposed biomarkers in JDM are von Willebrand factor VIII-related antigen, flow cytometry of peripheral blood lymphocyte subsets, neopterin, and interferon

(IFN)-regulated proteins. However, abnormalities of a measure in isolation may not be accurate (Rider 2002; Baechler et al. 2007; Griffin and Reed 2007). MRI of the upper leg or shoulder muscles can be helpful. Short tau inversion recovery (STIR) or fat-suppressed images on T2-weighted sequences assess the degree of muscle edema or inflammation. T1-weighted images are useful in assessing the degree of muscle atrophy and fibrosis (see Fig. 19.3). However, the reliable application of these imaging techniques across medical centers is currently lacking.

Myth: The rash of JDM is relatively benign. Treatment strategies should be directed toward the underlying muscle disease.

Reality: Many different types of rashes occur in JDM. The heliotrope rash, marked by red or purple discoloration of the upper eyelids, often associated with edema, occurs in 80% of patients (see Fig. 19.1). Gottron's papules, raised erythematous patches that appear over the extensor surfaces of joints are each seen in about 80% of patients with JDM (see Fig. 19.2).

Cutaneous ulcerations, which are present in fewer than 10% of all JDM patients, portend a difficult illness course. The periungual nailfold capillaries typically demonstrate vessel dilation, avascularity, and morphologic changes (Fig. 19.4). These correlate with active skin disease. An erythematous appearance of the skin at either the sites of classic lesions (the eyelids, knuckles) or elsewhere (the face, shoulders, etcetera) often indicates active cutaneous disease. However, this must be distinguished from poikiloderma atrophicans, post-inflammatory dyspigmentation, and cutaneous atrophy, all of which are consistent with skin damage.

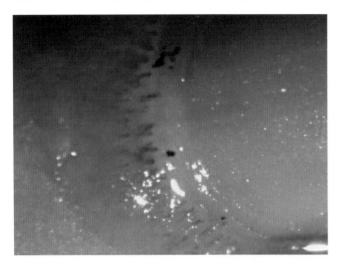

Fig. 19.4 Periungual nailfold capillary changes. Dilated periungual capillaries, with bushy loop formation, capillary dropout and subungual hemorrhage also evident, under magnification

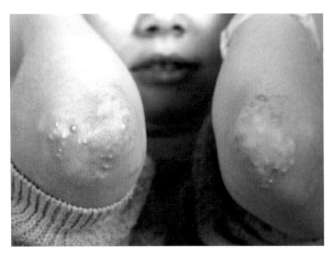

Fig. 19.5 Calcinosis. Small subcutaneous nodules extruding from the skin over the elbows in the region of overlying Gottron's papules

Active, severe rash even in a JDM patient who does not have muscle weakness is an indication for systemic treatment. Agents that may be effective are enteral or parenteral glucocorticoids, methotrexate, hydroxychloroquine, mycophenolate mofetil, intravenous immunoglobulin, and cyclosporine. These agents may be prescribed individually, but are often used in combination. Active rashes also frequently benefit from the use of topical therapies, including topical glucocorticoids or topical tacrolimus/pimecrolimus.

Pearl: The rash of JDM is photosensitive.

Comment: The purpose of treatment for rash is to prevent the scarring damage of JDM, including the chronic rashes mentioned earlier and, most importantly, calcinosis (Fig. 19.5). Protection from ultraviolet A and B (UVA and UVB) light is hypothesized to help control skin and potentially muscle

disease. In this regard, photoprotective measures may be helpful, including the use of sunscreen or sunblock that decreases exposure to ultraviolet A and B (UVA and UVB) light, use of wide brimmed hats and photoprotective clothing, and avoidance of sun exposure during peak day-light hours.

Pearl: A rash that persists despite therapy heralds a chronic course of illness.

Comment: Rash can be a persistent manifestation of JDM. In our experience, the presence of persistent rash and periungual nailfold capillary changes after 3 months of systemic therapy predicts a chronic course of disease.

Myth: *Autoantibodies in JDM are phenomenology that has little bearing on patients' clinical features and prognosis.*

Reality: Myositis-specific autoantibodies (MSA) are autoantibodies that are found in many adult patients who have specific idiopathic inflammatory myopathies. These autoantibodies are also detected in children and adolescents with these disorders, but less often than in adults. Anti-Jo1 autoantibodies, detected in 5–8% of patients with juvenile myositis, are associated with anti-synthetase syndrome. The anti-synthetase syndrome consists of arthritis, Raynaud's phenomenon, mechanic's hands, fevers, and interstitial lung disease in the setting of moderate to severe muscle weakness and high serum CK levels (Rider and Miller 1997; Wedderburn et al. 2007a). Other autoantibodies, though less common than anti-synthetase antibodies, help predict disease subset and treatment response (Rouster Stevens 2008; Rider et al. 1994).

Patients with juvenile myositis often have anti-nuclear antibodies of unknown specificity. A novel autoantibody that immunoprecipitates 155- and 140-kD proteins has been found in the sera of up to 30% of JDM patients (Targoff et al. 2006; Gunawardena et al. 2008). JDM patients with anti-p155 autoantibodies have more cutaneous involvement and a prolonged illness course (Gunawardena et al. 2008). This autoantibody has also been associated with generalized rather than localized lipodystrophy (Bingham et al. 2008).

Myth: Dystrophic calcifications are associated with a good outcome.

Reality: Dystrophic calcification can develop in either the muscle or the skin of a patient with JDM. One of the first publications concerning the outcome of JDM in the era before the advent of glucocorticoids presented the concept that if the child with JDM lived to develop calcifications, the outcome was "good". Approximately 30% of patients fell into that category (Bitnum 1964). In the glucocorticoid era, 20–40% of JDM patients still develop dystrophic calcification, although the extent and severity of calcification may be less than those observed before the availability of current therapies (Huber et al. 2000; Sheshadri et al. 2008).

Calcifications are often accompanied by a significant loss of range of motion, physical dysfunction, as well as infection. They are a major contributor to the morbidity and mortality of JDM (Huber et al. 2000). The development of calcifications is associated with a young age at diagnosis (Pachman et al. 2006), delay in the institution of effective therapy, and a genetic predisposition to increased production of TNF-α(alpha). The use of high-dose intravenous glucocorticoids at diagnosis may decrease the development of calcifications (Fisler et al. 2002), but the deposits may appear later in the disease course, if unsuppressed inflammation persists or recurs.

A variety of treatments have been reported anecdotally, including the use of calcium channel blockers, probenecid, aluminum hydroxide, and bisphosphonates, but none appears consistently effective in the dissolution of calcifications once they have formed. Calcinosis can regress, sometimes without treatment, but not in a predictable manner. It can also develop even as medical treatments are being administered (McCann et al. 2006). In short, contrary to the earliest publications on outcomes in JDM, calcifications are not associated with good clinical outcomes.

Pearl: There is no definitive treatment for calcinosis.

Comment: Current approaches to the treatment of calcinosis associated with JDM are largely based on anecdotal reports. Regression of calcinosis or retardation of progression has been observed in case reports following treatment with colchicine, hydroxychloroquine, IVIG, cyclosporine, intralesional steroid and most recently with infliximab (Rider and Miller 1997; Riley et al. 2008; Hazen et al. 1982). One problem with these uncontrolled studies is that the natural history of calcinosis is unpredictable: spontaneous regression may occur, making positive successes difficult to interpret.

The first aim of therapy in patients with JDM is to prevent calcinosis. Several reports suggest that the early initiation of intensive anti-inflammatory therapy for JDM is effective in preventing calcinosis. This strategy includes the early administration of daily oral glucocorticoid therapy in adequate doses, as well as the early introduction of methotrexate or intravenous methylprednisolone (Fisler et al. 2002).

Other therapeutic approaches have aimed to inhibit the deposition of calcinosis through mechanisms intended to disrupt calcium-phosphorous homeostasis. The following medications have been attempted for this purpose:

- Diltiazem, a calcium channel-blocker
- Aluminum hydroxide, which decreases the intestinal absorption of phosphate and lowers the serum calcium-phosphate product, thereby decreasing the likelihood of calcium deposition in tissues
- Probenecid, which increases the renal excretion of phosphate, thereby diminishing the calcium-phosphorus product in the serum

- Bisphosphonates, which inhibit calcium hydroxyapatite formation, macrophage function, and the mobilization of bone calcium.

For some patients with tumorous deposits, surgical removal is indicated. This includes patients with chronic or severe pain, loss of function, recurrent infections, or non-healing ulcers. The optimal timing of surgery is when myositis is quiescent.

Myth: Treatment of children with JDM can be standardized.

Reality: The variability of JDM mitigates efforts to propose single therapeutic strategies that might apply to all patients. Patients can present with a variety of rashes, arthritis, joint contractures, esophageal disease leading to dysphagia, mesenteric vasculitis, fatigue, dystrophic calcification, and varying degrees of weakness and functional disability (Rider 2007; Feldman et al. 2008). The duration of the inflammatory process, the age of the child at disease onset, autoantibody status, and genetic factors all contribute to the disease's heterogeneity (Pachman et al. 2006; Rider 2007).

Genetic markers such as certain major histocompatibility complex class II alleles, tumor necrosis factor-alpha-308 and interleukin-1-alpha polymorphisms all appear to contribute to JDM (Wedderburn et al. 2007a; Pachman et al. 2000; Mamyrova et al. in press). Preliminary results of novel immune activation markers suggest molecular biomarkers from the IFN and IL-17 pathways predict disease resistant and drug responsive phenotypes (Baechler et al. 2007).

Myth: Most children with JDM do not have long-term complications of their illness.

Reality: Disease damage, defined as irreversible manifestations of illness present at least 6 months and attributed to previously active disease, medication side effects, or other concurrent illnesses, occurs in many patients with JDM. Cutaneous scarring or atrophy, joint contractures, persistent muscle dysfunction or weakness, dysphagia, and dysphonia are frequently reported in long-term outcome studies. Endocrine complications are also observed, including growth failure (10% of JDM patients) and osteoporosis with fractures (Huber et al. 2000; Ramanan et al. 2005).

Metabolic abnormalities, including insulin resistance and hyperlipidemia, are frequent sequelae of JDM. Metabolic abnormalities reported in JDM are:

- Lipodystrophy, loss of subcutaneous fat
- Insulin resistance, with a visible clue being acanthosis nigricans (Fig. 19.6)
- Diabetes mellitus

Patients with partial and generalized lipodystrophy have a high prevalence of metabolic abnormalities, including glucose intolerance, insulin resistance, and hypertriglyceridemia

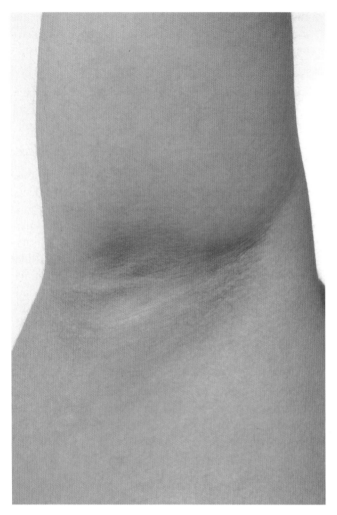

Fig. 19.6 Acanthosis nigricans. Increased pigmented skin in the axilla, which is a sign of insulin resistance

(Bingham et al. 2008). Non-alcoholic steatohepatitis (NASH), testosterone elevation, and menstrual irregularities are also frequently present in patients with total or generalized lipodystrophy (Bingham et al. 2008).

Pearl: The presenting signs and symptoms of JDM can be subtle.

Comment: Many patients with JDM are symptomatic for many months before a diagnosis is made. The duration of untreated disease is a poor prognostic factor: longer duration is associated with increased long-term damage and a greater likelihood of developing calcinosis (Pachman 1998). Physicians may miss the early symptoms and signs of JDM, as they are often subtle and slow to evolve.

Muscle weakness may be mild and often presents as fatigue. In younger children, clumsiness, more frequent falls, and inability to keep up in play activities may become evident. The serum CK level may be normal in up to 40% of JDM patients at the time of diagnosis, even those with evident weakness.

Gottron's papules (see Fig. 19.2) may be misdiagnosed as flat warts, psoriasis, or be missed altogether. When Gottron's lesions are not raised, they are termed "Gottron's sign".

In fair-skinned children, mild heliotrope or malar rashes can be confused with their normal complexion, facial flushing, or allergies. Up to 70% of patients with JDM have a photosensitive rash; only a minority of these are malar rashes. In dark-skinned children, mildly erythematous rashes with hyperpigmentation may be difficult to discern from surrounding skin.

Periungual capillary changes, most easily visible at the nailfold using oil or water-soluble gel and an otoscope or other magnified light source, are almost always present in patients with JDM (see Fig. 19.4). The most sensitive finding, however, is a reduction in the capillary density, which can be difficult to appreciate without a measuring microscope. Nonetheless, this is an important sign to look for and may be a diagnostic clue in the presence of otherwise subtle signs and symptoms.

Pearl: Nailfold capillary end row loops are important markers of JDM disease activity.

Comment: JDM patients frequently have periungual capillary drop-out. The remaining capillaries are often dilated and bushy, as seen under magnification using an ophthalmoscope or DermLite™. The quantitative decrease in the number of end row capillary loops in untreated children with JDM at diagnosis correlates with skin inflammation rather than muscle involvement. In a 36-month longitudinal study of JDM, 40% of JDM patients regenerated their end row capillary loops as they responded to therapy. Persistent capillary loss was highly associated with a delay in starting effective medical therapy and was related to chronically active cutaneous inflammation rather than muscle Christian-Zäch et al., 2008. Decreased nailfold end row capillary loops may also correlate with impaired intestinal absorption.

Pearl: Oral glucocorticoid therapy alone is not always sufficient to control active disease in patients with JDM.

Comment: Our understanding of effective treatments for JDM comes from observational studies and clinical experience. Standard treatment for JDM has been high-dose daily oral glucocorticoids (e.g., up to 2 mg/kg/day of prednisone, at times in divided doses), which is continued until clinical and laboratory improvements are evident and then reduced slowly over a 2-year period (at least). With this regimen, however, most patients develop treatment-related side-effects. Many patients are now treated with adjunctive immunosuppressive medications in an attempt to spare high doses of daily glucocorticoids.

Some children with more severe myositis or those unable to swallow safely are treated with pulse intravenous methylprednisolone (usually 30 mg/kg/day, to a maximum of 1 g daily).

Intravenous methylprednisolone is proposed to minimize the daily oral exposure. However, studies of mild to moderate JDM patients have not shown that long-term outcome is altered by intravenous glucocorticoid treatment (Sheshadri et al. 2008).

The introduction of steroid-sparing agents, such as methotrexate, cyclosporine, azathioprine, or intravenous immune globulin may limit the total glucocorticoid exposure and results in fewer steroid-related side effects. The introduction of methotrexate at the start of treatment does not impact muscle strength outcomes or JDM activity, but does limit the duration and total amount of glucocorticoid exposure and attenuates problems related to weight gain and growth failure (Ramanan et al. 2005). Methotrexate is now widely used by pediatric rheumatologists at the start of the illness.

Standard therapy for the initial treatment of children with JDM now ranges from oral glucocorticoids alone to oral glucocorticoids preceded by a 3-day pulse of methylprednisolone, with or without methotrexate, cyclosporine, or another agent. Hydroxychloroquine is often employed specifically for the treatment of skin disease (Feldman et al. 2008).

Pearl: Children with JDM may require the use of several medications to achieve disease control.

Comment: The aim of treatment in JDM patients is to control the disease completely and achieve remission off therapy, with few or no sequelae. Responses to treatment vary widely:

- Disease that is relatively easy to control in all respects
- Myositis that is difficult to control, with residual unacceptable weakness or functional impairment
- Persistently active skin disease
- Recalcitrant systemic manifestations such as dysphagia, interstitial lung disease, or gastrointestinal ulceration
- Smoldering, mildly active disease complicated by the development of calcinosis.

Most treatment-refractory patients do not respond simply to increasing dosage of disease-modifying drugs. Their symptoms may improve somewhat with glucocorticoids, but usually only on a short-term basis accompanied by unacceptable side-effects. These patients inevitably require a combination of immunosuppressive or immunomodulatory drugs. Disease-modifying anti-rheumatic drugs (DMARDS), including cyclophosphamide, mycophenolate mofetil, cyclosporine, tacrolimus, TNFα(alpha) inhibitors, and rituximab, have been employed in treatment-resistant myositis or potentially life-threatening organ involvement (Pilkington and Wedderburn 2005; Reed 2002). Anecdotal treatment successes have been reported, but controlled studies of these agents have not been reported.

Pearl: There may be a role for sun protection in the management of JDM.

Comment: Exposure to UVA and UVB light is of concern with JDM patients. A subset of patients report significant worsening of their rash and possibly their muscle disease following exposure to the sun. Many of the rashes of DM are also photodistributed, suggesting a role for sun exposure in their activity. Sun protection decreases the extent and severity of skin rash in these patients.

These findings of a role for UV radiation, although preliminary, suggest a potential benefit in using photoprotective measures as an adjunct to therapy. This includes avoiding sun exposure during peak hours of the day; using sunscreen or sun blocks (containing titanium dioxide and zinc oxide) with a high sun protective factor (SPF) daily; reapplying them several times a day; and using wide-brimmed hats and photoprotective clothing.

Pearl: Bone health is important in JDM.

Comment: Children with active JDM symptoms are at risk for bone fracture. They often have markedly diminished bone mineral density on dual x-ray absorptiometry studies and decreased serum levels of osteocalcin (reflecting reduced bone synthesis). Several factors contribute to decreased bone density in JDM:

- A history of prolonged inflammation
- Decreased calcium absorption because of glucocorticoid use
- An intake of calcium and vitamin D that is insufficient for proper bone maintenance and repair

Children with JDM often have less UV exposure and therefore less natural vitamin D, because photoprotective measures are often recommended. Consequently, JDM patients should be provided with supplemental vitamin D and calcium. Supplemental dosing needs to be individualized, but general guidelines suggest 1,200 mg/day of calcium and 800 IU/day of vitamin D for older children and 600 mg calcium/400 IU vitamin D for younger ones.

Pearl: Delays in skeletal growth and the onset of puberty suggest uncontrolled disease or the effects of chronic glucocorticoid administration.

Comment: JDM patients whose disease is controlled in a sustained, effective manner grow and develop normally. A patient with growth delay should be investigated for subtle, uncontrolled JDM disease activity or the presence of another autoimmune condition, e.g., thyroid disease or inflammatory bowel disease. Chronic glucocorticoid use also leads to growth delay.

Successful DMARD use permits the control of JDM and glucocorticoid tapering. In one study of methotrexate, children who received 15 mg/m²/week either orally or subcutaneously from the time of diagnosis had half the cumulative glucocorticoid exposure and weight gain, improved height velocity, and equivalent disease control when compared to patients treated with glucocorticoids alone (Ramanan et al. 2005).

Pearl: Acutely ill patients with JDM require aggressive treatment.

Comment: Serious complications of JDM include acute gastrointestinal ulceration or other acute bowel involvement pneumatosis intestinalis; aggressive interstitial lung disease; acute respiratory insufficiency caused by severe respiratory muscle weakness or air leaks such as pneumomediastinum or pneumothorax; myocarditis; severe muscle weakness with an inability to rise from bed; profound dysphagia leading to aspiration risk; and (rarely) central nervous system vasculitis.

The management of such complications requires the initiation of aggressive therapies, often in combination, to reverse these manifestations quickly. Medications of potential utility in such scenarios include methylprednisolone 30 mg/kg/day thrice (maximum dose: 1,000 mg), intravenous immune globulin, and intravenous cyclophosphamide. The monthly dose of cyclophosphamide may be divided into a weekly dose (10–15 mg/kg) for more rapid effect.

Pearl: JDM patients may have an overlap syndrome or another autoimmune condition.

Comment: Up to 25% of patients with JDM meet classification criteria for another autoimmune disease, e.g., systemic sclerosis (scleroderma), systemic lupus erythematosus, juvenile idiopathic arthritis, inflammatory bowel disease, type I diabetes mellitus, or celiac disease (Pilkington and Reed 2007). Patients with JDM, in association with scleroderma features, are (on average) older than those without scleroderma features; more likely to be girls; have a lengthy diagnostic delay; and manifest a higher frequency of myositis-specific or myositis-associated autoantibodies (Wedderburn et al. 2007a).

Mixed connective tissue disease (MCTD) is characterized by the presence of a high-positive titer of anti-U1-RNP autoantibody in the setting of symptoms and signs of rheumatic conditions such as Raynaud's phenomenon and arthritis. Children with MCTD often present with features of JDM, including Gottron's papules or heliotrope rashes, proximal weakness, and elevated serum muscle enzyme levels.

Juvenile idiopathic arthritis can be associated with muscle inflammation. However, the histopathological features of such cases differ from those of classic JDM. Conversely, 60% of JDM subjects have arthritis, usually as a non-erosive joint condition that responds well to immunosuppressive therapy (Feldman and Ravelli 2007; Lindehammar and Lindvall 2004).

Other gastrointestinal conditions such as active hepatitis, chronic biliary cirrhosis, inflammatory bowel disease, and celiac disease have been described in association with juvenile myositis. Endocrine conditions such as type-1 diabetes and autoimmune thyroid disease are seen at an increased frequency in association with JDM.

Pearl: Children with JDM do not require a routine evaluation for malignancy.

Comment: DM and PM in adult patients have a strong association with malignancy (see Chapter 18). In contrast, the association of JDM and malignancy is much weaker than in adult dermatomyositis (Rider and Miller 1997). Because of the rarity of events in which JDM and malignancy occur together, patients with JDM whose diagnoses appear straightforward do not require malignancy evaluation.

References

Baechler EC, Bauer JW, Slattery CA, et al An interferon signature in the peripheral blood of dermatomyositis patients is associated with disease activity. Mol Med 2007; 13(1–2):59–68

Bingham A, Mamyrova G, Rother KI, et al Predictors of acquired lipodystrophy in juvenile-onset dermatomyositis and a gradient of severity. Medicine (Baltimore) 2008; 87(2):70–86

Bitnum S, Daeschner CW, Jr., Travis LB et al Dermatomyositis. J Pediatr 1964; 64:101-31

Bohan A, Peter JB. Polymyositis and dermatomyositis (first of two parts). N Engl J Med 1975a 292(7):344–347

Bohan A, Peter JB. Polymyositis and dermatomyositis (second of two parts). N Engl J Med 1975b; 292(8):403–407

Brown VE, Pilkington CA, Feldman BM, Davidson JE. An international consensus survey of the diagnostic criteria for juvenile dermatomyositis (JDM). Rheumatology (Oxford) 2006; 45(8):990–993

Christen-Zäch S, Seshadri R, Sundberg J et al Pathological nailfold capillaroscopy changes in juvenile dermatomyositis: association with duration of untreated disease, skin involvement over 36 months and a non-unicyclic disease course. Arthritis Rheum 2008; 58:571-576

Feldman BM, Ravelli A. Maintaining flexibility: Joints and other considerations. In: LG Rider, LM Pachman, FW Miller, H Bollar (eds) Myositis and you: A guide to juvenile dermatomyositis for patients, families and health care providers. The Myositis Association; 2007:269–274

Feldman BM, Rider LG, Reed AM, Pachman LM. Juvenile dermatomyositis and other idiopathic inflammatory myopathies of childhood. Lancet 2008; 371(9631):2201–2212

Fisler RE, Liang MG, Fuhlbrigge RC, Yalcindag A, Sundel RP. Aggressive management of juvenile dermatomyositis results in improved outcome and decreased incidence of calcinosis. J Am Acad Dermatol 2002; 47(4):505–511

Griffin TA, Reed AM. Pathogenesis of myositis in children. Curr Opin Rheumatol 2007; 19(5):487–491

Gunawardena H, Wedderburn LR, North J, et al Clinical associations of autoantibodies to a p155/140 kDa doublet protein in juvenile dermatomyositis. Rheumatology (Oxford) 2008; 47(3):324–328

Guzman J, Petty RE, Malleson PN. Monitoring disease activity in juvenile dermatomyositis: The role of von Willebrand factor and muscle enzymes. J Rheumatol 1994; 21:739–743

Hazen PG, Walker AE, Carney JF, Stewart JJ. Cutaneous calcinosis of scleroderma. Successful treatment with intralesional adrenal steroids. Arch Dermatol 1982; 118(5):366–367

Huber AM, Lang B, LeBlanc CM, et al Medium- and long-term functional outcomes in a multicenter cohort of children with juvenile dermatomyositis. Arthritis Rheum 2000; 43(3):541–549

Lindehammar H, Lindvall B. Muscle involvement in juvenile idiopathic arthritis Rheumatology (Oxford) 2004; 43(12):1546–1554

Lopez de Padilla CM, Vallejo AN, McNallan KT, et al Plasmacytoid dendritic cells in inflamed muscle of patients with juvenile dermatomyositis. Arthritis Rheum 2007; 56(5):1658–1668

Mamyrova G., O'Hanlon TP, Sillers L, et al, for the Childhood Myositis Heterogeneity Collaborative Study Group. Cytokine gene polymorphisms as risk and severity factors for Juvenile Dermatomyositis. Arthritis Rheum 2008; 58(12):3941-50

McCann LJ, Juggins AD, Maillard SM, et al The Juvenile Dermatomyositis National Registry and Repository (UK and Ireland)–clinical characteristics of children recruited within the first 5 yr. Rheumatology (Oxford) 2006; 45(10):1255–1260

Miles L, Bove KE, Lovell D, et al Predictability of the clinical course of juvenile dermatomyositis based on initial muscle biopsy: A retrospective study of 72 patients. Arthritis Rheum 2007; 57(7):1183–1191

Miller, FW. Inflammatory myopathies: Polymyositis, dermatomyositis, and related conditions. In: Koopman W, Moreland L (eds) Arthritis and allied conditions - A textbook of rheumatology (15th edn, volume 2). Philadelphia, PA, Lippincott Williams & Wilkins, 2005, pp. 1593–1620

Pachman LM, Hayford JR, Chung A et al Juvenile dermatomyositis at diagnosis: clinical characteristics of 79 children. J Rheumatol 1998; 25:1198-1204

Pachman LM, Abbott K, Sinacore JM, et al Duration of illness is an important variable for untreated children with juvenile dermatomyositis. J Pediatr 2006; 148(2):247–253

Pilkington C, Reed AM. When your child has more than one autoimmune disease. In: Rider LG, Pachman LM, Miller FW, Bollar H (eds) Myositis and you (1st edn), Addition. Washington DC, The Myositis Association, 2007, pp. 321–326

Pilkington CA, Wedderburn LR. Paediatric idiopathic inflammatory muscle disease: Recognition and management. Drugs 2005; 65(10): 1355–1365

Ramanan AV, Campbell-Webster N, Ota S, et al The effectiveness of treating juvenile dermatomyositis with methotrexate and aggressively tapered corticosteroids. Arthritis Rheum 2005; 52(11): 3570–3578

Reed AM, Lopez M. Juvenile dermatomyositis: Recognition and treatment. Paediatr Drugs 2002; 4(5):315–321

Rider L, eed A, James-Newton L, Feldman B, Ravelli A, Cabalar I, Villalba M, Rider LG, Miller FW. New perspectives on the idiopathic inflammatory myopathies of childhood. Curr Opin Rheumatol 1994; 6(6):575–582

Rider LG. Outcome assessment in the adult and juvenile idiopathic inflammatory myopathies. Rheum Dis Clin North Am 2002; 28(4):935–977

Rider LG. The heterogeneity of juvenile myositis. Autoimmun Rev 2007; 6(4):241–247

Rider LG, Miller FW. Classification and treatment of the juvenile idiopathic inflammatory myopathies. Rheum Dis Clin North Am 1997; 23(3):619–655

Riley P, McCann LJ, Maillard SM, Woo P, Murray KJ, Pilkington CA. Effectiveness of infliximab in the treatment of refractory juvenile dermatomyositis with calcinosis. Rheumatology 2008; 47(6): 877–880

Rouster-Stevens KA, Pachman LM. Autoantibody to signal recognition particle in African-American girls. J Rheumatol 35:927-929, 2008

Sheshadri R, Feldman BM, Ilowite N, Cawkwell G, Pachman LM. The role of aggressive corticosteroid therapy in patients with juvenile dermatomyositis: A propensity score analysis. Arthritis Rheum 2008; 59(7):989–995

Targoff IN, Mamyrova G, Trieu EP, et al A novel autoantibody to a 155-kd protein is associated with dermatomyositis. Arthritis Rheum 2006; 54(11):3682–3689

Wedderburn LR, McHugh NJ, Chinoy H, et al HLA class II haplotype and autoantibody associations in children with juvenile dermatomyositis and juvenile dermatomyositis-scleroderma overlap. Rheumatology (Oxford) 2007a; 46(12):1786–1791

Wedderburn LR, Varsani H, Li CK, et al International consensus on a proposed score system for muscle biopsy evaluation in patients with juvenile dermatomyositis: A tool for potential use in clinical trials. Arthritis Rheum 2007b; 57(7):1192–1201

Vasculitic Neuropathy

20

David A. Chad and Peter Siao

20.1 Vasculitic Neuropathy Overview

> Vasculitic neuropathy results from inflammation within the blood vessel walls of the vasa nervorum, the blood vessels that supply peripheral nerves.

> The forms of systemic vasculitis most likely to be associated with vasculitic neuropathy are polyarteritis nodosa, microscopic polyangiitis, the Churg–Strauss syndrome, Wegener's granulomatosis, and mixed cryoglobulinemia.

> Large-vessel vasculitides such as giant cell arteritis and Takayasu's arteritis seldom cause vasculitic neuropathy. Similarly, vasculitic neuropathy is seldom (if ever) a complication of the types of vasculitis that involve the smallest blood vessels, e.g., cutaneous leukocytoclastic angiitis (hypersensitivity vasculitis) and Henoch–Schönlein purpura. Rather, vasculitic neuropathy tends to be caused by systemic vasculitides that have the ability to target medium-sized blood vessels.

> Vasculitic neuropathy can also occur as a disease process that is limited to the peripheral nerves, sparing other organs. Such cases are sometimes referred to as "isolated vasculitis of the peripheral nervous system" or "nonsystemic vasculitic neuropathy."

> Vasculitic neuropathy is generally a "length-dependent" disease process. Thus, the distal extremities tend to be involved more extensively than are the proximal extremities and trunk importantly, vasculitic neuropathy can also present initally as a multifocal, nonlength dependent process (arms affected earlier than legs).

> Vasculitic neuropathy has the potential to cause serious morbidity (persisting weakness) through the resultant infarctions of peripheral nerves.

> The combination of cyclophosphamide and high doses of glucocorticoids is an appropriate treatment regimen for most patients with vasculitic neuropathy.

20.2 Presentation

Pearl: Although mononeuritis multiplex is the best known pattern of presentation of vasculitic neuropathy, other clinical expressions of neuropathy are in fact more common.

Comment: Mononeuropathy multiplex is defined as some combination of sensory loss, weakness, or both in the territory of two or more specific, clearly defined peripheral nerves. This pattern of disease is the most widely recognized presentation for vasculitic neuropathy. However, mononeuropathy multiplex occurs in only a minority of patients with vasculitic neuropathy (Kissel and Mendell 1992). In fact, this condition can present with a wide range of clinically defined neurological patterns. Two patterns are relatively common:

- The most common pattern of presentation is a distal, symmetrical polyneuropathy. This is a length-dependent disorder, characterized by sensory loss, motor weakness, or both. It begins in the feet and extends proximally.
- The second most common pattern is an overlapping mononeuropathy multiplex, defined as an asymmetrical polyneuropathy that blends neurological deficits of similar character in adjacent nerve territories.

Two additional manifestations of polyneuropathy are observed less often:

- A pure sensory neuropathy, predominantly involving large nerve fibers (Seo et al. 2004).
- A painful, small-fiber sensory polyneuropathy that targets the thinly myelinated and unmyelinated sensory nerve fibers (Lacomis et al. 1997).

Many patients have a pattern of distal symmetrical polyneuropathy when they are first evaluated. This pattern might be secondary to widespread, fulminant vasculitic involvement of many peripheral nerves (Schaumburg et al. 1992). It may also be caused by the involvement of individual peripheral nerves and nerve trunks in a step-wise, asymmetrical fashion, such that the neuropathy has evolved through a pattern of overlapping multiple mononeuropathies by the time the patient is evaluated. In such cases, it is only by careful review of the history and a painstaking neurological examination that subtle asymmetries can be detected. These asymmetries suggest a stuttering, multifocal process, underlying what appears to be a typical distal symmetrical polyneuropathy.

Pearl: A careful, detailed history (often followed by electrodiagnostic studies) of the onset and progression of polyneuropathy is the are important first steps in the evaluation of a patient with possible vasculitic neuropathy.

Comment: Mononeuropathy multiplex is the most distinctive feature of vasculitic neuropathy. For patients with known systemic vasculitides, such as polyarteritis nodosa, Churg–Strauss syndrome, Wegener's granulomatosis, microscopic polyangiitis, or cryoglobulinemic vasculitis, any neuropathic complaints alert the clinician to consider the possibility of vasculitic neuropathy. However, when evaluating patients with no known history of systemic vasculitis or any condition associated with vasculitic neuropathy, e.g., systemic lupus erythematosus, Sjögren's syndrome, hepatitis C, or HIV infection, the situation is different. In this circumstance, a stepwise progression and accumulation of neurologic deficits of multiple mononeuropathies may be the only clue for the clinician to suspect the presence of a vasculitic neuropathy.

The accumulation of multiple individual peripheral nerve deficits may coalesce into a picture of a relatively "symmetrical," "stocking-glove," "axonal," or the so-called "length-dependent" sensorimotor polyneuropathy (Fig. 20.1). At this stage, even a careful neurologic examination may not reveal any asymmetry of the sensorimotor deficits. Only a detailed history can alert the clinician about the possibility of vasculitic neuropathy.

The timing of the neurological examination and electrodiagnostic studies (nerve conduction studies and needle electromyographic examination) in relationship to the onset and progression of the neurologic symptoms is critical. The importance of bilateral nerve conduction studies with side-to-side comparison of sensory and motor responses cannot be overemphasized. When electrodiagnostic studies are performed at a stage when asymmetry is still demonstrable, it supports the clinical suspicion of vasculitic neuropathy and helps the clinician choose the appropriate nerve for biopsy.

Pearl: Vasculitic neuropathy has a predilection for some nerves or nerve distributions over others. Lower extremity involvement is more common than upper extremity involvement, and cranial nerve involvement is rare.

Comment: In a series of 200 patients with necrotizing vasculitis, the peroneal division of the sciatic nerve was the most commonly affected distribution (62.5% unilaterally, 33% bilaterally) (Said 1997). The posterior tibial nerve was the next most commonly involved nerve (27.5% unilaterally, 5%

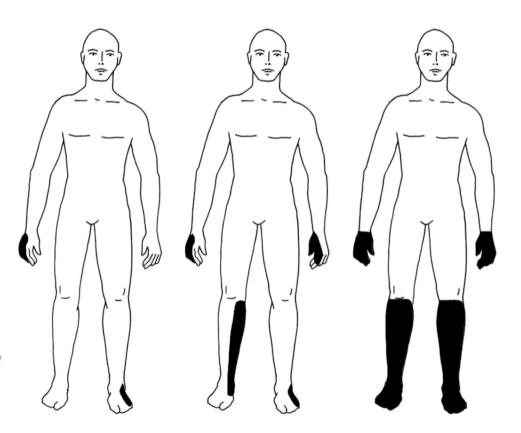

Fig. 20.1 The figure on the *left* shows the sensory deficits in the right ulnar and left sural nerve distributions. The *middle* figure shows additional sensory deficits in the right saphenous and left radial nerves distributions. The figure on the *right* shows the merging or summation of sensory deficits of different nerves giving the picture of a distal, symmetrical, "length-dependent" axonal polyneuropathy

bilaterally). In the upper limbs, the ulnar nerve was most commonly involved (25.5% unilaterally and 8% bilaterally), followed by the median nerve (21.5% bilaterally, 3% unilaterally) and the radial nerve (8% unilaterally and 2% bilaterally). Involvement of more proximal nerves was less common. Unilateral disease of the femoral and sciatic nerves was found in only 6 and 3% of patients, respectively.

A review of four case series of vasculitic neuropathy noted that the sural nerve was involved in 84% of patients and that the radial nerve was involved in up to 44% of cases (Lacomis and Zivkovic 2007). Thus, the precise percentages vary from series to series but the general principles of lower extremity involvement being more common than upper extremity involvement and distal disease more common than proximal are consistent.

Cranial vasculitic neuropathies were rare, with the trigeminal and facial nerves involved in only one patient each. However, cranial nerve involvement may be more common in Wegener's granulomatosis than in other forms of systemic vasculitis. Nearly 20% of the patients with Wegener's granulomatosis had evidence of cranial neuropathies (Said 1997). This finding may relate to the extension of inflammation from the cavernous sinus or meninges (Said 1997).

Myth: Vasculitic neuropathy is a manifestation of systemic necrotizing vasculitis or connective tissue disease. Thus, it always presents in the context of clinical signs of systemic illness with constitutional symptoms (fever, anorexia, weight loss) along with laboratory abnormalities that indicate immune activation.

Reality: The most common presentation of a vasculitic neuropathy is in the context of a known systemic disorder such as polyarteritis nodosa, an ANCA-associated disease, or a paraneoplastic syndrome (Oh 1997). In most cases, a variety of laboratory abnormalities occur, including elevated acute phase reactants; the presence of antineutrophil cytoplasmic antibodies, rheumatoid factor, or other autoantibodies; and the finding of active hepatitis B or C infections. However, 30–40% of patients presenting with a vasculitic neuropathy have isolated involvement of the peripheral nervous system and no sign of disease beyond peripheral nerve and muscle. This vasculitic syndrome is designated nonsystemic vasculitic neuropathy (Dyck et al. 1987; Burns et al. 2007).

Nonsystemic vasculitic neuropathy tends to run a protracted, indolent course. Its prognosis is considerably better than that of vasculitic neuropathy occurring in the context of a systemic disease. Patients with nonsystemic vasculitic neuropathy may have arthralgias, constitutional signs, and elevations of the acute phase reactants, but major organ involvement of the kidneys, lungs, skin, and bowel does not occur (Kissel et al. 1992). Hence, establishing the diagnosis of nonsystemic vasculitic neuropathy poses a challenge to even the most experienced clinicians.

Pearl: Patients diagnosed with nonsystemic vasculitic neuropathy are unlikely to experience systemic spread of the vasculitic process.

Comment: When patients with suspected nonsystemic vasculitic neuropathy are evaluated thoroughly and not found to have symptoms, signs, or serological features of a systemic vasculitis and when immunosuppressive treatment is instituted at an appropriate time, there is a low risk of systemic dissemination of the vasculitic pathology. One study of patients followed for more than 5 years indicated that disease beyond the peripheral nerves and muscles evolved in only 6% of patients (Collins and Periquet 2004).

Other investigators have reported a higher conversion rate from nonsystemic to systemic disease (34%) (Said et al. 1988). The likelihood of the emergence of systemic symptoms undoubtedly varies from center to center and depends to a large extent on how thorough the initial examination has been. The principal point, however, is that a large percentage of patients (indeed, a majority or even a large majority) of patients who have nonsystemic vasculitic neuropathy at diagnosis do not develop clinical disease in other organs, despite lengthy periods of follow-up.

Pearl: In the absence of trauma, the abrupt onset of pain and paresthesias followed by weakness in the territory of a specific peripheral nerve is a clinical presentation that should raise the suspicion of an emerging vasculitic neuropathy.

Comment: When the involvement of one nerve is followed by an evolution of several peripheral neurological deficits in a relatively short time frame that ranges from days to months, a vasculitic etiology must be considered. As described above, vasculitic neuropathy may evolve over a period of months and present as a polyneuropathy, but it is not unusual for it to come on abruptly and evolve rapidly, with deficits that accrue over days to weeks. This rapid onset can be associated with multiple ischemic lesions in different nerve trunks and nerve roots, leading to pronounced asymmetrical weakness. Distal disease, e.g., of the feet or hands, is generally prominent, as is sensory loss and hyporeflexia in affected limbs.

Electrodiagnostic studies are consistent with axon loss and a sensorimotor polyneuropathy, characterized by asymmetric motor and sensory responses and normal or low-normal nerve conduction velocities. A given nerve in one limb might be affected while its fellow nerve on the opposite side is relatively spared.

Other rapidly progressive neuropathies that must be considered in the differential diagnosis include immune-mediated, demyelinating neuropathies classified as Guillain–Barre syndrome (GBS), toxic neuropathies, infectious neuropathies (e.g., West Nile virus infection). In GBS, the time-course to the nadir of weakness is typically only days to weeks. In contrast to vasculitic neuropathy, the weakness is usually symmetrical, present in distal and proximal muscle groups, involves the legs and arms, and is accompanied by cranial mononeuropathies. Bilateral facial nerve involvement is typical of GBS. Respiratory compromise occurs in 25% of patients with GBS. An elevated cerebrospinal fluid protein in the absence of a pleocytosis is a hallmark of GBS, and electrodiagnostic features underscore demyelination rather than axonal loss as the predominant pathologic process.

Patients with toxic neuropathies generally have a clear cut history of exposure to a potential culprit toxin, e.g., saxitoxin from the ingestion of shell fish in red tide season or ciguatoxin from the ingestion of predatory fish. Infectious neuropathies are often revealed by accompanying systemic features of infection (for example, headache and fever in West Nile virus infection).

Myth: The patient presenting with multiple mononeuropathies should be considered to have a vasculitic neuropathy until proven otherwise.

Reality: There is a kernel of truth to this statement. Certainly, one cannot afford to miss the diagnosis of vasculitic neuropathy because of its potential to progress to further nerve damage or systemic disease if left untreated. The point of this Myth, however, is that other neuropathic conditions can present as multifocal peripheral nerve disorders and mimic closely the clinical phenotype of a vasculitic neuropathy.

A major mimicker of vasculitic neuropathy is a variant of chronic inflammatory demyelinating polyneuropathy known as "multifocal acquired demyelinating sensory and motor neuropathy" (Lewis et al. 1982). This disorder initially affects the arms and later spreads to distal nerves in the legs in a manner that conforms to discrete peripheral nerve distributions. The onset of this condition is insidious and slow in its progression (over several months). It often presents with pain and paresthesias. The demyelinating character of this neuropathy is revealed by electrodiagnostic studies. A nerve biopsy is generally not necessary. The treatment response to intravenous gamma globulin and corticosteroids is generally good.

A second major mimicker of vasculitic neuropathy is multifocal motor neuropathy (Pestronk 1998). This condition typically has only motor manifestations and tends to affect the upper limb nerves (radial, median, ulnar) in an asymmetric manner. The condition evolves slowly over months to years. Electrodiagnostic testing discloses multiple regions of motor nerve conduction block and points to the demyelinating nature of this condition. It too has an often gratifying response to intravenous immune globulin.

Finally, patients with glucose intolerance or frank diabetes can present with an asymmetric distribution of sensory loss, pain, and weakness in the territories of the lumbosacral roots, plexuses, and large nerve trunks of the lower extremities (Bradley et al. 1984). This presentation simulates vasculitic overlapping multiple mononeuropathies. The character of the illness is typically revealed by identifying the metabolic abnormality and by electrodiagnostic features that point more to a lumbosacral polyradiculoplexopathy rather than an asymmetrical polyneuropathy. Whether this condition responds to immunosuppressive therapy is uncertain.

20.3 Diagnosis: Electrodiagnostic Studies and Biopsy

Myth: Normal sensory and motor nerve conduction studies exclude vasculitic neuropathy with a high degree of confidence.

Reality: "Normal" nerve conduction studies reduce the likelihood of vasculitic neuropathy but certainly do not rule it out. The normal range of sensory and motor nerve conduction values is broad. As an example, the amplitude of a normal sural sensory potential ranges from 4 to 50 μV or higher. If one finds a sural sensory potential amplitude of 10 μV, the value is "normal" but should not be interpreted as such if it was 30 μV only 1 year before. The biopsy of a nerve that was electrophysiologically normal is shown in Figs. 20.2 and 20.3.

Of course, most patients do not have prior nerve conduction studies for comparison, and the electromyographer must therefore regard the sural sensory potential of 10 μV to be normal or, more accurately, within normal limits. In a series of 40 patients with biopsy-proven vasculitic neuropathy, 5 patients (12.5%) had normal nerve conduction studies of the nerve that was biopsied (Živković et al. 2007).

Follow-up nerve conduction studies often yield important information. The first study may reveal "normal" sural sensory potentials, but subsequent studies may demonstrate significant reductions or even absence of a sensory nerve potential.

Pearl: Bilateral nerve conduction studies for side-to-side comparison are often helpful.

Comment: A sural sensory potential amplitude of 10 μV is "within normal limits" but should be considered abnormal if the contralateral side shows an amplitude of 20 or 30 μV. In general, an amplitude asymmetry of more than 50% is considered significant.

The nerve conduction studies must be directed by the clinician so that the appropriate nerves are studied. As an example, if the patient presents with radial sensory symptoms, the finding of normal median, ulnar, superficial peroneal, and sural sensory potentials does not exclude a radial sensory neuropathy.

Pearl: Examination of the flexor hallucis brevis muscle with electromyography and nerve conduction studies is critical in the evaluation of length-related axonopathies.
Comment: A study of the flexor hallucis brevis may establish the presence of motor involvement that is not otherwise

apparent. The finding of motor nerve involvement may alter the differential diagnosis substantially.

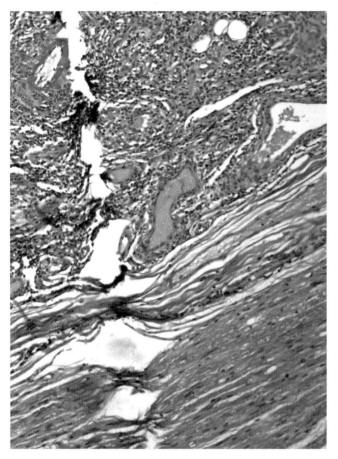

Fig. 20.2 Low power magnification of the sural nerve. The nerve fibers are seen in the *lower right corner*. The epineurial blood vessel in the *upper left corner* showed marked lymphocytic infiltrates and fibrinoid necrosis of the vessel wall, characteristic of vasculitic neuropathy. Hematoxylin and eosin

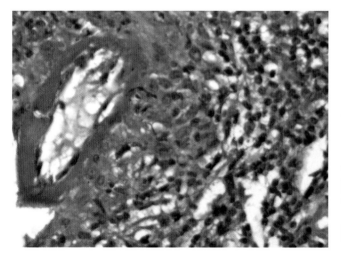

Fig. 20.3 High power magnification of an epineurial blood vessel with fibrinoid necrosis of the vessel wall and intense inflammatory infiltrates characteristic of vasculitic neuropathy. Hematoxylin and eosin

Although nerve conduction studies alone may suggest a pure sensory axonopathy (with normal motor conduction velocities and absent sensory nerve action potentials in the lower limbs), fibrillation potentials in both flexor hallucis brevis muscles indicate subclinical involvement of motor fibers. This points to a sensorimotor multiple mononeuropathy, thereby broadening the differential diagnosis and placing vasculitic neuropathy front and center as a cause of the patient's symptoms (Vallat et al. 2007).

Pearl: It is important to understand the difference between clinical and neurophysiologic presentations of vasculitic neuropathy.

Comment: Multiple mononeuropathies are the most distinctive clinical and neurophysiologic pattern of abnormality in vasculitic neuropathy. However, the most common neurophysiologic finding is a diffuse polyneuropathy (symmetric or asymmetric). This pattern is observed in more than half of all cases of vasculitic neuropathy (Živković et al. 2007). In contrast, neurophysiologic evidence of multiple mononeuropathies is detected in approximately 30% of cases. The different neurophysiologic patterns of injury that occur in vasculitic neuropathy are shown in Table 20.1. With time, multiple mononeuropathies often merge into a picture of distal symmetric or asymmetric sensorimotor polyneuropathy, as illustrated in Fig. 20.1.

Most patients with vasculitic neuropathy (90%) have sensorimotor involvement, but 8% have a pure sensory involvement. Two percent of patients have neurophysiologic evidence of a demyelinating polyneuropathy, even though the nerve biopsy confirms an axonal pattern of injury (Živković et al. 2007).

Pearl: The performance of a muscle biopsy simultaneously with a sensory nerve biopsy increases the diagnostic yield in patients with vasculitic neuropathy.

Comment: In a group of 83 patients with vasculitic neuropathy with or without multisystem disorders who underwent both muscle and nerve biopsies, the muscle biopsy was diagnostic for necrotizing arteritis in 80% and the nerve biopsy was diagnostic in 55% (Said et al. 1988). Even among the 32 patients with clinical features that suggested an isolated vasculitic neuropathy, 26 (81%) had necrotizing arteritis demonstrated within their muscle biopsy. Only 13 patients (41%) showed

Table 20.1 Neurophysiologic patterns of injury in vasculitic neuropathy

Diffuse polyneuropathy (symmetrical or asymmetrical)
Mononeuritis multiplex
Mononeuropathies
Brachial plexopathy
Multilevel lumbosacral radiculopathy
Abnormalities of the upper extremity nerves that are out of proportion to the lower extremity nerves
Disproportionate abnormality of two neighboring nerves

necrotizing arteritis in the nerve specimen. Necrotizing arteritis in both muscle and nerve occurred in seven patients (22%).

Biopsy of the superficial peroneal sensory nerve has the advantage of its proximity with the peroneus brevis muscle. The surgeon can biopsy the nerve and muscle with a single incision. Otherwise, the patient may need one incision for the sural nerve and another incision for the gastrocnemius muscle biopsy.

Myth: In the evaluation of a patient with possible vasculitic neuropathy, the finding of an absent sural sensory potential should direct the clinician to biopsy another nerve.

Reality: When choosing the nerve for biopsy, the finding of an absent sural sensory potential does not mean that sural sensory nerve biopsy would not reveal any useful information, especially if the symptoms are recent or subacute.

Pathologic confirmation of vasculitic neuropathy is very important prior to embarking on long-term immunosuppressant or immunomodulating treatments. Selection of the optimal sensory nerve or sensory nerve/muscle combination to target is therefore critical to establishing the diagnosis. Motor nerves are not biopsied because muscle weakness would be the inevitable consequence of the biopsy. Biopsies of nerve fascicles rather than the entire nerve (so as to avoid significant weakness or sensory loss from the procedure) are possible, but this technique is generally available only in a few academic centers.

In practice, one has relatively few candidate sensory nerves from which to choose. The patient will have residual sensory loss in the distribution of the biopsied sensory nerve. The usual target selected in the lower extremities is either the sural or the superficial peroneal sensory nerve. In the upper extremities, one may choose the superficial radial sensory nerve or the lateral and medial antebrachial cutaneous sensory nerves. The residual sensory loss in the upper extremities may be more bothersome to patients than the residual sensory loss in the lower extremity. Patients should be warned about the possibility of pain syndromes or neuroma formation after nerve biopsy.

20.4 Pathophysiology

Pearl: The tissue targeted by the pathological process of vasculitic neuropathy is the neural vasculature. Nerve damage and axonal degeneration are mediated by ischemia.

Comment: The vasa nervorum provide conduits for nourishing peripheral nerve tissue. When its elements are damaged, the stage is set for nerve ischemia and ultimately the clinical manifestations of peripheral neuropathy. In vasculitic neuropathy, the predominant nerve pathology is axonal degeneration, with the process of segmental demyelination much less prevalent.

The blood supply of the peripheral nerves is profuse, derived from a plethora of nutrient arteries that penetrate the nerve from nearby arterial trunks. Vascular branches divide and subdivide to establish an anastamosing vascular network in the epineurium and perineurium – a reticular endoneurial vascular plexus with frequent interconnections. In the face of this richly collateralized blood supply, nerve ischemia is difficult to produce. Thus, a key prerequisite for nerve ischemia is a disease process such as a vasculitis that targets and damages (in an extensive manner) blood vessels that range in diameter from 50 to 300 µm. It is blood vessels of this caliber that constitute the vasa nervorum.

The most vulnerable portion of the peripheral nerves is at proximal locations – the mid-humerus and mid-thigh – where the nerve trunks lie between the distributions of major nutrient arteries (i.e., in watershed areas). The nerve fascicles that comprise the nerve trunks and contain motor and sensory fibers are most vulnerable in their central regions (Dyck et al. 1972). Hence, axon loss is most notable in what has been called a central-fascicular location.

Because sural nerve biopsies are far downstream from the site of the axonal degeneration lesion and because of branching and inter-mixing of nerve fibers that occurs between fascicles as they descend through the nerves of the limbs, a central-fascicular pattern of degeneration is seldom observed in sural nerve biopsies. Rather, the appearance of the fascicles at the level of the sural nerve that often emerges is one of preferential fascicular involvement (see below).

Pearl: A multifocal pattern of axon loss in a nerve biopsy, characterized by the selective depletion of myelinated nerve fibers in some nerve fascicles more than others, is strongly suggestive of a vasculitic neuropathic process.

Comment: The nerve fiber pathology in vasculitic neuropathy is characterized by axonal degeneration that appears as myelin ovoids in longitudinal sections (representing the disintegration of the axons and their myelin sheaths). The loss of myelinated fibers sometimes involves all of the nerve fascicles within a biopsy specimen. More often, however, a proportion of the total number of nerve fascicles is much more depopulated of myelinated fibers than others, leading to a pattern of a patchy, asymmetrical nerve fiber loss among the fascicles (Kissel and Mendell 1992; Said 1997; Lacomis and Zivkovic 2007). This type of pattern, termed preferential fascicular involvement, is typical of vasculitic neuropathy.

Myth: The diagnosis of vasculitic neuropathy is established by the finding of perivascular inflammatory infiltrates involving epineurial blood vessels.

Reality: The brunt of damage in vasculitic neuropathy stems from the involvement of muscular-walled arteries within the epineurium that constitute the vasa nervorum. However, perivascular inflammation alone is not sufficient to support a definitive diagnosis of vasculitis. Rather, the characteristic and diagnostic findings include necrosis of all components of the vessel wall (transmural necrosis), often with the deposition of fibrin (fibrinoid change), thrombotic occlusion of the lumen, and infiltration of the vessel wall by inflammatory cells. The inflammatory cells are principally polymorphonuclear leukocytes, but eosinophils and mononuclear cells also occur occasionally.

Pearl: Electrodiagnostic studies (nerve conduction and electromyographic studies) play an important role in the diagnosis of vasculitic neuropathy.

Comment: The clinical presentation, physical examination findings, and laboratory results often suggest the possibility of a vasculitic neuropathy, and the analysis of a nerve and muscle biopsy specimens can provide confirmation of that diagnosis. Electrodiagnostic studies also have a major place in the evaluation of patients with possible vasculitic neuropathy, and fulfill two main functions. First, electrodiagnostic studies are a critical intermediate step between the clinical evaluation and tissue biopsy, serving to support the diagnosis of vasculitic neuropathy or to cast doubt on that clinical impression before a nerve/muscle biopsy is undertaken. Second, electrodiagnostic studies help select the most appropriate nerve for biopsy.

Electrodiagnostic studies can confirm the clinical suspicion that the patient's weakness is secondary to axon loss rather than to demyelination. (Demyelination is a relatively minor component of vasculitic neuropathy.) In addition, these investigations define the pattern of nerve involvement – for example, discerning a multifocal, asymmetric process by identifying examining side-to-side differences in the motor and sensory responses.

The most commonly biopsied nerves are the sural and superficial peroneal nerves. The diagnostic yield of nerve biopsy is increased enormously when electrodiagnostic studies demonstrate abnormalities of the target nerve (Wees et al. 1981; Kissel and Mendell 1992). The cutaneous branch of the radial nerve is also a candidate nerve to biopsy for histological confirmation of the diagnosis, particularly if the neuropathic manifestations occur prominently in the upper limbs (Kissel and Mendell 1992).

Pearl: The combination of nerve and muscle biopsy increases the chances of identifying vascular histopathology diagnostic of a vasculitic neuropathy.

Comment: In most cases of suspected vasculitic neuropathy, either the sural nerve or the superficial peroneal nerve is deemed suitable for biopsy. A positive biopsy is more likely if the nerve biopsied is the one from the more symptomatic side, if the area of skin supplied by the nerve in question is hypesthetic, and if the nerve is found to be compromised by electrodiagnostic testing. However, even when these

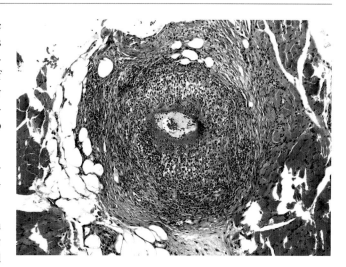

Fig. 20.4 Vasculitis within skeletal muscle. Intramuscular, medium-sized artery from a patient with a overlapping multiple mononeuroapathies, showing severe transmural mononuclear cell inflammation and fibrinoid necrosis, indicative of vasculitis. Surrounding muscle fibers, seen in cross section, are angulated and atrophic consistent with the process of neurogenic atrophy. [Courtesy of Professor Thomas W. Smith, University of Massachusetts, Worcester, MA]

conditions are met, the likelihood that a nerve biopsy specimen will reveal diagnostic histopathology is only approximately 60% (Burns et al. 2007).

Several studies have shown that the addition of a muscle biopsy (Fig. 20.4) increases the chance of visualizing characteristic arterial lesions (Said et al. 1988; Vital et al. 2006). When the superficial peroneal nerve is deemed an acceptable candidate for biopsy, the subjacent peroneus brevis muscle should also be sampled because no additional incision is required. When the sural nerve is selected, a second incision should be performed to obtain a muscle biopsy from either the gastrocnemius or the vastus lateralis.

20.5 Treatment

Pearl: The combination of cyclophosphamide and glucocorticoids is more effective in the treatment of vasculitic neuropathy that occurs in the context of systemic vasculitis than is treatment with glucocorticoids alone.

Comment: There are no controlled treatment trials for the management of vasculitic neuropathy. However, published clinical experience suggests strongly that more than two-thirds of patients with systemic vasculitic syndromes treated early in their clinical course with cyclophosphamide in addition to glucocorticoids have favorable outcomes. Patients treated with cyclophosphamide and glucocorticoids have a greater degree of improvement in their neuropathic symptoms and a reduced rate of relapse compared with those who receive glucocorticoids alone (Kissel and Mendell 1992; Mathew et al. 2007).

For patients with nonsystemic vasculitic neuropathy, no adequate clinical studies exist to serve as a guide to pharmacotherapy (Vrancken et al. 2007). Consequently, the management of these patients is controversial (Collins and Periquet 2004; Kissel and Mendell 1992; Burns et al. 2007). Methotrexate and azathioprine have both been proposed as alternatives to cyclophosphamide, but there are insufficient data on which to judge this recommendation.

For patients with hepatitis C-associated nonsystemic vasculitic neuropathy, antiviral therapy might increase the likelihood of a favorable outcome for peripheral nerve recovery and lessens the risk of cirrhosis (David et al. 1996).

Myth: The development of a new nerve infarction dictates the need for intensification of therapy in the treatment of vasculitic neuropathy.

Reality: The response to a new nerve deficit all depends on the context. New nerve infarctions can occur in distributions of extensive vascular compromise even up to several weeks after the institution of high-dose glucocorticoids and cyclophosphamide. The development of a new nerve infarction shortly after starting immunosuppression does not necessarily signal the need to intensify treatment, particularly if other indicators of disease activity suggest disease control.

References

Bradley WG, Chad D, Verghese JP, Liu HC, Good P, Gabbai AA, Adelman LS. Painful lumbosacral plexopathy with elevated erythrocyte sedimentation rate: a treatable inflammatory syndrome. Ann Neurol. 1984;15:457–64

Burns TM, Schaublin GA, Dyck PJ. Vasculitic neuropathies. Neurol Clin. 2007;25:89–113

Collins MP, Periquet MI. Non-systemic vasculitic neuropathy. Curr Opin Neurol. 2004;17:587–98

David WS, Peine C, Schlesinger P, Smith SA. Nonsystemic vasculitic mononeuropathy multiplex, cryoglobulinemia, and hepatitis C. Muscle Nerve. 1996;19:1596–602

Dyck PJ, Benstead TJ, Conn DL, et al Nonsystemic vasculitic neuropathy. Brain 1987;110:843–54

Dyck PJ, Conn DL, Okazaki H. Necrotizing angiopathic neuropathy: three dimensional morphology of fiber degeneration related to sites of occluded vessels. Mayo Clin Proc. 1972;47:461–75

Kissel JT, Mendell JR. Vasculitic neuropathy. Neurol Clin. 1992;10: 761–81

Lacomis D, Giuliani MJ, Steen V, et al Small fiber neuropathy and vasculitis. Arthritis Rheum. 1997;40:1173–7

Lacomis D, Zivkovic SA. Approach to vasculitic neuropathies. J Clin Neuromusc Dis. 2007;9:265–76

Lewis RA, Sumner AJ, Brown MJ, Asbury AK. Multifocal demyelinating neuropathy with persistent conduction block. Neurology 1982; 32:958–64

Mathew L, Talbot K, Love S, et al Treatment of vasculitic peripheral neuropathy: a retrospective analysis of outcome. QJM. 2007; 100:41

Oh SJ. Paraneoplastic vasculitis of the peripheral nervous system. Neurol Clin. 1997;15:849–63

Pestronk A. Multifocal motor neuropathy: diagnosis and treatment. Neurology 1998;51:S22–24

Said G, Lacroix-Ciaudo C, Fujimura H, Blas C, Faux N. The peripheral neuropathy of necrotizing arteritis: a clinicopathological study. Ann Neurol. 1988;23:461–5

Said G. Necrotizing peripheral nerve vasculitis. Neurol Clin. 1997; 15: 835–48

Seo J-H, Ryan HF, Claussen GC, Thomas TD, Oh SJ. Sensory neuropathy in vasculitis: a clinical, pathological, and electrophysiologic study. Neurology 2004;63:874–8

Schaumburg HH, Berger AR, Thomas PK. Disorders of peripheral nerves (Contemporary Neurology Series 36). 2nd ed. Philadelphia: FA Davis; 1992. p. 130–5

Vallat J-M, Cros DP, Hedley-White ET. Case 9-2007: a 27 year-old woman with pain and swelling of the legs. N Engl J Med. 2007; 356:1252–9

Vital C, Vital A, Canron MH, Jaffre A, Viallard JF, Ragnaud JM, Brechenmacher C, Lagueny A. Combined nerve and muscle biopsy in the diagnosis of vasculitic neuropathy. A 16-year retrospective study of 202 cases. J Peripher Nerv Syst. 2006;11 :20–9

Vrancken AF, Hughes RA, Said G, et al Immunosuppressive treatment for non-systemic vasculitic neuropathy. Cochrane Database Syst Rev. 2007;24(1):CD006050

Wees SJ, Sunwoo IN, Oh SJ. Sural nerve biopsy in systemic necrotizing vasculitis. Am J Med. 1981;71:525–32

Živković SA, Ascherman D, Lacomis D. Vasculitic neuropathy: electrodiagnostic findings and association with malignancies. Acta Neurol Scand. 2007:115;432–6

Pediatric Vasculitis

21

Anne H. Rowley, Seza Ozen, Robert P. Sundel, and Frank T. Saulsbury

Overview

> Based on surverys of providers, vasculitis in children appears to have an incidence of about 50 cases per 100,000 children per year. Only HSP and KD are more common in children than in adults, with each one affecting at least 10-20/100,000 pediatric patients per year. Takayasu arteritis and ANCA-positive vasculitides, on the other hand, strike approximately one child in a million each year.

> Differences between adult and pediatric vasculitides are generally subtle, though they may have important implications. Since these conditions are so rare in the pediatric age group, diagnosis may be significantly delayed, leading to more disease-related damage at the time therapy is initiated. In addition, unlike adults, children may suffer irreversible effects on their physical and mental development both from the disease and from the medications used to treat it.

> On the other hand, children tend to have fewer comorbidities and they are therefore more tolerant of potentially toxic therapies. This often results in better outcomes for children than adults, especially in conditions like Takayasu arteritis and PAN.

> Kawasaki disease (KD) has replaced acute rheumatic fever as the leading cause of acquired heart disease among children in developed nations. Since IVIG became the standard treatment for KD in 1986, the mortality rate of the disease has decreased from 1-2% to <0.1%, and the incidence of coronary artery aneurysms has decreased by 75%.

> Henoch-Schonlein purpura, also known as anaphylactic purpura, is a benign condition in the vast majority of affected children. Nonetheless, in rare cases, children affected by HSP may develop hypertension (especially during pregnancy) or renal failure long after the acute syndrome has resolved.

> One-third or more of children with PAN have the cutaneous form, largely limited to skin and joint involvement. While mortality is rare, aggressive control of the systemic inflammation and end-organ involvement is nonetheless needed if significant long-term morbidity is to be avoided.

21.1 Kawasaki Disease

Myth: Kawasaki's disease is a rare illness.

Reality: Kawasaki's disease is a very common illness in Japan. Approximately 1 in 150 Japanese children develop Kawasaki's disease by the age of 5 years incidence of 175,100,00 children (Yanagawa et al. 2001). The incidence is about tenfold lower among Caucasian children (15–20/100,000 children <5 years) (Holman et al. 2003) and is intermediate among African-Americans. The incidence also varies by age and gender (Table 21.1). Thus, the incidence of Kawasaki's disease in U.S. children is slightly higher than the incidence of invasive *Haemophilus influenzae* type b (Hib) in that population prior to the introduction of Hib conjugate vaccine (13.9/100,000 children <5 years) (Centers for Disease Control 1998). No one considered Hib to be a "rare" condition in those days.

Pearl: Neck swelling is the most dramatic clinical symptom in some children with Kawasaki's disease.

Comment: A diagnosis of Kawasaki's disease should be considered in any child with prolonged fever and neck swelling that does not respond to antibiotics. Other Kawasaki's disease features can remain unrecognized for days after neck swelling develops, or begin afterward. Neck swelling in Kawasaki's disease can represent superficial adenitis or, more rarely, inflammation within the deeper tissue planes of the neck, including the retropharyngeal or parapharyngeal spaces (Stamos et al. 1994). Despite the intensity of inflammation in these spaces and the decreased attenuation that can

J. H. Stone (ed.), *A Clinician's Pearls and Myths in Rheumatology,*
DOI:10.1007/978-1-84800-934-9_21, © Springer Science + Business Media B.V. 2009

Table 21.1 Approximate incidence of Kawasaki's disease in U.S. and Japanese population by age[a] (adapted from Holman (2003) and Yanagawa (2001))

Age	U.S.		Japan	
	Male	Female	Male	Female
<1 year	25	14	225	140
1–4 years	20	13	100	75
>4 years	1–4	1–4	10	10

[a]Per 100,000 children

be observed on CT scan (suggesting an abscess), true abscesses do not develop in these areas. Surgical drainage does not yield purulent material and is generally not indicated, as most patients improve dramatically with intravenous gammaglobulin (IVIG) therapy.

Myth: A positive rapid test for respiratory syncytial virus (RSV) or parainfluenza virus (PIV) from the nasopharynx excludes Kawasaki's disease.

Reality: A statement included in classic diagnostic criteria for Kawasaki's disease is that "the illness cannot be explained by a known disease process." Some clinicians have taken this to mean that a positive test for a known pathogen from any site rules out the diagnosis of Kawasaki's disease. This is only true if that pathogen is known to produce clinical findings that truly mimic Kawasaki's disease.

Because RSV and PIV produce respiratory symptoms but not the other clinical features of Kawasaki's disease, they are unlikely to be responsible for an illness compatible with Kawasaki's disease. Because Kawasaki's disease cases occur with greater frequency in winter–spring in nontropical climates, the same time that RSV and some strains of PIV are circulating, Kawasaki's disease patients will occasionally be coinfected with RSV, PIV, or other respiratory pathogens. Such patients should be promptly treated for Kawasaki's disease.

Pearl: Conjunctival injection can be the most persistent Kawasaki's disease manifestation, persisting long after IVIG therapy has led to the improvement of other symptoms and signs.

Comment: Persistent conjunctival injection can be observed in Kawasaki's disease patients who have experienced resolution of fever and other clinical signs following the institution of IVIG and aspirin therapy. If the patient is otherwise doing well, persistent conjunctival injection does not necessarily indicate treatment failure.

Pearl: Kawasaki's disease is a particularly difficult diagnosis to make in young babies.

Comment: Young babies seldom get autoimmune or idiopathic inflammatory disorders, perhaps because their immune systems remain quite immature for the first several months of life. Kawasaki's disease is an exception to this rule.

Infections must be considered first in any febrile infant. However, if no organism has been identified after a week of fever, Kawasaki's disease should receive serious consideration. The disease in infants tends to be both less typical, often without other signs of mucocutaneous inflammation, and more morbid, causing aneurysms in up to 35% of patients despite treatment with IVIG.

The need for a heightened concern for Kawasaki's disease in young babies is reflected in recommendations that children under 6 months of age with at least 7 days of fever receive an echocardiogram, even if other classic manifestations of Kawasaki's disease are absent (Newburger et al. 2004a).

Myth: Any patient who develops Kawasaki's disease should have periodic echocardiograms performed for life.

Reality: Kawasaki's disease is an acute vasculitis; coronary artery abnormalities typically are visible by echocardiography at 3–4 weeks after the onset of fever. There is no convincing evidence that coronary artery disease will develop in a Kawasaki's disease patient if it has not developed within the first 2 months after the onset of Kawasaki's disease.

A patient who develops coronary artery abnormalities needs to be followed with periodic echocardiograms. Other studies may also be indicated, depending upon the severity of the coronary artery disease (Newburger et al. 2004a). However, the child who has normal echocardiograms at diagnosis, 2–3 weeks after onset, and 6–8 weeks after onset generally does not require additional echocardiograms.

Pearl: In a toddler with some clinical features of Kawasaki's disease, refusal to walk should heighten suspicion of the diagnosis.

Comment: Conditions that mimic Kawasaki's disease, such as adenovirus or enterovirus infections or scarlet fever, generally do not manifest this sign. Children with Kawasaki's disease frequently develop small-joint arthritis in the hands and feet, which is painful and limits their willingness to walk or to pick up small objects. Swelling of the hands and feet is also common in Kawasaki's disease but rarely observed in other illnesses that comprise the usual differential diagnosis (excluding measles).

Myth: A normal ESR rules out the diagnosis of acute Kawasaki's disease.

Reality: The ESR is influenced by numerous factors, and can be falsely lowered by a very high white blood cell count, hypofibrinogenemia, or other factors (Jurado 2001). The CRP is not affected by these factors, and should therefore be determined in a patient presenting with possible acute Kawasaki's disease. Discrepancy between the ESR and CRP in acute Kawasaki's disease has been reported (Anderson et al. 2001). CRP normalizes faster than the ESR following acute Kawasaki's disease.

The ESR can be particularly useful in evaluating a child for possible "missed" Kawasaki's disease between the second and fourth weeks after fever onset. During that time period following acute Kawasaki's disease, the ESR would likely remain elevated while the CRP may have normalized.

Pearl: The ESR is not useful in monitoring clinical progress for at least 7–10 days after IVIG therapy.

Comment: The ESR is dependent upon the levels of several plasma proteins, including IgG (van Leeuwen and van Rijswijk 1994). Thus, the ESR rises transiently following IVIG infusion even as the disease begins to come under control in most patients. In contrast to the ESR, C-reactive protein (CRP) levels are useful in monitoring disease responses to IVIG, because the CRP level is not altered directly by the constituents of this therapy.

Myth: A child who develops an illness with some features of Kawasaki's disease in association with a finding not compatible with Kawasaki's disease has "atypical Kawasaki's disease."

Reality: A patient with prolonged fever, red lips, rash, and a lobar pneumonia is much more likely to have bacterial infection than Kawasaki's disease, because lobar pneumonia is not characteristic of acute Kawasaki's disease. The terms "atypical" and "incomplete" Kawasaki's disease refer to illnesses in which the patient has some but not all features of classic Kawasaki's disease. They were not intended to describe patients whose clinical features are inconsistent with that diagnosis. In such patients, additional testing to determine the correct diagnosis should be performed.

Myth: Dilation of coronary arteries in a febrile child is presumptive evidence of a diagnosis of Kawasaki's disease.

Reality: Coronary artery ectasia and aneurysmal dilation can be caused by a variety of illnesses. Kawasaki's disease is the most widely recognized of these conditions and the one that is most important to diagnose acutely to improve outcomes. However, systemic-onset JRA (Still's disease), systemic lupus erythematosus, polyarteritis nodosa, and EBV infection should also be considered in the differential diagnosis of a child with dilated coronary arteries (Binstadt et al. 2005).

Pearl: A child with Kawasaki's disease who develops influenza or chickenpox should discontinue aspirin.

Comment: The discontinuation of aspirin in the setting of an influenza or varicella infection is essential to reduce the possibility of Reye syndrome. Children with Kawasaki's disease on aspirin therapy should be immunized with the inactivated influenza vaccine. There is considerable overlap between influenza season and the peak of acute Kawasaki's disease incidence in nontropical climates (winter–spring). As a result, patients with both conditions are observed on occasion.

A child with Kawasaki's disease and chickenpox or a varicella-susceptible Kawasaki's disease patient with a significant exposure should discontinue aspirin, and another antiplatelet agent be administered until varicella has resolved or the incubation period has passed. Clopidogrel offers an option for antiplatelet therapy, especially in a child deemed to be at particularly high risk for thrombosis (Newburger et al. 2004a).

Myth: If a child with suspected Kawasaki's disease is not cranky, he probably does not have Kawasaki's disease.

Reality: The cause of irritability in children with Kawasaki's disease is not known. Many clinicians suspect subclinical meningoencephalitis and, indeed, many children with Kawasaki's disease are found to have abnormalities of the CSF when a lumbar puncture is performed (Dengler et al. 1998).

Crankiness is typical of children with Kawasaki's disease but is not present invariably. Older children, for example, are more likely to be somnolent or lethargic than irritable, but even young children are not always cranky. Thus, if Kawasaki's disease is suspected because of certain clinical features, the presence or the absence of crankiness should not influence clinical thinking significantly one way or the other.

Pearl: A diagnosis of Kawasaki's disease is unlikely in children with splenomegaly, discrete intraoral lesions, or a lymphocytic predominance in the peripheral blood.

Comment: Differentiation of Kawasaki's disease from viral conditions is often difficult. Indeed, the manifestations of atypical measles (i.e., measles following vaccination against measles) can be clinically indistinguishable from Kawasaki's disease. Similarly, EBV, adenovirus, parvovirus, and other conditions can mimic Kawasaki's disease. Splenomegaly, discrete oral lesions (as opposed to diffuse oral erythema), and a lymphocytic predominance in the peripheral blood all suggest one of the viral mimics of Kawasaki's disease rather than Kawasaki's (Burns et al. 1991).

Pearl: Kawasaki's disease should be considered in the differential diagnosis of prolonged fever and aseptic meningitis of unknown etiology in infants and in young children.

Comment: Infants present with incomplete Kawasaki's disease more commonly than do older children. In an infant or young child with prolonged fever and aseptic meningitis, the diagnosis of Kawasaki's disease should be considered if enterovirus and herpes simplex virus infections have been excluded (Dengler et al. 1998). Aseptic meningitis is occasionally the most significant clinical manifestation of the illness, but other findings potentially related to Kawasaki's disease must be sought carefully.

Pearl: Peribronchial infiltrates and mild interstitial infiltrates can be observed on chest radiographs in children with acute Kawasaki's disease and should not dissuade the clinician from that possible diagnosis.

Comment: Peribronchial and interstitial infiltrates are more common in Kawasaki's disease than generally appreciated, because many Kawasaki's disease patients do not have chest radiographs performed. One study reported radiographic abnormalities in 15% of acute Kawasaki's disease patients (Umezawa et al. 1989). These consisted primarily of reticulogranular infiltrates, peribronchial cuffing, pleural effusion, and atelectasis. Autopsy studies of acute Kawasaki's disease patients reveal that pneumonitis and bronchial inflammation are observed in the majority of fatal acute Kawasaki's disease cases (Amano et al. 1980).

Pearl: In a child with prolonged fever, the presence of tachycardia even when fever has temporarily abated should heighten suspicion of acute Kawasaki's disease.

Comment: Because myocarditis is present to some degree in the majority of acute Kawasaki's disease patients, the presence of tachycardia even when fever is not present is common, and may provide a clue to the diagnosis. Myocarditis and its associated cardiac dysfunction improve following IVIG therapy (Newburger et al. 1989).

Myth: If the platelet count is not elevated and there is no peeling of the fingers and toes, then acute Kawasaki's disease is unlikely.

Reality: Thrombocytosis and peeling of the hands and feet are characteristic features of the subacute phase of Kawasaki's disease. They usually occur 2–3 weeks after the onset of fever, and are therefore not useful for the diagnosis of acute Kawasaki's disease. The optimal approach to caring for a patient with Kawasaki's disease is to make the diagnosis and begin treatment with IVIG before either thrombocytosis or peeling has developed. Treatment does not affect the occurrence of either finding.

Thrombocytopenia during the acute phase of Kawasaki's disease, although uncommon, is a well-recognized risk factor for the development of coronary artery disease as a complication of the illness (Niwa et al. 1995).

Pearl: Erythema in the groin area might be the result of a Candida infection – but also possibly a manifestation of Kawasaki's disease.

Comment: When prolonged fever accompanies groin erythema and peeling, a simple cutaneous fungal infection may not be the true diagnosis. Clinicians sometimes miss a case of incomplete Kawasaki's disease in an infant or young child when a groin rash is mistakenly diagnosed as candidal dermatitis. Knowledge of the many clinical presentations of acute Kawasaki's disease, combined with a high index of suspicion, is needed to make the diagnosis and prevent the potentially severe coronary artery sequelae of the illness.

Myth: Kawasaki's disease does not occur in infants younger than 6 months of age.

Reality: Kawasaki's disease is uncommon but does occur in this age group (Rosenfeld et al. 1995; Burns et al. 1986). Infants with acute Kawasaki's disease have prolonged fever, but other clinical findings of Kawasaki's disease can be absent or subtle. Unfortunately, young infants can have severe coronary artery sequelae following acute Kawasaki's disease.

Myth: Kawasaki Disease is not observed in older children and adolescents.

Reality: Kawasaki's disease can occur in older children and teenagers, and these patients can be at risk for developing coronary artery disease. Older children are likely to experience a delay in diagnosis (Stockheim et al. 2000; Momenah et al. 1998; Muta et al. 2004). A high index of suspicion is needed to make the diagnosis.

Pearl: The clinical features of Kawasaki's disease can appear discontinuously (i.e., all may not be present at the same time).

Comment: Obtaining a complete history of all physical findings from the family is often critical in establishing the diagnosis of Kawasaki's disease. A history of a maculopapular rash that lasted for more than a day or of swollen hands and feet that lasted several days but have since resolved could be helpful clues to establishing a diagnosis of Kawasaki's disease. Consensus criteria for the classification of Kawasaki's disease are shown in Table 21.2.

Myth: Kawasaki's disease and infantile periarteritis nodosa are two different illnesses.

Reality: Children in the U.S. and throughout the world die of unrecognized acute Kawasaki's disease. In the years before Dr. Kawasaki reported the characteristic clinical features of the illness, the only cases of Kawasaki's disease reported in the literature were the fatal ones. Pathologists used the term "infantile periarteritis nodosa" to describe these cases. Studies comparing the pathologic features of acute fatal Kawasaki's disease cases and cases of infantile periarteritis

Table 21.2 Criteria for the classification of Kawasaki's disease (modified from Ozen 2006)

Mandatory criterion: fever persisting for at least 5 days
Additional criteria (four of five features required)
Skin changes in the peripheral extremities or perineal region
Polymorphous exanthema
Bilateral conjunctival injection
Changes of lips and oral cavity, with injection of oral and   pharyngeal mucosa
Cervical lymphadenopathy

In the presence of coronary artery involvement (detected onechocardiography) and fever, fewer than four of the remaining five criteria are sufficient (the exact number of criteria required is to be defined in an ongoing study)

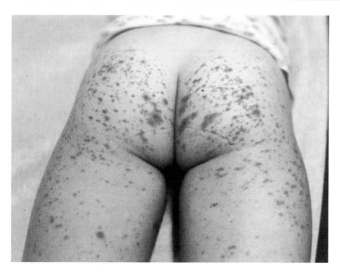

Fig. 21.1 Typical rash of HSP concentrated on buttocks and lower extremities (Figure courtesy of Dr. Frank Saulsbury)

nodosa indicate that these two conditions are, in fact, one (Landing and Larson 1977; Tanaka et al. 1976).

Myth: Kawasaki's disease only strikes children who were previously healthy.

Reality: The vast majority of children with acute Kawasaki's disease are previously healthy. However, the illness can occur in children with underlying medical conditions. Kawasaki's disease may not be recognized in these children, because the condition is not even considered in the differential diagnosis. One example is a patient who developed fever, conjunctival injection, and rash 1 year following an autologous stem cell transplantation for another illness. Adenovirus infection was the leading diagnosis, but the virus was not identified by culture from any site. Fevers eventually resolved, but the patient presented 3 months later with a myocardial infarction, and had aneurysms of multiple coronary arteries.

21.2 Henoch–Schönlein Purpura

Myth: Henoch–Schönlein purpura (HSP) is the only small vessel vasculitis that affects children.

Reality: HSP is the most common form of small-vessel vasculitis in children, but not the only one. Other vasculitides, including infection-induced vasculitis, hypersensitivity vasculitis, microscopic polyangiitis, and Wegener's granulomatosis, can cause a similar clinical picture (Ozen et al. 2007). In addition, HSP or HSP-like vasculitis can occur as a part of other conditions. For example, HSP occurs in 5–10% of patients with familial Mediterranean fever (Ozdogan et al. 1997). It has also been reported in some children with the

hyper-IgD syndrome, another hereditary periodic fever syndrome (Wickiser et al. 2005).

Myth: A skin biopsy is necessary for the diagnosis of HSP.

Reality: The vast majority of patients with HSP can be diagnosed on clinical grounds alone (Ozen et al. 2007). The typical rash of HSP consists of palpable purpuric lesions 2–10 mm in diameter. The lesions are concentrated on the buttocks and lower extremities, but not confined exclusively to those areas (Fig. 21.1). A skin biopsy is helpful if the rash is atypical. For example, only 2% of children with HSP have bullous lesions; thus, a biopsy should be considered if bullous lesions are present. A biopsy should be considered if there is evidence of tissue necrosis, since this complication is extremely uncommon in children with HSP.

A skin biopsy should also be considered if the patient has unusual or atypical symptoms, such as nasal or sinus inflammation or pulmonary disease, all of which suggest other disorders. Of course, if a biopsy is performed, the point is not to demonstrate leukocytoclastic vasculitis (this could be inferred from the finding of palpable purpura). Rather, the goal of the biopsy is to either demonstrate IgA deposition in small blood vessels or to exclude the finding. Although HSP is just one cause of small vessel leukocytoclastic vasculitis, it is the only form of vasculitis that is always associated with granular IgA deposition in vessel walls.

Because 80% of HSP cases occur in children younger than 10 years of age, a skin biopsy should be considered in teenagers, particularly those in their late teen years. Finally, a skin biopsy should be considered in patients with high fever or prolonged fever.

Pearl: Joint symptoms precede the onset of purpura in up to one quarter of patients with HSP.

Comment: Among HSP patients whose presentation consists of joint symptoms alone, purpura – a sine qua non of HSP – almost always appears within 1 week (Saulsbury 1999; Trapani et al. 2005). In general, cutaneous purpura develops before the results of the laboratory studies that were ordered when the patient presented with joint complaints. The joint swelling associated with HSP may not represent a true synovitis, but rather periarticular soft tissue edema. The swelling often extends beyond the joint boundaries (e.g., to include the dorsum of the feet in addition to the ankles, or the dorsum of the hand in addition to the wrists) (Fig. 21.2). The joint involvement of HSP always involves the lower extremities (knees, ankles, or feet), but one half of the patients also have upper extremity involvement, usually the wrists and hands (Saulsbury 1999; Trapani et al. 2005).

Pearl: Gastrointestinal symptoms precede the onset of purpura in up to 20% of patients.

Comment: Colicky abdominal pain, vomiting, and gastrointestinal bleeding precede the onset of purpura by up to 2 weeks

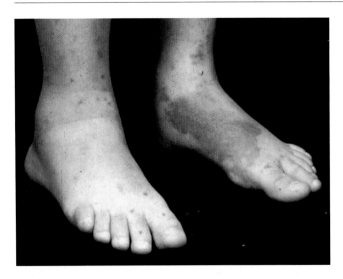

Fig. 21.2 Swelling of the ankles and dorsum of the foot in a patient with HSP (Figure courtesy of Dr. Frank Saulsbury)

in a sizeable subset of patients: nearly one-fifth (Saulsbury 1999; Trapani et al. 2005). Gastrointestinal symptoms in the absence of the characteristic rash can mimic a surgical abdomen, an infectious enteritis, or inflammatory bowel disease. More than one surgeon has been fooled by HSP.

Pearl: Most intussusceptions in patients with HSP are confined to the small bowel.

Comment: Only 1–5% of patients with HSP develop intussusception. Intussusceptions are confined to the small bowel in 60% of patients with HSP. This contrasts with the usual ileo-colic location in children without HSP who develop idiopathic intussusception (Choong and Beasley 1998). Thus, abdominal computerized tomography or ultrasound, rather than air contrast enema, is the preferred diagnostic modalities if intussusception is suspected in a child with HSP. Surgical reduction of the intussusception is often necessary.

Pearl: Nephritis rarely precedes the appearance of cutaneous purpura.

Comment: Unlike arthritis and gastrointestinal symptoms, nephritis rarely develops before the appearance of the characteristic rash. In fact, the onset of nephritis may be delayed for up to 3 months in a substantial minority of patients.

Myth: Nonsteroidal anti-inflammatory agents (NSAIDs) are an effective treatment for the joint pain and abdominal pain associated with HSP.

Reality: There has never been a properly conducted study examining the efficacy of NSAIDs in the treatment of HSP. Moreover, there is little anecdotal evidence that NSAIDs are effective. Nevertheless, NSAIDs are often recommended for the treatment of HSP. One should be circumspect about using

drugs with gastrointestinal and renal side effects to treat a disease in which the major complications are gastrointestinal bleeding and nephritis.

Myth: Early administration of glucorticoids prevents the development of nephritis.

Reality: Approximately 40% of children with HSP develop nephritis. The majority of patients develop nephritis within the first 4 weeks of the illness, but the onset of nephritis is delayed for up to 3 months in 25% of patients. There is little evidence that initiation of glucocorticoid therapy at the onset of symptoms prevents the acute or delayed onset of nephritis. Indeed, there is substantial evidence to the contrary (Saulsbury 1993; Ronkainen et al. 2006).

Pearl: Glucocorticoids are beneficial in the treatment of some aspects of HSP.

Comment: A recent randomized, double-blind, placebo-controlled study showed that prednisone in a dose of 1 mg/kg/day for 2 weeks, then tapered over the subsequent 2 weeks, is effective in treating the joint and abdominal pain associated with HSP (Ronkainen et al. 2006). These results confirmed previous retrospective studies, anecdotal reports, and many unpublished clinical observations. However, glucocorticoids do not shorten the duration of purpura, prevent nephritis, or forestall disease recurrences (Ronkainen et al. 2006).

Pearl: Renal function may deteriorate years after an episode of HSP nephritis in a child.

Comment: Nephritis is the one feature of HSP that may have chronic consequences, and the long-term prognosis is heavily dependent upon the severity of nephritis at presentation. Approximately 30–50% of patients with nephritis have persistent urinary abnormalities for months or years, but only 1–3% of patients progress to end-stage renal disease (Saulsbury 1999; Trapani et al. 2005).

In general, patients with microscopic hematuria and trivial proteinuria have an excellent prognosis (Narchi 2005). By contrast, nephritis complicated by nephrotic syndrome has a poor prognosis (Ronkainen et al. 2003). In addition, the histopathologic finding of crescents in more than 50% of glomeruli on renal biopsy is associated with a poor prognosis. However, neither the clinical presentation nor the biopsy findings serve as precise predictors of the ultimate outcome in all patients.

Two long-term follow-up studies of children with HSP nephritis showed worsening renal disease as adults. Renal deterioration was seen in some patients who had relatively mild nephritis as children (Goldstein et al. 1992; Ronkainen et al. 2002). Both studies also showed that pregnancy was complicated by proteinuria and hypertension in 40–60% of women who had HSP nephritis as children. One half of the women had mild nephritis that had completely resolved when they were children. Thus, long-term monitoring of patients is necessary, and particular vigilance is warranted in pregnant women.

Pearl: The vast majority of patients have a disease duration of less than 12 weeks.

Comment: One should not classify patients as having prolonged disease until they have experienced persistent symptoms lasting greater than 12 weeks (Saulsbury 1999; Trapani et al. 2005). A variety of infections appear able to precipitate HSP, and it is possible that others are also capable of prolonging the disease process, as well. If an infection is present, a course of antibiotic therapy is often successful in bringing the condition to a halt. Thus, a careful search for underlying infection is warranted. A few anecdotal reports suggest that dapsone and colchicine are effective in treating prolonged symptoms, but neither drug has been studied in a systematic fashion.

Myth: HSP is always a self-limited disorder.

Reality: HSP can appear with a frightening, multi-organ system presentation in previously healthy patients. Fortunately, in the large majority of cases, the process is self-limited and does not require immunosuppressive therapy. (Indeed, it is not entirely clear that immunosuppressive therapy helps some of the clinical manifestations.)

In a small minority of cases – particularly those in adults – HSP appears to be a more chronic condition or at least one that requires months or years to resolve. These cases can be characterized by recurrent or even virtually continuous cutaneous purpura, with intermittent arthritis or other disease manifestations.

Pearl: If HSP is not self-limited, "mega" doses of prednisone may work.

Comment: In a small minority of patients, palpable purpura (Fig. 21.3) and sometimes other major disease manifestations (joint complaints and abdominal pain) recur regularly and respond poorly to series of conventional treatment approaches: glucocorticoids at doses of up to 60 mg/day, colchicine, dapsone, azathioprine, and others. Limited anecdotal experience suggests that rituximab is also ineffective in this setting.

For reasons that remain unclear, "mega" doses of glucocorticoids appear to work in a significant number of these cases. A 3-day methylprednisolone pulse (1 g/day) can lead to disappearance of the purpura for a year or more. In some cases, HSP returns after that time, but typically responds again to mega doses of glucocorticoids. Because glucocorticoids have 100% oral bioavailability, anecdotal experience has also shown that oral pulses of prednisone can be effective: prednisone 960 mg (sixteen 60 mg tablets) once daily for 3 days. This is appropriate, because most cases of recurrent purpura related to HSP do not require hospitalization.

Pearl: In adult cases of refractory HSP, patients should be evaluated for the presence of an IgA paraproteinemia.

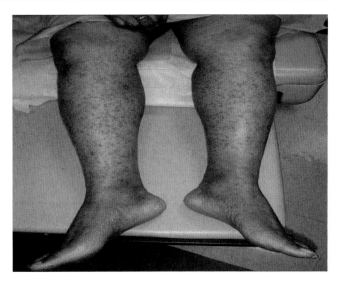

Fig. 21.3 Palpable purpura: the *sine qua non* of HSP. This patient is a 30-year-old man who experienced months of recurrent, diffuse purpura, refractory to conventional doses of prednisone (e.g., 1 mg/kg/day) and other therapies. He responded dramatically to 3 days of pulse methylprednisolone (1 g/day three times) and entered a year-long remission before a recurrence, which responded again to pulse methylprednisolone (Figure courtesy of Dr. John Stone)

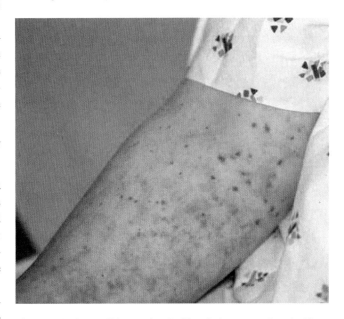

Fig. 21.4 IgA vasculitis associated with an IgA paraproteinemia. There are cutaneous findings of both small- and medium-vessel vasculitis. Small-vessel: purpura; medium-vessel: livedo reticularis (racemosa) (Figure courtesy of Dr. John Stone)

Comment: Patients with IgA paraproteinemia and vasculitis have involvement of larger caliber vessels than do patients with typical HSP, and often present with livedo reticularis (indicative of medium-vessel vasculitis) as well as purpura (Fig. 21.4). The natural history of this disorder and its optimal treatment remain unclear. Evolution to multiple myeloma has been reported (Birchmore et al. 1996).

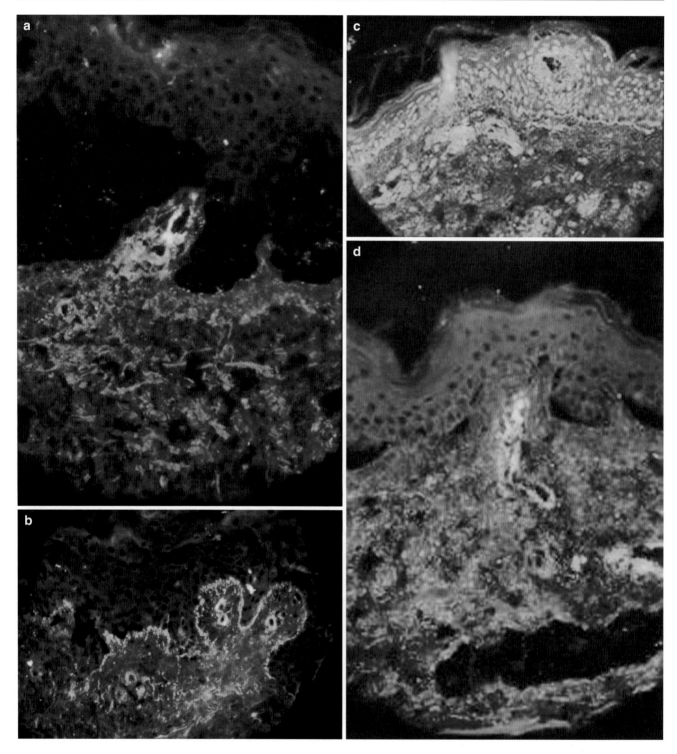

Fig. 21.5 Direct immunofluorescence studies in four types of cutaneous vasculitis: (**a**) HSP; (**b**) hypocomplementemic urticarial vasculitis; (**c**) connective tissue disease; and (**d**) type II cryoglobulinemia secondary to hepatitis C (from Stone and Nousari (2001); reprinted with kind permission from *Current Science*)

Myth: Performing direct immunofluorescence (DIF) studies on skin biopsies from patients with cutaneous vasculitis is usually unnecessary.

Reality: Failure to perform DIF squanders the opportunity to collect important data about the etiology of cutaneous vasculitis. Not only is DIF the only way of confirming the diagnosis of HSP (Fig. 21.5a), proper interpretation of the pattern of immunoreactant deposition may also yield clues to the diagnosis and underlying pathophysiology of other conditions. For example, DIF studies in hypocomplementemic urticarial vasculitis show striking IgG deposition around blood vessels and at the basement membrane zone (Fig. 21.5b). In cutaneous vasculitis associated with connective tissue disorders, the phenomenon of the "in vivo ANA" is also observed in keratinocytes and dermal cells in DIF studies (Fig. 21.5c). In cryoglobulinemia, DIF reveals IgM, IgG, and complement deposition (Fig. 21.5d).

Pearl: Prolonged standing sometimes triggers a flare of cutaneous vasculitis in patients whose disease is not entirely controlled.

Comment: Purpura resolves more quickly with bed rest. This pressure-related phenomenon partly explains the most common distribution of purpura: over the dependent lower extremities and buttocks. Patients who have recently begun therapy for cutaneous vasculitis should be advised to avoid prolonged periods of standing, as this may cause new purpuric eruptions.

Pearl: Immunofluorescence studies of skin biopsies may yield a diagnosis of vasculitis even when H&E stains are nondiagnostic.

Comment: This is a sampling issue that is obvious to pathologists but not appreciated by many clinicians. The skin biopsy is divided and sent to separate laboratories for processing. One sample may contain diagnostic information that is absent in the other. Even if the H&E stain is nondiagnostic, the immunofluorescence study may demonstrate the characteristic immunoreactants within blood vessel walls (i.e., IgA).

Incidentally, the same phenomenon is true for other kinds of tissue biopsies. Kidney biopsy samples sent for H&E and immunofluorescence studies in renal disease may lack the all-important glomeruli, yet the electron microscopy study can reveal crescentic and necrotizing changes, findings that are critical to rendering the diagnosis.

Pearl: The immunopathogenesis of HSP involves IgA1, not IgA2.

Comment: IgA plays a pivotal role in the pathogenesis of HSP, even though the precise details surrounding the etiology of this disease remain unclear. There are two subclasses of IgA: IgA1 and IgA2. Only IgA1 is involved in the pathogenesis of HSP. The clinical manifestations of HSP are a consequence of deposition of IgA1 in vessel walls and the renal mesangium.

The reasons for the exclusive involvement of IgA1 in HSP are not known for certain. However, IgA1, unlike IgA2, contains a hinge region with multiple O-linked glycosylation sites. Two studies have demonstrated aberrant glycosylation of the hinge region of IgA1 in patients with HSP (Saulsbury 1997; Allen et al. 1998). IgA1 molecules with diminished glycosylation of the hinge region are prone to aggregate into macromolecular complexes have delayed clearance from the circulation, activate the alternative pathway of complement, and deposit in vessel walls and renal mesangium (Saulsbury 2001). Understanding the mechanisms of aberrant glycosylation of IgA1 may shed light on the fundamental cause of HSP.

21.3 Polyarteritis Nodosa

Myth: The outcome of polyarteritis nodosa (PAN) in childhood is poor.

Reality: Childhood PAN is a curable disease (as in PAN in adults [see polyarteritis nodosa]). In fact, a recent international study of 110 children with PAN showed that the prognosis in children compared favorably with that of adults reported in the literature. Relapses were rare following the induction of remission in children, and the overall mortality was only 1.1% (Ozen et al. 2004). Like March, PAN can come in like a lion, but if treated with prudent aggression it is subject to taming.

Pearl: Hepatitis B-related PAN is now vanishingly rare.

Comment: Thanks to the hepatitis B vaccine, this type of PAN has almost become an extinct disease in childhood. In an international registry of 110 PAN patients (Ozen et al. 2004), only 4.6% of the children had hepatitis B-related cases. In all of those patients, their diagnosis antedated the time when vaccination became mandatory.

Because hepatitis C virus (HCV) is usually mentioned in the same breath as hepatitis B, it is worth noting here that HCV-associated cryoglobulinemic vasculitis is also almost never encountered in children. This is probably because of the long latency observed between the acquisition of HCV infection and the appearance of cryoglobulinemic vasculitis in the minority of patients who develop that complication. By the time a pediatric patient has had HCV long enough to develop cryoglobulinemic vasculitis; the child has become an adult.

Myth: The American College of Rheumatology (ACR) classification criteria for Takayasu's arteritis (TA) cover the pediatric manifestations of this disease adequately.

Reality: An important hole in the ACR classification criteria is the failure to acknowledge that most childhood cases of TA present with hypertension (Golding et al. 1977; Ozen et al. 2007; Cakar et al. 2008). Hypertension, usually caused by the development of intra- or extra-renal arterial or arteriolar stenoses (Fig. 21.6), is not numbered among the ACR criteria, which were based principally upon adult cases. In contrast, the European League Against Rheumatism/Paediatric Rheumatology European Society criteria include hypertension as a feature (Ozen et al. 2006).

Pearl: Subglottic stenosis is more common among children with Wegener's granulomatosis (WG) than it is in adult patients.

Comment: Pediatric case series highlights the greater frequency of subglottic stenosis among children with WG (Rottem et al. 1993; Frosch and Foell 2004). In addition to subglottic stenoses, tracheal and endobronchial lesions are probably also more common in pediatric cases of WG. Subglottic, tracheal, and endobronchial stenoses comprise a

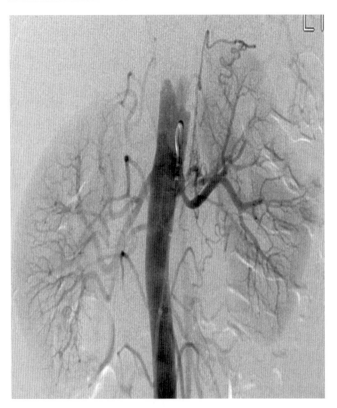

Fig. 21.6 Renal angiogram in a pediatric patient with Takayasu's arteritis. Several arteriolar stenosis in an intra-renal vessel has led to dramatic collateral circulation and high serum renin levels. Efforts to revascularize this patient's kidney through stent placements were not successful. The blood pressure was control effectively with an angiotensin converting enzyme inhibitor (Figure courtesy of Dr. John Stone)

Table 21.3 Consensus classification criteria for Wegener's granulomatosis in children[a]

Three of the following six features should be present:
Abnormal urinalysis[b]
Granulomatous inflammation on biopsy[c]
Nasal sinus inflammation
Subglottic, tracheal, or endobronchial stenosis
Abnormal chest radiograph or CT
PR3-ANCA[d] or C-ANCA staining

[a]European League Against Rheumatism/Paediatric Rheumatology European Society (adapted from Ozen 2006)
[b]Hematuria and/or significant proteinuria
[c]Kidney biopsy typically shows necrotizing pauci-immune glomerulonephritis
[d]ANCA: antineutrophil cytoplasmic antibodies

separate criterion in the EULAR/PReS classification criteria for WG (Table 21.3). A high index of suspicion is required for the diagnosis of all three of these types of lesions.

Myth: Cutaneous PAN is always at risk for progression to the systemic form of the disease.

Reality: Classic PAN can cause painful skin nodules and horrific cutaneous ulcerations, but within the universe of skin ulcers caused by medium-vessel vasculitis there are distinct disease entities. One of these is cutaneous PAN, a disorder that affects primarily the medium-sized arteries and muscular arterioles of the skin.

The progression of cutaneous PAN to a severe systemic form is unusual, and it is likely that cutaneous PAN is different from classic PAN from the start (Daoud et al. 1997; Kumar et al. 1995). Cutaneous PAN is characterized by a relapsing and remitting course that responds to glucocorticoids and other immunosuppressive agents, but tends to flare when the prednisone is discontinued or the dose tapered to a sufficiently low level. Cutaneous PAN has also been associated with streptococcal infections, albeit the precise relationship between this organism and at least some cases of the disease is not clear (Kumar et al. 1995; Ozen et al. 2004).

Patients with cutaneous PAN occasionally have musculoskeletal complaints in addition to skin ulcers. Some also have a sensory peripheral neuropathy, but the size and type of nerve fibers involved in this entity remain poorly defined. The potentially devastating sensorimotor mononeuritis multiplex that often complicates classic PAN is not characteristic of cutaneous PAN, and if present this finding puts the diagnosis squarely into the classic PAN basket.

Myth: PAN is more common in boys than in girls.

Reality: The origin of this myth is not clear, but it is a myth. Girls are equally likely to be affected by childhood PAN as are boys (1997; Ozen et al. 2004).

Pearl: Genetic associations have been defined in systemic vasculitis.

Comment: A number of genetic associations have been reported in systemic vasculitides, suggesting leads for further understanding of these complex genetic traits that certainly involve other factors (particularly environmental) in their pathogenesis. A study in ANCA associated vasculitis found an association between an IL-10 polymorphism (−1082) and ANCA-associated vasculitis (Bártfai et al. 2003). Disease susceptibility and clinical course in WG may be associated with polymorphisms in genes of certain cytokines and CTLA4 genes (Spriewald et al. 2005). In children with vasculitis and PAN, mutations in the MEFV gene have been reported as risk factors for the disease (Ozen et al. 2003; Yalçinkaya et al. 2007). In Kawasaki's disease, genetic variation in the gene of IL4 appears to play a role in disease susceptibility (Burns et al. 2005). The genetic epidemiology of the vasculitides remains a wide open field.

Myth: The vasculitis damage index can be applied readily to pediatric cases.

Reality: The vasculitis damage index has significant shortcomings, even in adult patients (Seo et al. 2007). Its use in children highlights additional shortcomings. For example, "growth failure" due to either the underlying disease or the effects of long-term glucocorticoids use is a major source of damage in children with vasculitis. Other items that are scored commonly in adults (e.g., myocardial infarction) almost never apply to children with vasculitis.

In short, children are not "just little adults." Their cases have distinct nuances that require special expertise in the interest of proper management. A new classification of childhood vasculitis is shown in Table 21.4.

Pearl: The von Willebrand factor antigen is a useful biomarker in small-vessel vasculitis in children.

Comment: Assays for the von Willebrand factor antigen are used most commonly for evaluating boys with a bleeding diathesis. This antigen is also an acute phase reactant that is released by both platelets and endothelial cells following cellular injury or death. Conditions such as small-vessel vasculitides (e.g., HSP, PAN, and microscopic polyangiitis) and microangiopathic disorders (dermatomyositis and systemic sclerosis) can be associated with von Willebrand levels that are elevated up to four times the upper limit of normal (Tse et al. 1998).

Elevated levels of von Willebrand factor antigen do not distinguish primary vasculitic disorders from those associated with vasculopathy, but serial measurements of the levels of this antigen may be helpful in tracking disease activity in individual patients.

Table 21.4 Classification scheme for pediatric vasculitis (adapted from Ozen (2006))

Predominantly large-vessel vasculitis
  Takayasu's arteritis
Predominantly medium-vessel vasculitis
  Childhood polyarteritis nodosa
  Cutaneous polyarteritis
  Kawasaki's disease
Predominantly small-vessel vasculitis
Granulomatous
  Wegener's granulomatosis
  Churg–Strauss syndrome
Non-granulomatous
  Microscopic polyangiitis
  HSP
  Isolated cutaneous leucocytoclastic vasculitis
  Hypocomplementemic urticarial vasculitis
Other vasculitides
  Behcet disease
  Vasculitis secondary to infection (including hepatitis B-associated polyarteritis nodosa), malignancies, and drugs, including hypersensitivity vasculitis
  Vasculitis associated with connective tissue diseases
  Isolated vasculitis of the central nervous system
  Cogan syndrome

References

Allen AC, Willis FR, Beattie TJ, et al Abnormal IgA glycosylation in Henoch–Schönlein purpura restricted to patients with clinical nephritis. Nephrol Dial Transplant. 1998;13:930–4

Amano S, Hazama F, Kubagawa H, et al General pathology of Kawasaki disease. Acta Pathol Jpn. 1980;30(5):681–94

Anderson MS, Burns J, Treadwell TA, et al Erythrocyte sedimentation rate and C-reactive protein discrepancy and high prevalence of coronary artery abnormalities in Kawasaki disease. Pediatr Infect Dis J. 2001;20(7):698–702

Bártfai Z, Gaede KI, Russell KA, et al Different gender-associated genotype risks of Wegener's granulomatosis and microscopic polyangiitis. Clin Immunol. 2003;109(3):330–7

Binstadt BA, Levine JC, Nigrovic PA, et al Coronary artery dilation among patients presenting with systemic-onset juvenile idiopathic arthritis. Pediatrics 2005;116:e89–93

Birchmore D, Sweeney C, Choudhury D, et al IgA multiple myeloma presenting as HSP/Polyarteritis nodosa overlap. Arthritis Rheum. 1996;39:698–703

Burns JC, Wiggins JW, Toews WH, et al Clinical spectrum of Kawasaki disease in infants younger than 6 months of age. J Pediatr. 1986;109:759–63

Burns JC, Mason WH, Glode MP, et al Clinical and epidemiologic characteristics of patients referred for evaluation of possible Kawasaki disease. United States Multicenter Kawasaki Disease Study Group. J Pediatr. 1991;118:680–6

Burns JC, Shimizu C, Shike H, et al Family-based association analysis implicates IL-4 in susceptibility to Kawasaki disease. Genes Immun. 2005;6(5):438–44

Cakar N, Yalcinkaya F, Duzova A, et al Takayasu arteritis in children. J Rheumatol. 2008;35(5):913–19

Centers for Disease Control. Haemophilus influenzae invasive disease among children age <5 years–California, 1990–1996. MMWR. 1998;47:737–40

Choong CK, Beasley SW. Intra-abdominal manifestations of Henoch-Schönlein purpura. J Paediatr Child Health. 1998;34:405–9

Daoud MS, Hutton KP, Gibson LE. Cutaneous periarteritis nodosa: a clinicopathological study of 79 cases. Br J Dermatol. 1997;136:706–13

Dengler LD, Capparelli EV, Bastian JF, et al Cerebrospinal fluid profile in patients with acute Kawasaki disease. Pediatr Infect Dis J. 1998;17:478–81

Frosch M, Foell D. Wegener granulomatosis in childhood and adolescence. Eur J Pediatr. 2004;163:425–34

Golding RL, Perri G, Cremin BJ. The arteriographic manifestations of Takayasu's arteritis in children. Pediatr Radiol. 1977;5:224–30

Goldstein AR, White RHR, Akuse R, et al Long-term follow-up of childhood Henoch-Schönlein nephritis. Lancet 1992;339:280–2

Holman RC, Belay ED, Curns AT, et al Kawasaki syndrome hospitalizations among children in the United States, 1988–1997. Pediatrics 2003;111:e448

Jurado RL. Why shouldn't we determine the erythrocyte sedimentation rate? Clin Infect Dis. 2001;33:548–9

Kumar L, Thapa BR, Sarkar B, Walia BN. Benign cutaneous PAN in children below 10 years of age: a clinical experience. Ann Rheum Dis. 1995;54:134–6

Landing BH, Larson EJ. Are infantile periarteritis nodosa with coronary artery involvement and fatal mucocutaneous lymph node syndrome the same? Comparison of 20 patients from North America with patients from Hawaii and Japan. Pediatrics 1977;59:651–62

Momenah T, Sanatani S, Potts J, et al Kawasaki disease in the older child. Pediatrics 1998;e102(1):e7

Muta H, Ishii M, Sakaue T, et al Older age is a risk factor for the development of cardiovascular sequelae in Kawasaki disease. Pediatrics 2004;114:751–4

Narchi H. Risk of long term renal impairment and duration of follow up recommended for Henoch–Schönlein purpura with normal or minimal urinary findings: a systematic review. Arch Dis Child. 2005;90:916–20

Newburger J, et al Diagnosis, treatment, and long-term management of Kawasaki disease: a statement for health professionals from the committee on rheumatic fever, endocarditis, and Kawasaki disease, council on cardiovascular disease in the young, Am Heart Assoc Pediatr. 2004a;114:1708–33

Newburger JW, Sanders SP, Burns JC, et al Left ventricular contractility and function in Kawasaki syndrome. Circulation 1989;79:1237–46

Newburger JW, Takahashi M, Gerber MA, et al Diagnosis, treatment, and long-term management of Kawasaki disease. Circulation 2004a;110:2747–71

Niwa K, Aotsuka H, Hamada H, et al Thrombocytopenia: a risk factor for acute myocardial infarction during the acute phase of Kawasaki Disease. Coron Artery Dis. 1995;6(11):857–64

Ozdogan H, Arisoy N, Kasapcapur O, et al Vasculitis in familial Mediterranean fever. J Rheumatol. 1997;24:323–7

Ozen S, Bakkaloglu A, Yilmaz E, Duzova A, Balci B, Topaloglu R, Besbas N. Mutations in the gene for familial Mediterranean fever: do they predispose to inflammation? J Rheumatol. 2003;30(9):2014–8

Ozen S, Anton J, Arisoy N, et al Juvenile polyarteritis: results of a multicenter survey of 110 children. J Pediatr. 2004;145:517–22

Ozen S, Ruperto N, Dillon MJ, et al EULAR/PReS endorsed consensus criteria for the classification of childhood vasculitides. Ann Rheum Dis. 2006;65:936–41

Ozen S, Duzova A, Bakkaloglu A, et al Takayasu arteritis in children: preliminary experience with cyclophosphamide induction and corticosteroids followed by methotrexate. J Pediatr. 2007;150:72–6

Ronkainen J, Nuutinen M, Koskimies O. The adult kidney 24 years after childhood Henoch–Schönlein purpura: a retrospective cohort study. Lancet 2002;360:666–70

Ronkainen J, Ala-Houhala M, Huttunen NP, et al Outcome of Henoch-Schoenlein nephritis with nephrotic-range proteinuria. Clin Nephrol. 2003;60:80–4

Ronkainen J, Koskimies O, Ala-Houhala M, et al Early prednisone therapy in Henoch–Schönlein purpura: a randomized, double-blind, placebo-controlled trial. J Pediatr. 2006;149:241–7

Rosenfeld EA, Corydon KE, Shulman ST. Kawasaki disease in infants less than one year of age. J Pediatr. 1995;126:524–49

Rottem M, Fauci AS, Hallahan CW, et al Wegener granulomatosis in children and adolescents: clinical presentation and outcome. J Pediatr. 1993;122(1):26–31

Saulsbury FT. Corticosteroid therapy does not prevent nephritis in Henoch–Schönlein purpura. Pediatr Nephrol. 1993;7:69–71

Saulsbury FT. Alterations in the O-linked glycosylation of IgA1 in children with Henoch–Schönlein purpura. J Rheumatol. 1997;24:2246–9

Saulsbury FT. Henoch–Schönlein purpura in children: report of 100 patients and review of the literature. Medicine 1999;78:395–409

Saulsbury FT. Henoch–Schönlein purpura. Curr Opin Rheumatol. 2001;13:35–40

Seo P, Luqmani R, Flossmann O, et al The future damage assessment in vasculitis. J Rheumatol. 2007;34:1357–71

Spriewald BM, Witzke O, Wassmuth R, et al Distinct tumour necrosis factor alpha, interferon gamma, interleukin 10, and cytotoxic T cell antigen 4 gene polymorphisms in disease occurrence and end stage renal disease in Wegener's granulomatosis. Ann Rheum Dis. 2005;64:457–61

Stamos JK, Corydon K, Donaldson J, Shulman ST. Lymphadenitis as the dominant manifestation of Kawasaki disease. Pediatrics 1994;93(3):525–8

Stockheim JA, Innocentini N, Shulman ST. Kawasaki disease in older children and adolescents. J Pediatr. 2000;137:250–2

Stone JH, Nousari HC. Essential cutaneous vasculitis: everything a rheumatologist needs to know about vasculitis of the skin. Curr Opin Rheumatol. 2001;13:23–34

Tanaka N, Sekimoto K, Naoe S. Kawasaki disease. Relationship with infantile periarteritis nodosa. Arch Pathol Lab Med. 1976;100:81–6

Trapani S, Micheli A, Grisolia F, et al Henoch–Schonlein purpura in childhood: epidemiological and clinical analysis of 150 cases over a 5-year period and review of the literature. Semin Arthritis Rheum. 2005;35:143–53

Tse WY, Cockwell P, Savage CO. Assessment of disease activity in systemic vasculitis. Postgrad Med J. 1998;74:1–6

Umezawa T, Saji T, Matsuo N, Odagiri K. Chest X-ray findings in the acute phase of Kawasaki disease. Pediatr Radiol. 1989;20(1–2):48–51

van Leeuwen MA, van Rijswijk MH. Acute phase proteins in the monitoring of inflammatory disorders. Baillieres Clin Rheumatol. 1994;8(3):531–52

Wickiser JE, Saulsbury FT. Henoch–Schönlein purpura in a child with hyperimmunoglobulinemia D and periodic fever syndrome. Pediatr Dermatol. 2005;22:138–41

Yalçinkaya F, Ozçakar ZB, Kasapçopur O, et al Prevalence of the MEFV gene mutations in childhood PAN. J Pediatr. 2007;151:675–8

Yanagawa H, Nakamura Y, Yashiro M, et al Incidence survey of Kawasaki disease in 1997 and 1998 in Japan. Pediatrics 2001; 107(3):e33

Behçet's Syndrome

Hasan Yazici and Yusuf Yazici

22

22.1 Disease Overview

> The prevalence of Behçet's syndrome is highest in countries of the eastern Mediterranean, the Middle East, and East Asia.

> Aphthous oral ulcers are usually the first and most persistent clinical feature of Behçet's syndrome. Aphthous ulcers also occur frequently on the genitals (e.g., the scrotum or vulva).

> Uveitis – most frequently a bilateral panuveitis is common in Behçet's syndrome. Eye disease constitutes a major source of morbidity.

> Many forms of central nervous system disease may occur in Behçet's syndrome. These include dural sinus thrombi and white matter lesions in the midbrain and brainstem. Unlike other vasculitides, however, peripheral nervous system disease is rare.

> HLA-B51 is a risk factor for Behçet's syndrome.

Myth: Behçet's syndrome is very rare.

Reality: This certainly is not so in Turkey, where the prevalence of the disorder is one in every 250 adults (Azizlerli et al. 2003). A recent survey from France showed that Behçet's syndrome is several times more common than Wegener's granulomatosis, microscopic polyangiitis, the Churg-Strauss syndrome, and polyarteritis nodosa (Mahr et al. 2004, 2008).

Although the diagnosis of Behçet's syndrome is probably more common in many geographic areas than generally believed, there appear to be important differences in the clinical expression of Behçet's syndrome across different regions. In general, the severity of Behçet's syndrome is lower in regions where the disease is least prevalent (e.g., in the United States and Western Europe). For example, among 300 patients collected in New York City, a region of low prevalence when compared to Turkey, no patients with complete visual loss secondary to Behçet's syndrome were observed (Yazici and Moses 2007). Mild disease was also the

rule among a cohort of patients reported from northern Italy (Pipitone et al. 2004).

Myth: Neutrophil hypermotility is a cardinal characteristic of Behçet's syndrome.

Reality: Neutrophil hypermotility is often referred to as a central feature in the pathogenesis of Behçet's syndrome. Statements about the importance of neutrophil hypermotility are usually accompanied by assertions that colchicine achieves its effectiveness through the inhibition of neutrophil motility.

In fact, there is little evidence that any of this is true. We are not aware of any studies that demonstrate greater neutrophil motility in Behçet's syndrome when compared with other inflammatory conditions. On the contrary, one controlled study revealed no such differences in a study of Behçet's syndrome and other disorders (Tüzün et al. 1999). Moreover, colchicine has rather limited utility in the treatment of Behçet's syndrome.

Myth: Colchicine is an effective agent for the treatment of oral ulcers in Behçet's disease.

Reality: Colchicine remains one of the most widely used medications for the treatment of Behçet's syndrome, yet, objective data do not suggest tremendous efficacy for this drug. Neither of the two randomized, controlled trials of this agent in Behçet's syndrome demonstrated efficacy for the treatment of oral ulcers (Aktulga et al. 1980; Yurdakul et al. 2001). Although one trial reported efficacy for colchicine in the management of genital ulcers, this effect was observed only in female patients (Yurdakul et al. 2001).

In short, the putative efficacy of colchicine in Behçet's syndrome is significantly overblown. Patients tend to tolerate the drug well, but clinicians should not delay long before moving on to another strategy if the positive effects of colchicine are slow in appearing.

Myth: Behçet's syndrome is a form of spondyloarthropathy.

Reality: The origin of this Myth stems from the early 1970s, when the newly described HLA-B27 antigen was believed to be the seat of the soul of many rheumatic conditions. Behçet's syndrome was classified as a seronegative spondyloarthropathy

J. H. Stone (ed.), *A Clinician's Pearls and Myths in Rheumatology,*
DOI:10.1007/978-1-84800-934-9_22, © Springer Science + Business Media B.V. 2009

because of certain characteristics that were reminiscent of ankylosing spondylitis, reactive arthritis, and other HLA-B27-associated conditions: e.g., uveitis, oral and genital ulcers, and oligoarthritis. Although additional investigations demonstrated that sacroiliitis is not a part of the spectrum of Behçet's syndrome and that the strong HLA association for this disorder is with B51 rather than B27, the notion that Behçet's syndrome is a form of spondyloarthropathy has somehow persisted in the minds of some.

Behçet's syndrome and seronegative spondyloarthropathies belong to separate kettles, but there is an additional disease manifestation that these conditions sometimes share: enthesopathy. The finding of enthesopathy in Behçet's syndrome tends to cluster in patients who have both acne and arthritis (Tunc et al. 2002; Hatemi et al. 2008).

Pearl: Behçet's syndrome is not a "connective tissue disorder".

Reality: Although non-rheumatologists frequently tar Behçet's syndrome with the same brush as they do systemic lupus erythematosus, rheumatoid arthritis, and scleroderma, the fundamental differences exist between Behçet's syndrome and the other rheumatic conditions. They share little, other than the need for the involvement of a rheumatologist in their care.

Behçet's syndrome differs from the classic "connective tissue disorders" in several respects. For example, it is often especially helpful to remember that:

- Behçet's syndrome is not associated with either Raynaud's phenomenon or digital ulceration.
- Behçet's syndrome is not associated with secondary Sjögren's syndrome (Günaydin et al. 1994).
- Behçet's syndrome is often complicated by unique eye findings, genital ulcerations, and papulopustular lesions that occur beyond the sites where acne is usually found (e.g., the buttocks) (Fig. 22.1) (Hatemi et al. 2004).
- Behçet's syndrome tends to be more severe in men. This marks a noticeable departure from the pattern of disease generally observed in connective tissue diseases such as lupus.
- Behçet's syndrome does not appear to carry a long-term risk of atherosclerosis development. The frequency of coronary calcifications, atherosclerotic plaques, angina pectoris, and myocardial infarction are not increased in Behçet's syndrome (Kural-Seyahi et al. 2003; Seyahi 2004; Urgurlu 2008).

Myth: Behçet's syndrome is an "autoinflammatory disorder (Yazici and Fresko 2005)".

Reality: Behçet's syndrome is an idiopathic inflammatory condition, but differs substantially from the emerging group of diseases with which it is sometimes lumped, known as the autoinflammatory disorders (see Chap. 45). The major

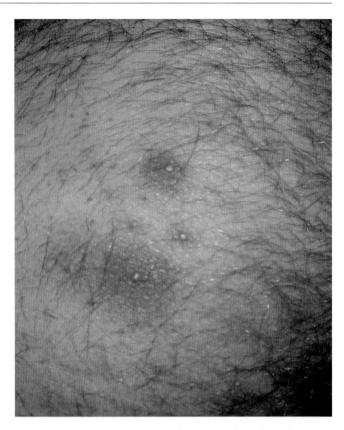

Fig. 22.1 Papulopustular lesions on the buttocks of a patient with Behçet's syndrome. Acneiform lesions tend to occur in unusual areas in patients with Behçet's syndrome

Table 22.1 Differences between autoinflammatory diseases and Behçet's syndrome

	Autoinflammatory diseases	Behçet's syndrome
Age group affected	Pediatric	Adult
Areas of highest prevalence	Mostly Europe and North America	Silk Route
Monogenic heritability	Yes	No
Relapsing fever	Very common	Very rare
Disease course	Relentless unless treated	Abates in time

differences between Behçet's syndrome and autoinflammatory disorders are shown in Table 22.1.

Particular links have been drawn between Behçet's syndrome and the hyper IgD syndrome (Sakane et al. 1999). In fact, IgD levels are not elevated in Behçet's syndrome (Brezniak et al. 1998).

Myth: All clinical manifestations of Behçet's syndrome are caused by vasculitis.

Reality: Many Behçet's syndrome lesions are associated with perivascular inflammation in the absence of true vascular wall destruction. Examples of such manifestations are the oral ulcers, genital lesions, and brain findings (Hirohata 2008). Acne lesions and their associated pustules have also been considered to represent cutaneous vasculitis, but it is now known that they are indistinguishable histopathologically from acne vulgaris (Ergun et al. 1998).

Tissue biopsies in Behçet's syndrome generally yield no pathological findings that are pathognomonic of that condition. Clinicians must bear in mind that unless there are compelling reasons for biopsy to exclude other disorders, the diagnosis of Behçet's syndrome usually rests upon its clinical features alone.

Myth: The pustules of Behçet's syndrome are sterile.

Reality: Bacteria are present in the cultures of pustules in Behçet's syndrome patients, just as they are in acne vulgaris (Hatemi et al. 2004). However, the bacteriology of Behçet's syndrome differs from that of acne vulgaris. *Staphylococcus aureus*, common in the lesions of Behçet's syndrome, is unusual in acne vulgaris.

Knowledge of the bacteriology of non-pustular lesions in Behçet's syndrome remains poorly described. Impairments of innate immunity may explain some of the findings within the acne pustules associated with Behçet's syndrome, including *Staphylococcus aureus* growth. One piece of evidence supporting defects in innate immunity is the fact that decreased mannose binding lectin levels (MBL) correlate with more severe Behçet's syndrome (Inanc et al. 2005). MBL plays an important role in complement activation and the opsonization of pathogens. Deficiency in this molecule heightens a person's susceptibility to infection.

Myth: The diagnosis of Behçet's syndrome is untenable without a history of oral ulcers.

Reality: Oral ulcers are often viewed as a sine qua non of Behçet's syndrome. Although oral ulcers occur in the overwhelming majority of Behçet's patients, there is a small subset that has classic disease features in every other way but do not manifest oral ulcers.

During the development of the International Study Group's 1990 classification criteria (International Study Group 1990), 28 such patients were identified among the 914 patients included in the study. Thus, 3% of patients diagnosed by Behçet's syndrome experts as having that disorder did not have oral ulcers. At times, some of those patients developed the classic oral lesions, but others remained ulcer-free even as other manifestations of Behçet's syndrome persisted or recurred.

Myth: Tender red lesions that occur on the lower extremities in Behçet's syndrome are inevitably erythema nodosum.

Reality: Erythema nodosum (EN), a septal panniculitis, does occur in Behçet's syndrome and presents as it does in other

conditions with tender, nodular lesions. However, the EN of Behçet's syndrome bears some important differences to that observed, for example, in sarcoidosis and inflammatory bowel disease. The following major distinctions can be drawn:

- Many EN lesions in Behçet's syndrome are accompanied by a medium-vessel vasculitis. Vasculitis is not a component of the EN found in sarcoidosis and inflammatory bowel disease.
- Permanent pigmentation of the overlying skin can complicate the EN associated with Behçet's syndrome. This finding is reminiscent of the hyperpigmentation that occurs frequently following the resolution of medium-vessel vasculitides involving the skin (e.g., polyarteritis nodosa; Fig. 22.2).

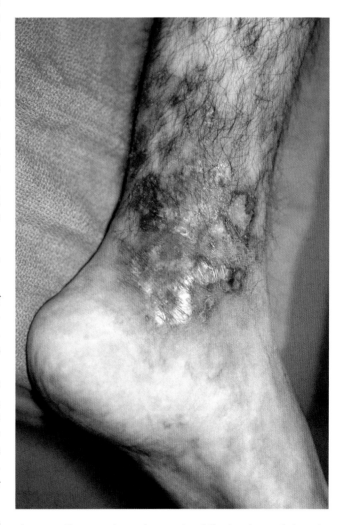

Fig. 22.2 Cutaneous hyperpigmentation following the resolution of a medium-vessel vasculitis (in this case, polyarteritis nodosa). The same phenomenon can be observed in cases of erythema nodosum that occur in Behçet's syndrome, because these lesions are often associated with a medium-vessel vasculitis

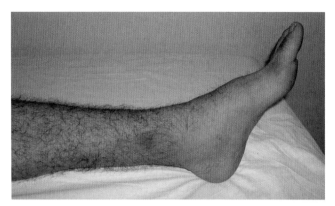

Fig. 22.3 Superficial thrombophlebitis in a patient with Behçet's syndrome. Biopsy may be required to distinguish this lesion from erythema nodosum

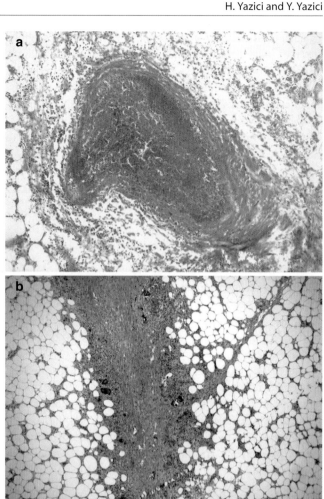

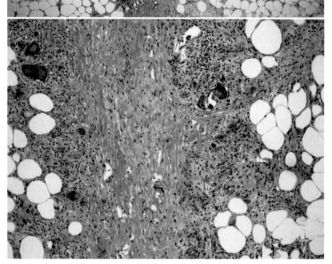

Superficial thrombophlebitis (STP) is another important cause of painful red lesions in Behçet's syndrome (Fig. 22.3). STP is observed much more commonly among men with Behçet's syndrome. In contrast, EN lesions are more common among female patients. Making the distinction between EN and STP is important, because STP is associated with a different subset of severe disease manifestations, e.g., inflammation within large veins that can lead to intraluminal thrombosis (Tunc 2002). In many instances, a biopsy is required for differential diagnosis (Fig. 22.4a, b).

Myth: Behçet's syndrome is an unrelenting disorder that generally leads to blindness among patients with ocular involvement.

Reality: Several decades ago, uveitis of Behçet's syndrome had an extremely poor prognosis, particularly if the process was advanced at the time of diagnosis. Although posterior uveitis still poses significant challenges in therapy, its prognosis is not inevitably dire. Tumor necrosis factor inhibitors and interferon-alpha have both found important niches in the treatment of ocular Behçet's syndrome.

Pearl: Males with Behçet's syndrome tend to have a more severe disorder than females with the disease.

Comment: Disease-related mortality is significantly higher among males than females. Ocular disease is particularly severe in male patients. Differences in the expression of Behçet's syndrome according to sex are summarized in Table 22.2.

In contrast to the typically more severe disease in male patients, Behçet's syndrome is often a mild condition among women and the elderly. Moreover, in many patients, the disease goes into complete remission with the passage of time (Kural-Seyahi et al. 2003).

Pearl: Genital ulcers in male patients with Behçet's syndrome are usually found on the scrotum.

Fig. 22.4 Histology of superficial thrombophlebitis (**a**) and erythema nodosum lesions (**b**) (**a**). An intraluminal thrombus (**b**). Septal panniculitis. Also see Fig. 22.2

Comment: This feature helps distinguish the ulcers of Behçet's syndrome from those of reactive arthritis and venereal diseases, which tend to occur on the penis. In female patients with Behçet's syndrome, genital ulcers usually occur on the

Table 22.2 Sex differences in the disease phenotype of Behçet's syndrome

	Same frequency in males and females	More common among men	More common among women
Oral ulceration, genital ulceration and arthritis	+		
Erthema nodosum			+
Superficial thrombophlebitis		++	
Eye disease		++	
Unilateral eye disease			+
Pulmonary artery aneurysms		++++	
Venous disease		++	
Peripheral arterial disease		+++	
Central nervous system disease		++	

labia – the embryological equivalent of the scrotum in men. Another helpful point in sorting through the differential diagnosis of genital lesions is that the scrotal ulcers of Behçet's syndrome usually leave scars (Fig. 22.5). Urethritis is also uncommon in Behçet's syndrome and suggests either a sexually-transmitted disease or a complication of reactive arthritis.

Pearl: Intermittent claudication can be a feature of Behçet's syndrome, but the mechanism appears to be independent of atherosclerosis.

Comment: Intermittent claudication is observed in patients with peripheral venous disease rather than arterial involvement (Ugurlu et al. 2008). It is thought to be due to severe venous outflow impairment, but the precise mechanism remains unclear.

Pearl: If a Behçet's syndrome patient presents with hemoptysis, aneurysms of the pulmonary artery must be excluded.

Comment: Pulmonary arterial aneurysms comprise the most deadly complication of this condition (Fig. 22.6). They normally present with hemoptysis, and in the absence of aggressive therapy (typically involving cyclophosphamide), the 1-year patient mortality associated with this complication is in the order of 50% (Hamuryudan et al. 2004).

Pulmonary arterial aneurysms are associated with thrombosis of the big veins, i.e. vena cavae, in 80% of the cases. The so-called "Hughes-Stovin syndrome", which consists of aneurysms of the pulmonary artery in the absence of other stigmata of Behçet's syndrome, probably represents an incomplete form of Behçet's syndrome (Erkan et al. 2004).

Pearl: Parenchymal lung disease can also occur in Behçet's syndrome.

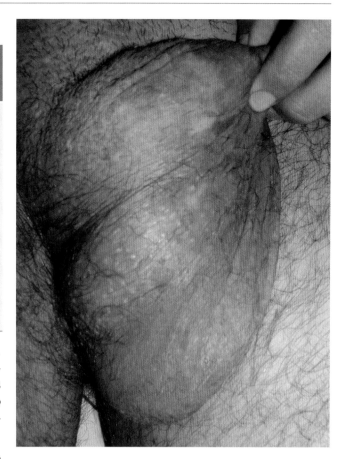

Fig. 22.5 Scars on the scrotum of a patient with Behçet's syndrome, occurring at the sites of previous genital ulcers

Comment: Some Behçet's syndrome patients develop nodular pulmonary lesions that have a tendency to cavitate. These nodules may be seen independently of pulmonary artery aneurysms. Such lesions, often seen in association with pulmonary arterial aneurysms, are often mistaken for opportunistic infections (see Fig. 22.6). They can also create diagnostic confusion vis-à-vis Wegener's granulomatosis.

Myth: Behçet's syndrome patients who suffer deep venous thromboses should be anti-coagulated for life.

Reality: The optimal management of deep venous thromboses in Behçet's syndrome remains a source of debate. Indeed, it is not clear whether patients who develop deep venous thrombosis require anti-coagulation at all. Deep venous thromboses in Behçet's syndrome are believed to result from vascular inflammation rather than from a hypercoagulable tendency per se. In addition, deep venous clots that occur in Behçet's syndrome are believed to adhere tightly to the blood vessel wall. Thus, embolization is rare. Although there remains little data to support this practice, the general approach to the management of deep venous thrombosis in Behçet's syndrome is to intensify immunosuppression rather than to begin anti-coagulation.

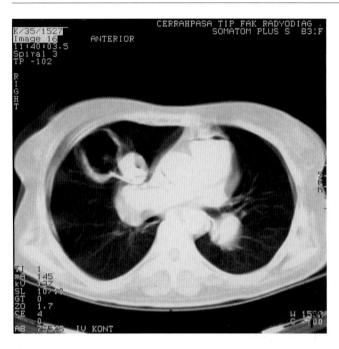

Fig. 22.6 Cavitating pulmonary artery aneurysms

Myth: Behçet's syndrome patients with thrombophlebitis should be anti-coagulated until the acute event is resolved.

Reality: There is also a debate about the optimal management of thrombophlebitis in Behçet's syndrome. Formal data showing that anti-coagulation is not useful are sparse (Kahraman et al. 2003; Ahn et al. 2008). Superficial thrombophlebitis in Behçet's syndrome is often associated with pulmonary arterial aneurysms, and anti-coagulation in this setting can lead to catastrophic bleeding events. If anti-coagulation is contemplated for a patient with superficial thrombophlebitis, it seems prudent to perform computed tomography scans of the chest to exclude pulmonary artery aneurysms first. Most Behçet's syndrome experts do not anti-coagulate patients with superficial thrombophlebitis, but rather employ immunosuppressive agents such as azathioprine along with brief courses of glucocorticoids for treatment.

Pearl: Azathioprine is frequently underdosed in the treatment of Behçet's syndrome.

Comment: Azathioprine has salutary effects on the course of Behçet's syndrome, but is frequently administered in doses that are too low. Azathioprine decreases the frequency of hypopyon uveitis attacks; the development of new eye disease; the occurrence of new genital ulcers; arthritis; and the likelihood of thrombophlebitis (Hatemi et al. 2008).

Despite its potential efficacy in Behçet's syndrome, azathioprine is frequently dosed in regimens that are too low to be effective. Doses approaching 2.5 mg/kg/day should be employed in Behçet's syndrome before concluding that the medication is

ineffective (Yazici et al. 1990; Hamuryudan et al. 1997). Guidelines on the use of azathioprine and the importance of testing for thiopurine methyltransferase alleles are discussed elsewhere (see ANCA-associated vasculitis Chap. 24).

Pearl: Azathioprine should not be employed together with interferon-alpha.

Comment: Interferon-alpha has a number of potential uses in Behçet's syndrome. However, the use of interferon-alpha is frequently associated with leukopenia. Because of the possibility of a synergistic effect on bone marrow suppression, interferon-alpha and azathioprine should not be employed together.

Pearl: Although multiple sclerosis shares the tendency of Behçet's syndrome to involve the central nervous system white matter, distinguishing these two conditions is usually straightforward.

Comment: The following points are useful in distinguishing between multiple sclerosis and Behçet's syndrome:

- Sensory symptoms are common in multiple sclerosis but extremely rare in Behçet's syndrome.
- Optic neuritis and spinal involvement are also uncommon in Behçet's syndrome, but occur frequently in multiple sclerosis.
- On neuroimaging, multiple sclerosis lesions tend to occur in a periventricular distribution (Fig. 22.7a). In contrast, the typical brain lesions of Behçet's syndrome have a subcortical location and extend into the midbrain and brainstem (Fig. 22.7b).
- Brainstem lesions in multiple sclerosis are usually small. In contrast, both brainstem and cerebellar atrophy are often prominent in chronic Behçet's syndrome.
- An inflammatory cerebrospinal fluid strongly favors Behçet's syndrome (Siva and Yazici 2004).

Pearl: If vasculitic neuropathy is present, the diagnosis is probably not Behçet's syndrome.

Comment: Although Behçet's syndrome has a predilection for the nervous system, it rarely involves the peripheral nervous system. This helps considerably in differentiating Behçet's syndrome from other primary forms of vasculitis, e.g., polyarteritis nodosa, microscopic polyangiitis, or Wegener's granulomatosis.

Pearl: Clusters of clinical manifestations are observed to occur among individual patients in Behçet's syndrome.

Comment: Three studies have confirmed the high frequency with which acne, arthritis, and enthesopathy occur together in Behçet's syndrome (Tunc 2002; Diri et al. 2001 Hetami 2008). A second recognized clinical cluster is the association of superficial and deep vein thrombosis, with the

Figs. 22.7 Contrasting magnetic resonance imaging features in multiple sclerosis (**a**) and Behçet's syndrome (**b**). (**a**). Multiple periventricular, T2 hyperintense white matter lesions in a patient with multiple sclerosis. (**b**). A single lesion starting at basal ganglia and extending into the midbrain in a patient with Behçet's syndrome. Widespread central nervous system lesions can also occur (Figures courtesy of Professor S. Saip)

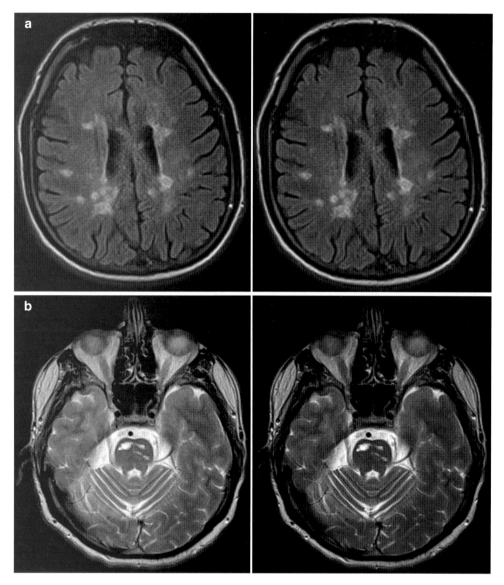

development of dural sinus thrombi (Tunc et al. 2004). A third possible cluster is that of the presence of antibodies to anti-saccharomyces, a hallmark of Crohn's disease, only among those patients with gut disease (Fresko et al. 2005).

Apart from their obvious clinical implications, the presence of such clusters suggests that there might be more than one disease mechanism in Behçet's syndrome and hence, the designation "syndrome" is more appropriate than "disease".

References

Ahn JK, Lee YS, Jeon CH, et al. Treatment of venous thrombosis associated with Behçet's disease: Immunosuppressive therapy alone versus immunosuppressive therapy plus anticoagulation. Clin Rheumatol 2008; 27:201–205

Aktulga E, Altac M, Muftuoglu A, et al A double blind study of colchicine in Behçet's disease. Haematologica 1980; 65:399–402

Azizlerli G, Kose AA, Sarica R, et al Prevalence of Behçet's disease in Istanbul, Turkey. Int J Dermatol 2003; 42:803–806

Brezniak N, Shtrasburg S, Langevitz P, et al Serum IgD as a discriminator between the two periodic febrile syndromes hyperimmunoglobulinaemia D syndrome and Behçet's disease. Ann Rheum Dis 1998; 57:255–256

Diri E, Mat C, Hamuryudan V, et al Papulopustular skin lesions are seen more frequently in patients with Behçet's syndrome who have arthritis: A controlled and masked study. Ann Rheum Dis 2001; 60:1074–1076

Ergun T, Gurbuz O, Dogusoy G, et al Histopathologic features of the spontaneous pustular lesions of Behçet's syndrome. Int J Dermatol 1998; 37:194–196

Erkan D, Yazici Y, Sanders A, et al Is Hughes-Stovin syndrome Behçet's disease? Clin Exp Rheumatol 2004; 22(4 Suppl 34):S64–S68

Fresko I, Ugurlu S, Ozbakir F, et al Anti-Saccharomyces cerevisiae antibodies (ASCA) in Behçet's syndrome. Clin Exp Rheumatol 2005; 23(4 Suppl 38):S67–S70

Günaydin I, Ustündağ C, Kaner G, et al The prevalence of Sjögren's syndrome in Behçet's syndrome. J Rheumatol 1994; 21:1662–1664

Hamuryudan V, Ozyazgan Y, Hizli N, et al Azathioprine in Behçet's syndrome: Effects on long-term prognosis. Arthritis Rheum 1997; 40:769–774

Hamuryudan V, Er T, Seyahi E, et al Pulmonary artery aneurysms in Behçet syndrome. Am J Med 2004; 117:867–870

Hatemi G, Bahar H, Uysal S, et al The pustular skin lesions in Behçet's syndrome are not sterile. Ann Rheum Dis 2004; 63:1450–1452

Hatemi G, Fresko I, Tascilar K, et al Increased enthesopathy among Behçet's syndrome patients with acne and arthritis: An ultrasonography study. Arthritis Rheum 2008; 58:1539–1545

Hirohata S. Histopathology of central nervous system lesions in Behçet's disease. J Neurol Sci 2008; 267:1–2

Inanc N, Mumcu G, Birtas E, et al Serum mannose-binding lectin levels are decreased in Behçet's disease and associated with disease severity. J Rheumatol 2005; 32:287–291

International Study Group for Behcet's disease. Criteria for diagnosis of Behcet's disease. Lancet 1990; 335:1078–1080

Kahraman O, Celebi-Onder S, Kamali S, et al Long-term course of deep venous thrombosis in patients with Behçet's disease. Arthritis Rheum 2003; 48 (Suppl):S385

Kural-Seyahi E, Fresko I, Seyahi, et al The long-term mortality and morbidity of Behçet syndrome: AN 2-decade outcome survey of 387 patients followed at a dedicated center. Medicine (Baltimore) 2003; 82:60–76

Mahr A, Guillevin L, Poissonnet M, et al Prevalences of polyarteritis nodosa, microscopic polyangiitis, Wegener's granulomatosis, and Churg-Strauss syndrome in a French urban multiethnic population in 2000: A capture-recapture estimate. Arthritis Rheum 2004; 51:92–99

Mahr A, Belarbi L, Wechsler W, et al Population-based study of Behçet's disease: Differences by ethnic origin and low variation by age at migration. Arthritis Rheum 2008; 58:3951-9 (in press)

Pipitone N, Boiardi L, Olivieri, et al Clinical manifestations of Behçet's disease in 137 Italian patients: Results of a multicenter study. Clin Exp Rheumatol 2004; 22(Suppl 36):S46–S51

Seyahi E, Memisoglu E, Hamuryudan, et al Coronary atherosclerosis in Behçet's syndrome: A pilot study using electron-beam computed tomography. Rheumatology (Oxford) 2004; 43: 1448–1450

Sakane T, Takeno M, Suzuki N, et al Behçet's disease. N Engl J Med 1999; 341:1284–1291. Arthritis Rheum 2008 (in press)

Siva A, Yazici H. Behcet's Disease. In: Levine S, Doruk E (eds) Handbook of systemic autoimmune diseases, neurology volume [The Neurologic Involvement in Systemic Autoimmune Disorders]. New York, Elsevier Science, 2004, pp. 193–216

Tunc R, Keyman E, Melikoglu M, et al Target organ associations in Turkish patients with Behçet's disease: A cross sectional study by exploratory factor analysis. J Rheumatol 2002; 29: 2393–2396

Tunc R, Saip S, Siva A, et al Cerebral venous thrombosis is associated with major vessel disease in Behçet's syndrome. Ann Rheum Dis 2004; 63:1693–1694

Tüzün B, Tüzün Y, Yurdakul, et al Neutrophil chemotaxis in Behçet's syndrome. Ann Rheum Dis 1999; 58:658

Ugurlu S, Seyahi E, Yazici H. Prevalence of angina, myocardial infarction and intermittent claudication assessed by Rose Questionnaire among patients with Behçet's syndrome. Rheumatology (Oxford) 2008; 47(4):472–475

Yazici Y, Moses N. Clinical manifestations and ethnic background of patients with Behçet's syndrome in a US cohort. Arthritis Rheum 2007; 56:S502

Yazici H, Pazarli H, Barnes CG, et al A controlled trial of azathioprine in Behçet's syndrome. N Engl J Med 1990; 322: 281–285

Yurdakul S, Mat C, Tuzun Y, et al. Double-blind trial of colchicine in Behçet's syndrome. Arthritis Rheum 2001; 44:2686–2692

The Churg–Strauss Syndrome

23

Andrew Churg, Ulrich Specks, and John H. Stone

23.1 Overview of the Churg–Strauss Syndrome

> The Churg–Strauss Syndrome (CSS) is a form of necrotizing vasculitis characterized by eosinophilic infiltration of small- and medium-sized blood vessels.

> The initial disease manifestation is usually the development of asthma in an individual who did not suffer previously from reactive airway disease. Allergic rhinitis is another manifestation of atopy, often identified in retrospect as the first sign of CSS.

> The extra-pulmonary organs commonly involved in the CSS are the peripheral nerves, skin, joints, and heart. The brain, eyes, gastrointestinal tract, and kidneys are involved less often.

> Vasculitic neuropathy occurs in 80% of patients with CSS and can lead to devastating complications through paralysis of the distal extremities. Nerve infarctions generally lead to an asymmetric, axonal sensorimotor neuropathy.

> The clinical features of CSS overlap in many ways on those of two other forms of necrotizing vasculitis, Wegener's granulomatosis, and microscopic polyangiitis. However, patients with CSS are less likely to have antineutrophil cytoplasmic antibodies (ANCA) than those with other conditions.

> When patients with CSS are ANCA-positive, the antigen specificity is directed more often against myeloperoxidase than against serine proteinase-3. Anti-myeloperoxidase ANCA produces a perinuclear ("P-ANCA") pattern of staining in immunofluorescence studies of serum.

> CSS must be distinguished from a group of non-vasculitic conditions associated with hypereosinophilia. Among these are the hypereosinophil syndrome, eosinophilic leukemia, eosinophilic fasciitis, and parasitic infections.

Pearl: CSS tends to unfold in three stages.

Comment: It is often possible to recognize three distinct phases of CSS (Lanham et al. 1984):

• A prodromal phase characterized by allergic disease (typically asthma or allergic rhinitis). This phase may last from months to many years.

• An eosinophilia/tissue infiltration phase, in which remarkably high peripheral eosinophilia may occur and tissue infiltration by eosinophils is observed in the lung, gastrointestinal tract, and other tissues.

• A vasculitic phase, in which systemic vasculitis afflicts a wide range of organs, ranging from the heart and lungs to the peripheral nerves and skin.

With the onset of the vasculitic phase of CSS, patients' asthma may improve substantially, even before therapy for vasculitis is begun.

Myth: CSS requires the combination of three histopathologic findings for confirmation of the diagnosis: vasculitis, granulomas, and eosinophils in the tissue.

Reality: CSS granulomas were present in all patients reported in the original case series published in 1951 (Churg and Strauss 1951). However, this publication preceded the widespread availability of glucocorticoids. Glucocorticoid therapy has altered both the clinical and histopathological presentation of CSS: fewer than half of the cases in which the diagnosis is confirmed by either tissue biopsy or autopsy have granulomas (Lanham et al. 1984).

In the early phase of CSS, tissue biopsies often reveal eosinophilic infiltration but neither granulomas nor vasculitis (Churg 2005). The absence of histopathological evidence of vasculitis correlates with a good response to treatment.

Myth: Necrotizing vasculitis on biopsy is the sine qua non of CSS.

Reality: The morphologic appearance of vasculitis in CSS is highly variable. Some cases demonstrate necrotizing vasculitis

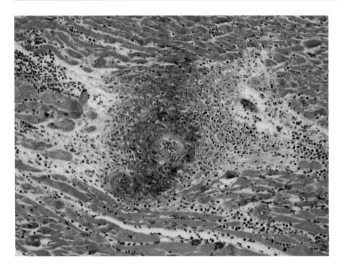

Fig. 23.1 Classic necrotizing vasculitis in the heart in a fatal case of the Churg–Strauss syndrome. Note the eosinophils infiltrating the tissue (Figure courtesy of Dr. Andrew Churg)

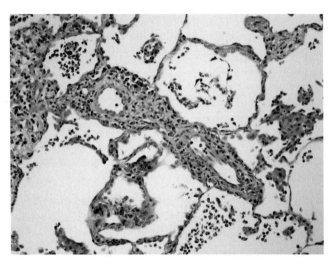

Fig. 23.2 Non-necrotizing vasculitis in a small vessel in the lung in the Churg–Strauss syndrome. Collections of eosinophils are also present in the airspaces (the biopsy has caught the edge of an eosinophilic pneumonia-like area) (Figure courtesy of Dr. Andrew Churg)

(Fig. 23.1), but others document only the infiltration of eosinophils into the vascular walls (Fig. 23.2). In a large series of patients from France, only half of the cases proved histopathologically had necrotizing vasculitis (Guillevin et al. 1999). Insistence on the presence of necrotizing vasculitis for the label of CSS leads to under-diagnosis.

Myth: CSS is caused by the use of leukotriene inhibitors.

Reality: This Myth, approximately as old as leukotriene inhibitors themselves, is a classic case of confounding by indication. Leukotrienes are highly effective asthma medications and permit the taper of prednisone in glucocorticoid-dependent asthma. The majority of patients with CSS have asthma as their presenting feature and are usually misdiagnosed

initially as having simple reactive airway disease. Leukotriene inhibitors often permit the tapering of prednisone and, in a minority of patients with "asthma", to the unmasking of CSS (Wechsler et al. 2000).

CSS-related vasculitis recurs in only about 25% of all patients. Unfortunately, after the vasculitic phase of CSS has been treated effectively, most CSS patients are left with glucocorticoid-dependent asthma and are unable to taper their prednisone below 8 mg/day (Pagnoux et al. 2007). Managing this refractory reactive airway disease is a major challenge in caring for CSS patients over the long-term. Some clinicians who are also experienced in the care of CSS patients are sufficiently comfortable with the fact that leukotriene inhibitors do not cause the disease, and they actually use these agents to treat glucocorticoid-dependent asthma of CSS (Keogh and Specks 2003).

Pearl: CSS often involves lymphadenopathy.

Comment: Godman and Churg noted that CSS, Wegener's granulomatosis, and microscopic polyangiitis are linked (Godman and Churg 1954). These three diseases, observed those investigators, "group themselves into a compass, (ranging from) necrotizing and granulomatous processes with angiitis to vasculitis without granulomata" (with mixed forms in between). These disorders share intriguing similarities, but also have features that mark them individually.

One interesting difference between CSS and the other forms of ANCA-associated vasculitis is the frequency with which CSS is associated with lymphadenopathy (Churg 2001), which is rarely a feature of either WG or MPA. CSS can also cause striking salivary gland enlargement (Boin et al. 2006).

Myth: CSS is an "ANCA-associated vasculitis".

Reality: Despite the undeniable connections between CSS, Wegener's granulomatosis, and microscopic polyangiitis, a substantial percentage of CSS patients – more than 50% in some studies – are ANCA negative (Guillevin et al. 1999). To some extent, the ANCA status of CSS patients may depend on when the testing is performed during the course of therapy (Keogh and Specks 2003), but in general, it seems that CSS patients are significantly less likely to be ANCA positive than those with WG or MPA. ANCA negativity should not dissuade one from the diagnosis of CSS if other clinical findings fit.

The presence or absence of ANCA may also influence clinical phenotype in CSS, but the literature is mixed on this point. In one study (Keogh and Specks 2003), central nervous system involvement was more common among ANCA-positive patients (20 vs. 5%). In another (Sablé-Fourtassou et al. 2005), ANCA-positive patients were significantly more likely to have glomerulonephritis and neurologic disease, but ANCA-negative patients were more likely to have cardiac involvement. ANCA

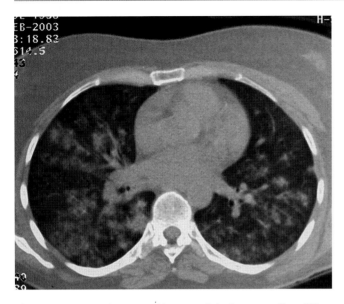

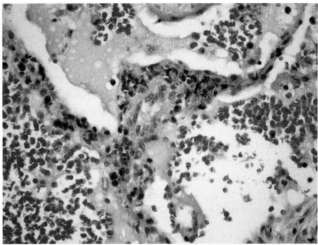

Fig. 23.4 Capillaritis in the Churg–Strauss syndrome, associated with hemorrhage. In this example, there is not only infiltration of the alveolar walls by eosinophils, but considerable eosinophil degranulation as well (Figure courtesy of Dr. Andrew Churg)

Fig. 23.3 Computed tomographic scan of the lung revealing diffuse pulmonary infiltrates caused by alveolar hemorrhage in a patient with the Churg–Strauss syndrome (Figure courtesy of Dr. John H. Stone)

status did not appear to affect either mortality or the likelihood of relapse.

Myth: Pulmonary capillaritis and diffuse alveolar hemorrhage do not occur in CSS.

Reality: The frequency with which pulmonary capillaritis and lung hemorrhage occur in CSS is a point of some contention. These complications have been documented to occur in CSS (Fig. 23.3), but they are substantially more common in Wegener's granulomatosis and microscopic polyangiitis than in CSS. In one series of 96 patients, alveolar hemorrhage occurred in three (Guillevin et al. 1999).

Some data suggest that ANCA positivity is a risk factor for alveolar hemorrhage in CSS: In a series of 93 patients, seven of 35 patients with CSS (20%) who were ANCA-positive had alveolar hemorrhage, but none of the 58 patients who were ANCA-negative experienced this complication (Sinico et al. 2005). However, in contrast to these results, a series of 99 patients reported no cases of diffuse alveolar hemorrhage despite the fact that 70% were ANCA positive if tested before initiation of immunosuppressive therapy (Keogh and Specks 2003).

Thus, the largest series of CSS patients to date indicate that alveolar hemorrhage is less common in this disorder than in Wegener's granulomatosis and microscopic polyangiitis. The reason for this must relate in part to the differing cellular nature of these diseases' inflammatory infiltrates. The inflammatory infiltrate that invades small blood-vessel walls in CSS can be purely eosinophilic (Fig. 23.4). This is not observed in Wegener's granulomatosis and microscopic polyangiitis, although substantial eosinophilic infiltration may accompany either of those disorders.

Myth: The finding of neutrophils on tissue biopsy is not a feature of CSS vasculitis and should suggest another diagnosis.
Reality: Neutrophils can be observed in some cases of CSS, particularly those complicated by leukocytoclastic vasculitis of the skin. However, such neutrophils are usually mixed with a liberal sprinkling or even an abundance of eosinophils.

Myth: CSS always involves the lung parenchyma.

Reality: Although almost all CSS patients have asthma, a significant fraction of patients have no other indication of pulmonary disease. Approximately 30% of the patients reported by Lanham had no pulmonary disease apart from reactive airway disease (Lanham et al. 1984). These findings were confirmed in a larger study from France, in which 27% of the cohort had no lung disease other than asthma (Pagnoux et al. 2007). Thus, the absence of lung involvement does not detract from the diagnosis.

Pearl: Glucocorticoid therapy can alter the histopathologic findings in CSS lung substantially.

Comment: Glucocorticoid therapy suppresses the tissue infiltration of eosinophils and often renders the diagnosis of CSS difficult on the basis of pathologic features alone. In this situation, vasculitis without eosinophils and with or without necrosis can be observed. These findings are difficult to distinguish from Wegener's granulomatosis, microscopic polyangiitis, vasculitis associated with a collagen vascular disease, or other forms of vasculitis. Close clinico-pathological correlation, with questions about the patient's history of asthma, allergic rhinitis, or blood eosinophilia, points the way to the correct diagnosis.

Pearl: Patients with CSS may develop "rheumatoid nodules".

Comment: Early in the disease course, CSS (as well as Wegener's granulomatosis) can be confused with rheumatoid arthritis. There are several reasons for this:

- Inflammatory arthritis, particularly involving large joints in a migratory fashion, is a common presentation of both CSS and WG.
- CSS and WG are often associated with positive serological assays for rheumatoid factor.
- Patients with CSS and WG often develop lesions over the extensor surfaces of the elbows that strongly resemble rheumatoid nodules (Fig. 23.5).

The occurrence of these lesions, sometimes termed "Churg–Strauss granulomas" was described by Dr. Jacob Churg and Dr. Lotte Strauss themselves in the earliest description of CSS (Churg and Strauss 1951). These lesions, also called cutaneous extravascular necrotizing granulomas, are histopathologically identical to the extravascular nodules reported by Churg and Strauss within other tissues in CSS (e.g., the heart, lungs, or spleen). They can be mistaken clinically and pathologically for rheumatoid nodules.

The misclassification of Churg–Strauss granulomas as rheumatoid nodules sometimes leads to severe disease manifestations such as mononeuritis multiplex or rapidly progressive GN before the correct diagnosis is established.

Pearl: CSS has a striking predilection for the peripheral nerves and myocardium.

Comment: Among all of the systemic vasculitides, none has a greater tendency than CSS to cause mononeuritis multiplex. The vasculitic neuropathy in CSS can be devastating. Recovery from severe cases, if recovery occurs, requires more than a year and is usually incomplete. Milder cases may improve more quickly, but the process is unpredictable and many patients have persistent distal sensory deficits that are troubling. These represent damage, not active disease, but sometimes lead to excessive treatment.

CSS is also distinguished (in a notorious sense) for its tendency to damage the myocardium, often fatally. In one study from France, congestive heart failure was a leading cause of death among patients with CSS (Guillevin et al. 1999). Compared with its cousins, Wegener's granulomatosis and microscopic polyangiitis, CSS is far more likely to cause clinically-evident cardiac disease.

Pearl: Although peripheral nerve biopsy is not always diagnostic in peripheral neuropathy, it nearly always tells you the information you need to know.

Comment: In one study of 106 patients with vasculitic neuropathy, 84 peripheral nerve biopsies were performed (82 sural nerve biopsies, 2 superficial radial nerve biopsies)

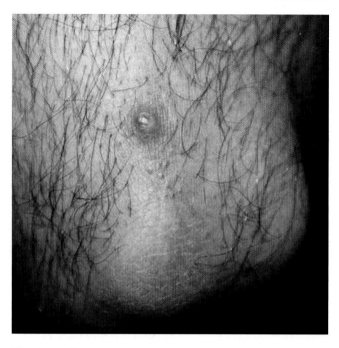

Fig. 23.5 "Churg–Strauss granulomas", also known as cutaneous extravascular necrotizing granulomas, in the Churg–Strauss syndrome Over the extensor surface of the elbow (Figures courtesy of Dr. John Stone)

(Mathew et al. 2007). In 49 of these cases (58%), the diagnosis of vasculitic neuropathy was confirmed. Thirty-one of the remaining biopsies demonstrated pathological findings "consistent with" but not diagnostic of vasculitic neuropathy; i.e., acute asymmetric axonal loss with differential fascicular involvement, with or without active Wallerian degeneration or regenerating fibers. Thus, 80 of 84 procedures (95%) led to findings compatible with or diagnostic of vasculitic neuropathy. In the proper clinical context, this is all the proof a clinician needs.

Myth: Nerve/muscle biopsies performed at the site of previous electromyography/nerve conduction studies (EMG/NCS) may be difficult to interpret because of artifact.

Reality: This is a Myth, as it relates to vasculitis and to NCS. The statement is closer to being correct with regard to inflammatory myopathies and EMG studies.

NCS are critical to identifying nerves involved in vasculitic neuropathy; subsequent biopsy may confirm the diagnosis. NCS studies do not involve needles and do not produce any artifacts that confound the diagnosis of vasculitis. In contrast, EMG needles cause injury to muscle and lead to inflammation, which may complicate the identification of a primary inflammatory myopathy. However, because of the starkly contrasting pathologies between vasculitis and muscle inflammation, previous EMGs should not pose a problem to the histopathological identification of vasculitis.

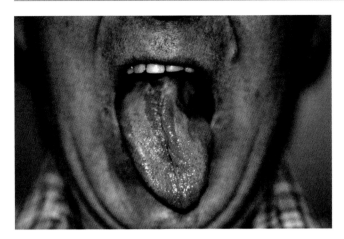

Fig. 23.6 Tongue wasting in a patient with CSS (Figure courtesy of Dr. John Stone)

Sural nerve biopsies are tolerated well by most patients. However, some patients experience several months of numbness or paresthesias. If the sensory symptoms of vasculitic neuropathy are severe, patients scarcely notice the biopsy afterwards. The incidence of permanent discomfort following a sural nerve biopsy is probably about 5%.

Myth: Nerve infarction in CSS signals the need to intensify treatment.

Reality: Active vasculitic neuropathy is one of the strongest indications for the use of cyclophosphamide in CSS. However, the development of a new nerve infarction shortly after starting immunosuppression does not necessarily signal the need to intensify treatment, particularly if other indicators of disease activity suggest disease control (Fig. 23.6). For example, nerve infarctions may manifest themselves even several weeks after the start of appropriate treatment (high-dose glucocorticoids and cyclophosphamide), with the abrupt occurrence of a foot or wrist drop or other nerve lesion.

In addition, the appearance of muscle wasting secondary to nerve infarctions may continue for weeks after the correct therapy is initiated. This is also not a sign of treatment failure and should not trigger an intensification of therapy.

Pearl: Compared with CSS, the eosinophil count in the hypereosinophil syndrome (HES) is more likely to be refractory to glucocorticoid therapy.

Comment: CSS and HES are difficult to differentiate. The two disorders have similar organ tropisms (heart, skin, peripheral nerves), and both are associated with striking eosinophilia. Making the distinction is crucial, however, because the treatments and prognoses of these two disorders differ substantially. While the eosinophil count in CSS usually drops dramatically upon the institution of glucocorticoids, HES can be refractory to this approach. A subset of patients with HES responds well to an anti-interleukin-5 monoclonal antibody

(Rothenberg et al. 2008; Wechsler 2008). Others respond well to imitinab (Dahabreh et al. 2007). A third subset requires hydroxyurea to lower the eosinophil count.

Myth: CSS never requires treatment with cytotoxic agents.

Reality: Although CSS is more likely than WG or MPA to respond adequately to glucocorticoids alone, a substantial number of patients with CSS do require cyclophosphamide. The complications of CSS most likely to require cyclophosphamide are vasculitic neuropathy, glucocorticoid-refractory glomerulonephritis, myocardial disease, severe gastrointestinal ischemia, and central nervous system disease. Confronted with any of these complications, it is probably better to treat aggressively with cytotoxic therapy from the outset.

Myth: Renal disease in CSS, when present, is mild.

Reality: Renal disease in CSS is typically less severe than that encountered in WG, but segmental necrotizing glomerulonephritis leading to a rapid decline in renal function is well-recognized (Clutterbuck et al. 1990). On renal biopsy, most of these patients have crescentic lesions and other findings indistinguishable from the renal pathology of its cousins, WG and MPA. Some CSS patients have marked eosinophilic interstitial nephritis in addition to the glomerular lesions.

Myth: Persistent asthma represents persistent CSS disease activity.

Comment: In the absence of helpful data, this remains a topic of contentious debate. The vasculitic disease manifestations of CSS usually respond readily to remission induction therapy with immunosuppressive regimens used for AAV. However, once these symptoms are controlled and glucocorticoid doses have been reduced, patients are frequently left with difficult to manage asthma, and they remain in need of significant systemic glucocorticoid doses to control the asthma. It remains unclear whether this truly represents persistent CSS as opposed to "simple" asthma. Long-term use of azathioprine or methotrexate may provide some glucocorticoid-sparing benefit in patients with severe residual reactive airway disease.

References

Boin F, Sciubba JJ, Stone JH. Churg-Strauss syndrome presenting with salivary gland enlargement and respiratory distress. Arthritis Rheum 2006; 55:167–170

Churg A. Recent advances in the diagnosis of Churg-Strauss syndrome. Mod Pathol 2001; 14:1284–1293

Churg A. Churg-Strauss syndrome, microscopic polyangiitis, and other forms of pulmonary vasculitis. In: Churg A, Myers J, Tazelaar H, Wright JL (eds) Thurlbeck's pathology of the lung (3rd edn). New York, Thieme Medical Publishers, 2005, pp. 391–412

Churg J, Strauss L. Allergic granulomatosis, allergic angiitis, and periarteritis nodosa. Am J Pathol 1951; 27:277–301

Clutterbuck E, Evans D, Pusey C. Renal involvement in Churg-Strauss syndrome. Nephrol Dial Transplant 1990; 5:161–167

Dahabreh IJ, Giannouli S, Zoi C, et al Management of hypereosinophilic syndrome: A prospective study in the era of molecular genetics. Medicine (Baltimore) 2007; 86(6):344–354

Godman G, Churg J. Wegener's granulomatosis: Pathology and review of the literature. Arch Pathol Lab Med 1954; 58:533–551

Guillevin L, Cohen P, Gayraud M, et al Churg-Strauss syndrome: Clinical study and long-term follow-up of 96 patients. Medicine (Baltimore) 1999; 78:26–37

Keogh KA, Specks U. Churg-Strauss syndrome: Clinical presentation, antineutrophil cytoplasmic antibodies, and leukotriene receptor antagonists. Am J Med 2003; 115:284–290

Lanham JG, Elkon KB, Pusey CD, Hughes GRV. Systemic vasculitis with asthma and eosinophilia: A clinical approach to the Churg-Strauss syndrome. Medicine (Baltimore) 1984; 63:65–81

Mathew L, Talbot K, Love S, et al Treatment of vasculitic peripheral neuropathy: A retrospective analysis of outcome. Q J Med 2007; 100:41

Pagnoux C, Guilpain P, Guillevin L. Churg-Strauss syndrome. Curr Opin Rheumatol 2007; 19:25–32

Rothenberg ME, Klion AD, Roufosse FE, et al Treatment of patients with the hypereosinophilic syndrome with mepolizumab. N Engl J Med 2008; 358(12):1215–1228

Sablé-Fourtassou R, Cohen P, Mahr A, et al Antineutrophil cytoplasmic antibodies and the Churg-Strauss syndrome. Ann Intern Med 2005; 143:632–638

Sinico RA, Di Toma L, Maggiore U, et al Prevalence and clinical significance of antineutrophil cytoplasmic antibodies in Churg-Strauss syndrome. Arthritis Rheum 2005; 52: 2926–2935

Wechsler ME. Combating the eosinophil with anti-interkeukin-5 therapy. N Engl J Med 2008; 358(12):1293–1294

Wechsler ME, Finn D, Gunawardena D, et al Churg-Strauss syndrome in patients receiving montelukast as treatment for asthma. Chest 2000; 117:708–713

ANCA-Associated Vasculitis

24

John H. Stone, Shoichi Ozaki, Karina Keogh, Ulrich Specks,
Carol A. Langford, Niels Rasmussen, Cees G.M. Kallenberg,
and Ingeborg M. Bajema

24.1 Overview of ANCA-Associated Vasculitis

> The majority of patients with Wegener's granulomatosis (WG) or microscopic polyangiitis (MPA) have antineutrophil cytoplasmic antibodies (ANCA) in their serum. This is particularly true of patients with "disseminated" disease, the great majority of whom are ANCA positive.

> WG and MPA are often termed "ANCA-associated vasculitides" (AAV), even though not all patients with these conditions have ANCA. The Churg–Strauss syndrome, another disorder classified as an AAV, is discussed in Chap. 23.

> Multiple antibodies may lead to positive immunofluorescence testing for ANCA in either perinuclear (P-ANCA) or cytoplasmic (C-ANCA) patterns. However, only antibodies to myeloperoxidase (MPO) and proteinase-3 (PR3) are associated with the AAV.

> Antibodies directed against PR3 and MPO are termed PR3-ANCA and MPO-ANCA, respectively.

> WG may be associated with destructive upper respiratory tract disease, including saddle-nose deformity, erosive sinusitis, and subglottic stenosis.

> A host of ocular lesions may occur in the AAV, including episcleritis, scleritis, peripheral ulcerative keratitis, and orbital pseudotumor. Most of these lesions are more common in WG than in MPA.

> Lung disease in the AAV ranges from nodular lesions with a tendency to cavitate (in WG), to interstitial lung disease (MPA), and to alveolar hemorrhage (both WG and MPA).

> Segmental, necrotizing glomerulonephritis commonly accompanies the AAV. Because of the paucity of immunoreactants such as immunoglobulins and complement components in kidney biopsies relative to the biopsies from patients with immune complex-mediated glomerulonephritis, the glomerulonephritis of the AAV is termed "pauci-immune."

The frequencies of clinical manifestations of WG in a clinical trial cohort of 180 patients are shown in Table 24.1.

24.2 Epidemiology

Pearl: WG is believed to be two or three times more common than MPA in western countries. This ratio is inverted in Japan.

Comment: Epidemiologic studies from Europe indicate that the annual incidence of WG is approximately three times higher than that of MPA. These figures are concordant with the experience of clinicians in the United States. For reasons that remain unclear, the ratio of these two diseases is flipped in Japan, where MPA appears to be substantially more common than WG. Japanese clinicians are far more likely to evaluate patients with MPO-ANCA than PR3-ANCA.

24.3 Nose, Sinuses, and Ears

Myth: The saddle nose is a diagnostic sign of active WG.

Reality: Yes and no. Active WG may lead to the well-known saddle-nose deformity (Fig. 24.1a, b) due to destruction of the nasal cartilages, especially the nasal septum. The nasal septum is particularly vulnerable to vasculitis as its blood supply is derived from terminal arteries.

Ironically, the partially effective therapies available for WG over the past few decades have led to an alternative route by which patients can develop saddle nose deformities. This is observed in patients who have constant pain localized to the nose and midfacial area. The examination of these patients is remarkable for crust formation and possibly superinfection, but a septal perforation is absent.

The "treatment-induced" saddle-nose deformity comes about in the following manner. Once it becomes clear that

J. H. Stone (ed.), *A Clinician's Pearls and Myths in Rheumatology,*
DOI:10.1007/978-1-84800-934-9_24, © Springer Science + Business Media B.V. 2009

Table 24.1 Clinical features of limited and severe Wegener's granulomatosis in a clinical trial cohort of 180 patients[a] (Modified from Stone and the WGET Research Group 2003)

	Limited (n = 52)	Severe (n = 128)	Overall (n = 180)	P-value[b]
General (%)	76.9	70.3	72.2	0.370
Arthralgias/Arthritis	69.2	64.8	66.1	
Fevers	7.7	21.1	17.2	
Cutaneous (%)	15.4	21.9	20.0	0.324
Purpura	13.5	18.8	17.2	
Ulcers	3.9	3.1	3.3	
Gangrene	0.0	0.8	0.6	
Mucous membranes/eyes (%)	25.0	27.3	26.7	0.747
Mouth ulcers	7.7	11.7	10.6	
Conjunctivitis/episcleritis	13.5	14.8	14.4	
Retro-orbital mass/proptosis	1.9	4.7	3.9	
Uveitis	0.0	0.0	0.0	
Scleritis	1.9	2.3	2.2	
Ear/Nose/Throat (%)	88.5	71.9	76.7	0.017
Bloody nasal discharge/nasal rusting/ulcer	67.3	56.3	59.4	
Sinus involvement	59.6	41.4	46.7	
Swollen salivary gland	1.9	3.1	2.8	
Subglottic inflammation	11.5	7.0	8.3	
Conductive deafness	25.0	22.7	23.3	
Sensorineural deafness	1.9	3.1	2.8	
Cardiovascular (%)	1.9	1.6	1.7	0.864
Pericarditis	0.0	0.8	0.6	
Gastrointestinal (%)	1.9	2.3	1.7	0.862
Mesenteric ischemia	0.0	0.8	0.6	
Pulmonary (%)	51.9	63.3	60.0	0.159
Pleurisy	7.7	7.0	7.2	
Nodules or cavities	38.5	28.1	31.1	
Other infiltrates	23.1	32.0	29.4	
Endobronchial involvement	3.9	3.1	3.3	
Alveolar hemorrhage	0.0	25.0	17.8	
Respiratory failure	0.0	2.3	1.7	
Renal (%)	28.9	64.1	53.9	<0.001
Hematuria	25.0	28.9	27.8	
RBC casts	3.9	35.9	26.7	
Elevated serum creatinine	3.9	28.1	21.1	
Nervous system (%)	0.0	12.5	8.9	0.017
Meningitis	0.0	0.0	0.0	
Cord lesion	0.0	0.0	0.0	
Stroke	0.0	0.0	0.0	
Cranial nerve palsy	0.0	2.3	1.7	
Sensory peripheral neuropathy	0.0	10.2	7.2	
Motor mononeuritis multiplex	0.0	2.3	1.7	
Other (%)[c]	46.2	39.1	41.1	0.244

[a]Organ involvement at enrollment, as recorded on the Birmingham Vasculitis Activity Score for Wegener's Granulomatosis (BVAS/WG) Form
[b]Chi-square or Fisher's Exact Test for categorical data
[c]Include lacrimal gland involvement (3 patients), supraglottic airway inflammation (2), aural chondritis (2), breast mass (2), peripheral 7th cranial nerve lesion (2), keratitis (2), optic neuropathy mimicking optic neuritis (1), splenic involvement - asymptomatic infarctions found on computed tomography (1), central nervous system involvement with parenchymal brain lesions and seizures (1), skull-based lesion in the infra-temporal fossa, misdiagnosed as a tumor (1), diabetes insipidus (1), pituitary involvement (1), hilar adenopathy (1), tongue ulcer (1), nodular vocal cord lesion (1), and hepatic transaminase elevation (1)[a]

the patient has active nasal disease and antiinflammatory treatment is commenced, the nasal septum can disappear rapidly—within days to weeks. This is probably due to the absorption of inflamed tissue and is profoundly unfortunate, because the patients are generally encouraged by this point that their disease is treatable and that the much-dreaded complication of a saddle-nose deformity can be avoided.

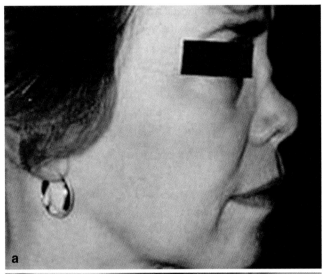

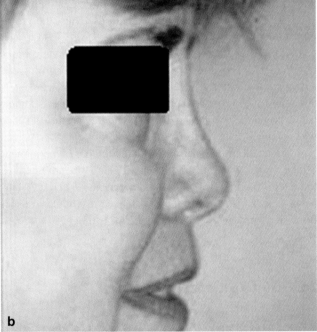

Fig. 24.1 Saddle-nose deformity repair, before (**a**) and after (**b**) (Figures courtesy of Dr. John Stone)

Pearl: To detect a nasal septal perforation, light is shone into one of the patient's nostrils through a nasal speculum while peering into the other nostril.

Comment: This is a simple test if the nose is relatively free of crusts. The light streams through the nasal septal defect if a perforation is present allowing the diagnosis to be made easily. If there are substantial crusts, bleeding, or purulent secretions, the nose must be cleaned (generally by an otolaryngologist) before a full examination is possible.

Inflammatory changes that are localized to the posterosuperior part of the nasal cavity can cause a septal perforation in the absence of a saddle nose deformity. Such cases are

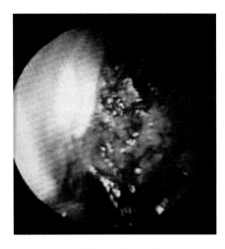

Fig. 24.2 Nasal crusting in Wegener's granulomatosis (Figure courtesy of Dr. Robert Lebovics)

often complicated by serous otitis media due to Eustachian tube involvement, and an endoscope is necessary to make the diagnosis.

Pearl: For patients with nasal crusting, irrigation of the nose with saline is a cornerstone of therapy.

Comment: There is a spectrum of responses to treatment in nasal disease. Some patients' noses clear up completely with immunosuppressive therapy. Others settle into a pattern of chronic nasal crusting that responds poorly to immunosuppressive therapy and is often difficult to parse according to active disease or damage (Fig. 24.2). Such patients often find that irrigation of the nose, performed by themselves once or twice daily, is the most effective intervention available for nasal crusting.

Isotonic saline is the preferred solution for nasal irrigation. WG patients devise ingenious solutions for irrigating their noses effectively, but generally an eyedropper or water pick is sufficient (Fig. 24.3). In addition to irrigation, antimicrobial therapy with trimethoprim-sulfamethoxazole or the local application of antimicrobial substances, such as mupirocin, has dramatic effects on crusting and rhinorhea in some patients.

Myth: Surgery on the nose or upper respiratory tract in WG may trigger a disease flare.

Reality: This contention is based entirely on anecdote. If surgery on the upper respiratory tract actually does increase the likelihood of a disease flare, the probable reason could be the preoperative tapering of patients' glucocorticoids that occurs due to wound healing concerns. Thus, in patients whose WG has been quiescent, particularly those who have been in remission on little or no immunosuppression, there is no reason to forgo elective repairs of saddle-nose deformities or subglottic stenoses.

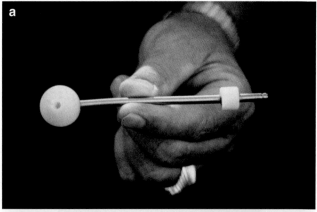

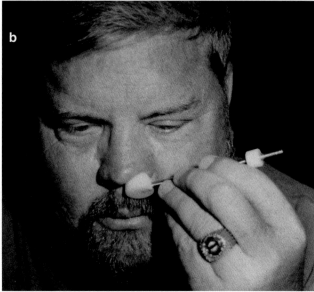

Fig. 24.3 (**a**, **b**) One patient's device for irrigating his nose (Figures courtesy of Dr. John Stone)

Ensuring that the disease is quiet both locally and systemically before surgery is important. Poor surgical outcomes, including severe fistulas, have occurred when nasal reconstruction is performed during a period of active disease. The cosmetic results of saddle-nose repairs can be spectacular (see Fig. 24.1a, b). Saddle-nose deformities may recur in the setting of a disease reactivation, but secondary and even tertiary repairs can be performed once disease control is restored.

Pearl: WG that is limited to the upper respiratory tract can remain subclinical or be misdiagnosed as a series of innocuous ailments for many months or even years.

Comment: WG should be suspected when mundane problems recur with excessive frequency or when they persist too long. Friedrich Wegener reported three patients in their 30s who presented with upper respiratory tract symptoms that had appeared harmless at first (Wegener 1936). Within 6 months, all three patients had died of renal failure.

Cases of WG "smoldering" in the upper respiratory tract, undiagnosed for years, are documented well in the literature. In many cases, the explanation for the chronic sinus dysfunction, nasal pain, bleeding, recurrent "otitis media," and other symptoms is understood only in retrospect, upon the occurrence of disease manifestions that threaten vital organs. The detection of ANCA can shorten the time to diagnosis by many months once the clinician thinks of ordering this test.

Pearl: Grommets (tubes) are helpful in WG-associated serous otitis media.

Comment: Yes—in the correct setting. In the initial disease phase, serous otitis media often develops because of inflammatory involvement of the Eustachian tube, leading to "Eustachian tube dysfunction." These acute symptoms often resolve without a mechanical intervention and are associated with a return of the hearing to normal after treatment with systemic immunosuppressive medications. Thus, the grommet should be spared in this phase.

Chronic serous otitis media, which occurs in later phases of WG, may benefit from the placement of grommets. Adequate audiometry testing before grommet placement is essential to ensure that the patient's hearing loss, as anticipated, is conductive rather than sensorineural in nature. (Tubes will not ameliorate sensorineural hearing loss.)

In cases of chronic serous otitis media, only a permanent T-tube can provide substantial benefit. Such tubes might have to be removed in cases of chronic infections. When that happens, permanent perforations of the eardrum may ensue. Bone-anchored hearing aids may be the ultimate solution.

24.4 Subglottic Stenosis

Pearl: Dyspnea on exertion in a WG patient whose disease has been quiescent suggests subglottic stenosis.

Comment: When WG patients present with decreased exercise tolerance, dyspnea on exertion, "asthma," or other similar complaints, clinicians must remember the propensity of WG to cause subglottic stenosis (see below).

Subglottic stenosis can develop even in patients who have been in apparent remission (Fig. 24.4). The reason for this can be either subclinical disease activity, progression to subglottic stenosis because of scarring rather than active disease, or both.

Pearl: Granulomatous subglottic stenosis responds easily to immunosuppressive treatment when it is an early manifestation of WG.

Comment: Subglottic stenosis is one of the more mysterious manifestations of WG. As illustrated in Fig. 24.5a, b,

Fig. 24.4 Subglottic stenosis in Wegener's granulomatosis (Figure courtesy of Dr. John Stone)

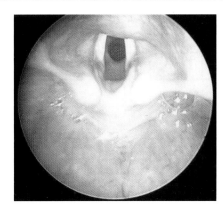

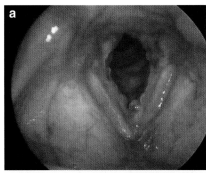

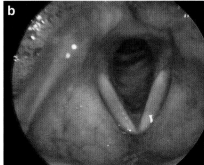

Fig. 24.5 (**a, b**) Prompt resolution of an early subglottic stenosis lesion following the institution of treatment (Figures courtesy of Dr. Niels Rasmussen)

subglottic stenosis may vanish completely within 2 weeks on standard immunosuppressive treatment if it is an early manifestation of inflammatory disease. Unfortunately, this favorable experience contrasts markedly with the course of subglottic stenoses later in the course of many patients, when the airway narrowing is sclerotic in nature and more refractory to medical interventions.

Pearl: Subglottic stenosis can be diagnosed over the telephone.

Comment: Subglottic stenosis can usually be detected by listening to patients as they speak. Because of their upper airway narrowing, they are forced to suck in air before beginning a sentence. This can be detected over the telephone as well as in the examining room. On chest auscultation, loud inspiratory sounds (sometimes audible without the stethoscope) are a finding consistent with subglottic stenosis.

Confirming the suspicion of subglottic stenosis can be challenging. The suspicion of a subglottic stenosis can be confirmed by endoscopic laryngoscopy using the flexible laryngoscope or a telescope as used for videostroboscopy. Thin-cut computed tomography scans of the trachea can be helpful to evaluate the extent of the stenosis, particularly if a surgical correction is planned.

Pearl: Pulmonary function testing with an inspiratory flow volume curve is helpful in the diagnosis and monitoring of large airway involvement in WG.

Comment: Subglottic stenosis classically causes a fixed obstruction with airflow limitation during both inspiration and expiration (Polychronopoulos et al. 2007). This results in plateaued or flattened inspiratory and expiratory flow volume curves (Fig. 24.6a, b).

Myth: Tracheostomies are usually good solutions for WG patients with difficult subglottic stenosis.

Reality: Tracheostomies should be avoided at all costs in WG. Even otolaryngologists who perform the procedure well in patients with WG concede that a tracheostomy generally makes the patient sicker than he or she was before the procedure. Avoiding a tracheostomy usually necessitates frequent endoscopic procedures to dilate stenotic segments of the trachea manually and to maintain the larger airway with glucocorticoids and mitomycin C injections.

When subglottic stenosis is associated with a significant degree of active inflammation, the narrowing may respond to an inhaled glucocorticoid powder. One regimen employed commonly in this setting is fluticasone (220 μg). This is administered initially as four puffs twice daily, then reduced to two puffs twice daily after several weeks. The success of this approach probably stems from the turbulence created by the stenosis, which makes the inhaled glucocorticoid settle locally and deliver the maximum medication dose at the site of the stenosis. After endoscopic dilatation of subglottic or endobronchial lesions, inhaled glucocorticoids may help to limit further scarring secondary to inflammation generated by the procedure itself. Regular nebulized saline is also recommended.

Pearl: Metal tracheal stents should not be used in WG.

Comment: Metal tracheal stents should not be used in patients with benign airway disorders, including WG. This was the subject of a Public Health Notification by the U.S. Food and Drug Administration (FDA Public Health Notification 2005). The Notification was based upon the high risk of complications from metal stents, including airway wall perforation and stent rupture.

When stenting of a large airway obstruction in WG is required, silicone stents are the preferred devise. The stenting procedure is performed with a rigid bronchoscope and

Fig. 24.6 Flow volume loops in the setting of subglottic stenosis in a 48 year-old woman with Wegener's granulomatosis (**a**). The inspiratory flow volume curve, graphed above the expiratory flow volume curve, is mildly flattened. This suggests a limitation of inspiratory flow and variable extrathoracic airway obstruction. (**b**). One year later, there was progression of her subglottic scarring. The flow volume curve demonstrates a fixed upper airway obstruction, evidenced by the more severe flattening of the inspiratory flow volume curve and the flattened expiratory flow volume curve (Figures courtesy of Dr. Karina Keogh)

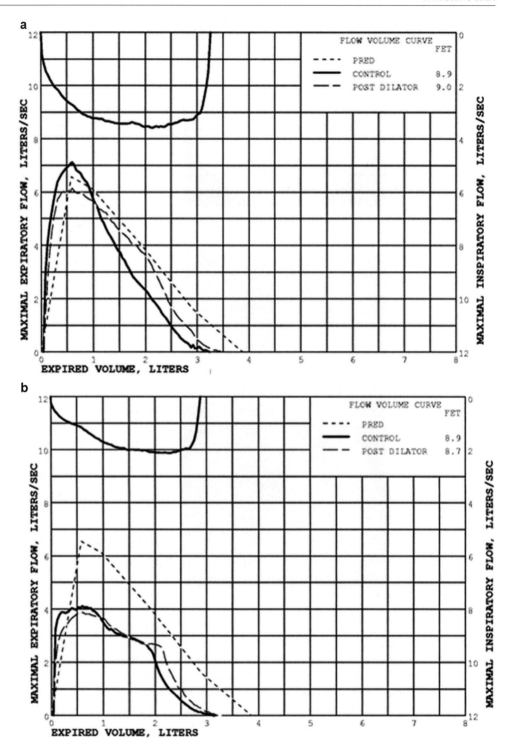

requires a general anesthetic. Silicone stents are generally tolerated well and are removable. They may migrate distally and require repositioning, which involves a repeat bronchoscopic procedure.

Stents may become obstructed by bronchial secretions. This can be prevented usually by the routine use of nebulized saline treatments. Granulation tissue sometimes develops around the stent and may require careful laser therapy to facilitate stent removal.

Myth: Laser therapy is a tissue-sparing method of intervention for subglottic stenosis in WG.

Reality: Medical therapy alone, especially in the chronic phase of the disease, is usually insufficient to control subglottic stenosis. This complication occurs to at least some degree in approximately 15% of WG patients, but the clinical features often reflect the development of scar tissue rather than active inflammation. Collaboration with an experienced otolaryngologist is required to manage this problem effectively.

Laser surgeries provide short-term relief in many cases but eventually become a self-defeating proposition: the resultant scar formation exacerbates the situation over the long term. This exuberant scarring that occurs in WG tissues following laser procedures makes laser interventions contraindicated for subglottic stenosis in this disorder (Langford et al. 1996).

Combined endoscopic dilatations and local glucocorticoid injections are the most effective approach to this problem. The injection of glucocorticoids decreases inflammation, impairs scar formation, and enhances resorption of the scar. Some patients need to undergo this procedure several times a year before stability of the lesion is achieved. The real key in addressing this problem effectively is having an alliance with an otolaryngologist who is willing to take on the problem energetically and provide close surveillance, with interventions as appropriate.

Pearl: Beware the "Boy Who Cried Wolf" effect, which clinicians can cause by submitting too many upper airway biopsies accompanied only by the question "Wegener's granulomatosis?"

Comment: Submitting biopsy specimens without detailed clinical information is a mistake. Clinicians sometimes believe they should not tell the pathologist too much, lest the pathologist be "led" to the diagnosis inappropriately. Failure to provide sufficient clinical information is particularly harmful in the case of upper-respiratory biopsies. Upper airway biopsies have a very low specificity for lesions that are characteristic of WG (i.e., granulomas, vasculitis, or both) (Devaney et al. 1990).

Most upper airway biopsies from patients who are diagnosed eventually with WG show nonspecific inflammation (D'Cruz et al. 1989). The type of inflammation present in combination with certain subtle features such as focal ulceration or a spot of necrosis may implicate WG. Understanding the full clinical history is important information for the pathologist.

The use of endoscopes to guide the bioptic procedures in the nasal cavity greatly enhances the diagnostic yield of biopsies, which should be obtained from inflamed but nonnecrotic areas. This calls for experience with obtaining these biopsies and at the same a restrictive policy on biopsying too often. Tissue damage may be increased by the biopsy, so biopsies should be performed only if their results have the potential to alter management.

24.5 Mouth

Pearl: Strawberry gums are a classic (if uncommon) sign of WG.

Comment: WG is unique among the vasculitides in its ability to cause extensive gum inflammation (Fig. 24.7). This complication responds well to WG treatment, but patients who have advanced gum inflammation at the time of diagnosis can be left with some recession of the gums.

Pearl: WG can cause painful oral lesions.

Comment: The prominence of oral ulcers in WG is often underappreciated (Fig. 24.8). Yet, oral ulcers (along with nasal ulcers) comprise one of the four American College of Rheumatology criteria for the classification of WG (Leavitt et al. 1990). The oral ulcers of WG typically involve the buccal mucosa or the tongue and heal quickly following the start

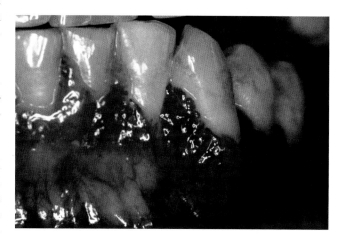

Fig. 24.7 Strawberry gums in Wegener's granulomatosis (Figure courtesy of Dr. John Stone)

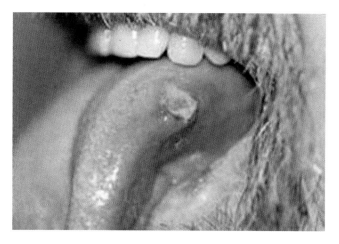

Fig. 24.8 Tongue ulcer in Wegener's granulomatosis (From Stone and Hoffman 2006)

of treatment, without scarring. In the WG Etanercept Trial (WGET), 14% of the patients had oral ulcerations that were attributed by the investigators to active disease over a mean follow-up of 2 years (Mahr et al. 2008).

Pearl: WG rarely erodes the roof of the mouth.

Comment: In contrast to the upper respiratory tract disease, oral lesions in WG are not destructive. When a patient has an oral lesion that destroys the roof of the mouth, a variety of other disorders must be considered, particularly cocaine use and T-cell lymphomas (once termed "lethal midline granuloma").

ANCA testing may be useful in differentiating cocaine-associated oral (and nasal) lesions from true WG (Wiesner et al. 2004). Cocaine-induced nasal destructive lesions have been associated with ANCA directed against human neutrophil elastase, which can result in a positive ANCA by commercial assays.

24.6 Eyes

Pearl: Chemosis, a common eye finding in AAV, is a complication of glucocorticoid therapy.

Comment: Patients are often concerned and clinicians puzzled by chemosis, the development of edema under the conjunctivae (Fig. 24.9). One might postulate many reasons for a patient with AAV to have chemosis: fluid overload, persistence of tears in the eye because of a blocked nasolacrimal duct, low-grade inflammation, and others. However, the common denominator is probably therapy with glucocorticoids.

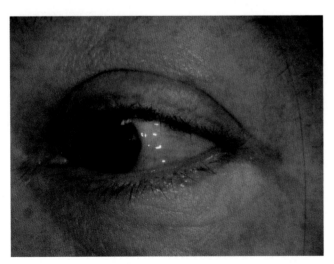

Fig. 24.9 Chemosis in a patient with microscopic polyangiitis (Figure courtesy of Dr. John Stone)

Glucocorticoid use is associated with edema at a variety of sites, e.g., the legs and the retina (cystoid macular edema). High-dose glucocorticoid use probably explains chemosis, as well, though the precise mechanism remains obscure.

Pearl: Orbital pseudotumor can be refractory to medical therapy.

Comment: Retrobulbar lesions are recalcitrant to conventional immunosuppression in some patients with WG, particularly those with longstanding, fibrotic lesions. Medical therapy is most likely to be effective for early inflammatory masses behind the eye. Radiographic persistence of orbital lesions is the rule, unfortunately, even if the masses appear to become dormant for a while after therapy.

For refractory orbital pseudotumors, surgical debulking can be an effective approach but is associated with a potential risk to vision. The biggest challenge is finding an ophthalmologist who is willing to undertake the procedure.

Pearl: The eyes of a patient with WG are much more likely to be wet than dry.

Comment: Nasal inflammation in WG can lead to nasolacrimal duct dysfunction, insufficient tear drainage, and watery eyes. In the setting of unilateral conjunctivitis in a patient who has WG, the underlying cause is probably nasolacrimal duct dysfunction.

Nasolacrimal duct obstruction (and accompanying dacryocystitis) is caused by active inflammation or damage to the nose. A dacrocystorhinostomy may ameliorate the problem, but the larger tear evacuation route often becomes occluded over time by inflamed tissue or scar. This is particularly likely when chronic *Staphylococcus aureus* infection is present and associated with nasal crusts. In some cases, a glass or plastic tube placed in the lacrimal duct may be beneficial.

Nasal disease in WG has other potential implications for extra-nasal symptoms. Serous otitis in WG is caused by problems that prevent ventilation of the middle ear through the Eustachian tube. As discussed earlier (see "Ears"), tympanostomy tubes (grommets) may provide prompt relief of this problem, but are used only in the context of chronic ear problems, not acute ones.

Pearl: There is a tarsal structure in the eye, and it can be a site of trouble in WG.

Comment: Most rheumatologists think of the foot when they hear the word "tarsus"; as in: "The first metatarsal joint is the most common initial site of gout." However, there is a tarsus in the eye, and it can cause a problem in WG....

The tarsus (plural *tarsi*) is the thick connective tissue plate within each of the eyelids that gives the eyelids their firm structure. When one describes the conjunctiva, the terms tarsal and bulbar conjunctivae are used to describe the regions of involvement of inflammatory processes. The tarsal conjunctiva refers to the conjunctiva that covers the interior surface of the eyelids. In contrast, the bulbar conjunctiva covers the globe.

Patients with WG can develop tarsal conjunctival inflammation and scarring. Tarsal conjunctival involvement in WG is characterized by inflammation of the palpebral conjunctiva and tarsus, followed by a fibrovascular proliferation and scar formation. The histopathological features of tarsal-conjunctival involvement in WG are granulomatous inflammation, focal necrosis, and areas of occlusive vasculitis in the tarsus and conjunctiva. WG patients who develop this complication also appear to be at risk for subglottic stenosis and nasolacrimal duct obstruction (Robinson et al. 2003).

Myth: Episcleritis is the most common eye lesion in WG.

Reality: Among the many ocular lesions of WG are scleritis, peripheral ulcerative keratitis, orbital pseudotumor, dacrocystitis, and (more rarely) uveitis. However, the most common eye problem in WG is episcleritis (Fig. 24.10), a painless ocular erythema that can occur in one eye or both. Episcleritis can cause diffuse eye redness or involve the eye in a more sectoral fashion. It can usually be managed by topical therapy, but may signal the presence of active disease in other organs that requires additional treatment.

Myth: The diagnosis of diffuse scleritis mandates the use of cyclophosphamide.

Reality: Scleritis is not a monolithic disorder. "Splitters" divide this form of ocular inflammation into at least five types: diffuse anterior scleritis, nodular scleritis, necrotizing anterior scleritis, posterior scleritis, and scleromalacia perforans (see Chapter 39). These forms of ocular inflammation are quite distinct clinically, and the individual types of scleritis rarely change categories. Whereas necrotizing anterior scleritis and posterior scleritis both require intensive immunosuppression with cyclophosphamide and high-dose glucocorticoids, the other forms may respond well to milder interventions (glucocorticoids alone, or even NSAIDs).

Although it is unusual for patients to morph from one type of scleritis to another, it is not uncommon for them to need to switch therapies. NSAID therapy for diffuse anterior scleritis may require ratcheting up to glucocorticoids if the initial therapy does not suppress the inflammation.

24.7 Lungs

Pearl: Interstitial fibrosis is frequently reported in MPA.

Comment: Interstitial lung disease is an important and under-recognized occurrence in MPA (Fig. 24.11) (Eschun et al. 2003; Homma et al. 2004; Birnbaum et al. 2007). This pulmonary complication is highly unusual among patients with AAV whose clinical phenotype is most consistent with WG (Table 24.2).

A study comprising 44 patients comparing two separate cohorts from Brescia, Italy, and the Mayo Clinic, respectively, revealed the same clinical, radiographic, and serologic manifestations of both MPA and the interstitial lung disease in both cohorts. The lung disease is radiographically and physiologically indistinguishable from usual interstitial pneumonia. It can precede other features of MPA and is usually present already at the time of MPA diagnosis. Additional studies are required to understand the response to treatment and long-term prognosis of patients with MPA who also have interstitial fibrosis.

Pearl: Patients with WG are at increased risk of venous thrombotic events (VTE).

Comment: During the Wegener's Granulomatosis Etanercept Trial (WGET), 16 of the 180 patients enrolled developed VTEs (Merkel et al. 2005). Moreover, 13 additional patients

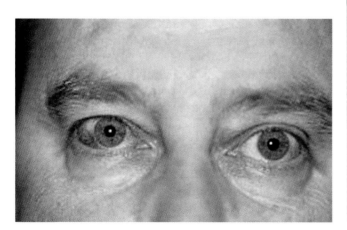

Fig. 24.10 Episcleritis in a patient with Wegener's granulomatosis (Figure courtesy of Dr. John Stone)

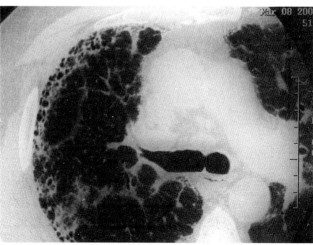

Fig. 24.11 Interstitial lung disease in microscopic polyangiitis (Figure courtesy of Dr. John Stone)

Table 24.2 Clinical phenotypes of Wegener's granulomatosis and microscopic polyangiitis

	WG	MPA
ANCA positive (%)	80–90%	75%
Typical ANCA pattern and antigen specificity	Cytoplasmic (C-ANCA) proteinase 3 (PR3)	Perinuclear (P-ANCA) Myeloperoxidase (MPO)
Upper respiratory tract	Nasal septal perforation Saddle-nose deformity Subglottic stenosis	Absent or mild
Lung	Nodules, infiltrates, or cavitary lesions Stenotic bronchial disease	Alveolar hemorrhage Interstitial lung disease
Kidney	Necrotizing, crescentic glomerulonephritis	Necrotizing, crescentic glomerulonephritis
Distinguishing features	Destructive upper airway disease, granulomatous inflammation	No granulomatous inflammation

(7%) had histories of VTE prior to enrollment. Thus, approximately one patient in six had a VTE either before or after trial entry. In a comparison of patients in the WGET cohort to patients in the Johns Hopkins Lupus Cohort, the incidence of VTE among patients in the WGET cohort was sevenfold higher. Moreover, the data on the timing of VTE occurrence were consistent with the concept that VTEs are a manifestation of active WG (Fig. 24.12). The median time from enrollment in WGET to VTE was 2 months.

The explanation for this finding probably relates to the distribution of blood vessel involvement in WG. In contrast to some other forms of vasculitis (e.g., PAN), WG involves both the venous and arterial sides of the circulation (Wegener 1939). Venous inflammation, combined with the low flow state in veins and possibly other more disease-specific factors, may explain this finding. Other ANCA-associated disorders such as MPA and the Churg-Strauss syndrome probably share this predisposition to venous thrombotic events.

Myth: Pulmonary-renal syndromes are caused by antiglomerular basement membrane (anti-GBM) disease most of the time.

Reality: AAV is substantially more common than anti-GBM disease as a cause of pulmonary-renal syndromes (Niles et al. 1996; Saxena et al. 1995; Gallagher et al. 2002). In a series of 88 patients with lung hemorrhage and glomerulonephritis, 48 (55%) had either MPO- or PR3-ANCA, 6 (7%) had antiglomerular basement membrane (GBM) antibodies, and 7 (8%) had both ANCA and anti-GBM antibodies (Niles et al. 1996). Among the 48 patients with ANCA only, 19 had antibodies to PR-3, and 29 had antibodies to MPO.

Myth: Most patients with MPA have pulmonary hemorrhage.

Reality: Pulmonary hemorrhage is the most dramatic manifestation of MPA, but only 12% of patients develop this complication (Fig. 24.13) (Guillevin et al. 1999). Far more common than pulmonary hemorrhage are glomerulonephritis (79%), weight loss (73%), mononeuritis multiplex (58%), and fever (55%). Thus, if one views MPA only as a pulmonary-renal syndrome and requires lung involvement before considering the diagnosis, detection of MPA will be delayed substantially or missed altogether.

Myth: Patients with alveolar hemorrhage always have hemoptysis.

Reality: Patients with MPA or WG can have substantial amounts of blood in their lungs without manifesting hemoptysis. Clinicians must have a low threshold for suspecting alveolar hemorrhage. Alveolar infiltrates on chest roentgenogram (typically in multiple lobes) that have a "ground glass" appearance on CT scans should raise suspicion of alveolar

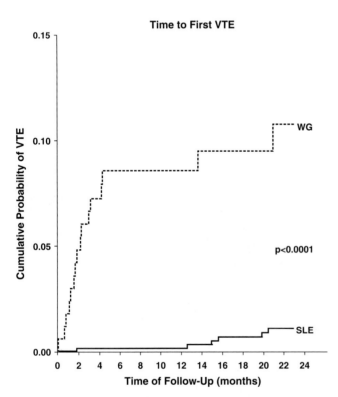

Fig. 24.12 Time to first venous thrombotic event (VTE). The incidence of venous thrombotic events in Wegener's granulomatosis patients is increased compared with that in patients with systemic lupus erythematosus (Merkel et al. 2005)

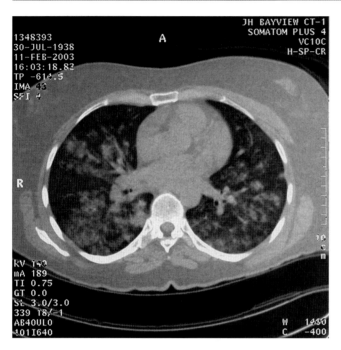

Fig. 24.13 Alveolar hemorrhage in microscopic polyangiitis (Figure courtesy of Dr. John Stone)

hemorrhage, particularly in patients with reduced or falling hemoglobin levels.

Bronchoscopy with bronchoalveolar lavage is the best approach to excluding alveolar hemorrhage. In the case of active alveolar hemorrhage, bronchoalveolar lavage yields progressively bloodier return with each successive aliquot. This is contrast to an endobronchial bleeding source, where successive aliquots clear. The presence of a high percentage (>30%) of hemosiderin-laden macrophages on BAL fluid cytology also indicative of blood in the alveoli that has been present for at least 24 h.

Hemosiderin-laden macrophages are an indication of hemorrhage even in the absence of bloody return on bronchoscopy. However, this finding does not identify the source of the blood as alveolar in origin. Active alveolar hemorrhage, even if mild at the time of presentation, should always be considered potentially life-threatening. Consequently, it needs to be treated promptly and aggressively, usually with high (pulse) doses of glucocorticoids and either cyclophosphamide or rituximab.

Pearl: In WG, chest radiography may reveal almost any abnormality *except* hilar adenopathy.

Comment: Hilar adenopathy is an unusual finding in WG. Evidence of hilar adenopathy on chest radiography vaults other diagnoses, particularly sarcoidosis, lymphoma, and tuberculosis, ahead of WG on the differential diagnosis. Computed tomography scans of the chest are more sensitive than chest radiography and often reveal pulmonary lesions

that are undetected on chest radiography, including modest hilar adenopathy.

Pearl: Tracheobronchial involvement of WG can be clinically silent.

Comment: Symptoms associated with tracheobronchial disease activity may be very minimal. As a result, this complication of WG is among the most difficult to diagnose and treat. The most common symptom of tracheobronchial disease is a cough, which is usually nonproductive. However, streaky hemoptysis may also occur. Dyspnea caused by tracheobronchial involvement usually requires significant mainstem bronchus narrowing or tracheal narrowing (usually in a subglottic location). Minor or localized (lobar or segmental) bronchial stenosis is usually asymptomatic but can lead to abnormalities of the shape of the expiratory flow volume loop on pulmonary function testing.

Symptoms and pulmonary function test abnormalities may progress during immunosuppressive therapy that successfully controls disease activity elsewhere. This may be because of persistent smoldering inflammatory activity of the tracheobronchial tree, bacterial (or rarely fungal) superinfection, or cicatricial narrowing of the lumen of affected bronchi.

Pearl: Inhaled glucocorticoids should be used in patients with documented endobronchial disease.

Comment: Tracheobronchial disease activity often is less responsive to methotrexate and at times even to cyclophosphamide than is necrotizing granulomatous inflammation in other locations. Glucocorticoids seem to be the most effective agent for the control of endobronchial disease activity in such patients. In order to minimize exposure to systemic glucocorticoids, high doses of inhaled glucocorticoids can provide substantial benefit for patients with endobronchial disease when used in conjunction with other therapies.

Pearl: Normal saline nebulizer treatment twice daily may be beneficial in WG patients who complain of cough and difficulties with the expectoration of thick secretions.

Comment: The bronchial epithelium is morphologically and functionally almost identical to the nasal mucosa. Consequently, inflammatory insults result in similar damage, which causes difficulties moisturizing and raising secretions (damaged ciliary mucous elevator function). Normal saline inhalations may partially compensate and provide symptomatic relief. Nasal mucosal damage also frequently requires the chronic administration of saline nasal spray.

Pearl: Progressive large airway obstruction does not necessarily represent disease activity.

Comment: Only bronchoscopy can allow differentiation of active inflammation from circumferential scarring as a cause of progressive bronchial narrowing (Polychronopoulos et al.

2007). In the case of circumferential scarring, additional systemic immunosuppression is not necessary. Bronchoscopic balloon dilation or silastic airway stent placement may be beneficial, depending on the specific location.

24.8 Kidneys

Myth: Granulomas in the renal biopsy of a patient with ANCA are pathognomonic of WG.

Reality: Granulomas occur in many different conditions and their histopathological features usually fail to reveal their specific cause. Granulomas in renal biopsies of patients with WG are a rare finding, but may occur in different forms. They can contain multinucleated giant cells, histiocytes, macrophages, fibroblasts, and areas of necrosis. They can occur around destroyed glomeruli, blood vessels, and tubes.

Granulomas were detected in 40 renal biopsies performed as part of a consecutive series between 1991 and 2004 (Javaud et al. 2007). Among these biopsies, 20 (50%) were from patient with sarcoidosis; seven (17.5%) were attributed to drug reactions; and three (7.5%) were related to tuberculosis (Javaud et al. 2007). Only two (5%) of the 40 biopsies were from patients with WG.

Even among patients with ANCA, the differential diagnosis for granulomas found within kidneys should include the full range of conditions in which granulomas occur, particularly if the glomerular lesions are not consistent with a small-vessel vasculitis (i.e., pauci-immune glomerulonephritis).

Myth: Wainright and Davson were the first to propose that fibrinoid necrosis in the glomerulus represents small-vessel vasculitis of the glomerular tuft.

Reality: Although the 1950 article by Wainright and Davson is often cited as the first to claim that fibrinoid necrosis represents small-vessel vasculitis in the glomerulus, it does not actually make this claim (Wainright et al. 1950). Fibrinoid necrosis of the glomerulus is a segmental lesion that consists largely of amorphic eosinophilic material, which is highlighted in trichrome stains as carmine red spots (Fig. 24.14).

The term "fibrinoid" was coined because of the fibrin-like structure of the lesion, but it is likely that the lesion is composed of constituents other than fibrin and fibrinogen (Bajema and Bruijn 2000). The relationship between ANCA in the serum and fibrinoid necrosis in the kidneys and other tissues is not clear.

Pearl: Crescentic necrotizing glomerulonephritis is often a focal, segmental disease. It can therefore be missed in renal biopsies that contain few glomeruli.

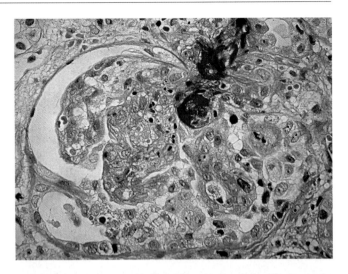

Fig. 24.14 Glomerulus with fibrinoid necrosis nearby the glomerular vascular pole, highlighted in this trichrome staining as carmine red spots (400 ×) (Figure courtesy of Dr. Ingeborg Bajema)

Comment: No one knows the minimum number of glomeruli that a renal biopsy should contain in order to be considered representative of overall disease extent within the kidneys. The issue has been debated for many years.

To some extent, the answer depends on the disease in question. In IgA nephropathy, for example, all glomeruli generally reveal mesangial IgA deposits by immunofluorescence. Thus, a limited number of glomeruli suffice to establish the diagnosis. (In the same way, the palpable purpura of Henoch-Schönlein purpura is generally more diffuse than is this finding in pauci-immune conditions such as WG.)

The pauci-immune immunofluoresence pattern that is characteristic of ANCA-associated vasculitis does not help to distinguish this disease in biopsies that lack the characteristic necrotic lesions, crescentic lesions, or both. In renal biopsies that show interstitial inflammation, the possibility of a glomerular disease such as pauci-immune crescentic glomerulonephritis should be considered. Deeper cuts through the biopsy block may be helpful. As is true with many disorders that require close clinicopathologic correlation for diagnosis, a dialog between the clinician and pathologist (often conducted most effectively over a microscope) is essential to getting the diagnosis right.

Myth: Fibrinoid necrosis must be present within a glomerulus if a crescent is evident.

Reality: This Myth stems from the notion that glomerular crescent formation is caused by fibrin leakage through disrupted glomerular basement membranes. It is not clear that this notion is correct. In a study of renal biopsies from patients with WG, 87 glomeruli were reconstructed in three dimensions and scored for the presence of crescents and fibrinoid necrosis (Hauer et al. 2000). Extracapillary proliferation (i.e., crescent formation) occurred in the absence of fibrinoid necrosis in 22% of the glomeruli.

These data do not disprove a relationship between crescent formation and fibrinoid necrosis. It is possible, for example, that the necrotic lesions resolved before the crescents came to "full bloom." Nevertheless, pathologists should use the term "necrotizing crescentic glomerulonephritis" only if both fibrinoid necrosis and crescents are actually detected in the biopsy.

Myth: Persistent hematuria in a patient with AAV under treatment is a signal to intensify immunosuppressive therapy.

Reality: Persistent hematuria in a patient with AAV is a common cause of clinician anxiety. Distinction between active disease and damage is essential in these patients. Disease-related hematuria results from rents in the glomerular basement membrane. As a result, red blood cells may persist in the urine for many months after the institution of appropriate treatment and the establishment of disease control. Red blood cell casts (Fig. 24.15) may also persist in the urine for many weeks and even months after arrest of the renal inflammation and systemic vasculitis. Thus, persistent red blood casts do not necessarily imply the failure of therapy, even if they are found still several months into treatment. (But they do make one worry, and look carefully for evidence of active disease in other organs.)

Patients with persistent hematuria and red blood cell casts must be observed very closely. They require other investigations, such as more frequent serial measurements of the glomerular filtration rate, the urine protein: creatinine ratio and even cystoscopy. However, more immunosuppression is an inappropriate knee-jerk response in this clinical scenario. Failure to recognize that hematuria and even red cell casts can persist in the urine even the achievement of clinical disease remission leads to misguided and excessive therapy.

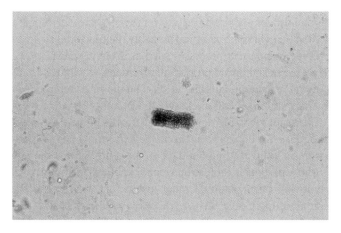

Fig. 24.15 Red blood cell casts in a patient with glomerulonephritis associated with microscopic polyangiitis (Figure courtesy of Dr. John Stone)

Hematuria in a cyclophosphamide treated patient can also occur as a result of drug-induced injury or a bladder malignancy, even if treatment was stopped many years ago. The presence of nonglomerular hematuria in a cyclophosphamide-treated patient should prompt cystocopy to examine for urothelial lesions or neoplasia (see "Bladder" below).

Pearl: ANCA positivity may correspond with a renal biopsy that reveals more than pauci-immune staining for immunoglobulins (i.e., >2 + for IgG, IgA, or IgM).

Comment: "Pauci-immunity" has been defined as 2 + staining or less (on a scale of 0 to 4+) for any immunoglobulin or complement component, as well as the absence of immune complex–type electron-dense deposits on electron microscopy. However, some renal biopsies from patients with ANCA-associated vasculitis patients stain > 2 + for immunoreactants. In one study of renal biopsies from 213 patients with ANCA-associated vasculitis, 30 (14%) had staining patterns for immunoglobulins that were more than pauci-immune (Harris et al. 1998).

Synergy between ANCA and the immune complexes could lead to more severe glomerular injury in some patients. This could also be the case for overlapping conditions in which AAV accompanies another form of glomerulonephritis. This phenomenon was underlined by the finding of extensive necrosis and crescent formation in a group of ten patients with lupus nephritis and ANCA positivity (Nasr et al. 2008).

The notion that electron-dense deposits are absent in ANCA-associated glomerulonephritis has also been called into question. In a study of 126 renal biopsies from patients with ANCA-associated vasculitis, immune complex deposits were detected via electron microscopy in 54% (Haas et al. 2004).

Pearl: Once renal involvement by WG begins, organ- or life-threatening disease may ensue swiftly.

Comment: Few diseases can cause renal deterioration as rapidly as WG. Once the serum creatinine begins to rise in WG, the disease often appears to accelerate, with rapidly progressive GN, swift progression to renal failure, and the appearance of "disseminated" involvement (alveolar hemorrhage, mesenteric vasculitis, and so on). In a patient with possible or known WG, a rising creatinine can't wait until Monday. Time is nephrons.

Pearl: The term "limited" WG should be used advisedly.

Comment: Contrary to the connotation of "limited," the prognosis of patients with limited WG is not benign in many patients to whom that appellation is applied. Patients with WG who did not have renal involvement were first reported in 1966 (Carrington and Liebow 1966). Many reports and studies in the literature now refer to such patients as having "limited" WG. This condition was once believed to correlate with a more favorable clinical outcome compared with that of the generalized form (Luqmani et al. 1994).

However, in a study of 180 patients with WG enrolled in a clinical trial, patients with limited disease tended to have longer disease duration, a greater likelihood of experiencing exacerbation of previous disease following a period of remission, and a higher prevalence of destructive upper respiratory tract disorders (WGET Research Group 2003). A careful examination of the patients described by Carrington and Liebow indicated that a number of those patients in fact had mild signs of renal involvement.

Clinicians and pathologists alike should bear in mind that renal biopsies from patients with only slightly elevated serum creatinine levels often reveal severe histological lesions. This is another reason that the term "limited" WG should be used with caution.

It should also be stressed that isolated alveolar hemorrhage in an ANCA-positive patient should never be labeled as "limited" disease. Even though the disease is "limited" to the lung at the time of presentation, this complication warrants remission induction therapy for life-threatening disease.

Myth: WG patients who present with end-stage renal disease who do not have severe pulmonary disease can be managed with prednisone alone.

Reality: WG, in contrast to lupus, does not "burn out" in patients whose kidneys fail. Therapy with a cytotoxic agent in addition to glucocorticoids is important to treat or prevent serious nonrenal disease in WG, e.g., alveolar hemorrhage. A second agent is usually required to control WG, even if salvaging useful renal function is no longer a possibility.

Among patients with disseminated WG treated with glucocorticoids alone, survival is approximately 50% at 12 months (Hollander 1967). Among WG patients in the longitudinal NIH series who were only treated with glucocorticoids, approximately 50% experienced some degree of clinical improvement, but only 4% (all of whom had mild disease) achieved remissions.

The second reason for aggressive (but judicious) treatment in WG patients who require dialysis is that aggressive therapy may lead to renal recovery. This point has also been emphasized in patients with MPA. Among 107 patients with MPA and GN in one study, 23 (21%) required dialysis at presentation. Of the 17 patients who received aggressive treatment, 9 no longer required dialysis after 3 months (Nachman 1996).

The caveat to treating AAV aggressively in patients with renal failure is that treatment must be administered with appropriate caution and adjustments of immunosuppression doses for renal dysfunction. These issues are discussed further below.

Pearl: The time around the start of dialysis is a hazardous one for patients with vasculitis.

Comment: Patients with end-stage or near end-stage renal disease are at increased risk for complications. In a randomized trial of plasma exchange in ANCA-associated vasculitis in which all patients had a serum creatinine of at least 5.7 mg/dL, 19 of the 137 patients died of infection within 1 year (Jayne et al. 2007). The overall mortality in that trial was 26%, underscoring the poor prognostic implications of presentation with end-stage renal disease.

The increased morbidity and mortality among patients with advanced renal dysfunction has multiple causes and several implications for therapy. The utmost precautions are required to prevent dialysis-related infections.

Pearl: Renal transplantation is an excellent option for treating patients with AAV who reach end-stage renal disease.

Comment: The patient and graft survival rates following renal transplantation in patients with ANCA-associated vasculitis are similar to those in patients with end-stage renal disease from other causes (Geetha and Seo 2007). In a recent study of 35 patients with ANCA-associated glomerulonephritis who received kidney transplants, the 5-year patient and death-censored allograft survival rates were 94% and 100%, respectively (Gera et al. 2007).

Standard transplant immunosuppression does not preclude a relapse of AAV, but not all relapses affect the transplanted kidney. In one study, 40% of relapses were extrarenal (Nachman et al. 1999). If a renal relapse does occur, it is characterized by a crescentic necrotizing glomerulonephritis, which can be distinguished easily from a transplant glomerulitis.

Pearl: Prognostication about renal function early in the treatment course of WG is risky.

Comment: The kidneys are often the last organ to respond to therapy in WG. Even if aggressive treatment begins when patients appear to have relatively good renal function (e.g., a serum Cr of 1.4 mg/dL), a small minority of patients march directly to end-stage renal disease despite the use of intensive immunosuppression. The reasons for the delay in renal response to treatment in some cases are probably multifactorial and may include intercurrent processes such as acute tubular necrosis. However, a significant proportion of patients who require dialysis in this setting are able to discontinue renal replacement therapy within several weeks to a few months.

It is not clear that any types of treatment alter the renal prognosis in such patients. Some centers would add plasmapheresis in this setting but data on the utility of that therapy for this particular indication remain unclear. "Sitting tight," removing other potential renal insults, and waiting for the immunosuppressive therapy to take effect may be the best course of action.

Pearl: Co-occurrence of ANCA and anti-GBM antibodies is associated with a worse renal prognosis.

Comment: Up to 30% of patients diagnosed with anti-GBM disease also have ANCA, most often MPO-ANCA (Bosch et al. 2006). Conversely, up to 10% of patients with AAV also have anti-GBM antibodies. Both types of autoantibodies should be sought in pulmonary-renal syndromes. The presence of anti-GBM antibodies is an indication for plasma exchange in addition to immunosuppressive agents.

Myth: Patients with AAV on the renal transplant list must be ANCA negative in order to be suitable candidates for a renal allograft.

Reality: The currently available evidence does not support this practice (Rostaing 1997; Geetha and Seo 2007). Patients with AAV and end-stage renal disease can undergo renal transplantation even if they remain ANCA positive, provided their disease has been quiescent clinically for a reasonable length of time (e.g., 6 months).

24.9 Bladder

Pearl: Drug-induced cystitis caused by cyclophosphamide can occur within several weeks of treatment initiation.

Comment: One important cause of hematuria in patients with WG that is not related to either active disease or damage is drug-induced cystitis caused by cyclophosphamide. The degree of symptomatology in cyclophosphamide-induced cystitis is highly variable. Some patients, a minority, present with profound symptoms of dysuria. On the other hand, many patients with this complication of therapy do not have urinary symptoms (urinary frequency, dysuria), but present rather with asymptomatic microscopic hematuria. Gross hematuria is less common.

Pearl: Self monitoring by patients for recurrent hematuria by regular urine dipsticks is an excellent early warning system for the detection of recurrent disease.

Comment: This Pearl is useful for patients whose hematuria has resolved after treatment. Patients can learn easily to dipstick their urine every 1–2 weeks. Patients whose urine dipstick shows evidence of hematuria should immediately undergo a full urinalysis with microscopy on a fresh urine specimen to exclude the presence of red blood cell casts.

Pearl: WG can involve the genitourinary tract.

Comment: In this protean disease, even the genitourinary tract is not spared. WG involvement of the cervix, vulva, uterus, penis, prostate gland, and other parts of this organ system have been described (Stone 1996; Bean and Conner 2007). If a patient with WG develops peculiar problems in these organs, WG must be excluded with appropriate biopsies.

24.10 Skin

Myth: Vasculitic lesions in AAV are always "pauci-immune."

Reality: Most vasculitic skin lesions in AAV have a histology of leukocytoclastic vasculitis. However, "leukocytoclastic vasculitis" does not distinguish AAV from Henoch-Schönlein purpura, mixed cryoglobulinemia, erythema elevatum diutinum, and a host of other conditions that cause vasculitis of the skin. Immunofluorescence studies of skin biopsies are frequently used to narrow the diagnostic possibilities further. Positive findings, especially for IgA and complement, are often used to exclude AAV. However, a substantial number of skin biopsies in AAV that reveal leukocytoclasis are not pauci-immune in nature. These can reveal substantial IgA, IgM, and complement staining, and may create diagnostic confusion (Brons et al. 2001).

Pearl: Scurvy can mimic AAV, particularly MPA.

Comment: Scurvy can cause perifollicular petechiae that mimic purpura, extensive gum inflammation, and alveolar hemorrhage, all of which can be confused with MPA (Duggan et al. 2007). Think of scurvy when a severely malnourished patient is suspected of having an AAV.

24.11 Joints

Pearl: Arthritis is a common presentation of a flare in AAV.

Comment: Arthritis and arthralgias are a frequently overlooked manifestation in AAV, perhaps because they improve so quickly after the institution of therapy. The arthritis commonly involves large joints in a migratory, asymmetric, oligoarticular pattern, 1 day involving a knee and an ankle, the next day a shoulder or wrist (Fig. 24.16). Small joints may also be involved. Arthritis and arthralgias are a very common tip-off to a disease flare in AAV.

24.12 Peripheral and Cranial Nerves

Pearl: Even a frail, elderly woman should not have "breakable" foot dorsiflexion strength.

Comment: Vasculitic neuropathy can become lost in the shuffle of other organ system involvement and remain subclinical (i.e., undiagnosed) if the clinician does not ask about symptoms of numbness, pain, and burning in the feet and hands. In addition, a careful physical examination for foot dorsiflexion weakness must be performed, because this is the most common peripheral nerve lesion in vasculitic

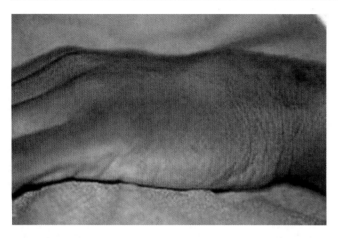

Fig. 24.16 Wrist arthritis in a patient with Wegener's granulomatosis (WG). When frank arthritis occurs in WG, involvement of one major joint (often with an effusion, as in this case) is common. Diffuse, migratory arthralgias are often the presenting feature of a disease flare (Figure courtesy of Dr. John Stone)

Pearl: Vasculitic neuropathy is more common in MPA than in WG.

Comment: This statement is correct: MPA has a greater propensity to involve peripheral nerves than does WG. However, devastating vasculitic neuropathy can occur in either disorder and is associated with either PR3-ANCA or MPO-ANCA positivity.

Pearl: A facial droop may result from granulomatous inflammation within the middle ear in WG.

Comment: The seventh cranial nerve courses through the middle ear cavity (see Fig. 39.1 in Chap. 39, I). If middle ear inflammation is sufficiently severe in WG and leads to an expanding, compressive lesion, both conductive hearing loss and a seventh nerve palsy can result (Fig. 24.18). Such lesions may heal completely through medical treatment alone.

24.13 Central Nervous System

Pearl: WG can present with headaches that mimic giant cell arteritis (GCA).

Comment: The principal characteristic of a GCA headache is that it is new; i.e., the patient has not experienced such

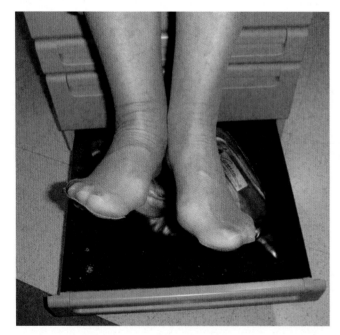

Fig. 24.17 Examination of the foot for dorsiflexion weakness. In mild cases of foot dorsiflexion weakness, the most common manifestation of vasculitic neuropathy, the lesion is often unrecognized by patients with more severe manifestation of disease in other organs and is also often overlooked by clinicians. This patient had substantial bilateral foot dorsiflexion weakness, left greater than right, which even she had not appreciated. She had, however, noted pain from sensory neuropathy, which almost always accompanies motor neuropathy in vasculitic neuropathy (Figure courtesy of Dr. John Stone)

neuropathy (Fig. 24.17). Even a strong examiner should not be able to overcome the foot dorsiflexion strength of a patient whose distal muscle strength is intact.

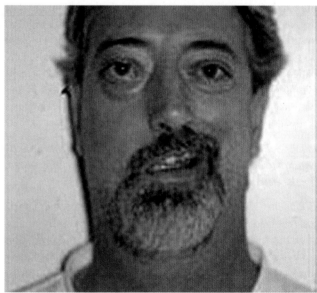

Fig. 24.18 Peripheral seventh cranial nerve palsy in Wegener's granulomatosis. The patient has a facial droop on the affected side and is unable to wrinkle the ipsilateral forehead. This lesion results from granulomatous inflammation within the middle ear, leading to compression of the portion of the seventh cranial nerve that runs through that cavity. Middle ear surgery places the patient at risk for irreversible damage to the nerve if granulomatous tissue it. Thus, if the diagnosis can be established in other ways, the middle ear should be left alone

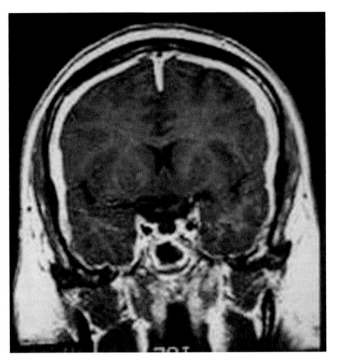

Fig. 24.19 Meningeal involvement in Wegener's granulomatosis (Figure courtesy of Dr. John Stone)

headaches before. WG can cause intense, unrelenting headaches that are new for the patient and mimic GCA. There are several potential sources of headache in WG: sinusitis, chronic osteitis in the mid-facial bones, meningeal inflammation (Fig. 24.19), ocular disease (posterior scleritis, which may require ocular ultrasound to diagnose (Sadiq et al. 2003)), and temporal artery inflammation (Small and Brisson 1991; Genereau et al. 1999).

24.14 Spleen

Myth: Splenic involvement in WG is rare.

Reality: Splenic involvement was actually recognized by Friedrich Wegener in his first paper on this disease (Wegener 1936). Wegener's paper was illustrated with a pathologic figure of splenic infarctions, which he termed *Fleckmilz* ("spotted spleen").

Because of the decrease in the number of WG patients who die from their illness and the declining frequency of deaths studied by autopsy, splenic involvement is underrecognized in WG (and its clinical implications, if any, are unclear). Cross-sectional imaging studies have reminded us that splenic involvement can occur in WG, and that it usually presents with splenic infarctions.

24.15 ANCA

Myth: A rise in ANCA titer predicts a disease flare.

Reality: This has been one of the most hotly debated issues in AAV since the mid-1980s. Several prospective studies have shown that the temporal association between ANCA titer elevations and the occurrence of disease flares is poor (Table 24.3) (Finkielman et al. 2007; Boomsma et al. 2000; Jayne et al. 1995). Many patients flare after elevations in ANCA titer, but these events are seldom linked tightly enough in time for clinical decisions to be based upon ANCA serologies.

Data from prospective studies on whether or not the achievement of a negative ANCA protects against future disease flares are mixed. Two studies from the Netherlands reported that patients who became ANCA-negative were less likely to flare than those who remained ANCA positive (Boomsma et al. 2000; Stegeman et al. 1994). However, in the Wegener's Granulomatosis Etanercept Trial, the achievement of ANCA-negative status did not protect patients against subsequent disease flares (Finkielman et al. 2007).

Pearl: There is considerably more overlap than dissimilarity between patients who have MPO- as opposed to PR3-ANCA.

Comment: Various studies have investigated whether the clinical and pathological parameters differ between patients with anti-MPO and anti-PR3 ANCA. One investigation of 46 anti-MPO positive patients and 46 anti-PR3 positive patients concluded that extrarenal organ manifestations and respiratory tract granulomas were more common in patients with anti-PR3 ANCA than in those with anti-MPO antibodies, and that anti-PR3–positive patients are predisposed to more dramatic deteriorations in renal function (Franssen et al. 1998). Earlier studies had found that these patient groups have similar prognoses (Geffriaud-Ricouard et al. 1993).

In renal biopsies, there is a tendency toward more chronic lesions in anti-MPO positive patients (Hauer et al. 2002).

Table 24.3 ANCA titers correlate poorly with the timing of disease flares

Study	Patients	PR3-ANCA positive (no.)	Serum collection	ANCA increases (no.)	Relapses (no.)
Boomsma[b]	100	85	2	38	22[a]
				30	15[a]
Jayne[c]	60	39	1	27	13[a]
Kyndt[d]	43	17	1–3	14	4
				17	2

[a]Within the following year after the increase in ANCA
[b]Boomsma et al 2000
[c]Jayne et al. 1995
[d]Kyndt et al. 1999

This may be related to the timepoint at which the biopsy is performed: patients with PR3-ANCA are likely to have earlier renal biopsies because upper respiratory tract disease calls the patient to medical attention.

Pearl: Seek, and ye shall find ANCA.

Comment: All large studies of "ANCA-associated vasculitis" have reported small numbers of patients who are ANCA-negative despite the presence of generalized disease. These patients, who normally comprise up to 10% of most studies, stand as a compelling argument against the pathogenicity of ANCA.

By combining all ANCA testing methods (indirect immunofluorescence, direct ELISA, and capture ELISA), the number of patients with severe clinical disease who remain ANCA negative can be reduced to a minimum of 4%. This was demonstrated in a study of 180 patients with WG, of whom 128 had severe disease and 52 had limited disease (Finkielman et al. 2007).

There are very few data regarding the histomorphology of ANCA-negative patients. Eisenberger et al. reported a group of 20 patients with pauci-immune, crescentic, necrotizing renal vasculitis who were ANCA negative (Eisenberger et al. 2005). The occurrence of crescents, fibrinoid necrosis, and interstitial infiltrates was similar to that found in PR3- and MPO-positive patients. Renal biopsies of ANCA-negative patients tended to show more interstitial fibrosis and glomerulosclerosis, probably a consequence of later diagnosis because of their ANCA negativity (Hauer et al. 2002).

Pearl: Antithyroid medications are the most common cause of drug-induced AAV.

Comment: Drug-induced AAV provides a compelling model for studying the role of ANCA in disease pathogenesis. The strongest associations between medications and ANCA production involve antithyroid drugs such as proplthiouracil (Gunton et al. 2000). ANCA positivity develops in up to 25% of patients treated with PTU, but clinically evident vasculitis is found in only a small minority (Gunton et al. 2000). Far less robust relationships have been reported between the development of ANCA and the use of medications such as penicillamine, alloprinol, procainamide, phenytoin, cefotaxime, isoniazid, and indomethacin (Sakai et al. 1999; Feriozzi et al. 2000; Bienaime et al. 2007).

In a study of 209 patients with hyperthyroidism, 13 (6%) became positive for MPO-ANCA, PR3-ANCA, or antielastase ANCA (Slot et al. 2005). Among the ANCA-positive patients, the odds ratio for previous treatment with antithyroid medications was 11.8. Some data suggest that the likelihood of developing clinically significant AAV (e.g., glomerulonephritis) correlates with length of time on antithyroid medications.

24.16 Treatment and Course

Pearl: "Refractory WG" is an opportunistic infection until proven otherwise.

Comment: During the first 3–4 months of therapy, patients who improve and enter remission on cyclophosphamide and glucocorticoids are more likely to suffer serious complications of this treatment than an exacerbation of WG. Patients with "disseminated" or generalized WG who are refractory to high doses of conventional immunosuppression are truly rare. Thus, a WG patient who "worsens" after being on cyclophosphamide and prednisone for a while probably has an opportunistic infection or another complication of treatment. The most common site of an opportunistic infection in AAV is the lung. In critically ill patients, bronchoscopy with bronchoalveolar lavage should be performed immediately.

The upper respiratory tract is another challenging site. A sensible approach to distinguishing chronic sinusitis from smoldering WG is to treat vigorously with antimicrobial agents for an appropriate length of time. If this strategy does not achieve control of the problem, it may be assumed that the disease is active. If neither antimicrobial agents nor an increased dose of prednisone helps, then the patient may need a surgical intervention to clean damaged sinuses.

Pearl: A little bit of prednisone goes a long way toward sustaining disease remissions in AAV.

Comment: An important lesson from the major clinical trials in AAV published since 2003 is that keeping patients on a small glucocorticoid dose has a dramatic impact on the flare rate. This is highlighted in Table 24.4. Patients enrolled in protocols that called for tapering glucocorticoid doses to zero in the months after remission had dramatically higher rates of disease flare compared with patients whose treatment protocols permitted ongoing doses equivalent to between 5 and 10 mg of prednisone (Goek et al. 2005).

Myth: Cyclophosphamide should be continued until the patient has been in a clinical remission for 1 year.

Table 24.4 Relationship between maintenance glucocorticoid dose and disease flare in three randomized clinical trials

	CYCAZAREM[b] (*n* = 144)	NORAM[c] (*n* = 100)	WGET[d] (*n* = 180)
Prednisolone dose 6 months	>10 mg	7.5 mg	Off
Prednisolone dose 12 months	7.5 mg	Off	Off
Flare rate (%)	15%	70% (Methotrexate arm) 47% Cyclophosphamide arm)	51%

Reality: Cyclophosphamide revolutionized the treatment of WG. The use of this medication (first employed regularly at the National Institutes of Health [NIH] in the late 1960s) changed an illness that was almost universally fatal within 1 year to one in which remission is achieved, at least temporarily, in the great majority of cases. Patients and physicians alike were reluctant to discontinue cyclophosphamide following early successes with this medication. It became standard practice to continue cyclophosphamide for at least 1 year after the patient had achieved disease remission.

The downside of using cyclophosphamide in this fashion became apparent in the 1990s. In a report of the longitudinal NIH series of patients with WG, the mean duration of cyclophosphamide use was approximately 2 years. More than 40% of the patients suffered permanent treatment-related morbidity, including drug-induced cystitis, bladder cancer, an increased risk of leukemia/lymphoma, opportunistic infection, and others (Hoffman et al. 1992).

Subsequent studies have demonstrated that the acceptable risk: benefit ratio for the continuation of cyclophosphamide is exceeded long before the 2-year mark. Shorter courses of cyclophosphamide are equally effective in inducing remission. The standard of care for remission induction in patients with severe AAV now is to use cyclophosphamide for 3–6 months along with high-dose glucocorticoids, and then to discontinue cyclophosphamide in favor of either azathioprine or methotrexate. This standard of care may be altered by conclusions from the ongoing Rituximab in ANCA-associated Vasculitis (RAVE) trial (Specks et al. 2009).

Pearl: Patients tolerate less and less cyclophosphamide as time goes by.

Comment: Regular monitoring for toxicity is required for patients on cyclophosphamide. The need for dose adjustments may be apparent after only 1 or 2 weeks in some patients, but more often signs of bone marrow toxicity become apparent after several months on the drug. It is a rare patient who can tolerate full doses of cyclophosphamide without a decline in bone marrow function for more than 1 year.
The bone marrow never forgets that it has seen cyclophosphamide. Patients tolerate second courses of cyclophosphamide less well than their first. Moreover, the use of azathioprine or methotrexate after an induction course of cyclophosphamide can be associated with precipitous declines in cell counts shortly after the start of the remission maintenance regimen. Vigilance must remain high for cytopenias even after the patient is off cyclophosphamide.

The white blood cell line is usually affected first by cyclophosphamide toxicity. A minority of patients become thrombocytopenic quickly, before an effect is evident on leukocytes. The red blood cell line is typically affected last.

Pearl: The effect of cyclophosphamide on lymphocytes persists for months after the drug has been discontinued.

Comment: The effects of cyclophosphamide on lymphocyte counts persist for many months after the drug has been discontinued (Fauci 1974). This has direct implications for the duration of Pneumocystis jiroveci pneumonia prophylaxis (Suryaprasad 2008). No one knows precisely how long Pneumocystis prophylaxis should be continued in patients after cyclophosphamide (or other immunosuppressive medications) has been stopped. However, it seems prudent to monitor CD4 lymphocyte counts and to continue Pneumocystis prophylaxis until the total lymphocyte count is greater than 200/mm^3.

The take home lesson is that *Pneumocystis* prophylaxis may need to continue in some patients for some months, even after cyclophosphamide and other intensive immunosuppressive agents have been discontinued. Fatal *Pneumocystis* infections have been reported months after the discontinuation of cyclophosphamide.

Myth: The induction of neutropenia is essential to the successful treatment of WG.

Reality: Neutropenia (and lymphopenia) is precisely what leads to many of the adverse events associated with the conventional treatment of WG. Nearly, all patients' disease can be controlled without the induction of neutropenia (white blood counts below 4,000/mm^3). This concept was promulgated in the 1970s in one of the early papers from the NIH on WG: "*Granulocyte kinetics were measured… we found that marked suppression of granulocytopoiesis was not necessary for a favorable response…*" (Fauci 1974). Despite this observation, too many practitioners target neutropenia or lymphopenia as a therapeutic target, believing that this is necessary for the induction of disease remission.

Pearl: Watch not only the absolute neutrophil count but also the trend in values in cyclophosphamide-treated patients.

Comment: Although a total white blood cell count of 5.0 × 10^3/mm^3 sounds fine for a patient on cyclophosphamide, it signals a worrisome trend if the previous week's count was 9.0 × 10^3/mm^3 and measurement the week before that was 12.4 × 10^3/mm^3. Appropriate steps in the management of this patient would be to hold the cyclophosphamide for a few days and repeat the white blood cell count, or at a minimum to reduce the daily dose (and repeat the count).

Blood counts drawn on 1 day reflect the dose of cyclophosphamide taken roughly 1 week earlier. This makes following *trends* as important as following absolute numbers. In a patient with a declining white blood cell count, consideration should be made for dosage reduction or even drug holding in certain instances.

Myth: Cyclophosphamide is more effective if given twice a day.

Reality: Splitting the dose of cyclophosphamide offers no pharmacokinetic advantages and increases the medication risks. Acrolein, a metabolite of cyclophosphamide, is toxic to the urothelium and can lead to drug-induced cystitis. To minimize this risk, daily cyclophosphamide should always be taken all at once and in the morning, with a large amount of fluid to maintain frequently voided, dilute urine. Cyclophosphamide should never be taken before bedtime because this increases the potential for acrolein to be in contact with the urothelium.

Pearl: Disease-associated morbidity usually occurs within the first 3 months.

Comment: The CYCAZAREM trial compared the abilities of cyclophosphamide and azathioprine to maintain remission in 155 patients with ANCA-associated vasculitis (WG = 95 patients; MPA = 60 patients) (Jayne et al. 2003). Eighteen severe or life-threatening adverse events occurred during the first 3 months of therapy. In contrast, only 27 such events occurred during the remission-maintenance phase, which lasted five times longer. Seven patients died during the remission-induction phase (two from pneumonia, three from pulmonary vasculitis and infection, and two from stroke), but only one died during the remission-maintenance phase (from a stroke).

These data were echoed also in findings from the Wegener's Granulomatosis Etanercept Trial, in which a disproportionate number of adverse events occurred in the first 6 months (remission induction) as opposed to the subsequent remission maintenance phase (WGET 2005).

There are several explanations for the high incidence of adverse events shortly after the initiation of treatment:

- The patients are generally sickest at the start of remission induction.
- A sizeable percentage of patients experience significant renal dysfunction (and even end-stage renal disease) at this time.
- The doses of immunosuppression are highest just after therapy has begun.

Pearl: Make sure your patient also knows that methotrexate and daily double-strength TMP/SMZ should not be used together.

Comment: Because both methotrexate and TMP/SMZ are folate antagonists, daily administration of double-strength TMP/SMZ should be avoided. Prolonged courses of double-strength TMP/SMZ and methotrexate can be disastrous, leading to bone marrow aplasia.

Primary-care doctors who do not prescribe methotrexate regularly may not recall this detail but are inclined to prescribe double-strength TMP/SMZ for a variety of complaints: urinary tract infections, upper respiratory disturbances, and other problems that might not come to the attention of the patient's rheumatologist. Moreover, patients may also get one medicine from one pharmacy and the other from another pharmacy, thereby reducing the likelihood that the potential for drug interaction will be caught. Thus, patients themselves should be aware of this potential interaction.

On the other hand, *Pneumocystis* prophylaxis is crucial for all patients receiving immunosuppressive regimens comprised of high-dose glucocorticoids and another immunosuppressive regimen, including methotrexate. A daily single-strength TMP/SMZ tablet (or a double-strength tablet every *other* day) given for that purpose appears to be well-tolerated by patients on methotrexate, provided that folic acid supplementation (1 mg/day orally) is given at the same time.

Myth: Vaccination is contraindicated in patients with AAV because it can trigger disease flares.

Reality: The results of a large cohort study of individuals vaccinated with the influenza vaccine indicated this vaccination did not lead to disease flares in patients with AAV (Stassen et al. 2008). In addition, contrary to popular perception, patients with these diseases are able to mount adequate antibody responses to influenza vaccination despite active or previous immunosuppressive therapy (Holvast et al. 2008).

Pearl: The dose of cyclophosphamide needs to be modified in the setting of renal dysfunction.

Comment: Cyclophosphamide should be dosed for renal failure (Haubitz et al. 2002). The dose should be reduced by 50% for those on dialysis (i.e., 1 mg/kg/day should be administered rather than 2 mg/kg/day). Cyclophosphamide dose reductions are also advisable in the elderly, even those with "normal" renal function as reflected by their serum creatinine.

Pearl: Cyclophosphamide is dialyzed.

Comment: This is another way that renal failure complicates the management of WG. In addition to the importance of dosing cyclophosphamide for renal failure, as described above, cyclophosphamide must be given back to the patient after dialysis on the day when dialysis occurs. An approved practice is to administer the patient's morning dose as usual and then to give a half-dose later in the day after the dialysis session (Haubitz et al. 2002).

Pearl: Methotrexate is contraindicated in patients with a serum creatinine > 2.0 mg/dL.

Comment: Methotrexate is cleared in part through renal metabolism. The use of this medication in the setting of significant renal dysfunction can lead to severe bone marrow toxicity. Although most clinicians get this right when prescribing methotrexate initially, methotrexate doses must also be adjusted in the setting of subsequent renal function declines. The case of herpes zoster depicted in Fig. 24.20 illustrates this point.

Pearl: Be extra careful about monitoring for cytopenias during times of glucocorticoid dose reductions or during

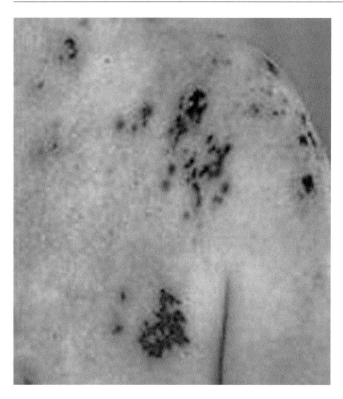

Fig. 24.20 Zoster that occurred in a neutropenic patient with Wegener's granulomatosis on methotrexate (MTX). The patient's serum creatinine was 1.7 mg/dL when MTX therapy began. However, his renal function declined slowly during follow-up and his serum creatinine rose to 2.4 mg/dL. He presented with disseminated herpes zoster in the setting of a peripheral white blood cell count of $1.2 \times 10^3/mm^3$

periods of transitioning from cyclophosphamide to another immunosuppressive agent.

Comment: When cyclophosphamide is administered orally, the WBC has a tendency to fall once the prednisone dose is reduced below 20 mg/day.

Because the action of cyclophosphamide on bone marrow function lasts for many months beyond the last dose, the initial period when another agent is begun (e.g., azathioprine or methotrexate) is a time when the patient may suffer bone marrow suppression from the effects of both cyclophosphamide and the new agent.

Avoid the tendency to "loosen up" on blood count monitoring once the patient is off cyclophosphamide. The usual starting doses of azathioprine (2 mg/kg/day), methotrexate (15–25 mg/week), and mycophenolate (2,000 mg/day) are sufficient to cause cytopenias by themselves and require especially close monitoring when these medications are given after cyclophosphamide.

Pearl: MPA is less likely than WG to flare.

Comment: In the CYCAZAREM trial (Jayne et al. 2003), disease flares occurred in 17 of the 92 patients with WG (18%), compared with 4 of 52 (8%) of those with MPA. In a case series of 85 patients with MPA with longer follow-up, disease flares occurred in approximately 33% (Guillevin et al. 1999). In contrast, up to 80% of patients with WG flare over time (WGET Research Group 2005; Reinhold-Keller et al. 2000).

As WG is more frequently associated with antibodies against PR3 than to MPO, while the opposite is true for MPA, it may be the ANCA specificity that is associated with the risk of flares. In addition to the data from the CYCAZAREM trial, some retrospective data suggest that this is the case, as within a group of patients with WG the relapse risk was found to be significantly higher in PR3-ANCA than in MPO-ANCA associated patients (Stegeman 2002).

Pearl: Check a patient's thiopurine methyltransferase status before starting azathioprine.

Comment: Azathioprine is commonly used as a remission maintenance drug in ANCA-associated vasculitis. Although the medication has been around for half a century, only recently has it been realized that people are born with (or without) genes necessary to metabolize the drug properly.

Azathioprine metabolism is governed largely by thiopurine methyltransferase (TPMT) genes, which are inherited in an autosomal fashion. Approximately 90% of individuals are born with two TPMT alleles and have no problem with azathioprine metabolism. Approximately 9% of patients are heterozygous for the TPMT mutation. In these patients, a "start low and go slow" is reasonable, even though many heterozygotes are able to tolerate large doses of azathioprine (Stassen et al. 2008). Fifty milligrams per day is a reasonable starting dose for TPMT heterozygotes. Less than 1% of individuals are homozygous negative for TPMT and are at risk for disastrous bone marrow toxicity if they receive azathioprine.

Pearl: The syndrome of azathioprine hypersensitivity has nothing to do with TPMT alleles.

Comment: TPMT alleles go a long way toward determining patients' susceptibility to bone marrow toxicity but do not affect the likelihood of certain other AZA side effects. For example, azathioprine hypersensitivity reactions can occur quite severely even in patients with two TPMT alleles. Similarly, gastrointestinal tract toxicity – severe nausea that commences shortly after taking the medication – is not affected by the patient's number of TPMT alleles.

References

Antineutrophil cytoplasmic autoantibody-associated pauci-immune glomerulonephritis and vasculitis, and other vasculitides. In: D'Agati VD, Jennette JC, Silva FG (eds) Non-neoplastic kidney diseases (1st edn). Silver Spring, MD, ARP, 2005, pp. 385–424

Bajema IM, Bruijn JA. What stuff is this! A historical perspective on fibrinoid necrosis. J Pathol 2000; 191:235–238

Bean SM, Conner MG. Wegener's granulomatosis of the uterine cervix: A case report and review of the literature. Int J Gynecol Pathol 2007; 26:95–98

Bienaime F, Clerbaux G, et al D-Penicillamine-induced ANCA-associated crescentic glomerulonephritis in Wilson disease. Am J Kidney Dis 2007; 50(5):821–825

Birnbaum J, Danoff S, Askin FB, Stone JH. Microscopic polyangiitis presenting as a 'pulmonary-muscle' syndrome: Does alveolar hemorrhage contribute to the mechanism of pulmonary fibrosis?. Arthritis Rheum 2007; 56(6):20–71

Boomsma MM, Stegeman CA, van der Leij MJ, et al Prediction of relapses in Wegener's granulomatosis by measurement of antineutrophil cytoplasmic antibody levels. A prospective study. Arthritis Rheum 2000; 43:2025–2033

Bosch X, Guilabert A, Font J. Antineutrophil cytoplasmic antibodies. Lancet 2006; 368:404–418

Brons RH, de Jong MC, de Boer NK, et al Detection of immune deposits in skin lesions of patients with Wegener's granulomatosis. Ann Rheum Dis 2001; 60:1097–1102

Carrington CB, Liebow A. Limited forms of angiitis and granulomatosis of Wegener's type. Am J Med 1966; 41:497–527

D'Cruz DP, Baguley E, Asherson RA, et al Ear, nose, and throat symptoms in subacute Wegener's granulomatosis. BMJ 1989; 299: 419–422

Devaney KO, Travis WD, Hoffman G, et al Interpretation of head and neck biopsies in Wegener's granulomatosis. A pathologic study of 126 biopsies in 70 patients. Am J Surg Pathol 1990; 14:555–564

Duggan CP, Westra SJ, Rosenberg AE. Case records of the Massachusetts General Hospital. Case 23-2007. A 9-year-old boy with bone pain, rash, and gingival hypertrophy. N Engl J Med 2007; 357:392–400

Eisenberger U, Fakhouri F, Vanhille P, et al ANCA-negative pauci-immune renal vasculitis: histology and outcome. Nephrol Dial Transplant 2005; 20:1392–1399

Eschun GM, Mink SN, Sharma S. Pulmonary interstitial fibrosis as a presenting manifestation in perinuclear antineutrophilic cytoplasmic antibody microscopic polyangiitis. Chest 2003; 123:297–301

FDA Public Health Notification: Complications from metallic tracheal stents in patients with benign airway disorders. http://www.fda.gov/cdrh/safety/072905-tracheal.html

Feriozzi S, Muda AO, et al Cephotaxime-associated allergic interstitial nephritis and MPO-ANCA positive vasculitis. Ren Fail 2000; 22(2):245–251

Finkielman JD, Lee AS, Hummel AM, et al ANCA are detectable in nearly all patients with active severe Wegener's granulomatosis. Am J Med 2007; 120:643.e9–e14

Finkielman JD, Merkel PA, Schroeder D, et al for the WGET Research Group. Antineutrophil cytoplasmic antibodies against proteinase 3 do not predict disease relapses in Wegener's granulomatosis. Ann Intern Med 2007 147(9):611–9

Franssen C, Gans R, Kallenberg C, et al Disease spectrum of patients with antineutrophil cytoplasmic autoantibodies of defined specificity: Distinct differences between patients with anti-proteinase 3 and anti-myeloperoxidase autoantibodies. J Intern Med 1998; 244: 209–216

Gallagher H, Kwan JT, Jayne DR. Pulmonary renal syndrome: A 4-year, single-center experience. Am J Kidney Dis 2002; 39:42–47

Geetha D, Seo P. Renal transplantation in the ANCA-associated vasculitides. Am J Transplant 2007; 7:2657–2662

Geffriaud-Ricouard C, Noël LH, Chauveau D. Clinical significance of ANCA in 98 patients. Adv Exp Med Biol 1993; 336:273–279

Genereau T, Lortholary O, Pottier M, et al Temporal artery biopsy. A diagnostic tool for systemic necrotizing vasculitis. Arthritis Rheum 1999; 42:2674–2681

Gera M, Griffin MD, Specks U, et al Recurrence of ANCA-associated vasculitis following renal transplantation in the modern era of immunosupression. Kidney Int 2007; 71:1296–1301

Goek ON, Stone JH. Randomized controlled trials in ANCA-associated vasculitis. Curr Opin Rheumatol 2005; 17:257–264

Guillevin L, Durand-Gasselin B, Cevallos R. Microscopic polyangiitis: Clinical and laboratory findings in eighty-five patients. Arthritis Rheum 1999; 42:421–430

Gunton JE, Stiel J, et al Prevalence of positive anti-neutrophil cytoplasmic antibody (ANCA) in patients receiving anti-thyroid medication. Eur J Endocrinol 2000; 142(6):587

Haas M, Eustace JA. Immune complex deposits in ANCA-associated crescentic glomerulonephritis: A study of 126 cases. Kidney Int 2004; 65:2145–2152

Harris AA, Falk RJ, Jennette JC. Crescentic glomerulonephritis with a paucity of glomerular immunoglobulin localization. Am J Kidney Dis 1998; 32:179–184

Haubitz M et al Cyclophosphamide phramacokinetics and dose requirements in patients with renal insufficiency. Kidney Int 2002; 61: 1495–1501

Hauer HA, Bajema IM, de Heer E, et al Distribution of renal lesions in idiopathic systemic vasculitis: A three-dimensional analysis of 87 glomeruli. Am J Kidney Dis 2000; 36:257–265

Hauer HA, Bajema IM, van Houwelingen HC, et al Renal histology in ANCA-associated vasculitis: Differences between diagnostic and serologic subgroups. Kidney Int 2002; 61:80–89

Hoffman G, Kerr G, Leavitt R, et al Wegener's granulomatosis: An analysis of 158 patients. Ann Intern Med 1992; 116:488–498

Holvast A, Stegeman CA, Benne CA, et al Wegener's granulomatosis patients show an adequate antibody response to influenza vaccination. Ann Rheum Dis 2008 July 14. [Epub ahead of print]

Hollander D, Manning RT. The use of alkylating agents in the treatment of Wegener's granulomatosis. Ann Intern Med 1967; 67:393-8

Homma S, Matsushita H, Nakata K. Pulmonary fibrosis in myeloperoxidase antineutrophil cytoplasmic antibody-associated vasculitides. Respirology 2004; 9(2):190–196

Javaud N, Belenfant X, Stirnemann J, et al Renal granulomatoses: A retrospective study of 40 cases and review of the literature. Medicine (Baltimore) 2007; 86:170–180

Jayne D, Rasmussen N, Bacon, et al Randomised trial of cyclophosphamide versus azathioprine during remission in ANCA-associated systemic vasculitis. N Engl J Med 2003; 349: 36–44

Jayne DR, Gaskin G, Pusey CD, Lockwood CM. ANCA and predicting relapse in systemic vasculitis. QJM 1995; 88:127–133

Jayne DR, Gaskin G, Rasmussen N, et al Randomized trial of plasma exchange or high-dosage methylprednisolone as adjunctive therapy for severe renal vasculitis. J Am Soc Nephrol 2007; 18:2180–2188

Kyndt et al Serial measurements of antineutrophil cytoplasmic autoantibodies in patients with systemic vasculitis. Am J Med 1999; 106:527–533

Langford C, Talar-Williams C, Barron K, et al A staged approach to the treatment of Wegener's granulomatosis: Induction of remission with glucocorticoids and daily cyclophosphamide switching to methotrexate for remission maintenance. Arthritis Rheum 1999; 42: 2666–2673

Leavitt RY, Fauci AS, Bloch DA, et al The American College of Rheumatology 1990 criteria for the classification of Wegener's granulomatosis. Arthritis Rheum 1990; 33:1101–1107

Luqmani RA, Bacon PA, Beaman, et al Classical versus non-renal Wegener's granulomatosis. Q J Med 1994; 87:161–167

Mahr AD, Neogi T, LaValley MP, et al Assessment of the item selection and weighting in the Birmingham Vasculitis Activity Score for Wegener's Granulomatosis (BVAS/WG) (submitted)

Merkel PA, Lo GH, Holbrook JT, et al for the WGET Research Group. Incidence of venous thrombotic events among patients with Wegener's granulomatosis. Ann Intern Med 2005; 142:620–626

Nachman PH, Hogan SL, Jennette JC, Falk RJ. Treatment response and relapse in antineutrophil cytoplasmic autoantibody-associated microscopic polyangiitis and glomerulonephritis. J Am Soc Nephrol 1996; 7(1):33-9

Nachman PH, Segelmark M, Westman K, et al Recurrent ANCA-associated small vessel vasculitis after transplantation: A pooled analysis. Kidney Int 1999; 56:1544–1550

Nasr SH, D'Agati VD, Park, et al Necrotizing and crescentic lupus nephritis with antineutrophil cytoplasmic antibody seropositivity. Clin J Am Soc Nephrol 2008; 3:682–690

Niles JL, Böttinger EP, Saurina GR, et al The syndrome of lung hemorrhage and nephritis is usually an ANCA-associated condition. Arch Intern Med 1996; 156:440–445

Polychronopoulos VS, Prakash UB, Golbin JM, et al Airway involvement in Wegener's granulomatosis. Rheum Dis Clinics N America 2007; 33:755–775

Reinhold-Keller E, Beuge N, Latza U, et al An interdisciplinary approach to the care of patients with Wegener's granulomatosis. Long term outcome in 155 patients. Arthritis Rheum 2000; 43(5):1021–1032

Robinson MR, Lee SS, Sneller MC, et al Tarsal-conjunctival disease associated with Wegener's granulomatosis. Ophthalmology 2003; 110:1770–1780

Rostaing L, Modesto A, Oksman F et al Outcome of patients with antineutrophil cytoplasmic autoantibody-associated vasculitis following cadaveric kidney transplantation. Am J Kidney Dis 1997; 29(1):96-102

Sadiq Z, Shepherd R, Vardy S. Posterior scleritis: An unusual presentation of facial pain. Br J Oral Maxillofac Surg 2003; 41:62–63

Sakai N, Wada T, et al Tubulointerstitial nephritis with anti-neutrophil cytoplasmic antibody following indomethacin treatment. Nephrol Dial Transplant 1999; 14(11):2774

Saxena R, Bygren P, Arvastson B, Wieslander J. Circulating autoantibodies as serological markers in the differential diagnosis of pulmonary renal syndrome. J Intern Med 1995; 238:43–52

Slot MC, Links TP, et al Occurrence of antineutrophil cytoplasmic antibodies and associated vasculitis in patients with hyperthyroidism treated with antithyroid drugs: A long-term followup study. Arthritis Rheum 2005; 53(1):108–113

Small P, Brisson M-L. Wegener's granulomatosis presenting as temporal arteritis. Arthritis Rheum 1991; 34:220–223

Sneller MC, Hoffmann GS, Talar-Williams C, et al An analysis of forty-two Wegener's granulomatosis patients treated with methotrexate and prednisone. Arthritis Rheum 1995; 38:608–613

Specks U et al Design of the rituximab in ANCA-associated vasculitis (RAVE) trial. 2009 (in press)

Stassen PM, Sanders JS, Kallenberg CG, Stegeman CA. Influenza vaccination does not result in an increase in relapses in patients with ANCA-associated vasculitis. Nephrol Dial Transplant 2008; 23:654–658

Stassen PM, Derks RPH, Kallenberg CGM, Stegeman CA. Thiopurinemethyltransferase (TPMT) genotype and TPMT activity in patients with anti-neutrophil cytoplasmic antibody-associated vasculitis: relation to azathioprine maintenance treatment and adverse effects. Ann Rheum Dis Ann Rheum Dis 2009; 68(5):758–9

Stegeman CA, Cohen Tervaert JW, Sluiter WJ, Manson WL, de Jong PE, Kallenberg CGM. Association of nasal carriage of Staphylococcus aureus and higher relapse in Wegener's Granulomatosis. Ann Intern Med 1994; 120:12–17

Stegeman CA. Anti-neutrophil cytoplasmic antibody (ANCA) levels directed against proteinase-3 and myeloperoxidase are helpful in predicting disease relapse in ANCA-associated small-vessel vasculitis. Nephrol Dial Transplant 2002; 17(12):2077-80

Stone J, Millward C, Criswell L. Two Unusual Genitourinary Manifestations Of Wegener's Granulomatosis. The Journal of Rheumatology 1997; 24(11): 1846-1848

Stone JH: and the Wegener's Granulomatosis Etanercept Trial Research Group. Limited versus severe Wegener's granulomatosis: Baseline data on patients in the Wegener's granulomatosis etanercept trial. Arthritis Rheum 2003; 48:2299–2309

Stone JH, Hoffman GS, Wegener's Granulomatosis. In: Hochberg MC, Smolen JS, Weinblatt ME, Weisman MH (eds) Rheumatology (4th edn). London, Elsevier, 2006, pp. 72.1–72.25

Suryaprasad A, Stone JH. When is it safe to stop Pneumocystis carinii (jiroveci) prophylaxis? Insights from cases complicating autoimmune diseases. Arthritis Care & Research 2008; 59(7):1034-9

The WGET Research Group. Design of the Wegener's Granulomatosis Etanercept Trial (WGET). Controlled Clinical Trials 2002; 23: 450–468

The WGET Research Group. Etanercept plus standard therapy in patients with wegener's granulomatosis. N Engl J Med 2005; 352:351–361

Wainright J, Davson J. The renal appearances in the microscopic form of periarteritis nodosa. J Pathol Bacteriol 1950; 62:189–196

Wegener F. Uber generalisierte, septische Gefasserkrankungen. Verh Dtsch Ges Pathol 1936; 29:202

Wegener F. Über eine eigenartige rhinogene Granulomatose mit besonderer Beteiligung des Arteriensystems und der Nieren. Beitr Pathol 1939; 102:36

Wiesner O, Russell KA, Lee AS, et al Antineutrophil cytoplasmic antibodies reacting with human neutrophil elastase as a diagnostic marker for cocaine-induced midline destructive lesions but not autoimmune vasculitis. Arthritis Rheum 2004; 50:2954–2965

Cryoglobulinemia

25

Dimitrios Vassilopoulos

25.1 Overview of Cryoglobulinemia

> Cryoglobulins are immunoglobulins that precipitate from serum under laboratory conditions of cold. The usual laboratory temperature used to precipitate cryoglobulins is 4°C.

> Cryoglobulinemia is divided into three clinical subsets (types I, II, and III). This classification is based on two features: (1) the clonality of the IgM component and (2) the presence of rheumatoid factor activity.

> In its clinical manifestations, type I cryoglobulinemia is usually quite distinct from types II and III. In contrast, substantial clinical overlap exists between types II and III.

> Type I cryoglobulinemia is associated with a monoclonal component and is typically associated with a hematopoietic malignancy.

> Type II and III cryoglobulinemia are often termed "mixed" cryoglobulinemias, as they are comprised of both IgG and IgM components.

> Vasculitis associated with mixed cryoglobulinemia involves both small- and medium-sized blood vessels. Small-vessel disease is more common than medium-vessel disease.

> Vasculitis associated with mixed cryoglobulinemia is caused by hepatitis C virus (HCV) infections in approximately 90% of the cases. In such patients, the antigens involved in cryoglobulinemic vasculitis are portions of the (HCV) virion. The relevant antibodies are both IgG and IgM, leading to the designation "mixed" cryoglobulinemia.

> Virtually, all patients with mixed cryoglobulinemia are rheumatoid factor positive.

> The treatment of cryoglobulinemia of any of the three types is directed whenever possible at the underlying cause. In some cases, the broad-spectrum immunosuppression and other measures must be employed with glucocorticoids, cytotoxic therapies, and plasma exchange.

Myth: The majority of patients with mixed cryoglobulinemia develop clinical manifestations of cryoglobulinemic vasculitis.

Reality: Although circulating mixed cryoglobulins (type II or III) are detected in a number of infectious, autoimmune, or malignant diseases, the development of cryoglobulinemic vasculitis occurs in only a small minority. For example, in patients who have chronic HCV infections, cryoglobulins are detected in approximately 40% using traditional methods of detection (Vassilopoulos et al. 2002). Despite the high prevalence of cryoglobulins, the syndrome of cryoglobulinemic vasculitis occurs in less than 5% of cases (Vassilopoulos et al. 2002).

Pearl: The likelihood of cryoglobulinemic vasculitis increases in proportion to the length of time the patient has been infected with HCV.

Comment: Patients have usually been infected with HCV for many years by the time cryoglobulinemic vasculitis appears. A common scenario is for a patient who received a blood transfusion 25 years ago to present with palpable purpura of the lower extremities, heralding the diagnosis of cryoglobulinemia (and HCV).

The relationship between the length of time a patient has been infected with HCV and the likelihood of cryoglobulinemic vasculitis is reflected in the peak age at presentation with vasculitis, which is generally between the ages 50 and 70 years (Vassilopoulos et al. 2002). In this regard, HCV and cryoglobulinemia differ substantially from hepatitis B viral (HBV) infections and polyarteritis nodosa. With HBV, polyarteritis nodosa typically develops either during the acute HBV infection or in the early stages of chronic HBV infection. Thus, most cases of HBV-associated polyarteritis nodosa present within 1 year of HBV infection.

Pearl: False-negative results in testing for cryoglobulins are common.

Comment: Sensitive testing for cryoglobulins requires an experienced laboratory that is set up to perform the collection in the proper conditions. While the patient is fasting (lipids can interfere with the assay), at least 20 mL of blood should

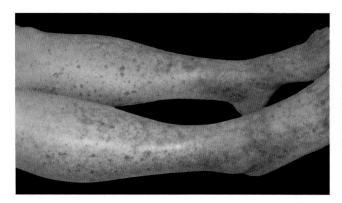

Fig. 25.1 Characteristic purpuric lesions in a patient with chronic HCV infection and associated type II cryoglobulinemic vasculitis. New erythematous lesions and old hyperpigmented lesions are evident in the lower extremities of this patient (Figure courtesy of Dr. Vassilopoulos)

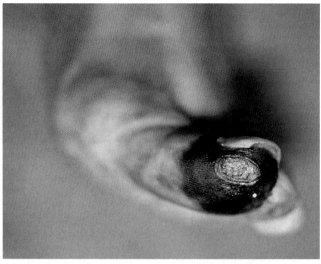

Fig. 25.2 Severe digital ischemia in a patient with type I cryoglobulinemia. Although most patients with symptomatic type I cryoglobulinemia manifest features of hyperviscosity, digital ischemia can occur in some. The precise basis of this digital ischemia is not always clear. This patient had multiple myeloma and a cryocrit of 48%. She responded well to melphalan and prednisone, and entered a remission sustained by thalidomide for several years (Figure courtesy of Dr. John Stone)

be drawn into a tube that has not been treated with anticoagulant. The specimen should be transported and centrifuged at 37°C, and then kept for more than 72 h at 4°C, to allow for the precipitation of cryoglobulins (Musset et al. 1992).

Persistence (i.e., repeat testing and coordination with the laboratory) may be required to obtain a good assay. Clues that suggest a harder look for cryoglobulins is in order include positive HCV serologies and a serum C4 level that is depressed out of proportion to the decrease in C3.

Myth: Purpura is a persistent manifestation of patients with type II or III cryoglobulinemic vasculitis.

Reality: In most patients with cryoglobulinemic vasculitis, purpura is the presenting symptom. It is usually located on the lower extremities and is not associated with pruritus (Gorevic et al. 1980; Vassilopoulos et al. 2002). In the majority of cases of HCV-related cutaneous vasculitis, purpura has an intermittent pattern of appearance – even *without* specific treatment. In patients, with chronic purpura, residual hyperpigmentation of the lower extremities is a common finding (Fig. 25.1).

Pearl: Type I cryoglobulinemia is more likely to be associated with syndromes of hyperviscosity than with vasculitis.

Comment: Symptoms of sludging within the central nervous system are typical in type I cryoglobulinemia because of the burden of cryoproteins in that disorder. (Type I cryoglobulinemia is often associated with an extremely high cryocrit). In contrast, diffuse, confluent purpura is atypical of type I cryoglobulinemia. Type I cryoglobulinemia can cause intense digital ischemia, however, as shown in Fig. 25.2.

Myth: Cryoglobulinemic symptoms are exacerbated by winter and other conditions of cold.

Reality: The cryoglobulins associated with HCV (types II and III) are immune complexes that precipitate in cold *laboratory conditions* (e.g., refrigeration for several days at 4°C). This is

a condition that does not occur under physiologic conditions because of the maintenance of body temperature at approximately 35–37°C, even in the acral extremities.

In contrast, type I cryoglobulins *can* precipitate at temperatures achieved in the distal extremities, nose, ears, and elsewhere. Type I cryoglobulins often present with cold-induced symptoms, and are then termed "cryoprecipitating monoclonal gammopathies."

Pearl: A disproportionate decrease in C4 levels provides an important clue to the diagnosis of cryoglobulinemia.

Comment: The presence of significant levels of cryoglobulins is often associated with very low or undetectable levels of C4 and normal levels of C3. This is most common in type II cryoglobulinemia. Low complement levels may also be seen in association with type II cryoglobulinemia complicating Sjögren's syndrome or, rarely, in type III cryoglobulinemia in patients with HCV infection, rheumatoid arthritis, vasculitis, or SLE (Kallemuchikkal and Gorevic 1999). Interestingly, the C4 level may be persistently low, even when cryoglobulins have become undetectable following treatment. Presumably there are sufficient immune complexes to activate complement, but not enough to be detected as cryoglobulins.

Myth: Renal disease is often detectable in the early stages of cryoglobulinemia.

Reality: In contrast to other forms of immune-complex mediated glomerulonephritis such as lupus and Henoch–Schönlein purpura, renal involvement in the form of membranoproliferative glomerulonephritis (MPGN) is usually a late manifestation of cryoglobulinemia. MPGN typically appears 3–5 years after the onset of purpura (D'Amico 1998; Roccatello et al. 2007).

The presentation of MPGN in cryoglobulinemia is usually associated with asymptomatic hematuria or proteinuria (Roccatello et al. 2007). In approximately 20% of cases, proteinuria in cryoglobulinemia-associated MPGN reaches the nephrotic range. Flares of glomerulonephritis during long-term follow-up are common. However, the overall prognosis of renal disease is good, with only about 15% of patients developing end-stage renal disease over long-term follow-up (D'Amico 1998). Nevertheless, renal involvement at presentation is an independent variable associated with poor survival (Ferri et al. 2004; Roccatello et al. 2007).

Myth: Arteritis is a common finding in renal biopsies of patients with HCV-associated cryoglobulinemia.

Reality: Renal involvement occurs in approximately 30% of patients with HCV-associated cryoglobulinemia, usually (as noted) in the form of MPGN (Ferri et al. 2004). Renal biopsy also shows mesangial proliferative or focal membranoproliferative glomerulonephritis in some patients (Roccatello et al. 2007). Arteritis involving small- or medium-sized vessels is an uncommon finding, occurring in less than 10% of patients (Roccatello et al. 2007). In this way, cryoglobulinemic glomerulonephritis resembles lupus nephritis, another form of immune-complex-mediated renal disease in which the finding of arteritis in the kidney is rare.

Pearl: True inflammatory arthritis is a rare manifestation of cryoglobulinemia.

Comment: Many patients with cryoglobulinemia are misdiagnosed early in their course as having rheumatoid arthritis. There are two reasons for this: (1) the high prevalence of joint complaints in cryoglobulinemia and (2) the rheumatoid factor activity demonstrated by the IgM component of the cryoglobulins.

Although symmetric polyarthralgias are common in patients with cryoglobulinemia (70–80%), frank synovitis is unusual (2–5%) (Rosner et al. 2004; Vassilopoulos and Calabrese 2003). The small joints of the hands are the joints most commonly affected by arthralgias, followed by the knees. The absence of true synovitis, the absence of erosive changes on joint radiographs, and the absence of antibodies to cyclic citrullinated peptides (anti-ccp) are all useful in distinguishing cryoglobulinemia from rheumatoid arthritis (Vassilopoulos and Calabrese 2003).

Myth: Disappearance of HCV from the serum of patients with HCV-associated cryoglobulinemia is always associated with clinical remission.

Reality: It is generally accepted that chronic HCV viremia is responsible for the appearance of serum cryoglobulins and the clinical manifestations of cryoglobulinemia in patients who have HCV-associated disease. Most patients with HCV-associated cryoglobulinemia who clear the virus after antiviral treatment demonstrate disappearance of the cryoglobulins from the serum and clinical remission (Vassilopoulos et al. 2002).

However, a number of recent studies have indicated that some patients with HCV-associated cryoglobulinemia continue to have vasculitic symptoms and to maintain cryoglobulins in their serum, despite the absence of detectable virus (HCV RNA) in the blood or bone marrow (Landau et al. 2008; Levine et al. 2005). An underlying non-Hodgkin lymphoma (NHL) could be responsible for the persistent cryoglobulinemia in some of these cases. Thus, a thorough evaluation to exclude NHL is recommended in this setting (Landau et al. 2008).

Myth: The cryocrit correlates well with disease activity in cryoglobulinemic vasculitis.

Reality: This is particularly incorrect in the setting of type I cryoglobulinemia, where clinical responses (e.g., improvement in digital ischemia) may occur in the face of cryocrits that continue to be frighteningly high. When forced to use immunosuppression to treat cryoglobulinemia, the cryocrit is just like almost every biomarker ever described: treat the patient and not the cryocrit.

Pearl: NHL is a known complication of cryoglobulinemia.

Comment: Patients with cryoglobulinemia with or without HCV infection have a higher than normal risk of developing hematologic malignancies, particularly NHLs. NHL in this setting, reported in approximately 5% of patients with cryoglobulinemia, usually belong to the lymphoplasmacytic or diffuse large cell type (Ferri et al. 2004; Trejo et al. 2003).

NHL presents with extra-nodal involvement in 70% of cases associated with cryoglobulinemia (Trejo et al. 2003). The usual extra-nodal sites are the liver, salivary glands, and stomach (Trejo et al. 2003). NHL accounts for approximately 15% of the deaths in patients with cryoglobulinemia (Ferri et al. 2004).

Myth: Mononeuritis multiplex is the most common form of neuropathy in cryoglobulinemic vasculitis.

Reality: Peripheral nerve involvement is very common in cryoglobulinemic vasculitis, occurring eventually in up to 80% of cases. The most common type of nerve dysfunction is a distal symmetric sensory polyneuropathy that has a predilection for the lower extremities. Mononeuritis multiplex is the second most common form of peripheral nerve involvement.

A number of pathologic lesions are found in nerve biopsies from affected patients, including vasculitis of the small- and/or medium-sized vessels or perivascular infiltrates

(Authier et al. 2003). The neuropathy of cryoglobulinemic vasculitis is less responsive to antiviral and immunosuppressive therapy than are some other manifestations of cryoglobulinemic vasculitis (e.g., purpura and nephropathy). This is probably a consequence of the fact that peripheral nerves, once injured, require many months to recover and continue to be symptomatic for long periods of time.

Some data suggest that mononeuritis multiplex responds better than the distal polyneuropathy to therapy (Saadoun et al. 2006). Encouraging results in the treatment of cryoglobulinemic neuropathy have been reported using rituximab either alone or in combination with antiviral therapy in patients with HCV-associated cryoglobulinemic neuropathy (Cacoub et al. 2008; Saadoun et al. 2008).

Pearl: HCV-associated cryoglobulinemia can present with a pulmonary–renal syndrome.

Comment: A proliferative glomerulonephritis is a well-known complication of cryoglobulinemic vasculitis. Less common complications of HCV infection can involve the lung. Both pulmonary hemorrhage and interstitial fibrosis have been reported in patients with HCV infection (Prasad et al. 2006). The potential association between HCV and lung dysfunction is worth keeping in mind when the pieces of a puzzling pulmonary case do not quite add up.

Myth: Immunosuppressive therapy is frequently associated with flares of the underlying hepatitis in patients with HCV-associated cryoglobulinemia.

Reality: In patients with severe manifestations of cryoglobulinemic vasculitis, immunosuppressive therapy with high-dose glucocorticoids and cyclophosphamide is employed frequently (Vassilopoulos et al. 2002). This type of treatment was used for years, even prior to the discovery of HCV as the principal etiology of cryoglobulinemia (Vassilopoulos et al. 2002).

In contrast to HBV infection, in which immunosuppressives (especially glucocorticoids) frequently lead to rebound viremia and hepatitis flares, a number of observational studies over the years have shown that such complications of immunosuppression are uncommon events in patients with HCV-associated cryoglobulinemia (Vassilopoulos et al. 2002). This is true also for the newer modalities of treatment (e.g., rituximab), which can cause a transient increase in HCV RNA levels without immediate harmful effects on liver function (Saadoun et al. 2008).

Although these observations on the short-term safety of immunosuppression are reassuring, the full impact of long-term immunosuppression on liver function in HCV-infected cryoglobulinemic patients is not known. It is always important to employ immunosuppressive therapy only when necessary and to minimize the length of time that patients are exposed to these potentially toxic agents.

Pearl: Interferon-alpha can exacerbate HCV-associated cryoglobulinemic vasculitis.

Comment: Interferon-alpha (IFN-α) in either its standard or pegylated form remains the cornerstone of treatment for chronic hepatitis C. In patients with HCV-associated cryoglobulinemia, IFN-based regimens have been associated with favorable virologic and clinical outcomes in patients when administered either with ribavirin or in combination with immunosuppressive agents (Saadoun et al. 2006, 2008; Vassilopoulos et al. 2002).

However, clinicians should be aware that IFN-a can exacerbate every single manifestation of cryoglobulinemia including purpura, glomerulonephritis, or peripheral neuropathy (Vassilopoulos et al. 2002). This is of particular clinical importance when treatment decisions are made for patients with severe disease manifestations such as severe renal disease, gastrointestinal vasculitis, or digital necrosis. In such cases, immunosuppressive therapy (glucocorticoids, cyclophosphamide, rituximab) should be administered first to suppress the immune response of the host. After control of the immune response, antiviral therapy can be initiated with less concern about a worsening of clinical manifestations.

Myth: HBV is a common etiologic factor for cryoglobulinemia.

Reality: Although studies in the early 1980s suggested that HBV causes a substantial proportion of cryoglobulinemic vasculitis cases, these data have been refuted in subsequent investigations. One must wonder if the cases of cryoglobulinemic vasculitis linked to HBV in those early studies were not examples of patients coinfected with both HBV and "non-A/non-B hepatitis virus," as HCV was known before its identification in the late 1980s. HBV now accounts for less than 5% of cryoglobulinemic vasculitis cases (Ferri et al. 2004).

Nevertheless, a search for HBV infection is obligatory for patients who present with cryoglobulinemia, because HBV often coincides with HCV (and human immunodeficiency virus) infections in high risk groups. An early diagnosis of HBV infection has significant clinical implications because its treatment can prevent the detrimental effects of immunosuppression in that patient population.

Pearl: Ribavirin can cause significant hemolysis in patients with HCV-associated cryoglobulinemia and renal dysfunction.

Comment: The combination of ribavirin and IFN-a (in either its standard or pegylated form) is the standard of care for the treatment of chronic hepatitis C. This regimen is also effective for patients with HCV-associated cryoglobulinemia (Saadoun et al. 2006). However, extreme caution is required when using ribavirin in patients with renal dysfunction. In its usual dose (800–1,200 mg/day), ribavirin can cause severe hemolytic anemia during the first 2 weeks of its administration.

Ribavirin is contraindicated in patients whose creatinine clearance is less than 50 mL/min. In patients with borderline renal function, a slow upward titration of the dose accompanied by close monitoring of the hematocrit is imperative. In many cases, patients cannot tolerate even low doses of ribavirin and the medication must be stopped.

Pearl: Use plasmapheresis when patients present with severe systemic vasculitis.

Comment: Physicians vary in their threshold for resorting to plasmapheresis, an intervention that has potential side-effects (particularly infection) and is unproven for the treatment of most of the disorders in which it is employed. However, the absence of evidence does not constitute evidence of absence, and there are certain clinical situations in which the application of plasmapheresis makes good sense. Overwhelming systemic vasculitis associated with cryoglobulinemia is one such instance. In these cases, the removal of cryoglobulins and their associated immune complexes, as quickly as possible, is important. There is no quicker way to accomplish this than by plasmapheresis.

References

Authier FJ, Bassez G, Payan C, et al Detection of genomic viral RNA in nerve and muscle of patients with HCV neuropathy. Neurology 2003; 60:808–812

Cacoub P, Delluc A, Saadoun D, et al Anti-CD20 monoclonal antibody (rituximab) treatment for cryoglobulinemic vasculitis: Where do we stand? Ann Rheum Dis 2008; 67:283–287

D'Amico G. Renal involvement in hepatitis C infection: Cryoglobulinemic glomerulonephritis. Kidney Int 1998; 54:650–671

Ferri C, Sebastiani M, Giuggioli D, et al Mixed cryoglobulinemia: Demographic, clinical, and serologic features and survival in 231 patients. Semin Arthritis Rheum 2004; 33:355–374

Gorevic PD, Kassab HJ, Levo Y, et al Mixed cryoglobulinemia: Clinical aspects and long-term follow-up of 40 patients. Am J Med 1980; 69:287–308

Kallemuchikkal U, Gorevic P. Evaluation of cryoglobulins. Arch Pathol Lab Med 1999; 123:119–125

Landau DA, Saadoun D, Halfon P, et al Relapse of hepatitis C virus-associated mixed cryoglobulinemia vasculitis in patients with sustained viral response. Arthritis Rheum 2008; 58:604–611

Levine JW, Gota C, Fessler BJ, et al Persistent cryoglobulinemic vasculitis following successful treatment of hepatitis C virus. J Rheumatol 2005; 32:1164–1167

Musset L, Diemert MC, Taibi F, et al Characterization of cryoglobulins by immunoblotting. Clin Chem 1992; 38:798–802

Prasad M, Buller GK, Mena CI, Sofair AN. Sum of the parts. N Engl J Med 2006; 355:2468–2473

Roccatello D, Fornasieri A, Giachino O, et al Multicenter study on hepatitis C virus-related cryoglobulinemic glomerulonephritis. Am J Kidney Dis 2007; 49:69–82

Rosner I, Rozenbaum M, Toubi E, et al The case for hepatitis C arthritis. Semin Arthritis Rheum 2004; 33:375–387

Saadoun D, Resche-Rigon M, Thibault V, et al Antiviral therapy for hepatitis C virus-associated mixed cryoglobulinemia vasculitis: A long-term followup study. Arthritis Rheum 2006; 54:3696–3706

Saadoun D, Resche-Rigon M, Sene D, et al Rituximab combined with peg-interferon-ribavirin in refractory HCV-associated cryoglobulinemia vasculitis. Ann Rheum Dis 2008;67;1431–1436

Trejo O, Ramos-Casals M, Lopez-Guillermo A, et al Hematologic malignancies in patients with cryoglobulinemia: Association with autoimmune and chronic viral diseases. Semin Arthritis Rheum 2003; 33:19–28

Vassilopoulos D, Calabrese LH. Rheumatic manifestations of hepatitis C infection. Curr Rheumatol Rep 2003; 5:200–204

Vassilopoulos D, Calabrese LH. Hepatitis C virus infection and vasculitis. Implications of antiviral and immunosuppressive therapies. Arthritis Rheum 2002; 46:585–597

Polyarteritis Nodosa

26

John H. Stone

13.1 Overview of Polyarteritis Nodosa

> Polyarteritis nodosa (PAN) primarily affects medium-sized arteries that supply the skin, gut, nerve, and kidney. However, multiple other organs can be involved either clinically or subclinically.

> Microaneurysms of arteries to or within the kidneys, liver, or gastrointestinal tract are highly characteristic of PAN.

> Mononeuritis multiplex, an asymmetric sensory and motor neuropathy due to ischemia and infarction of peripheral nerves, occurs frequently in PAN.

> In mononeuritis multiplex, nerve conduction studies of peripheral nerves reveal a distal, asymmetric, axonal neuropathy involving both motor and sensory nerves.

> PAN is characterized pathologically by patchy, transmural inflammation in medium- and small-sized muscular arteries, sparing large arteries, capillaries, and the venous system. The inflammation leads to fibrinoid necrosis, but is not associated with granulomatous features.

> High-dose glucocorticoids are the mainstay of therapy in PAN. In cases that are rapidly progressive or life or organ threatening, however, cyclophosphamide is added to glucocorticoid treatment.

Myth: PAN is sometimes associated with antineutrophil cytoplasmic antibodies (ANCA).

Reality: This Myth is a holdover from the early days of ANCA testing, when reliable enzyme immunoassays for antibodies to proteinase-3 (PR3) and myeloperoxidase (MPO) were not available. Classic PAN is an ANCA-negative disease, meaning that it is neither associated with PR3- nor with MPO-ANCA.

Many types of disorders, even many types of nonvasculitic diseases, are associated with ANCA when only immunofluorescence testing is used (Stone et al. 2000). However, positive ANCA assays in patients with PAN, inflammatory bowel disease, sarcoidosis, and liver or thyroid dysfunction are not caused by antibodies directed against PR3 or MPO, but rather by antibodies to antigens such as lactoferrin, bactericidal permeability inhibitor, or others (Talor et al. 2007). If enzyme immunoassays for PR3- and MPO-ANCA are negative, then positive immunofluorescence assays are usually "false-positive" results, at least with regard to diagnoses of systemic vasculitis.

Pearl: The seronegative nature of PAN makes the diagnosis elusive.

Comment: Most cases of systemic lupus erythematosus (SLE) are not difficult to diagnose these days. Once the clinician considers the possibility of an autoimmune disease, the vast majority of patients with true SLE are found to be antinuclear antibody (ANA) positive and to have more specific serologic tests that clarify the diagnosis. (Unfortunately, the use of enzyme immunoassays with poor sensitivity has caused a resurgence of "ANA-negative lupus" in recent years.)

Similarly, even if clinicians overlook subtle signs of sclerodactyly, they may eventually get to the right diagnostic ballpark and think of scleroderma if they observe a strongly positive ANA assay and recognize that additional history, physical examination, and more detailed autoantibody testing are in order.

In contrast, many patients with PAN go undiagnosed for weeks or months because routine tests for "collagen vascular diseases" or "connective tissue disorders" are negative. PAN is not associated with ANA, rheumatoid factor, or other known autoantibodies. The fact is the task of teasing out the frequently subtle presentation of a subacute, multiorgan system disease or the detection of foot dorsiflexion weakness is much more difficult than checking off lists of assays on a laboratory slip.

Pearl: Classic PAN is often a curable illness.

Comment: In contrast to Wegener's granulomatosis (WG), giant cell arteritis (GCA), and some other forms of vasculitis, "classic" PAN – the disorder described by Kussmaul and Maier – is usually a *curable* disease. Approximately 50% of PAN cases can be cured with glucocorticoid treatment alone, usually in courses lasting a total of 9–12 months (Guillevin and Lhote 1998). The remainder of PAN patients requires cyclophosphamide to induce disease remission. Once classic PAN is in remission, however, it usually stays there and does not require long-term maintenance therapy.

The propensity of classic PAN to be cured was illustrated by a study from the French Vasculitis Study Group that evaluated the outcomes of 351 patients with classic PAN (Pagnoux et al. 2006). More than two-thirds of the patients were cured by their initial treatment courses.

Pearl: The development of mononeuritis multiplex in the absence of diabetes mellitus or multiple compression injuries strongly suggests the presence of vasculitis.

Comment: Mononeuritis multiplex is defined as a peripheral neuropathy in which named nerves are injured or infarcted one a time (Fig. 26.1). This syndrome is one of the great "eureka" signs in medicine, as its differential diagnosis is relatively brief and its identification also points the way to a potential diagnostic test: a nerve biopsy.

Peripheral nervous system vasculitis is a form of nerve dysfunction in which vascular inflammation is confined to the vasa nervorum. The disorder can occur in an isolated fashion, involving only the peripheral nerves, or in the context of a multiorgan system disorder such as several primary vasculitides. Inflammatory disorders associated with autoimmunity such as rheumatoid arthritis, SLE, Sjögren's syndrome, and a variety of hematopoietic malignancies can also cause mononeuritis multiplex (Gorson 2001). However, these other disorders usually cause vasculitic neuropathy only months or years after the underlying disease has already been diagnosed. With PAN, in contrast, mononeuritis multiplex typically occurs early in the disease course, and may be a primary feature of the disease by the time the patient gets to medical attention.

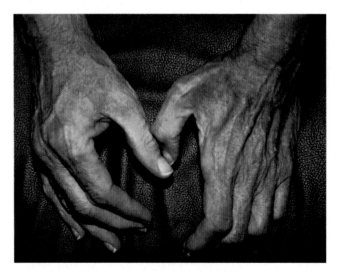

Fig. 26.1 The effects of vasculitic neuropathy

Table 26.1 Forms of vasculitis most likely to cause vasculitic neuropathy

Polyarteritis nodosa
Microscopic polyangiitis
Churg--Strauss syndrome
Wegener's granulomatosis
Cryoglobulinemia

Pearl: When selecting a peripheral nerve for biopsy, target an affected nerve but not a dead one.

Comment: Several forms of systemic vasculitis have particular predilections for causing vasculitic neuropathy (Table 26.1). Which nerve offers the highest yield for making the diagnosis through biopsy? Biopsies of peripheral nerves that are electrophysiologically normal are rarely useful: such nerves are histologically normal, too. The surgeon should biopsy a nerve that is affected but not "dead." If the sural nerves demonstrate no action potentials, the superficial peroneal nerve and peroneus brevis muscle are other potential targets (Collins et al. 2000). In addition, upper extremity nerves (e.g., the lateral antebrachial cutaneous nerve or other nerves in the upper extremities) are also candidates for biopsy. A contiguous muscle should be biopsied during the same procedure.

Myth: Biopsy of a peripheral nerve that is demonstrably abnormal by EMG/NCV has a high likelihood of yielding diagnostic tissue.

Reality: Don't be overly optimistic about this. Useful information is gained in the great majority of peripheral nerve biopsies performed under such circumstances, and the procedure is very worthwhile under the proper clinical circumstances. Nevertheless, even when a given nerve is demonstrably abnormal on electrophysiologic testing, the chance that a nerve biopsy will provide incontrovertible histologic proof of the diagnosis is only about 50%. Careful clinicopathological correlation is required.

Nevertheless, a peripheral nerve biopsy usually provides important clues to the presence of a vasculitic neuropathy. This was illustrated by a study of 93 cases of vasculitic neuropathy (Mathew et al. 2007). The following observations were made:

- Eighty-four peripheral nerve biopsies were performed. Eighty-two of these were sural nerve biopsies. Two were biopsies of superficial radial nerves.
- The diagnosis of vasculitic neuropathy was confirmed in 49 of the 84 biopsies (58%).
- In an additional 31 cases (37%), the histopathological results were "consistent with" but not diagnostic of vasculitic neuropathy. Most of those cases demonstrated an acute, asymmetric loss of axons and differential involvement of nerve fascicles.

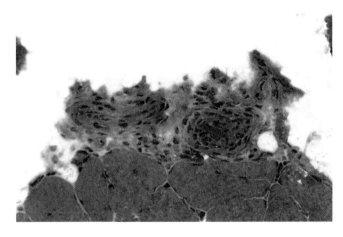

Fig. 26.2 Muscle biopsy showing necrotizing vasculitis

Thus, 95% of nerve biopsies (58 plus 37%) contributed information critical to the diagnosis of vasculitic neuropathy. In the absence of another clear site to biopsy, it is usually worth biopsying a peripheral nerve that has been demonstrated to be abnormal by NVCs.

In many cases, the diagnosis can be inferred from a highly consistent clinical history, NCVs that reveal an asymmetric, length-dependent process, and compatible pathological findings, even if the histology is not diagnostic.

Pearl: Gastrocnemius muscle biopsies augment the yield of sural nerve biopsies.

Comment: Biopsies of skeletal muscle increase the yield of tissue sampling substantially, even in the absence of symptoms, signs, or laboratory abnormalities that suggest skeletal muscle involvement. Serum creatine kinase levels, for example, can be entirely normal even in the face of a raging vasculitis that involves the arteries of muscles. Skeletal muscle is a highly vascular tissue, and biopsies in the search for vasculitis often "hit paydirt" (Fig. 26.2).

Pearl: Examination of the flexor hallucis brevis muscle on electrophysiologic testing is important in the evaluation of length-dependent axonopathies.

Comment: Length-dependent axonopathies are those diseases of nerve that affect first the longest nerves in the body, i.e., usually those of the feet. Vasculitic neuropathy is one type of a length-dependent axonopathy. Others include diabetes mellitus, sarcoidosis, leprosy, and connective tissue diseases such as SLE or Sjögren's syndrome.

EMG/NCVs of the flexor hallucis brevis can establish the presence of motor involvement that is not otherwise apparent. This finding can alter the differential diagnosis substantially. Fibrillation potentials of the flexor hallucis brevis muscle indicates subclinical involvement of motor fibers – thereby pointing to a sensorimotor multiple mononeuropathy if sensory nerve action potentials are also absent in the lower extremities (Vallat and Cros 2007).

When evaluating a patient for vasculitic neuropathy, the electromyographer must perform EMGs of the flexor hallucis brevis. Requesting this part of the examination specifically will also probably buy you a more careful procedure and a more thoughtful interpretation, as the request implies greater than average insight of the test orderer.

Pearl: The greatest challenge in vasculitic neuropathy lies in managing the phase after the start of therapy.

Comment: Management of the long-term sequelae of nerve infarctions in PAN – painful sensory neuropathies and residual muscle weakness – poses major challenges. This is true for vasculitic neuropathy caused by any form of vasculitis. Pain control and physical and occupational therapy modalities assume the highest priority once remission has been induced.

A variety of newer agents have been employed to treat the pain associated with peripheral nerve injury in recent years. For example, gabapentin and related medications have become popular and widely used, particularly by neurologists. Tricyclic antidepressants (TCAs) should not be discarded too quickly in the rush to embrace the new. These drugs remain the most effective medication for the treatment of painful vasculitic neuropathy. TCAs should be regarded as the cornerstone of therapy for this type of pain, the treatment to which other interventions are added.

Pearl: Observing a patient's recovery from severe vasculitic neuropathy is like watching grass grow, only much slower.

Comment: Although the vasculitic process in PAN responds readily to therapy, damage from the disease may be slower to resolve. Indeed, most patients do not recover full function of both sensory and motor nerves that have been affected severely. To the extent that recovery occurs, it takes many months and often continues over a year or more (thus, considerably slower than grass).

The pain of chronic nerve injury and the painfully slow time to recovery underscore the importance of preventing this complication whenever possible through early diagnosis and the appropriate application of aggressive immunosuppression. In this day and age, the presence of an active vasculitic neuropathy related to PAN is an indication for cyclophosphamide. It is not clear whether any biologic agent on the horizon will change that any time soon.

Myth: Punch biopsies of the skin are an easy way to make the diagnosis of PAN.

Reality: Classic PAN involves muscular, medium-sized arterioles and arteries. The cutaneous location of such blood vessels is in the deep dermis or subcutaneous fat (Fig. 26.3). No punch biopsy extends deeply enough to reach the culprit vessels and confirm the diagnosis of PAN (Stone and Nousari 2001).

In contrast, if the cutaneous lesion is one of a small-vessel vasculitides (e.g., palpable or nonpalpable purpura), a simple

Fig. 26.3 Depth of blood vessels involved in different forms of vasculitis

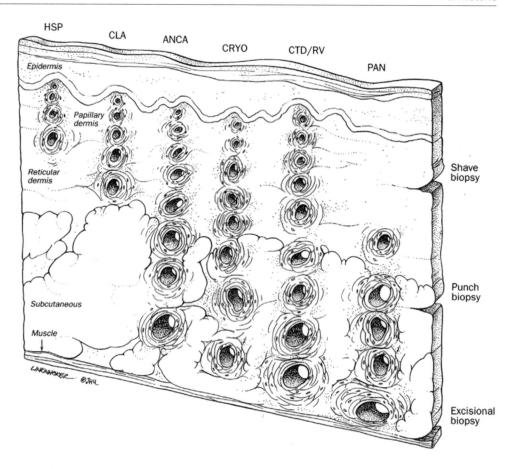

Fig. 26.4 Nodule from a patient with polyarteritis nodosa

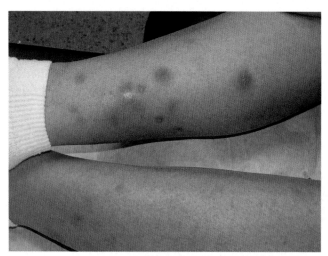

Fig. 26.5 Cutaneous ulcer in a patient with polyarteritis nodosa

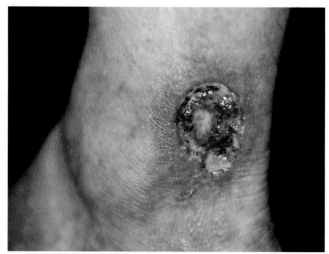

punch biopsy should suffice for diagnostic purposes. In addition to the standard hematoxylyn and eosin stains, immunofluorescence studies are critical in parsing the different forms of small-vessel vasculitis that involve the skin (Stone and Nousari 2001).

Pearl: Among the cutaneous lesions of medium-vessel vasculitis, nodular lesions are most likely to yield a diagnosis of vasculitis.

Comment: Medium-vessel vasculitis is associated with four primary skin lesions: nodules, ulcers, livedo reticularis, and digital ischemia. Nodules (Fig. 26.4) are the lesion most likely to yield a diagnosis of vasculitis. These should be biopsied in their center, deeply enough to capture subcutaneous fat in the sample.

Unfortunately, nodules in cutaneous vasculitis are usually short-lived; they quickly break down to form ulcers (Fig. 26.5). The best place to biopsy an ulcer is not in the center, but rather

Table 26.2 Differential diagnosis of ulcers on the legs and feet

Atherosclerosis
- Peripheral vascular disease

Ulcers due to arterial insufficiency typically occur on the toes, the heels, the anterior shin, and extend over the malleoli

Diabetes-related issues
- Neuropathic ulcers
- Necrobiosis lipoidica diabeticorum

Longstanding, poorly controlled diabetes mellitus is the rule

Vasculitis
- Polyarteritis nodosa
- ANCA-associated disorders
- Cryoglobulinemia (history of recurrent palpable purpura is usually strong. Lower extremities are characteristically hyperpigmented)
- Rheumatoid vasculitis (*occurs in patients with longstanding, severe rheumatoid arthritis*)
- Buerger's disease (predilection for digital ischemic lesions – necrotic fingers and toes – rather than leg ulcers)
- Erythema nodosum (rarely ulcerates – only in Behcet's disease)

Vasculitis mimickers
- Atrophie blanche (livedoid vasculopathy)
- Cholesterol embolization (history of vascular instrumentation within days to weeks is usually present)
- Pyoderma gangrenosum
- Sweet's syndrome
- Calciphylaxis (lesions tend to localize in fatty tissues of the buttocks and thighs rather than distal ones)

Connective tissue disorders
- Systemic sclerosis (digital ischemia and physical findings of sclerodactyly, telangiectasias, calcinoses, and dilated nailbed capillaries)
- Systemic lupus erythematosus
- Antiphospholipid syndrome

Stasis disease
- Venous disease with stasis

(venous ulcers typically occur above the lateral or medial malleoli)
- Lymphedema

Clotting problems
- Disseminated intravascular coagulation
- Heparin-induced thrombocytopenia (HIT)

HIT is associated with both venous and arterial thrombi
- Warfarin-induced skin necrosis

Hematologic disorders
- Polycythemia vera
- Essential thrombocythemia
- Therapy with hydroxyurea

Infections
- Osteomyelitis
- Necrotizing fasciitis
- Mycobacterium marinum
- Tuberculosis (erythema induratum)
- Fungal
- Cryptococcus
- Cocciodes
- Sporothrix

(London and Donnelly 2000; Arepally and Ortel 2006; Bazari et al. 2007).

at the edge. Again, a biopsy of sufficient depth must be performed. The differential diagnosis of leg ulcers is shown in Table 26.2. The clinical and laboratory approach to the evaluation of these lesions is shown in Table 26.3.

Compared with nodules or ulcers, livedo reticularis is associated with a significantly lower likelihood of yielding a diagnosis. In 19 of 26 patients with livedo reticularis from whom two biopsy specimens were available, no obvious pathologic change was detected in either biopsy, despite careful examination of multiple serial sections (Frances et al. 2005; Uthman and Khamashta 2006). When biopsies of livedo reticularis are attempted, the surgeon should take more than one deep punch biopsy (of a depth of 4 mm) from different areas of both the white and red areas. The sensitivity of three biopsies taken from white areas has been estimated to be as high as 80% (Stockhammer et al. 1993).

Lesions of digital ischemia are rarely biopsied because of their low yield and concerns about wound healing.

Table 26.3 Diagnostic evaluation of leg ulcers (Ha and Nousari 2003; Mimouni et al. 2003)

History and physical examination

Skin biopsy

- Three deep skin biopsies performed using a double trephine punch biopsy technique for sampling subcutaneous tissue. In short, after performing a 6 mm punch biopsy and before closing the surgical site, a 4 mm punch in introduced through the surgical defect in order to reach deeper subcutaneous tissue
- Both cylinders, 6 and 4 mm, are sent for
- From the center of the ulcer (one sample): The specimen is split, with one half going for routine histology and special stains and the other for DIF
- From the edge of the ulcer (two samples): One specimen is evaluated for routine histology and special stains and another is evaluated for bacterial (including mycobacterial) and fungal stains and cultures

Laboratory studies

- Complete blood count with differential
- Serum chemistries, including hepatic transaminases
- Acute phase reactants (erythrocyte sedimentation rate, C-reactive protein)
- Autoantibodies: ANCA, RF, cryoglobulins, C3/C4, ANA, dsDNA antibodies, antibodies to the Ro, La, Sm, and RNP antigens
- Clotting risk factor analysis, including anticardiolipin antibodies (IgG and IgM), Russell viper venom time, PT/PTT, antithrombin III, protein C & S, factor V Leiden, prothrombin gene mutation, homocysteine levels
- Paraproteinemia screen: SPEP, serum protein immunofixation, total serum immune globulins, UPEP, and urine protein immunofixation
- Assays for antibodies to hepatitis B, C, and the human immunodeficiency virus

Ancillary investigations

- Nerve conduction studies, compression duplex ultrasonography

Pearl: "Nodular vasculitis" is a confusing term that means medium-vessel arteritis.

Comment: The subject of cutaneous vasculitis is difficult enough by itself without the use of nonspecific nomenclature. "Nodular vasculitis" usually refers to biopsy-proven vasculitis of medium-sized muscular arteries and arterioles that causes a nodular skin lesion. Many forms of systemic vasculitis – e.g., PAN, the ANCA-associated disorders, and mixed cryoglobulinemia – can be associated with nodular cutaneous findings. Thus, "nodular vasculitis" is a syndrome, not a specific diagnosis. This term should be avoided by clinicians and pathologists alike.

Myth: Classic PAN involvement of the skin can be distinguished from important mimickers by its clinical appearance.

Reality: Diagnosing the cause of skin ulcers without histopathology is fraught with hazard. Cholesterol emboli, calciphylaxis lesions, the antiphospholipid syndrome, livedoid vasculopathy, pyoderma gangrenosum, and a host of other disorders can mimic PAN closely (see Table 26.2). A well-performed skin biopsy reviewed in person with an experienced dermatopathologist will shed light on many a confusing case – and often yield surprising results.

The common objection to biopsying a skin ulcer is concern about wound healing, but diagnostic confirmation and the ability to employ the correct therapy usually justify that risk, even if poor wound healing or extension of the lesion through pathergy are possible concerns.

Myth: The proper name for the lacy, purplish discoloration illustrated in Fig. 26.6 is livedo reticularis.

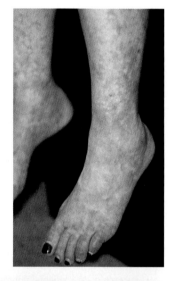

Fig. 26.6 "Livedo reticularis" from a patient with polyarteritis nodosa. The correct name of this cutaneous lesion is really livedo racemosa (Uthman and Khamashta 2006). This patient had vasculitic neuropathy with motor mononeuritis multiplex. She was cured with the combination of high-dose glucocorticoids (tapered off over 6 months) and 6 months of daily cyclophosphamide, followed by 6 months of azathioprine

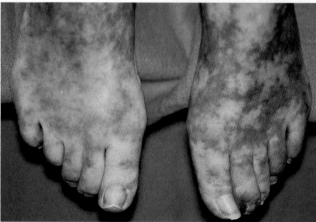

Fig. 26.7 Livedo racemosa

Reality: Purists note correctly the consistent sloppiness in the literature with regard to the terms "livedo reticularis" and "livedo racemosa." The literature is remarkably muddy here, and, frankly, at this point, it is probably not worth trying to change.

Livedo racemosa, named by Ehrmann (1907), is a more striking cutaneous finding than livedo reticularis (Fig. 26.7). Ehrmann described livedo racemosa as a *"tendril-like, bluish pattern reminiscent of forked lightening."*

Livedo racemosa differs from livedo reticularis in the following ways:

- Livedo racemosa is more generalized. Trunk or buttocks involvement is present in nearly all patients. Even the face can be involved in some patients.
- Livedo racemosa is bad news. It is nearly always associated with an underlying disease.
- In contrast, livedo reticularis often occurs in physiologic settings, e.g., a response to cold, rather than in the setting of a disease.

Disorders associated with livedo racemosa are not invariably vasculitic in nature. For example, in the antiphospholipid syndrome, livedo racemosa is frequently associated with cerebrovascular events, arterial thrombosis, and pregnancy morbidity (Frances et al. 1999). The constellation of cerebrovascular events, antiphospholipid antibodies, and livedo racemosa has been termed Sneddon's syndrome (Frances and Piette 2000). Other causes of livedo racemosa include essential thrombocythemia, polycythemia vera, pernicious anemia, disseminated intravascular coagulation, and cryofibrinogenemia.

Pearl: If leukopenia and thrombocytopenia are important components of the clinical presentation, a primary form of vasculitis is unlikely.

Comment: Leukopenia and thrombocytopenia are not usually associated with primary vasculitic syndromes. Their presence suggests other disorders, such as a connective tissue disorder in the spectrum of SLE, Felty's syndrome, or a malignancy.

Pearl: Classic PAN spares the lungs.

Comment: This observation goes back to the report of Kussmaul and Maier, who noted that in contrast to the *"peculiar, mostly nodular thickening (periarteritis nodosa) of countless arteries …in the bowel, stomach, kidneys, spleen, heart, and voluntary muscles…The lung artery remains unaffected, while the bronchial arteries, even if only in the mediastinum, were affected to a minor degree"* (Kussmaul and Maier 1866).

Even today, reports of pulmonary parenchymal involvement in classic PAN are virtually nonexistent. The diagnosis of *microscopic polyangiitis* is more likely if nongranulomatous, small- and/or medium-sized blood vessel involvement in the lung is detected. In the rare cases when pulmonary involvement is evident in PAN, it is the bronchial arteries that are involved (Matsumoto et al. 1993).

Myth: All patients with PAN should be treated with a cytotoxic agent.

Reality: Not true. Approximately half of all patients with PAN can be treated successfully with prolonged courses of glucocorticoids alone. However, certain disease manifestations strongly suggest the use of concomitant cyclophosphamide. These manifestations include mesenteric vasculitis, cardiac disease, and nervous system involvement (either central nervous system disease or vasculitic neuropathy of the peripheral nerves). The French Vasculitis Study Group has developed a "Five Factor Score" to specify which patients with PAN (and other forms of systemic vasculitis) are likely to benefit from the addition of cyclophosphamide from the outset of treatment (Guillevin et al. 2003).

The short- and long-term toxicities of high-dose glucocorticoid treatment are often underemphasized. Sometimes, physicians continue excessive doses of glucocorticoids for too long, much to the detriment of the patient. Using a cytotoxic agent concomitantly may decrease the quantity of glucocorticoid therapy required. In patients who are likely to tolerate glucocorticoids poorly because of weight gain, glucose intolerance, osteopenia, or other reasons, the simultaneous use of a cytoxic agent from the outset may be the wisest course.

If one waits too long to initiate a cytotoxic agent, then all too often the patient is "beaten up" already from heavy-handed glucocorticoid treatment. This only heightens the likelihood of complications from cyclophosphamide and concerns about using the medication in the first place. Inability to taper prednisone below 15 mg/day is a clear

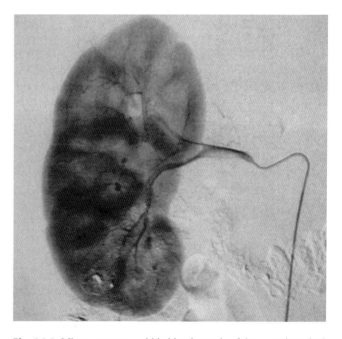

Fig. 26.8 Microaneurysms within blood vessels of the gastrointestinal tract in a patient with polyarteritis nodosa

signal that it is time to get another agent on board. The trick is not to use cyclophosphamide too long…

Myth: Visceral abdominal angiography is both specific and sensitive for PAN.

Reality: In the proper clinical setting, an angiogram that reveals multiple saccular aneurysms in more than one organ is quite specific for PAN (Fig. 26.8). For the purposes of roundsmanship, it is worth noting that microaneurysms can also be seen in conditions such as atrial myxoma, neurofibromatosis, the Ehlers–Danlos syndrome, endocarditis, and others. Thus, these findings are strongly suggestive but not diagnostic of PAN.

More common than multiple saccular aneurysms, unfortunately, are the vaguer luminal irregularities, vascular cut-offs, and fusiform changes — features that are not specific for PAN or any other type of vasculitis. These changes can be observed in a variety of vascular disorders, including atherosclerosis. Most data on the test characteristics of angiography result from relatively few case series, many of which are outdated and suffer from selection bias. The sensitivity of mesenteric angiography for the findings of PAN is not known with any reliability.

The upshot is that abdominal angiography should be performed in patients suspected of having classic PAN but in whom no symptomatic peripheral target organ is available for biopsy. Careful interpretation of these studies by both experienced clinicians and angiographers is essential.

Pearl: Don't be fooled by the turning of vessels "en fas" into thinking that a microaneurysm is present.

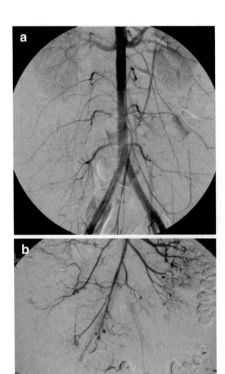

Fig. 26.9 Angiogram findings in a patient without (**a**) and with (**b**) polyarteritis nodosa

Comment: Figure 26.9a illustrates this point well. Although there is a rounding of the blood vessel and an intensification of color density that could represent a microaneurysm, this finding actually represents only a natural bending of the blood vessel back into the sagittal plane of the angiogram. This twist leads to an accentuation of the dye image, but is not a true outpouching of the blood vessel wall. The image in Fig. 26.9b is far more convincing.

Myth: If no microaneuryms are demonstrated in the renal or mesenteric vasculature by magnetic resonance angiography or computed tomographic angiography, then further study of those vascular beds is not indicated.

Reality: Despite the dramatic advances in imaging that have occurred, the resolution of magnetic resonance angiography and computed tomographic angiography still do not match that of conventional angiography. When the highest sensitivity for microaneurysms is required, conventional angiography remains essential. Clinicians should not draw false reassurances from less sensitive but noninvasive studies.

Pearl: A highly elevated serum renin level provides a hint that the answer may lie in further evaluation of the renal vasculature.

Comment: Renin is produced by the juxtaglomerular apparatus of the kidney in response to perceived hypotension (Coffman and Crowley 2008). In the setting of PAN that involves the kidney, lesions of the intrarenal arteries and muscular arterioles lead to renal hyperperfusion and elevated levels of renin. The hypertension characteristic of PAN is a renin-mediated process.

Although elevated serum renin levels are not diagnostic of PAN, this finding in the proper clinical context urges a more in-depth evaluation to exclude a medium-vessel vasculitis.

Pearl: PAN favors medium-sized muscular arteries, but spares veins.

Comment: This Pearl dates back to the original observations of Kussmaul and Maier: *"The most widespread and conspicuous change is that of the arteries. It is present….only in arteries whose media preferably have muscular elements and which do not exceed the caliber of the liver artery …and nowhere in the capillaries. A similar change like that of the arteries is not detectable in the veins…"* (Kussmaul and Maier 1866).

Many other forms of vasculitis do involve the venous circulation, however. Most forms of cutaneous vasculitis target the postcapillary venules. The lesions of the vasculitides that are commonly associated with ANCA often involve small- and medium-sized veins. Behçet's disease may affect veins of any size (including ones as large as the pulmonary veins and the vena cavae), and is associated with an increased risk of deep venous thrombosis. The posterior uveitis (retinal vasculitis) in Behcet's disease also consists primarily of a venulitis.

The reasons for this striking selectivity for different portions of the vascular bed remain unclear remain one of the great mysteries of vasculitis.

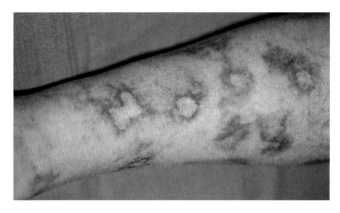

Fig. 26.10 Healed skin ulcers in a patient with polyarteritis nodosa

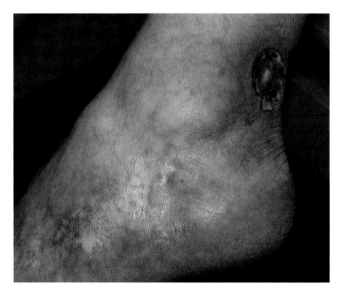

Fig. 26.11 Cutaneous lesions of livedoid vasculopathy, known as "atrophie blanche"

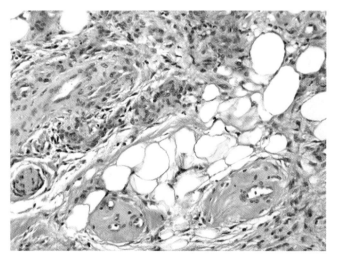

Fig. 26.12 Segmental hyalinizing vasculopathy. Livedoid vasculopathy is not a vasculitis per se but rather a vasculopathy associated with small-vessel thrombi and hyalinizing changes within the blood vessel walls. Note hyaline changes in the walls of these vessels that might be mistaken (by an amateur pathologist!) for fibrinoid necrosis.

Myth: Lower extremity ulcers that heal with the scars depicted in Fig. 26.10 are pathognomonic of atrophie blanche.

Reality: Atrophie blanche is the hallmark cutaneous lesion of livedoid vasculopathy, a bland vascular disorder of small blood vessels characterized by thrombosis (Kroshinsky et al. 2008). Livedoid vasculopathy is a thrombotic microangiopathy characterized clinically by lower extremity ulcerations and the stellate-shaped, porcelain-colored scars known as atrophie blanche (Fig. 26.11) (Maessen-Visch et al. 1999; Callen, 2006). Healed lesions of cutaneous PAN can mimic this clinical finding perfectly.

Livedoid vasculopathy is far less likely than is PAN to cause mononeuritis multiplex. However, mononeuritis multiplex has been reported in livedoid vasculopathy (Kroshinsky et al. 2008; Hairston et al. 2006). Thus, this feature does not differentiate reliably between these two conditions, and histopathological distinction must be sought. A good skin biopsy is usually sufficient to settle the question (Fig. 26.12).

References

Arepally GM, Ortel TL. Heparin-induced thrombocytopenia. N Engl J Med. 2006;355:809–17

Bazari H, Jaff MR, Mannstadt M, Yan S. Case 7-2007: a 59 year-old woman with diabetic renal disease and nonhealing skin ulcers. N Engl J Med. 2007; 356:1049–57

Callen JP. Livedoid vasculopathy: what it is and how the patient should be evaluated and treated. Arch Dermatol. 2006;142:1481–2

Coffman TM, Crowley SD. Kidney in hypertension: Guyton redux. Hypertension 2008;51:811–16

Collins MP, Mendell JR, Periquet MI, et al Superficial peroneal nerve/peroneus brevis muscle biopsy in vasculitic neuropathy. Neurology 2000;55:636–43

Ehrmann S. Ein Gefaessprozess Bei Lues. Wien Med Wochenschr. 1907;57:777

Frances C, Niang S, Laffitte E, et al Dermatologic manifestations of the antiphospholipid syndrome. Arthritis Rheum. 2005;52: 1785–93

Frances C, Piette JC. The mystery of Sneddon's syndrome: the relationship with antiphospholipid syndrome and systemic lupus erythematosus. J Autoimmun. 2000;15:139–43

Frances C, Papo T, Wechser B, et al Sneddon's syndrome with and without aPL. Medicine 1999;78:209–19

Gorson KC, Hedley-White ET, Skinner MM. Case records of the Massachusetts General Hospital. N Eng J Med. 2001;344: 917–23

Guillevin L, Lhote F. Treatment of polyarteritis nodosa and microscopic polyangiitis. Arthritis Rheum. 1998;41:2100–5

Guillevin L, Cohen P, Mahr A, et al Treatment of polyarteritis nodosa and microscopic polyangiitis with poor prognosis factors: a prospective trial comparing glucocorticoids and six or twelve cyclophosphamide pulses in sixty-five patients. Arthritis Rheum. 2003; 49:93–100

Ha C, Nousari, HC. Double trephine punch biopsy technique for sampling subcutaneous tissue. J Am Acad Dermatol. 2003;48:609–10

Hairston BR, Davis MD, Pittelkow MR, Ahmed I. Livedoid vasculopathy: further evidence for procoagulant pathogenesis. Arch Dermatol. 2006;142:1413–8

Kroshinsky D, Stone JH, Bloch D, Sepehr A. A 47 year-old woman with numbness and pain in the lower extremities. N Engl J Med. 2009; 360:711–20

Kussmaul A, Maier R. Über eine bisher nicht beschriebene eigenthumliche arterienerkrankung (periarteritis nodosa), die mit morbus brightii und rapid fortschreitender allgemeiner muskellahmung einhergeht. Dtsch Arch Klin Med. 1866;1:484–518

London NJ, Donnelly R. ABC of arterial and venous disease: ulcerated lower limb. BMJ 2000;320:1589–91

Maessen-Visch M, Koedam M, Hamulyak K, et al Atrophie blanche. Int J Dermatol. 1999;38:161–72

Mathew L, Talbot K, Love S, et al Treatment of vasculitic peripheral neuropathy: a retrospective analysis of outcome. QJM 2007; 100:41–57

Matsumoto T, Homma S, Okada M, et al The lung in polyarteritis nodosa: a pathologic study of 10 cases. Hum Pathol. 1993;24:717–24

Mimouni D, Ng PP, Rencic A, et al Cutaneous PAN in patients presenting with atrophie blanche. Br J Dermatol. 2003;148:789–94

Pagnoux C, Seror R, Mahr A, et al Polyarteritis nodosa: clinical description and long-term follow-up of the 351 patients from the French Vasculitis Study Group. Arthritis Rheum. 2006;49:S420

Stockhammer GJ, Felber SR, Zelger B, et al Sneddon's syndrome: diagnosis by skin biopsy and MRI in 17 patients. Stroke 1993;24 :685–90

Stone JH, Talor M, Stebbing J, et al Test characteristics of immunofluorescence and ELISA tests in 856 consecutive patients with possible ANCA-associated conditions. Arthritis Care Res. 2000;13: 424–34

Stone JH, Nousari HC. "Essential" cutaneous vasculitis: what every rheumatologist should know about vasculitis of the skin. Curr Opin Rheumatol. 2001;13:23–34

Talor MV, Stone JH, Stebbing JJ, et al Antibodies to selected minor target antigens in patients with anti-neutrophil cytoplasmic antibodies (ANCA) by immunofluorescence antibodies to minor target antigens in patients with anti-neutrophil cytoplasmic antibodies. Clin Exp Immunol. 2007;150:42–8

Uthman IW, Khamashta MA. Livedo racemosa: a striking dermatological sign for the antiphospholipid syndrome. J Rheumatol. 2006;33: 2379–82

Vallat J-M, Cros DP, Hedley-White ET. Case 9-2007: a 27 year-old woman with pain and swelling of the legs. N Engl J Med. 2007;356: 1252–9

Giant Cell Arteritis and Polymyalgia Rheumatica   27

James R. Stone, Misha Pless, Carlo Salvarani, Nicolo Pipitone, Simmons Lessell, and John H. Stone

Overview of Giant Cell Arteritis

> Giant cell arteritis (GCA) is a form a large- to medium-vessel vasculitis that involves the aorta and its branches.
> Polymyalgia rheumatica (PMR), a syndrome of muscle pain and stiffness in the neck, shoulders, and hips, often occurs with GCA but can occur independently.
> GCA predominantly affects the second- to fifth-order aortic branches, often in the extracranial arteries of the head.
> The mean age at diagnosis of GCA is approximately 72.
> The diagnosis of GCA is made usually by biopsy of the temporal artery.
> GCA associated with granulomatous inflammation within the blood vessel wall, but granulomatous changes are not always evident early in the disease. Giant cells occur in a slight majority of cases of positive temporal artery biopsies. Estimates of the frequency of giant cells in temporal artery biopsy tissues are on the order of 50-80%.
> In GCA, clinical symptoms of local vascular inflammation and vascular insufficiency are usually accompanied or preceded by a systemic inflammatory process.
> Visual loss is the most feared complication of GCA. Visual loss may occur through the syndrome of anterior ischemic optic neuropathy, caused by narrowing of the posterior ciliary artery, as well as through other arterial insufficiency syndromes.
> Glucocorticoids are the cornerstone of treatment for GCA and PMR. PMR occurring in the absence of GCA requires a lower dose of prednisone for disease control.

27.1 Symptoms and Signs

Pearl: GCA rarely (if ever) occurs among patients less than 50 years of age.

Comment: Biological and chronological age often correlate poorly with each other, but the statement that GCA does not occur in patients younger than 50 is remarkably robust. Of the 1,435 GCA patients with biopsy-proven disease included in a metaanalysis of 26 studies, only two patients were younger than 50 years of age (Smetana and Shmerling 2002).

One suspects that even those two patients might have had some form of systemic vasculitis other than GCA, as several other vasculitic conditions can involve the temporal arteries and mimic GCA. The ANCA-associated vasculitides are notorious for this (Small and Brisson 1991).

Pearl: GCA is rare among African-Americans, particularly African-American men.

Comment: This point is difficult to prove in the absence of a large, population-based study conducted in an area comprised of a substantial number of African-Americans. Olmsted County, Minnesota, and the Scandinavian countries, sites of much GCA research to date, are not such places.

A study from Baltimore, a city that is 65% African-American, evaluated 90 cases of biopsy-proven temporal arteritis and compared them with 90 controls (Regan et al. 2000). The cases included every single temporal artery biopsy-proven case of GCA at the Johns Hopkins Hospital between 1968 and 2000. The cases were matched to the controls on age, gender, and year of biopsy, but not race.

Among the controls, 26 of the 90 patients (28%) were African-Americans. However, among the cases, only five patients (6%) were African-Americans ($p < 0.001$). All five GCA patients who were African-American were female. Thus, at the Johns Hopkins Hospital, there was not a singe case of biopsy-proven GCA in an African-American man over a period spanning 32 years.

The upshot of these data is that, when considering the cause of an inflammatory illness in an African-American patient, diagnoses other than GCA should be weighed more heavily.

Myth: GCA is characterized by temporal arteries that are abnormal on physical examination.

Reality: Many patients who turn out to have biopsy-proven GCA do not have temporal arteries that are obviously

Table 27.1. Estimated likelihood ratios for the prediction of a positive temporal artery biopsy for findings on the history and physical examination

Symptom/sign	Number of patients with data on variable	Positive LR (95% CI)	Negative LR (95% CI)
Symptoms			
Anorexia	674	1.2 (0.96–1.4)	0.87 (0.75–1.0)
Weight Loss	1,417	1.3 (1.1–1.5)	0.89 (0.79–1.0)
Arthralgia	582	1.1 (0.86–1.4)	1.0 (0.92–1.1)
Diplopia	703	3.4 (1.3–8.6)	0.95 (0.91–0.99)
Fatigue	1,095	1.2 (0.98–1.4)	0.94 (0.86–1.0)
Fever	1,708	1.2 (0.98–1.4)	0.92 (0.85–0.99)
Temporal headache	386	1.5 (0.78–3.0)	0.82 (0.64–1.0)
Any headache	2,475	1.2 (1.1–1.4)	0.7 (0.57–0.85)
Jaw claudication	2,314	4.2 (2.8–6.2)	0.72 (0.65–0.81)
Myalgia	681	0.93 (0.81–1.1)	1.1 (0.87–1.3)
Polymyalgia rheumatica	1,383	0.97 (0.76–1.2)	0.99 (0.83–1.2)
Unilateral visual loss	341	0.85 (0.58–1.2)	1.2 (1.0–1.3)
Any visual symptoms	2,083	1.1 (0.93–1.3)	0.97 (0.9–1.0)
Vertigo	212	0.71 (0.38–1.3)	1.1 (0.93–1.2)
Signs			
Optic atrophy or ischemic optic neuropathy	142	1.6 (1.0–2.5)	0.8 (0.58–1.1)
Scalp tenderness	923	1.6 (1.2–2.1)	0.93 (0.86–1.0)
Synovitis	734	0.41 (0.23–0.72)	1.1 (1.0–1.2)
Beaded temporal artery	323	4.6 (1.1–18.4)	0.93 (0.88–0.99)
Prominent/enlarged temporal artery	508	4.3 (2.1–8.9)	0.67 (0.5–0.89)
Tender temporal artery	755	2.6 (1.9–3.7)	0.82 (0.74–0.92)
Absent temporal artery pulse	68	2.7 (0.55–13.4)	0.71 (0.38–0.75)

Adapted from Smetana and Shmerling (2002)

abnormal on physical examination. In approximately one third of cases, in fact, the physical examination of the temporal arteries is completely normal (Hall et al. 1983).

The classic physical examination finding of nodular, thickened temporal arteries is extremely helpful when present but, alas, is quite rare. (This is probably a good thing, as nodular temporal arteries suggest longstanding, undiagnosed disease.) Nodular thickening of the temporal artery on physical examination is associated with an odds ratio of 4.5 for biopsy-proven GCA (Smetana and Shmerling 2002). This makes it one of the most useful physical findings for the differentiation of patients who will have a positive biopsy from those who will not (Table 27.1).

Pearl: Patients with PMR have normal passive range of motion of the shoulder.

Comment: Patients with PMR can be moved to tears because of pain when attempting to raise their arms above their heads or abduct their shoulders through active movement. However, these same patients have full range of motion of the affected extremities if the examiner takes them through these motions passively.

Myth: Diplopia is a rare manifestation of GCA.

Reality: Many clinicians fail to recognize that diplopia, caused by ischemia of extraocular muscles, cranial nerves, or brainstem, can also be a feature of GCA. Diplopia occurs in up to 15% of patients with this disease (Gordon and Levin 1998). Diplopia was reported in 5 of 46 patients (11%) with biopsy-proven GCA from Olmsted County, Minnesota (Hall et al. 1983). Along with jaw claudication, diplopia is one of the most specific symptoms of GCA.

A variety of mechanisms can lead to diplopia in GCA.

- Branches of the ophthalmic artery supply ocular muscles within the orbit. Ischemia of the extraocular muscles is believed to be the etiology of diplopia in some cases.
- More proximal branches of the ophthalmic artery constitute the *vasa nervorum* of the cranial nerves, which direct ocular motor function. Involvement of the *vasa nervorum* by GCA can lead to discrete patterns of ophthalmoplegia, e.g., trochlear, oculomotor, or abducens nerve palsies.
- Finally, brainstem strokes caused by infarctions within the territories of the vertebral or posterior cerebral arteries are possible in GCA. Such lesions can affect the structures within the brainstem that serve binocular motor function, thereby leading to diplopia.

Pearl: A persistent dry cough can be a manifestation of occult GCA.

Comment: Cough is one of the many "occult" manifestations of GCA – disease features that are not considered classic for the diagnosis but which, when present, unveil the diagnosis to the astute clinician. The upper respiratory tract contains numerous "cough receptors." The etiology of cough in GCA is presumed to be irritation of the cough receptors by ischemia to surrounding tissues (Olopade et al. 1997).

Pearl: The most specific symptom of GCA is jaw claudication.

Comment: A 1983 study from the Mayo Clinic demonstrated this point nicely (Hall et al. 1983). Between 1965 and 1980, 134 Olmsted County residents underwent temporal artery biopsies, of which 46 (34%) were positive for GCA and 88 (66%) were negative. The symptoms of PMR, fever, headache of recent onset, scalp tenderness, and visual loss were all similar between the positive and negative biopsy groups (after all, the patients had to have symptoms compatible with GCA to prompt a biopsy). Jaw claudication, however, was present in 54% of the patients with positive biopsies, compared with only 3% of those whose biopsies were negative ($p < 0.001$).

When the patient tells you that she has jaw claudication, the diagnosis can be relatively straightforward. Of course, it never happens that way. Patients never complain of that buzzword – "jaw claudication" – but rather might note facial pressure while talking, the reluctance to eat meat because of difficulty chewing, the inability to open their mouths (reminiscent of trismus), difficulty speaking (Lee et al. 1999), pain in the tongue (Larson et al. 1984), and other similarly oblique confessions.

Pearl: Jaw claudication comes on fast.

Comment: It usually does not require a tough piece of steak to elicit jaw claudication. Patients with this symptom develop it quickly following the initiation of chewing, even of relatively soft foods. Jaw claudicators are seized characteristically with an angina-like pain in the cheek or jaw that gets their attention abruptly, usually after only a few seconds of chewing.

Pearl: New, unexplained pain located above the neck in a person older than 60 should suggest the possibility of GCA.

Comment: Headache and jaw claudication are classic manifestations of GCA. However, patients with GCA can present with many other less well-described pains above the neck, including pain over the nose, in the ears, along the jaw (not necessarily related to chewing), in the throat, in the mouth (e.g., tongue or "dental" like pain), or over the occiput. Indeed, many patients with these symptoms are first misdiagnosed as having "sinusitis," "otitis media," or "dental infections," even though physical signs of these disorders are absent.

Other facial manifestations described in GCA include odontogenic pain, chin numbness, glossitis, submandibular swelling, and necrosis of the scalp, tongue, and lips (Paraskevas et al. 2007; Ruiz-Masera et al. 1995; Porter, 1990).

Pearl: GCA is a common cause of fever of unknown origin (FUO) in the elderly.

Comment: Although GCA causes less than 2% of all cases of FUO, GCA is the culprit in 16% of FUO cases occurring

Table 27.2 Comparison of features of arteritic and nonarteritic anterior ischemic optic neuropathy (AION)

Feature	Arteritic	Nonarteritic
Age (mean years)	70	60
Gender distribution	Female: male = 3	Female: male = 1
Systemic complaints	Often	Uncommon
Visual acuity	Impaired (<20/20) in up to three-fourths	Preserved in the majority
Disc	Pale > hyperemic edema	Hyperemic > pale edema
Cup size	Normal	Small
Mean ESR (mm/h)	70	20–40
Natural history	Improvement rare	Improvement in up to 43%
Contralateral involvement	Fellow eye in 95%	Fellow eye in <30%
Treatment	Glucocorticoids	None proved

Adapted from Seo and Stone (2002)

among patients older than 65 years of age (Esposito and Gleckman 1978). In one study of fever in GCA, 15 of 100 consecutive cases of biopsy-proven GCA had fevers before diagnosis. The patients with fever all had normal white blood cell counts, but as a group they had significantly higher ESRs, platelet counts, and alkaline phosphatase levels than the other 85 patients, as well as lower hemoglobin concentrations. In four patients with no other symptoms or physical findings suggestive of GCA, temporal artery biopsies revealed arteritis.

Pearl: The most common cause of acute visual loss in GCA is anterior ischemic optic neuropathy.

Comment: Five known mechanisms of visual loss occur in GCA (Table 27.2).

- Arteritic anterior ischemic optic neuropathy (A-AION) is the most common mechanism of visual loss. A-AION involves vasculitic occlusion of the posterior ciliary arteries, which perfuse the vulnerable neuro-ocular junction at the optic nerve head (Fig. 27.1). The neuro-ocular junction contains 1.1 million axons that exit the globe posteriorly through the optic nerve. Approximately 80% of all cases of loss of vision from GCA occur through the mechanism of A-AION. The typical funduscopic finding 24 h after A-AION is swelling of the optic disc (Fig. 27.2).
- A subset of AION – posterior ischemic optic neuropathy (PION) – can also occur in GCA. In PION, the ischemic insult occurs in the retrobulbar portion of the optic nerve, through occlusion of the proximal posterior ciliary arteries. As a result, no disc edema is visible to the clinician upon funduscopy.
- Central or branch retinal artery occlusion (CRAO or BRAO) is the cause of visual loss in approximately 20% of GCA cases. The central and branch retinal arteries are both somewhat larger than the posterior ciliary artery.

Fig. 27.1 Arteritic anterior ischemic optic neuropathy (A-AION) is the most common mechanism of visual loss. A-AION involves vasculitic occlusion of the posterior ciliary arteries (LPCA and MPCA), which perfuse the vulnerable neuro-ocular junction at the optic nerve head. The neuro-ocular junction contains 1.1 million axons that exit the globe posteriorly through the optic nerve. Approximately 80% of all cases of loss of vision from GCA occur through the mechanism of A-AION. *ICA* internal carotid artery; *OA* ophthalmic artery; *CAR* central retinal artery; *LPCA* lateral posterior ciliary artery; *MPCA* medial posterior ciliary artery

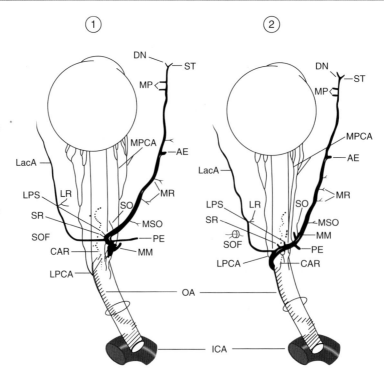

Width 25 pi
Height 24 pi

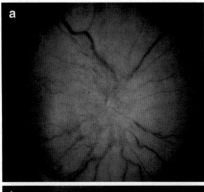

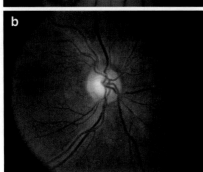

Fig. 27.2 Arteritic anterior ischemic optic neuropathy (A-AION). (**a**) The typical finding 24 h after the onset of vision loss within the eye is swelling of the optic nerve. (**b**) A normal optic nerve is shown for comparison

Myth: In patients with GCA who present with acute visual loss, funduscopy inevitably reveals abnormal findings.

Reality: Funduscopy yields findings consistent with GCA in most cases. However, the findings on funduscopy are never pathognomonic of GCA, and this examination can be normal even in patients with GCA who have lost vision. This is dictated by the precise site of the vascular lesion that has led to visual loss.

PION is the cause of visual loss in only a minority of GCA cases (Hayreh et al. 1998a, b). In contrast to AION, PION is associated with a normal optic disk in the acute phase of visual loss. Optic disk pallor ensues 4–6 weeks later (Rucker et al. 2004).

In extremely rare cases, blindness in GCA results from cortical ischemia. This is also associated with a normal optic disk.

Myth: It is possible to diagnose GCA by funduscopy.

Reality: It is impossible to distinguish arteritic from nonarteritic AION based on direct visualization of the optic nerve and/or ocular fundus. The optic nerve in AION of any type appears swollen and is often associated with papillary hemorrhages. In PION, the optic nerve appears normal in the context of acute loss of vision until atrophy sets in over a period of weeks. The optic nerve may look partially swollen within the background of retinal infarction in CRAO or BRAO.

Pearl: Pallid disc edema is helpful in diagnosing GCA.

- A rare mechanism of visual loss in GCA is ophthalmic artery occlusion. In such cases, the entire eye is ischemic, the orbit edematous, and there is ophthalmoplegia.
- Finally, a posterior circulation stroke involving the calcarine cortices can lead to visual field defects or cortical blindness by virtue of bilateral hemispheric involvement.

Comment: When the optic nerve has pallor in addition to edema at acute onset of visual loss, this implies there has been axonal loss before a more massive optic nerve head infarction. This is presumed to occur in GCA-associated AION more often than in a nonarteritic ischemic disorder of the optic nerve.

Pearl: GCA can cause visual hallucinations.

Comment: One highly intriguing ocular finding in GCA is the Charles Bonnet (pronounced "Bō nay'") syndrome. The Charles Bonnet syndrome is the occurrence of visual hallucinations – "release hallucinations" – in individuals who are psychologically normal (Razavi et al. 2004). Reversibility of these symptoms with glucocorticoid therapy has been reported.

The precise mechanism of these hallucinations is not defined, but the Charles Bonnet syndrome is believed to be a consequence of ischemia to parts of the visual pathways. This includes of the posterior circulation, i.e., the posterior cerebral arteries, leading to reversible ischemia in the calcarine cortex or the parietal subcortical white matter.

Pearl: GCA may present as noises in the head.

Comment: This disease feature is rarely mentioned in the literature, and its etiology is obscure. However, patients have reported a diversity of sounds appearing to come from within their heads. Examples of such sounds are turbine engines and tree frogs.

Myth: GCA does not affect the central nervous system (CNS).

Reality: If this Myth were reworded to read that "GCA seldom involves the intracerebral circulation yet can still affect the brain through causing extensive extracranial disease," then this statement would be correct. When transient ischemic attacks, vertigo, hearing loss, and stroke occur in GCA, they are usually the result of vertebral artery or internal carotid artery lesions that are extradural.

The rarity of intracerebral disease in GCA is a longstanding mystery. One frequently proffered explanation is the fact that once the extracranial arteries penetrate the dura they lose their external elastic laminae (Wilkinson and Russell 1972; Caselli et al. 1988). The full answer for the rarity of CNS vascular disease in GCA is probably more complicated.

Regardless of the reason, however, intracerebral GCA is very rare but well-documented in a small number of patients. In a study of 463 patients from the Mayo Clinic with clinical diagnoses of CNS vasculitis, only two had convincing evidence of intracranial GCA (Salvarani et al. 2006).

Myth: Acute unilateral vision loss in an elderly individual is likely to be GCA.

Reality: Only a minority of acute unilateral vision loss events in this setting are caused by GCA. Another entity with a tendency to occur in old age – nonarteritic anterior ischemic optic neuropathy (NAAION) – is approximately ten times more common than GCA as a cause of unilateral vision loss.

Table 27.3 Vascular lesions that can lead to vision loss in giant cell arteritis

Posterior ciliary artery occlusion
Anterior ischemic optic neuropathy (AION)
Posterior ischemic optic neuropathy (PION)
Retinal artery occlusion
Central retinal artery occlusion (CRAO)
Branch retinal artery occlusion (BRAO)
Ophthalmic artery occlusion
Posterior circulation stroke

With the exception of glaucoma, NAAION is the most common cause of optic neuropathy (Lessell 1999). NAAION tends to affect Caucasians older than 60 years of age, as is the case with GCA. Unlike GCA, however, NAAION is not an inflammatory disorder: constitutional symptoms and elevated acute phase reactants are usually absent.

NAAION is associated with funduscopic findings that help differentiate it from GCA: hyperemic disc swelling and a morphologically small optic disc with no cup in NAAION, compared with disc pallor, disc swelling, cotton-wool spots, and a normal optic cup size in GCA. Table 27.3 compares these two entities.

Pearl: GCA can cause facial swelling.

Comment: Facial swelling has been described as a complication of GCA (separate from prednisone-induced Cushingoid features) (Cohen et al. 1982). The pathogenesis of facial swelling in GCA is poorly understood. In one study, facial swelling was found to be associated with the risk of developing visual disturbances (Friedman and Friedman 1986), whereas in another study facial and neck swelling were found not to be linked to visual disturbances or to ischemic stroke (Liozon et al. 2006).

Pearl: Audiovestibular dysfunction may be a manifestation of GCA.

Comment: A syndrome of sensorineural hearing loss, often accompanied by vertigo and tinnitus, has been described in several immune-mediated disorders. These include vasculitides such as polyarteritis nodosa and Wegener's granulomatosis (WG) (Stone and Francis 2000). This syndrome, sometimes referred to as immune-mediated inner ear disease (IMIED), is frequently bilateral and is characterized by a clinical course that is more rapid than Meniere's syndrome, a disorder in which fluctuating hearing loss occurs over months to years (Papadimitraki et al. 2004).

A retrospective review of 271 GCA patients disclosed four who presented with sensineural hearing loss (Hausch and Harrington 1998). Audiovestibular dysfunction was found to be even more frequent in a prospective study on 44 patients with GCA (Amor-Dorado et al. 2003). This study investigated patients systematically for evidence of such dysfunction both by clinical interview and a battery of specific tests. More than one half of the patients complained of hearing loss, tinnitus, vertigo, or dizziness. Moreover, nearly 90% of the patients had objective evidence of vestibular dysfunction.

These symptoms were generally reversible after several days of glucocorticoid treatment. After 3 months of treatment, the percentage with vestibular dysfunction had declined to 30%, and after 6 months only one patient had persistently abnormal vestibular tests.

These data suggest that audiovestibular dysfunction – both sensorineural hearing loss and vestibular problems – is a feature of GCA. The audiovestibular manifestations of GCA appear to respond well to conventional GCA therapy, but their pathophysiologic basis remains obscure.

Pearl: GCA frequently affects large vessels, i.e., the aorta and its branches to the extremities.

Comment: Although the diagnosis of GCA is usually confirmed by biopsy of the temporal artery, this is only because of the convenience of sampling this vessel. In fact, the disease involves a wide range of other vessels, and sometimes appears to spare the temporal arteries altogether.

The frequency of aortic involvement in GCA was confirmed in 1995 by a population-based study conducted in Olmsted County (Evans et al. 1995). Sixteen of the 96 patients (17%) diagnosed with GCA between 1950 and 1985 developed either thoracic ($n = 11$) or abdominal ($n = 5$) aneurysms. Compared with all persons of the same age and gender living in the same county during that time period, patients with GCA were 17 times more likely to develop thoracic aneurysms, and 2.4 times more likely to develop abdominal aortic aneurysms.

Most aneurysms were detected several years after the diagnosis of GCA (median: 5.8 years). Less extensive inflammatory involvement of the aorta not sufficient to cause an aneurysm is likely to be even more common. Myocardial infarction, thoracoabdominal aortic dissections, and aortic regurgitation are all potential complications of GCA.

Patients who develop thoracic aortic aneurysms usually do not have histories of involvement of the subclavian arteries or other primary branches of the thoracic aorta (Evans et al. 1995). Thus, the group of patients with thoracic aortic aneurysms and the group with aortic arch syndromes may constitute two different GCA subsets.

Annual chest radiographs are recommended for patients with GCA, to screen for the development of thoracic aortic aneurysms (Bongartz and Metteson 2006). Patients with known aneurysms of the thoracic aorta require closer follow-up with other imaging modalities (e.g., echocardiography, MRI).

Pearl: Check the blood pressure in both arms in patients suspected of having GCA.

Comment: The primary branches of the thoracic aorta (carotid, vertebral, subclavian, and arteries) are involved clinically in about 15% of cases (Brack et al. 1999). Because patients with early involvement of these arteries may have neither local symptoms (e.g., arm claudication) nor stroke, the diagnosis may be suggested first by discrepancies detected between the blood pressures in the right and left arms, or auscultation over the brachial, subclavian, and axillary arteries.

Many GCA patients with aortic arch syndromes and findings of occlusive disease in the arms have few of the classic "temporal arteritis" symptoms such as headache, scalp tenderness, and jaw claudication. Thirty-one of the 74 GCA cases (42%) associated with aortic arch syndromes had negative temporal artery biopsies (Brack et al. 1999).

Pearl: If the patient has headaches, PMR symptoms, and calf pain, do not forget to check an ANCA.

Comment: Absent histopathologic confirmation of GCA by biopsy or unequivocal findings on imaging consistent with large-vessel vasculitis, checking an ANCA is a good idea anyway, calf pain or not. ANCA-associated disorders can present with headaches and PMR symptoms that are nearly perfect mimics of GCA. Calf pain is much more typical of vasculitides that involve small- to medium-sized vessels than it is of GCA. Thus, the ANCA-associated disorders, polyarteritis nodosa, and cryoglobulinemia must all be kept in mind. Among these, the ANCA-associated disorders are by far the most common to masquerade as GCA.

Myth: All GCA patients – even those without ocular symptoms – should be referred to an ophthalmologist.

Reality: When GCA affects the eyes, the symptoms are dramatic and not ignorable by the patient. CRAO and AION typically cause acute, severe vision loss. Patients who have transient amaurosis as a prelude to one of these ophthalmic catastrophes are usually aware that they have temporarily lost their vision. Patients with ophthalmoplegia from GCA (usually from sixth or third nerve palsy) have sudden binocular diplopia.

If a sentient GCA suspect has none of these symptoms, it is highly unlikely that the ophthalmologist will detect any abnormality that contributes to the diagnosis of GCA.

Myth: Ophthalmologists and rheumatologists should manage patients with GCA, who have ocular symptoms together.

Reality: In the absence of new eye symptoms, ophthalmic surveillance will not detect new disease activity in patients who do not have ocular complaints. The patient who is stable from the standpoint of visual health can be managed by the rheumatologist alone once the diagnosis has been established and treatment initiated. The occurrence of new or recurrent ocular symptoms is an indication to involve an ophthalmologist in the case again.

Myth: The eye is an important source of headache.

Reality: Popular lore holds that the eyes are an important "headache generator." This is not true. With regard to pain and common ocular syndromes, the following points are important:

- Open-angle glaucoma, a prevalent disease in the elderly, is not associated with either headaches or eye pain. Because open-angle glaucoma is asymptomatic, the diagnosis often goes unrecognized even during the evolution of irreversible peripheral vision loss. Thus, if headache is a major symptom, clinicians should not waste time referring patients for ocular pressure measurements.
- Primary angle-closure glaucoma, much rarer than open-angle glaucoma, *is* painful. However, acute angle closure is associated with red eye, severe ocular pain, and impaired vision. In such cases, the source of pain – the eye – is obvious to any physician, even if the mechanism remains obscure.
- Anterior uveitis and keratitis can occur at any age and are painful, but present acutely with prominent photophobia and external signs of inflammation. The pain in these patients is localized readily to the eye.
- Finally, miscellaneous disorders such as refractive error, cataracts, and eye muscle imbalance do not cause headaches.

Searches for "ocular causes" of headaches in patients without eye symptoms or signs are nearly always fruitless. They divert the clinician from etiologies that demand more urgent attention, such as GCA.

Myth: GCA does not cause vasculitic neuropathy.

Reality: Mononeuritis multiplex is most often associated with medium- to small-vessel vasculitis (medium much more so than small). The Churg–Strauss syndrome (CSS) and polyarteritis nodosa, for example, cause a potentially crippling vasculitic neuropathy in up to 80% of cases. GCA causes vasculitic neuropathy much less often, but well-documented cases are described (Caselli et al. 1988).

27.2 Laboratory Testing

Myth: GCA never presents with a low ESR.

Reality: A population-based study from Olmsted County, Minnesota, soundly repudiated this notion (Salvarani and Hunder 2001). In that report, eighteen of 167 patients (11%) with GCA had ESRs of less than 50 mm/h before receiving glucocorticoids. Nine of the 167 (5%) had ESRs less that 40 mm/h. All of the latter nine patients had positive temporal artery biopsies.

The C-reactive protein (CRP) level can also be normal in a minority of patients with biopsy-proven GCA. Relying upon acute phase reactants for the diagnosis of this disorder is merely one way that these tests can lead the clinician down the primrose path. PMR is even more likely than GCA to be associated with normal acute phase reactants.

Pearl: A normal ESR is more useful than an abnormal one when evaluating a patient for GCA.

Comment: A normal ESR is more useful in excluding GCA than a high result is in diagnosing it (Smetana and Shmerling 2002). In a metaanalysis that included 941 biopsy-proven GCA patients with sufficient information about the ESR, only 4% of the patients had normal values. A normal ESR diminished the probability of a positive temporal artery biopsy by a factor of five.

Even a sky-high ESR adds comparatively little to the likelihood of GCA. For example, an ESR > 100 mm/h is a less powerful predictor of a positive biopsy than are many elements of the history and physical examination, particularly jaw claudication, diplopia, and an abnormal (beaded or enlarged) temporal artery (Smetana and Shmerling 2002).

Myth: GCA headaches tend to focus over the temples.

Reality: There is no classic GCA headache. The chief distinguishing feature of headaches in GCA is that they mark a significant departure from normal for the patient. Thus, for patients who are not "headache people," the very presence of any headache at all is abnormal. For patients given to headaches in general, the headache associated with GCA constitutes a change from the usual pattern: a different location, greater or lesser severity, or a quality that is discrepant from the patient's baseline intermittent headaches.

GCA headaches can be of a boring, unrelenting quality that involves the entire head. They can be focused over the temples or the eyes. They can also be so trifling as to have the patient unaware of them unless asked specifically. But their cardinal feature is that they are different for that specific patient.

Pearl: Leukocytosis does not occur in GCA before the institution of glucocorticoid treatment.

Comment: Despite the often dramatic other indications of systemic inflammation, the white blood cell count is usually normal before the patient starts prednisone. This is true even in patients with fevers of unknown origin. Nonspecific laboratory abnormalities that can accompany GCA include a normochromic, normocytic anemia, thrombocytosis, polyclonal hypergammaglobulinemia, and hypoalbuminemia.

Myth: A rising ESR indicates the return of GCA.

Reality: This Myth is probably the most common error in the management of GCA. "Treating the sed rate" leads to substantial morbidity from excessive glucocorticoid therapy. An increase in the ESR should not trigger retreatment in the absence of clinical symptoms that recall the patient's presentation or which clearly signal the possibility of recurrent GCA. Remember: the ESR normally rises with each decade of life. In and of itself, an ESR of 48 mm/h in an 80-year-old is not worth spilling any more prednisone over unless there is compelling evidence of active disease.

Pearl: The serum alkaline phosphatase level can be elevated in GCA.

Comment: Approximately one quarter of patients with GCA with active disease have elevated levels of serum alkaline phosphatase (Kyle et al. 1991). The alkaline phosphatase level normalizes rapidly following the institution of glucocorticoid treatment. The cause for this abnormality is unknown, but it has been hypothesized that hepatic arteritis might be the underlying lesion.

Myth: A positive test for anticardiolipin antibodies is associated with an increased risk of ischemic complications in GCA.

Reality: Patients with GCA test positive for anticardiolipin antibodies more often than age- and gender-matched controls, but anticardiolipin antibodies do not increase the risk of thrombosis in these patients (Duhaut et al. 1998; Manna et al. 1998; Meyer et al. 1996). In a multicenter study, anticardiolipin antibodies were found in 21% of patients with GCA, compared with 3% of controls (Duhaut et al. 1998). However, no correlation was observed between positivity for anticardiolipin antibodies and thrombotic events in any of these studies.

27.3 Imaging

Myth: Ultrasonography is a useful procedure for the diagnosis of GCA in the community.

Reality: Ultrasonography made a splash when the idea of using this technology to diagnose GCA was introduced in the late 1990s. However, subsequent experience as revealed it to be a tool that is impractical for broad use in the community. In short, in the current state of its technology, ultrasound is unlikely to have a significant impact on the diagnosis or management of GCA.

Early studies of this imaging procedure were flawed by the failure to blind ultrasonographers to the clinical history and physical examination data of the patients. Subsequent studies have indicated that ultrasound of the temporal arteries adds no information to the evaluation of a patient with possible GCA, beyond that which can be gleaned from a thorough history and physical examination (Karahaliou et al. 2006; Salvarani et al. 2002b). The technique remains highly operator-dependent, and it seems unlikely that radiologists or other practitioners beyond specialty centers can be trained to use this technology in the diagnosis and management of GCA responsibly and well.

In the next few years, the emergence of a clinically useful imaging modality for the diagnosis and longitudinal management of GCA is a distinct possibility. However, that modality is more likely to be MRI than ultrasound.

Pearl: Ultrasound is not useful for the detection of disease flares in GCA.

Comment: Ultrasonography, notably color Doppler ultrasonography, is able to delineate both the vessel wall and the lumen of many arteries, including the temporal arteries. In GCA, the most specific and sensitive sign of temporal artery inflammation is a concentric hypoechogenic mural thickening ("halo" sign) (Schmidt et al. 1997). This probably represents vessel wall edema caused by inflammation. In the hands of a skilled and experienced ultrasonographer, the finding of a halo sign significantly increases the likelihood of a GCA diagnosis. Whether or not it precludes, the need for a temporal artery biopsy is a matter of debate.

However, even the most ardent devotees agree that ultrasound is not reliable as a gauge of disease activity or as a diagnostic technique for recurrent disease once glucocorticoids have been initiated. The utility of ultrasound is limited to the time of initial diagnosis.

Myth: Angiography is the most sensitive imaging study for GCA in its early stages.

Reality: Angiography is an excellent technique for the documentation of luminal irregularities such as stenoses or aneurysms in large-vessel vasculitis. However, angiography does not detect vessel wall thickening and mural edema, which represent vasculitic lesions in an earlier stage of the disease. Thus, angiography is not useful in diagnosing early large-vessel GCA.

Pearl: Among patients in whom GCA is suspected despite negative temporal artery biopsies, large-vessel imaging is an important adjunct to diagnosis.

Comment: MRI assists in the diagnosis of GCA in some settings (Fig. 27.3). In GCA with large-vessel involvement, MRI can demonstrate increased vessel wall thickness in the aorta, its primary branches, and even smaller blood vessels (the resolution of the technique improves continually) (Pipitone et al. 2008). Vessel wall thickening can suggest the diagnosis of GCA and, in the proper clinical setting, is virtually diagnostic of that entity. To date, however, no data from prospective studies have confirmed the utility of specific MRI findings (e.g., vessel wall edema or enhancement) for distinguishing active disease in large vessels from vascular remodeling, which can be associated with similar changes (Tso et al. 2002).

Preliminary data suggests that MRI at high field strength (1.5–3 T) is also be sensitive and specific for demonstrating inflammation within temporal arteries (Bley et al. 2005a, b). Thus, MRI studies of the temporal arteries might be useful one day in guiding the site of temporal artery biopsy. These

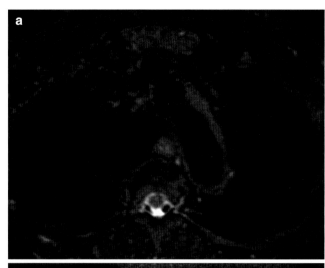

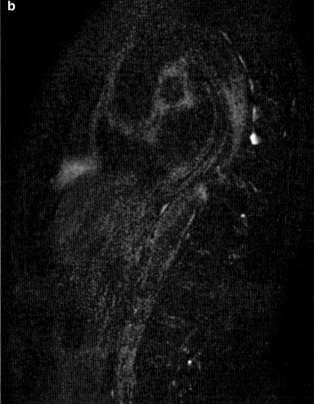

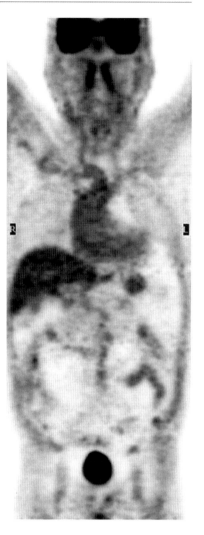

Fig. 27.4 Positron emission tomography (PET) scanning in giant cell arteritis. PET scan showing marked (>grade 1+) tracer uptake in the ascending aorta as well as in the supra-aortic vessels. The high tracer uptake, the smooth appearance of the lesions, and the vessel sites involved suggest the vasculitic nature of the alterations shown by PET

Fig. 27.3 Large-vessel involvement in giant cell arteritis. (a) Axial STIR MRI of the thoracic aorta showing vessel wall thickness with increased signal intensity corresponding to mural edema. (b) Sagittal STIR MRI of the thoracic aorta showing vessel wall thickness with increased signal intensity corresponding to mural edema, more marked in the ascending aorta and in the aortic arch

preliminary results must be confirmed in rigorous, prospective studies before examination of the temporal arteries by MRI becomes part of standard clinical practice.

The potential shortcoming of all currently available imaging modalities with regard to "temporal arteritis" is their failure to provide histopathologic specificity. Microscopic polyangiitis, WG, polyarteritis nodosa, and other forms of systemic vasculitis can also involve the temporal arteries. Although they do so less often than giant cell arteritis, their precise diagnosis is important because of their divergent implications for treatment, prognosis, and the involvement of other organ systems.

Myth: Positron emission tomography (PET) scans of the great vessels are superior to conventional acute phase reactants in the assessment of disease activity in large-vessel vasculitis.

Reality: Fluorodeoxyglucose PET (FDG-PET) scans make very pretty pictures when vasculitis involves large arteries (Fig. 27.4). This technology is helpful in making the diagnosis of GCA when temporal artery biopsies are negative but the focus of disease is within the great vessels (Meller et al. 2003). (No study to date has compared PET and MRI technologies head-to-head for the purpose of diagnosis in this setting). In a study of 35 patients with new-onset, untreated GCA, increased vascular [18]fluorodeoxyglucose uptake was observed in 83% of patients, mainly in the subclavian arteries (74%), in the aorta (>50%), and in the femoral arteries (37%) (Blockmans et al. 2006). FDG-PEt also sometimes reveals that patients believed to have PMR alone actually have GCA.

The utility of PET for following disease activity after the initiation of treatment remains unclear (Pipitone et al. 2008). It is appealing to believe that FDG-PET studies detect smoldering disease activity within the great vessels and their branches, but some data indicate that PET is no better than conventional acute phase reactants (i.e., the ESR and CRP) for this purpose – which is to say not very good (Blockmans 2008). Part of the reason for this is that the vascular remodeling process that the vessel undergoes following treatment is expected to be associated with inflammatory components and edema, as is active large-vessel vasculitis. Thus, distinguishing active disease from the healing process is not straightforward once treatment with glucocorticoids has begun. Additional investigations of FDG-PET as a mirror of disease activity in large-vessel vasculitis are required, and the use of serial PET studies as a gauge of disease activity is premature.

One limitation of FDG-PET is its inability to visualize the temporal arteries, which is due both to the high background signal of the neighboring brain and to the small diameter of the temporal arteries, which is below the resolution threshold of the PET scanners currently available (Blockmans, 2003; Bley et al. 2006).

27.4 Temporal Artery Biopsy

Myth: Temporal artery biopsy is an excellent way to make the diagnosis of giant cell arteritis.

Reality: Temporal artery biopsy is the best way to make the diagnosis of GCA. Unfortunately, it is far from perfect. Even when performed under rigorous circumstances, the false-negative rate of temporal artery biopsies is approximately 10% (Hall et al. 1983). The false-negative rate is probably considerably higher in many centers that do not perform as many temporal artery biopsies.

One reason is that "temporal arteritis" does not always clearly involve the temporal arteries (Horton et al. 1932, 1937). We merely use these vessels whenever possible to make the diagnosis because of their convenient location just under the skin. Sometimes, the diagnostic tissue is that of the occipital artery, not the temporal artery, but the occipital artery is less accessible (without shaving the patient's hair) and therefore is biopsied less often.

Myth: Bilateral negative temporal artery biopsies effectively exclude giant cell arteritis.

Reality: There are several potential explanations for false-negative temporal artery biopsies. First, skip lesions are known to occur in GCA such that the inflammatory changes do not affect the entire temporal artery. Clinicians should realize that the pathologists' procedure for the evaluation of temporal artery biopsies varies from center to center. In general, the entire pathological specimen submitted is not sectioned, therefore, leaving substantial tissue within the paraffin block that could harbor hidden GCA.

The second potential explanation for false-negative temporal artery biopsies is that GCA does not involve the temporal arteries in all patients. This is discussed earlier. Third, inadequate sampling might be the source of the problem. The skill of the operator who performs the biopsy is important. It is easier to biopsy a normal temporal artery than an abnormal one, but the abnormal ones are the ones one wants! More than one pathology report from a temporal artery biopsy procedure has been signed out as "Nerve," indicating that the surgical intern assigned to do the case missed the mark.

Finally, insufficient length of the surgical specimen can also cause the diagnosis of GCA to be overlooked. Although there is no definitive evidence to guide the optimal length of a temporal artery biopsy, a strong consensus of vasculitis experts – rheumatologists, ophthalmologists, and pathologists alike – supports the excision of at least two centimeters of temporal artery.

Myth: There are many contraindications to temporal artery biopsy.

Reality: There are actually very few contraindications to performing a temporal artery biopsy. The contraindications to this procedure are shown in Table 27.4. If necessary, temporal artery biopsy can be performed even while the patient is on warfarin therapy, although it is preferable to convert such patients to heparin before the biopsy.

One absolute contraindication to temporal artery biopsy is the potential need for pial synangiosis surgery (external-to-internal circulation bypass) in patients with severe intracranial or extracranial carotid or vertebral artery stenosis. In such cases, the temporal artery branches can be used to salvage severe intracranial arterial stenosis.

Myth: Temporal artery biopsies are not necessary in some cases because they will not alter the patient's management.

Reality: This rationalization for not performing the biopsy usually stems from one of two reasons: (1) reluctance on the part of the physician to put an elderly patient through a "procedure"; or, (2) anticipated difficulties in arranging a timely biopsy.

Many clinicians have misconceptions about how "invasive" a temporal artery biopsy is. The procedure is performed in an outpatient setting, under local anesthesia. The patient

Table 27.4 Contraindications to temporal artery biopsy

Scalp cellulites
Sepsis
Potential for nonhealing in patients with severe hematologic abnormalities
Severe skin conditions that preclude instrumentation along the scalp

leaves with dissolving sutures covered by a Band-aid. Within 2 weeks, it is often difficult to tell that the patient had the procedure done. Serious complications are vanishingly rare when the biopsy is performed by an experienced surgeon.

Thus, confronted with a patient with possible GCA at 4 p.m. on a Friday afternoon, the proper course is not to decide that a temporal artery biopsy is unnecessary – but rather to begin glucocorticoids at once and to arrange for a biopsy the following week. Starting glucocorticoids without making every effort to confirm the diagnosis by biopsy is a sin that often comes home to roost only months later, when the patient suffers side effects of glucocorticoids and the next physician to evaluate her is left to wonder whether or not she ever really had GCA at all. In such cases, the value of a positive biopsy is immense.

Myth: Unilateral temporal artery biopsies are generally sufficient for the diagnosis of GCA.

Reality: Unilateral biopsies in GCA are O.K., as long as one is content to miss between 20 and 40% of cases (Seo 2005; Boyev et al. 1999; Pless et al. 2000; Brass et al. 2008). Although a unilateral temporal artery biopsy can establish the diagnosis of GCA in many cases, at some institutions both temporal arteries are biopsied routinely.

Bilateral temporal artery biopsies were performed on 186 patients in one study (Boyev et al. 1999). Although only six patients had arteritis on only one side, this number represented 20% of the total number of GCA cases diagnosed through biopsy. In another study that involved 60 patients (Pless et al. 2000), eight (13%) had temporal arteritis on only one side. Those eight patients comprised 40% of the total number of patients diagnosed with GCA by biopsy.

Considering the potential consequences of a missed diagnosis and the very low morbidity of the procedure, the routine performance of bilateral temporal artery biopsies is prudent, especially at institutions where frozen sections cannot be examined intraoperatively to determine if the first biopsy is diagnostic.

Pearl: The diagnosis of GCA remains a clinical one in a significant number of cases, despite the best efforts of pathologists.

Comment: As noted elsewhere, even bilateral temporal artery biopsies performed in the most rigorous manner yield false-negative results in some cases – at least 10% but perhaps substantially higher than this in the community (Hall et al. 1983).

What does one do if bilateral biopsies are negative yet GCA still seems likely? The biopsies should be reviewed with the pathologist to confirm the adequacy of the specimens and the accuracy of the negative reading. Additional cuts of the available specimens might be informative, depending on the pathologist's procedure for reviewing biopsies initially. It is also important to ensure that a Congo red stain of the tissues was performed to exclude amyloid deposition,

since amyloidosis may mimic GCA closely. In some cases, large-vessel imaging (MRI or PET) is helpful.

Finally, if the biopsies are unequivocally normal yet there remains a strong case for the disease on clinical grounds, then the patient must be treated for GCA, fully assured that everything possible to confirm the diagnosis has been done.

Myth: Treatment of a patient suspected of GCA with glucocorticoids before the temporal artery biopsy renders the procedure worthless.

Reality: This myth was debunked by a paper from the Mayo Clinic in 1994 (Achkar et al. 1994). The investigators confirmed that diagnostic histopathological findings could be demonstrated readily by experienced pathologists, even 2 weeks (and as long as 11 months) after the institution of prednisone. Thus, concern about failing to establish the diagnosis because of prebiopsy treatment should *never* interfere with the institution of appropriate treatment.

Although it is still possible to make the diagnosis well after starting glucocorticoids, treatment does alter the histopathological features of GCA. "Atypical" temporal arteritis (e.g., the absence of giant cells or confinement of inflammation to the adventitia) was more common in the subset of patients treated with more than 14 days of glucocorticoids before undergoing biopsies (Achkar et al. 1994). Consequently, the temporal artery biopsy should be obtained as promptly as possible following the institution of glucocorticoids. Failing to do so within a few days, however, is not an opportunity irretrievably lost.

Myth: The surgeon can tell at the time of the biopsy what the pathologist will find.

Reality: No study has ever validated the notion that the surgeon can discern by the appearance and feel of the vessel whether or not the procedure will be diagnostic of GCA. In the case of a nodular, indurated vessel, the positive predictive value of such an examination while the skin is open is probably high. However, more subtle cases of GCA exist as well, and arteries that appear normal at the time of surgery frequently reveal inflammation consistent with GCA under the microscope.

Myth: Using lidocaine with epinephrine is contraindicated in temporal artery biopsy.

Reality: Epinephrine can cause a previously palpable temporal artery to constrict, thereby making it more difficult to identify during the dissection phase of the procedure. However, the benefit of diminishing blood loss is preferable in some cases, and therefore epinephrine should be used according to the discretion of the surgeon. If the artery is no longer readily apparent at dissection, a Doppler device is helpful.

Myth: Temporal artery biopsies should always be performed in the operating room.

Reality: If sterility can be ensured, a treatment room or a procedure room is a perfectly acceptable place to perform a temporal artery biopsy. Lack of timely access to a standard operating room should not delay this important procedure. The procedure is sufficiently simple that an experienced surgeon does not require a fully equipped operating room.

Pearl: Temporal artery biopsies should be performed in the scalp.

Comment: Some surgeons tend to perform biopsies in an area just anterior to the tragus of the ear. This vessel, the common (superficial) temporal artery, is *not* the right one to biopsy, even if a palpable pulse is present at that site. Branches of the facial nerve are vulnerable at a site that low, and facial paralysis can result from a misdirected scalpel.

The scalp is a much safer site at which to perform the biopsies. In the scalp, a rich blood supply promotes rapid healing of the surgical incision. The resulting scar is minimal and ultimately hard to detect, even in patients who are bald. Performance of a temporal artery biopsy in the scalp region requires shaving of a small region of hair, which grows back quickly.

The preferred site for the biopsy is the anterior temporal artery, also known as the frontal temporal artery. The posterior temporal artery, also termed the parietal temporal artery, is sometimes selected when the anterior branch is not readily found (Fig. 27.5a, b).

Pearl: The invasiveness of temporal artery biopsy procedure is overestimated.

Comment: Complications of temporal artery biopsies performed in the scalp region are very rare. As with any surgery, bleeding or infection may occur, but these are is unusual. On the other hand, if the surgeon is inexperienced, untoward results can occur. A facial nerve palsy is one example.

Pearl: Failure to locate the temporal artery is the biggest potential challenge faced in performing a biopsy.

Comment: Finding normal arteries, which are pulsatile, is much easier than identifying arteries that are narrowed or occluded by GCA. Patients should be informed about this possible difficulty. Before making an incision, the surgeon should be meticulous about locating and marking the vessel. A Doppler instrument should be available to help locate the artery if it is not readily identified by palpation. Owing to the scaphoid shape of surgical incisions, the skin incision should be "generous," as the breadth of the opening will gradually become smaller as the surgeon deepens the incision.

27.5 Pathology

Myth: Pathologists use standardized criteria when assessing temporal artery biopsies for GCA.

Reality: Some pathologists have outlined their individual opinions concerning minimal diagnostic criteria for GCA. However, there has never been a consensus statement by vascular pathologists that addresses this issue formally. Significant variability characterizes the criteria employed by different pathologists. As an example, some pathologists consider any adventitial inflammation sufficient for the diagnosis of GCA, but others demur.

This dilemma of variability among the opinions of pathologists is illustrated by the skip lesion shown in Fig. 27.6. Most pathologists would consider the right side of the image

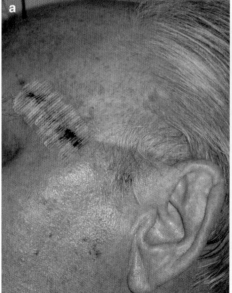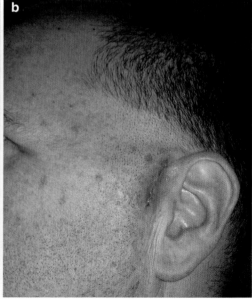

Fig. 27.5 Optimal and risky sites for temporal artery biopsies. The biopsy in (**a**) was taken from the anterior temporal artery and is generally the optimal site for biopsy. The biopsy in (**b**) was taken from the common temporal artery. Biopsy at this site runs the risk of facial nerve injury

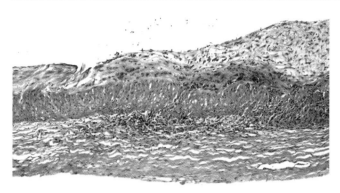

Fig. 27.6 Longitudinal section of a temporal artery biopsy with a skip lesion. On the *right* side of the sample, there is transmural inflammation composed of lymphocytes and macrophages, accompanied by intimal hyperplasia. Moving from *right* to *left*, there is progressively less inflammation. At the *far left* is a noninflamed segment of the artery. (Hematoxylin and eosin stained slide at 100× magnification)

to be diagnostic of GCA and the left side not. However, upon moving from right to left in the biopsy, the precise site at which criteria sufficient for a GCA diagnosis are met varies from pathologist to pathologist.

Clinicians must be conversant with the histopathological features of GCA themselves, conscious of the variability among pathologists, and willing to engage pathologists in a discussion about the final histopathologic diagnosis.

Myth: Transmural inflammation is required for a pathologic diagnosis of GCA.

Reality: GCA is a segmental disease that has "skip lesions." Figure 27.6 also demonstrates how GCA can cause a spectrum of severity within the same vessel: transmural inflammation is evident on the right side of the Figure. In contrast, the adventitia and internal elastic lamina are the sites of primary involvement in the center.

Some pathologists would classify the findings in the center portion of Fig. 27.6 as "atypical GCA" because of the restricted nature of the inflammatory infiltrates. In many such cases, the adventitial component is predominantly lymphocytic and the component located at the internal elastic lamina primarily contains macrophages.

Although transmural inflammation is not required for the diagnosis of active GCA, some degree of involvement of the arterial media or intima by macrophages and lymphocytes is typically present (Allsop and Gallagher 1981).

Myth: Giant cells are always present in lesions of active GCA.

Reality: Giant cells are neither required for a diagnosis of GCA, nor are they entirely specific for that condition. In fact, giant cells are present in approximately only one half of temporal artery biopsies that demonstrate active GCA (Lie 1990). Giant cells can also be detected in other conditions that involve temporal artery inflammation, such as WG and systemic amyloidosis.

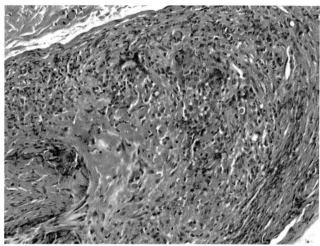

Fig. 27.7 Wegener's granulomatosis involving a temporal artery. There is extensive necrosis of the arterial wall with a mixed inflammatory infiltrate that contains lymphocytes, macrophages, and frequent neutrophils (Hematoxylin and eosin stained slide of a temporal artery biopsy at 200× magnification). This patient presented with recurrent amaurosis fugax but was found to be positive for antineutrophil cytoplasmic antibodies directed against proteinase-3 (i.e., PR3-ANCA). She also had pulmonary nodules that revealed granulomatous inflammation on biopsy

Pearl: In the temporal artery, the presence of extensive necrosis suggests involvement by a vasculitis distinct from GCA.

Comment: In the aorta, GCA can display large areas of necrosis. However, when GCA is present in the temporal arteries, the amount of necrosis is typically limited. Extensive necrosis in a temporal artery biopsy, particularly fibrinoid necrosis, suggests the presence of a different vasculitis such as WG, the CSS, microscopic polyangiitis, polyarteritis nodosa, or mixed cryoglobulinemia (Fig. 27.7).

Pearl: Amyloid deposition in the temporal artery can stimulate reactive inflammatory infiltrates that mimic GCA.

Comment: Amyloid deposits, particularly those caused by AL amyloidosis, can stimulate reactive inflammatory responses in multiple tissues, including the temporal artery (Fig. 27.8). The amyloid may not be appreciated without Congo red staining, and in such cases the inflammation could be misdiagnosed as GCA (Churchill et al. 2003).

Amyloidosis can also cause jaw claudication. One case series reported 22 patients with primary systemic amyloidosis who complained of typical jaw claudication. Some of these patients also had claudication of the upper and lower extremities. Appropriate staining of temporal artery biopsies often revealed amyloid deposits in the temporal arteries in patients who were clinically misdiagnosed as having GCA (Gertz et al. 1986).

Myth: A temporal artery biopsy revealing lymphocytic inflammation is diagnostic of GCA.

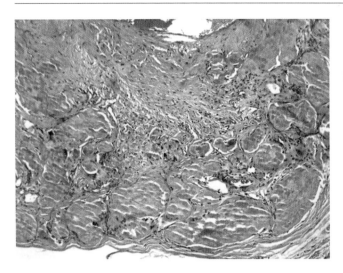

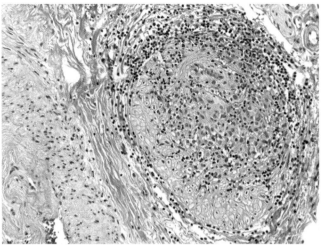

Fig. 27.8 Systemic amyloidosis involving a temporal artery. The patient was a 76 year-old woman who presented with jaw claudication and scalp tenderness. The biopsy shows numerous large, nodular deposits of amyloid within the wall of the vessel with a secondary reactive inflammatory infiltrate. Subsequent evaluation, including bone marrow biopsy, revealed the presence of multiple myeloma. (Hematoxylin and eosin stained section of a temporal artery biopsy at 200× magnification)

Fig. 27.9 Giant cell arteritis found incidentally in a hysterectomy specimen. The patient was a 76 year-old woman who underwent the procedure because of uterine prolapse. She had no history, symptoms, or signs to suggest vasculitis. (Hematoxylin and eosin stained section at 200× magnification)

Reality: The classic picture of granulomatous inflammation is detected in only approximately 50% of temporal artery biopsy specimens from symptomatic GCA patients. Most of the other 50% of cases demonstrate a panarteritis, with an infiltrate comprised primarily of lymphocytes, monocytes, and occasional other cells, e.g., neutrophils and eosinophils, but no giant cells.

Increasing numbers of reports have documented such pathological findings in patients with PAN, WG, CSS, and sarcoidosis (Small and Brisson 1991; Morgan and Harris 1978; Genereau et al. 1999). Headache, musculoskeletal pains, and a temporal artery biopsy demonstrating vasculitis are highly suggestive but not diagnostic of GCA. In the setting of upper airway disease, asthma, polyneuropathy, hilar adenopathy, or a positive serum assay for ANCA, one must remain suspicious of other entities.

Pearl: In temporal artery biopsies, atherosclerosis is less common than GCA.

Comment: Atherosclerosis can be associated with adventitial lymphocytic infiltrates within the temporal arteries. However, caution should be exercised before attributing these findings to atherosclerosis. GCA is more likely to be the cause. The superficial temporal arteries are relatively resistant to atherosclerosis.

Arteriosclerotic changes such as intimal hyperplasia and fragmentation of the internal elastic lamina are quite common in temporal artery biopsy specimens. (Disruption of the internal elastic lamina is not synonymous with GCA!). However, true atherosclerosis with lipid deposition and adventitial

lymphocytic infiltrates is only present in 4–5% of biopsies (Allsop and Gallaghar 1981).

Myth: The pathologic lesions of active GCA are always associated with a clinically apparent systemic vasculitis.

Reality: Large autopsy studies indicate that the GCA is ten times more prevalent pathologically than clinically. Thus, in 90% of patients who have pathologic lesions of GCA, the disease remains subclinical.

Pathologic lesions of GCA are observed unexpectedly on occasion in surgical specimens, particularly specimens from the ascending aorta and the female genital tract (Fig. 27.9). In a series of 1,204 patients from the Cleveland Clinic who underwent aortic surgery, 4% were found to have aortitis that was unsuspected prior to surgery (Rojo-Leyva et al. 2000). Some of these patients have no signs or symptoms of a systemic vasculitis, and many do well without systemic immunosuppression once the "nidus" of vasculitis has been removed.

Pearl: Immunohistochemistry can assist in the pathologic diagnosis of GCA.

Comment: Although lymphocytes are usually readily apparent on routine hematoxylin and eosin stained slides, subtle macrophage infiltrates can be overlooked (Fig. 27.10). Immunohistochemical staining for the macrophage marker CD68 assists in the diagnosis of GCA when these infiltrates are subtle (Gooi et al. 2008; Font and Prabhakaran 2007).

Myth: "Healed arteritis" – the presence of scarring in a temporal artery biopsy – is diagnostic of previously active GCA.

Reality: Scarring is a nonspecific response to injury. Scarring in a temporal artery can represent healed vasculitis, healed

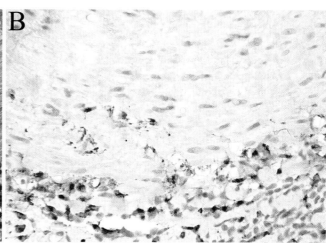

Fig. 27.10 Immunohistochemistry as an aid in evaluating temporal artery biopsies. In this temporal artery biopsy specimen, a lymphocytic infiltrate is clearly present in the adventitia of the hematoxylin and eosin stained slide (**a**). An immunohistochemistry stain for the mac- rophage marker CD68 reveals that numerous macrophages are also present in the adventitia, and that this macrophage infiltrate extends into the media (**b**). (Magnification for both images is 400×)

trauma, or the effects of some other injury. The superficial temporal arteries are particularly prone to traumatic injury because of their proximity to the skin, and scarring from traumatic injury cannot be distinguished from scarring from healed vasculitis. Moreover, even assuming that a systemic vasculitis caused the "healed arteritis," there is no pathologic means of pinning the precise diagnosis on GCA as opposed to some other form of systemic vasculitis.

"Healed arteritis" in a temporal artery is not synonymous with GCA. The term creates confusion for both pathologists and clinicians alike, and should be discarded.

Pearl: Frozen section analysis of a temporal artery biopsy can hinder or prevent a pathologic diagnosis of GCA.

Comment: The preferred method of examining temporal artery biopsies is through the assessment of cross sections of formalin-fixed, paraffin-embedded samples. The procedure of snap-freezing arteries significantly distorts the histology. In addition, significant amounts of tissue are lost during the processes of obtaining the frozen section, thawing and reprocessing it, and cutting new sections from the paraffin-embedded material. Both of these factors hinder the ability of the pathologist to diagnose GCA, albeit the diagnosis is still possible in many cases.

Diagnosing GCA is difficult enough without suboptimal processing of the sample. Communicate with the surgeon before the procedure and instruct him or her not to perform a frozen section unless the identity of the tissue at the time of the operation is in question.

Pearl: GCA can sometimes be identified in small branches of the temporal artery.

Comment: Diagnostic information can be present in the small branches of the temporal artery. As examples, sarcoidosis and WG have been diagnosed from histopathological findings within small blood vessels or connective tissue that is adherent to a normal temporal artery. In addition, GCA itself is sometimes present in branches smaller than the temporal artery (Esteban et al. 2001). The surgeon should not strive to remove tissue that is attached to the vessel.

The specimen should be placed in fixative and then sectioned and stained expeditiously. The technician should not strip or clean the specimen prior to embedding, lest one be deprived of potentially useful information from examination of the adherent tissues. Owing to the possibility of skip areas, sub-serial sectioning should be requested.

27.6 Treatment

Pearl: Alternate-day glucocorticoid tapers are ineffective in GCA.

Comment: For most patients, the worst part of GCA is the prednisone (Hellmann et al. 2003). But clinicians should resist the temptation to try alternate-day glucocorticoid therapy in GCA; it is less effective than daily prednisone. A randomized, controlled trial demonstrated this convincingly in the 1970s (Hunder et al. 1975). Moreover, there is little evidence that alternate-day glucocorticoids tapers lead to less toxicity. In the long run, patients and clinicians are better off controlling the disease with the lowest possible daily dose of prednisone.

Pearl: High doses of glucocorticoids can cause patients to hear voices.

Comment: Glucocorticoids can cause auditory hallucinations (Stone, 2006). Don't let the Psychiatry Liaison Consult Service be the ones to make the diagnosis of a glucocorticoids-induced psychosis.

Pearl: High doses of glucocorticoids can trigger major depressions.

Comment: Clinicians who are experienced in the use of glucocorticoids do not use this treatment cavalierly. High doses of prednisone can trigger life-threatening depression, particularly in individuals with histories of a depressed mood. Doses may need to be decreased more quickly than most clinicians are comfortable with in this setting.

Myth: PMR always improve within 24–48 h of the administration of prednisone.

Reality: Classic "PMR responses" to prednisone do occur and are enormously gratifying to the clinician. However, they do not always occur. In some patients with PMR, real clinical responses can require up to a week. Because the clinical response to prednisone can be less than dramatic over the first few days in patients who really have PMR, clinicians must do everything possible to design a clean clinical experiment:

- Start with 15 mg/day of prednisone. Ten mg/day may be too little to treat PMR, and more than 20 mg/day might be too much (i.e., it might treat other diseases entities effectively, too).
- Do not change more than one variable at once. Do not add an nonsteroidal antiinflammatory drug at the same time, do not give additional medications designed to relieve pain, and do not add an antidepressant or sleep medication, too. Let the prednisone act alone.
- See the patient again in 1 week. A longer period allows too many potential confounders to complicate the response to treatment.

Within 1 week of starting prednisone, a patient with PMR should feel like a new person. If not, you have got the wrong diagnosis.

Pearl: Aspirin is an important adjunct to glucocorticoids in the therapy of GCA.

Comment: The results of clinical trials designed to identify an effective steroid-sparing agent in GCA have been disappointing. However, two retrospective cohort studies demonstrated that a baby aspirin along with prednisone is more effective at preventing visual loss and cerebral ischemic events than is prednisone alone (Nesher et al. 2004; Lee et al. 2006). The consistency of these two studies and the strong reduction in the odds ratio for clinical events by aspirin make this

medication an important adjunct to glucocorticoids. A daily baby aspirin should be part of the standard therapy for GCA (Stone, 2007).

When GCA is suspected strongly, the patient can begin a baby aspirin even before the temporal artery biopsy is done. (The performance of a temporal artery biopsy in a patient on aspirin is safe.)

Myth: Judicious tapering of glucocorticoids can prevent disease flares in GCA.

Reality: Rapid tapering of glucocorticoids is associated with an increased risk of disease flares in both GCA and PMR (Pipitone et al. 2005). However, the converse is not necessarily true. In a sizeable number of patients, disease flares appear to have little relationship to the speed of the glucocorticoid tapering regimen. The issue for these patients relates more to a threshold dose of prednisone below which they cannot taper, no matter how slowly the prednisone is decreased. If a patient suffers repeated flares on 3 mg of prednisone a day, then she should remain on 4 mg of prednisone a day.

Myth: GCA always goes into remission if sufficient doses of glucocorticoids are given.

Reality: Patients with GCA usually demonstrate swift clinical responses following the institution of glucocorticoids, and the majority achieves disease remissions while on this treatment. However, in a small number of patients, GCA is not suppressed clinically despite large doses of glucocorticoids administered over prolonged periods (Caselli et al. 1988). In such cases, histopathological analysis of clinical samples (e.g., limb amputation specimens) shows chronic arteritis. The best treatment options for such patients are not clear. Fortunately, such patients are very rare, and nearly all patients respond clinically to glucocorticoids.

Myth: All patients with GCA can be weaned off glucocorticoids within 2 years of the start of treatment.

Reality: Many patients with GCA are able to discontinue glucocorticoid treatment within 6 months to 2 years. For instance, in a population-based study from Olmsted County, Minnesota, the median duration of glucocorticoid treatment was 7 months (Huston et al. 1978).

Unfortunately, ample other published experience confirms that this is by no means always the rule. In a study from Scandinavia of ninety patients with GCA, PMR, or both, 25% of those followed for 9 years were still on prednisone at an average dose of 5 mg/day (Andersson et al. 1986). Another study on ninety patients with biopsy-verified GCA reported that one third of the patients required low-dose glucocorticoid treatment indefinitely (Graham et al. 1981).

Pearl: Revascularization is rarely needed in large-vessel vasculitis, even if the artery appears to be narrowed beyond the point that blood can pass.

Fig. 27.11 Abundant collateral circulation in GCA. Exuberant collateral blood vessels that have formed to compensate for a severe stenosis at the junction of the subclavian and axillary arteries. An attempt at stent placement for a tight subclavian lesion failed (the stent clotted before the patient even left the radiology suite). The abundant collateral vessels make the point that the stent placement was probably ill-advised, anyway

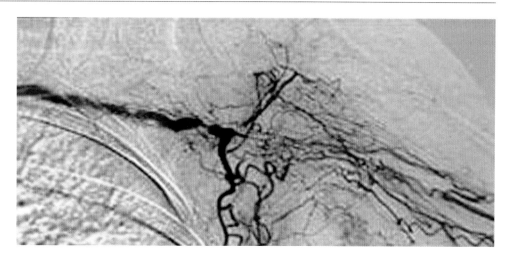

Comment: One of the striking angiographic features of GCA (and Takayasu's arteritis) is the exuberant neovascularization and collateral circulation that develops in patients with narrowing of the subclavian arteries and other large vessels (Fig. 27.11). Many patients with large-vessel GCA lose palpable pulses in one or both upper extremities. Despite this potentially frightening finding, such patients inevitably have sufficient blood flow to the extremity to maintain its viability. Many such patients, in fact, are asymptomatic.

Attempts at revascularization in patients with large-vessel GCA and stenotic lesions of primary branches of the aorta are frequently misguided. The collateral circulation that develops is not pulsatile – patients remain "pulseless" – but still have sufficient blood flow with stents, angioplasty, or bypass. In this sense, the purpose of prednisone is to suppress inflammation sufficiently that neovascularization can occur.

27.7 Outcomes

Myth: Prompt treatment with glucocorticoids prevents new visual loss in GCA.

Reality: Would that this were true! Although prompt treatment *usually* prevents further loss of vision and protects the fellow eye, there are numerous published examples in which there was not only further loss of vision in the eye originally affected, but also involvement of the second eye, normal at baseline.

The prevalence of vision loss in one randomized clinical trial of 98 patients with GCA was 18% at study entry (Hoffman et al. 2002). The incidence of new vision loss at 1 year was 14%, despite the fact that patients received high-dose daily prednisone for 3 months before transitioning to an alternate-day tapering regimen. There is wisdom in informing patients that although they are being properly treated, the threat of visual loss (or further visual loss) remains and may be higher than generally regarded by clinicians.

Myth: The prompt use of pulse glucocorticoids may restore vision lost in GCA.

Reality: This, unfortunately, is wishful thinking. Stuttering losses of vision may occur in which sight is gone for a second to minutes, but dense vision loss that has persisted for hours in GCA is usually permanent.

A carefully performed study that examined visual outcomes in GCA patients who had lost vision concluded that essentially all improvement in patients' ability to read eye charts was related to their accommodation of new visual difficulty rather than to qualitative improvement in ocular function (Hayreh et al. 2002).

In a patient who presents with the vision gone in one eye, a reasonable approach is to initiate treatment with methylprednisolone 1 g/day times three (plus a baby aspirin, if the patient is not already on it). The reason? There is no guarantee that even this will preserve vision in the other eye. If therapy fails, no clinician wants to be left wondering, "What if…?"

Myth: Reversible loss of vision is rare in GCA.

Reality: It is often stated that visual loss in GCA is permanent (see above). However, transient, fully reversible, visual obscurations and temporary monocular blindness occur frequently in GCA. These episodes may last up to hours, yet still be reversible.

Funduscopic examination in this setting may demonstrate a completely normal optic nerve and fundus, mild disc edema, hemorrhagic disc edema, branch retinal artery infarction, and/or cotton wool spots. The full reversibility of the visual disturbances underscores the intermittent disruptions in the blood supply of affected vasculitic territories.

Unfortunately, once visual loss has persisted for more than several hours, no recovery can be expected. The visual deficit will be permanent, indeed.

Pearl: Transient visual obscurations triggered by a Valsalva maneuver or change in body position indicate a GCA patient at risk for visual loss.

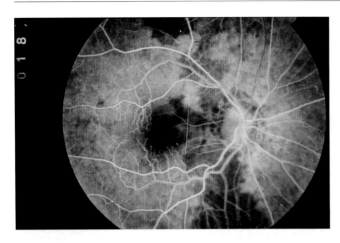

Fig. 27.12 Fluorescein Angiogram of the right eye in a patient with arteritic ischemic optic neuropathy. Note the areas of fluorescein hypoperfusion of the deep choroid along the superior and inferior retinal arterioles

Comment: A swollen optic nerve may experience transient disturbances of blood flow associated with Valsalva maneuvers (e.g., coughing). This can lead to a fully reversible loss of vision that is fleeting or persistent for up to several minutes. It is critical to recognize that transient visual loss with or without systemic symptoms might be a clue to the presence of GCA.

Pearl: Very dense loss of vision tends to occur more frequently in arteritic AION than in nonarteritic AION (NAAION).

Comment: Once in place, the vision loss that results from GCA tends to be dense and more often than not is associated with complete monocular blindness in the affected eye. Small, sectoral visual field defects or well-preserved visual acuity are more typical of NAAION, which is typically caused by an embolic lesion from an atheromatous source in the aorta or its primary branches.

Fluorescein angiography can be helpful in discriminating GCA from nonarteritic AION (Fig. 27.12). Large areas of nonperfusion in the posterior pole, choroidal nonperfusion, and circumferential optic nerve nonperfusion (as opposed to segmental nonperfusion) favor GCA.

Pearl: Patients with GCA and PMR have a longer disease course compared with those with GCA or PMR alone.

Comment: No reliable predictors of glucocorticoid treatment duration exist. Treatment regimens must be tailored to each individual patient and adjusted as needed on the basis of clinical course. Most attempts to discontinue prednisone altogether in less than 1 year, unfortunately, are met with treatment failure and disease flares at the lower doses.

The mean duration of therapy for patients with GCA is approximately 2 years, taking into consideration repeat courses of treatment necessitated by disease flares. There is some suggestion that patients with both GCA and PMR

require longer treatment courses compared with those with isolated GCA or PMR (Lundberg and Hedfors 1990; Kyle and Hazleman 1993).

One common error in treating GCA is the use of high doses of glucocorticoids for too long at the start of therapy. The general approach should be high doses of prednisone (e.g., 60 mg/day) for 1 month, followed by tapering to moderate daily doses by the end of month two (e.g., 20 mg/day). After that, the prednisone taper should be designed with a long "tail," such that patients are decreasing by 1 mg/month as the taper finishes (5 mg/day for 1 month, then 4 mg/day for 1 month, then 3 mg/day, etcetera).

Pearl: GCA is not associated with an increased mortality.

Comment: GCA is fraught with significant disease- and treatment-related morbidity. However, studies reveal no differences between GCA patients and age- and gender-matched controls in terms of mortality (Pipitone et al. 2006). The only disease subset known to have an increased risk of mortality is the group of patients with thoracic aorta aneurysms (Nuenninghoff et al. 2003). This complication carries a substantial risk of death from aortic dissection.

Myth: Orbital ischemia and proptosis are not seen in GCA.

Reality: Orbital ischemia may result in GCA from vasculitic involvement of the proximal ophthalmic artery branches that spares the posterior ciliary arteries. This pattern of vascular involvement can cause orbital pain, proptosis, ptosis, and diplopia, with or without vision loss.

Pearl: Distinguishing PMR from RA is often impossible at the patient's initial presentation.

Comment: Patients with PMR can have synovitis in peripheral joints. Sometimes only a period of observation determines whether PMR is the correct diagnosis or if the true cause of the patient's symptoms is RA. The availability of serologic tests for antibodies to anti-cyclic citrullinated peptides (anti-CCP antibodies) has facilitated this distinction in some cases, but some patients with RA are negative for both rheumatoid factor and anti-CCP antibodies at presentation.

In general, patients with RA improve on smaller doses of glucocorticoids than do patients with PMR, but they are less likely to enter complete remissions with prednisone alone.

Pearl: If a patient with PMR consistently requires more than 20 mg of prednisone a day to control the disease symptoms, the diagnosis is wrong.

Comment: A dose of 15 mg/day of prednisone is sufficient to control most cases of PMR. Failure of 20 mg of prednisone administered in divided doses to control the patient's symptoms should certainly make one rethink the diagnosis and consider such entities as GCA (which may require higher initial glucocorticoids doses), cancer (renal cell carcinoma, sarcoma, multiple myeloma and other hematopoietic malignancies), amyloidosis, fibromyalgia, and bursitis.

Pearl: Methotrexate is effective as steroid-sparing agent in GCA.

Comment: Truly, no one knows for certain whether this is a Pearl or a Myth. Three randomized controlled trials have assessed the efficacy of methotrexate (MTX) in recent-onset GCA, producing discordant results (Jover et al. 2001; Hoffman et al. 2002; Spiera et al. 2001). The results from these trials were pooled and analyzed (Mahr et al. 2007). According to this meta-analysis, MTX used as adjunctive treatment in GCA at a mean dosage of 11.1 mg per week led to a reduction of both first and second relapses of GCA, with hazard ratios of 0.65 and 0.49, respectively. However, despite a significant between-group difference in the cumulative GC dose by 842 mg at week 48, MTX use did not lead to a decreased incidence of glucocorticoid-related complications. In addition, the onset of action of MTX appeared to be slow.

At this point, one conclusion appears safe: If MTX has a beneficial effect in GCA, it is a small one relative to that of glucocorticoids. It is conceivable that a dose of MTX higher than that used in any of the three clinical trials to date might lead to greater efficacy than that demonstrated to date. The maximum dose used in any trial to date has been only 15 mg/week.

References

Achkar A, Lie J, Hunder G, et al How does previous corticosteroid treatment affect the biopsy findings in giant cell (temporal) arteritis? Ann Intern Med 1994;120:987–92

Allsop CJ, Gallagher PJ. Temporal artery biopsy in giant-cell arteritis: a reappraisal. Am J Surg Pathol 1981;5:317–23

Amor-Dorado JC, Llorca J, Garcia-Porrua C, et al Audiovestibular manifestations in giant cell arteritis: a prospective study. Medicine (Baltimore) 2003;82(1):13–26

Andersson R, Malmvall BE, Bengtsson BA. Long-term corticosteroid treatment in giant cell arteritis. Acta Med Scand 1986;220(5):465–9

Bley TA, Brink I, Reinhard M. [Imaging procedures for giant cell arteritis (Horton's disease)]. Ophthalmologe 2006;103(4):308–16

Bley TA, Weiben O, Uhl M, et al Assessment of the cranial involvement pattern of giant cell arteritis with 3 T magnetic resonance imaging. Arthritis Rheum 2005a;52(8):2470–7

Bley TA, Wieben O, Uhl M, et al High-resolution MRI in giant cell arteritis: imaging of the wall of the superficial temporal artery. AJR Am J Roentgenol 2005b;184(1):283–7

Blockmans D. The use of (^{18}F)fluoro-deoxyglucose positron emission tomography in the assessment of large vessel vasculitis. Clin Exp Rheumatol 2003;21(6 Suppl 32):S15–22

Blockmans D. PET in large-vessel vasculitis and polymyalgia rheumatica. In: Fourth International Conference on Giant Cell Arteritis and Polymyalgia Rheumatica, New York; 2008

Blockmans D, De Ceuninck L, Vanderschueren S, et al Repetitive 18F-fluorodeoxyglucose positron emission tomography in giant cell arteritis: a prospective study of 35 patients. Arthritis Rheum 2006;55(1):131–7

Bongartz T, Matteson EL. Large-vessel involvement in giant cell arteritis. Curr Opin Rheumatol 2006;18(1):10–7

Boyev LR, Miller NR, Green WR. Efficacy of unilateral versus bilateral temporal artery biopsies for the diagnosis of giant cell arteritis. Am J Ophthalmol 1999;128:211–5

Brack A, Martinez-Taboada V, Stanson A, Goronzy JJ, Weyand CM. Disease pattern in cranial and large-vessel giant cell arteritis. Arthritis Rheum 1999;42(2):311–7

Brass SD, Durand ML, Stone JH, et al A 59 year-old man with chronic daily headaches. N Engl J Med 2008; 359(21):2267–78.

Caselli RJ, Daube JR, Hunder GG, et al Peripheral neuropathic syndromes in giant cell (temporal) arteritis. Neurology 1988;38: 685–9

Caselli RJ, Hunder GG, Whisnant JP. Neurologic disease in biopsy-proven giant cell (temporal) arteritis. Neurology 1988; 38:352–9.

Churchill CH, Abril A, Krishna M, et al Jaw claudication in primary amyloidosis: unusual presentation of a rare disease. J Rheumatol 2003;30:2283–6

Cohen MD, Ginsburg WW, Allen GL. Facial swelling in giant cell arteritis. J Rheumatol 1982;9:325–7

Duhaut P, Berruyer M, Pinede L, et al Anticardiolipin antibodies and giant cell arteritis: a prospective, multicenter case-control study. Groupe de Recherche sur l'Arterite a Cellules Geantes. Arthritis Rheum 1998;41(4):701–9

Esposito AL, Gleckman RA. Fever of unknown origin in the elderly. J Am Geriatr Soc 1978;26:498–505

Esteban MJ, Font C, Hernandex-Rodriguez J, et al Small-vessel vasculitis surrounding a spared temporal artery: clinical and pathological findings in a series of twenty-eight patients. Arthritis Rheum 2001;44:1387–95

Evans J, O'Fallon W, Hunder G. Increased incidence of aortic aneurysm and dissection in giant cell (temporal) arteritis. Ann Int Med 1995;122:502–7

Font RL, Prabhakaran VC. Histological parameters helpful in recognizing steroid-treated temporal arteritis: an analysis of 35 cases. Br J Ophthalmol 2007;91:204–9

Friedman G, Friedman B. The sensation of facial swelling in temporal arteritis: a predictor for the development of visual disturbance. Postgrad Med J 1986;62(733):1019–20

Genereau T, Lortholary O, Pottier M, et al Temporal artery biopsy. A diagnostic tool for systemic necrotizing vasculitis. Arthritis Rheum 1999;42:2674–81

Gertz MA, Kyle RA, Griffing WL, et al Jaw claudication in primary systemic amyloidosis. Medicine 1986;65:173–9

Gooi P, Brownstein S, Rawlings N. Temporal arteritis: a dilemma in clinical and pathological diagnosis. Can J Ophthalmol 2008;43: 119–20

Gordon L, Levin L. Visual loss in giant cell arteritis. JAMA 1998; 280: 385–6

Graham E, Holland A, Avery A, Russell RW. Prognosis in giant-cell arteritis. Br Med J (Clin Res Ed) 1981;282(6260):269–71

Hall S, Lie J, Kurland L, et al The therapeutic impact of temporal artery biopsy. Lancet 1983;2:1217–20

Hausch RC, Harrington T. Temporal arteritis and sensorineural hearing loss. Semin Arthritis Rheum 1998;28(3):206–9

Hayreh SS, Podhajsky PA, Zimmerman B. Occult giant cell arteritis: ocular manifestations. Am J Ophthalmol 1998a;125(4):521–6

Hayreh SS, Podhajsky PA, Zimmerman B. Ocular manifestations of giant cell arteritis. Am J Ophthalmol 1998b;125(4):509–20

Hayreh SS, Zimmerman B, Kardon RH. Visual improvement with corticosteroid therapy in giant cell arteritis. Report of a large study and review of literature. Acta Ophthalmol Scand 2002;80:355–67

Hellmann DB, Uhlfelder ML, Stone JH, et al Domains of quality of life important to patients with giant cell arteritis. Arthritis Rheum 2003;49(6):819–25

Hoffman GS, Cid MC, Hellmann DB, et al A multicenter, randomized, double-blind, placebo-controlled trial of adjuvant methotrexate treatment for giant cell arteritis. Arthritis Rheum 2002;46(5):1309–18

Horton BT, Magath TB, Brown GE. Undescribed forms of arteritis of temporal vessels. Proc Staff Meet Mayo Clin 1932;7:700–1

Horton BT, Magath TB, Brown GE. Arteritis of temporal vessels: report of 7 cases. Proc Staff Meet Mayo Clin 1937;12:548–53

Hunder GG, Sheps SG, Allen GL, Joyce JW. Daily and alternate-day corticosteroid regimens in treatment of giant cell arteritis: comparison in a prospective study. Ann Intern Med 1975;82:613–8

Huston KA, Hunder GG, Lie JT, et al Temporal arteritis: a 25-year epidemiologic, clinical, and pathologic study. Ann Intern Med 1978; 88(2):162–7

Jover JA, Hernandez-Garcia C, Morado IC, et al Combined treatment of giant-cell arteritis with methotrexate and prednisone. a randomized, double-blind, placebo-controlled trial. Ann Intern Med 2001;134 (2):106–14

Karahaliou M, et al Colour duplex sonography of temporal arteries before decision for biopsy: a prospective study in 55 patients with suspected giant cell arteritis. Arthritis Res Ther 2006;8:R116

Kyle V, Hazleman B. Treatment of polymyalgia rheumatica and giant cell arteritis. II. Relation between corticosteroid dose and corticosteroid-associated diseases. Ann Rheum Dis 1989;48:662–6

Kyle V, Hazleman BL. The clinical and laboratory course of polymyalgia rheumatica/giant cell arteritis after the first two months of treatment. Ann Rheum Dis 1993;52(12):847–50

Kyle V, Wraight EP, Hazleman BL. Liver scan abnormalities in polymyalgia rheumatica/giant cell arteritis. Clin Rheumatol 1991;10(3):294–7

Larson T, Hall S, Hepper N, et al Respiratory tract symptoms as a clue to giant cell arteritis. Ann Intern Med 1984;101:594–7

Lee CC, Su WW, Hunder GG. Dysarthria associated with giant cell arteritis. J Rheumatol 1999;26:931–2

Lee MS, Smith SD, Gabor A. Antiplatelet and anticoagulant therapy in patients with giant cell arteritis. Arthritis Rheum 2006;54:3306–9

Lessell S. Nonarteritic anterior ischemic optic neuropathy: enigma variations. Arch Ophthalmol 1999;117:386–8

Lie JT. Illustrated histopathologic classification criteria for selected vasculitis syndromes. Arthritis Rheum 1990;33:1074–87

Liozon E, Roblot P, Paire D, et al Anticardiolipin antibody levels predict flares and relapses in patients with giant-cell (temporal) arteritis. A longitudinal study of 58 biopsy-proven cases. Rheumatology (Oxford) 2000;39(10):1089–94

Lundberg I, Hedfors E. Restricted dose and duration of corticosteroid treatment in patients with polymyalgia rheumatica and temporal arteritis. J Rheumatol 1990;17(10):1340–5

Mahr AD, Jover JA, Spiera RF, et al Adjunctive methotrexate to treat giant cell arteritis: an individual patient data meta-analysis. Arthritis Rheum 2007;56(8):2789–97

Manna R, Latteri M, Cristiano G, et al Anticardiolipin antibodies in giant cell arteritis and polymyalgia rheumatica: a study of 40 cases. Br J Rheumatol 1998;37(2):208–10

Meller J, Strutz F, Siefker U, et al Early diagnosis and follow-up of aortitis with [(18)F]FDG PET and MRI. Eur J Nucl Med Mol Imaging 2003;30(5):730–6

Meyer O, Nicaise P, Moreau S, et al Antibodies to cardiolipin and beta 2 glycoprotein I in patients with polymyalgia rheumatica and giant cell arteritis. Rev Rhum Engl Ed 1996;63(4):241–7

Morgan G, Harris E. Non-giant cell temporal arteritis. Arthritis Rheum 1978;21:362–6

Nesher G, Berkun Y, Mates M. Low-dose aspirin and prevention of cranial ischemic complications in giant cell arteritis. Arthritis Rheum 2004;50:1332–7

Nuenninghoff DM, Hunder GG, Christianson TJ, et al Mortality of large-artery complication (aortic aneurysm, aortic dissection, and/or large-artery stenosis) in patients with giant cell arteritis: a population-based study over 50 years. Arthritis Rheum 2003;48(12):3532–7

Olopade, CO, Sekosan, M, Schraufnagel, DE. Giant cell arteritis manifesting as chronic cough and fever of unknown origin. Mayo Clin Proc 1997;72:1048

Papadimitraki ED, Kyrmizakis DE, Kritikos I, Boumpas DT. Ear-nose-throat manifestations of autoimmune rheumatic diseases. Clin Exp Rheumatol 2004;22(4):485–94

Paraskevas KI, Boumpas DT, Vrentzos GE, Mikhailidis DP. Oral and ocular/orbital manifestations of temporal arteritis: a disease with deceptive clinical symptoms and devastating consequences. Clin Rheumatol 2007;26(7):1044–8

Pipitone N, Boiardi L, Bajocchi G, Salvarani C. Long-term outcome of giant cell arteritis. Clin Exp Rheumatol 2006;24(2 Suppl 41): S65–70

Pipitone N, Boiardi L, Salvarani C. Are steroids alone sufficient for the treatment of giant cell arteritis? Best Pract Res Clin Rheumatol 2005;19(2):277–92

Pipitone N, Versari A, Salvarani C. Role of imaging studies in the diagnosis and follow-up of large-vessel vasculitis: an update. Rheumatology (Oxford) 2008;47(4):403–8

Pless M, Rizzo JF III, Lamkin JC, Lessell S. Concordance of bilateral temporal artery biopsy in giant cell arteritis. J Neuroophthalmol 2000;20:216–8

Porter MJ. Temporal arteritis presenting as a submandibular swelling. J Laryngol Otol 1990;104(10):819–20

Razavi M, Jones, RD, Manzel, et al Steroid-responsive Charles Bonnet syndrome in temporal arteritis. J Neuropsychiatry Clin Neurosci 2004;16:505

Regan MJ, Green WR, Stone JH. Ethnic disparity in the incidence of temporal arteritis: a 32-year expereince at an urban medical center. Arthritis Rheum 2000;43:S128

Rojo-Leyva F, Ratliff N, Cosgrove D, et al Study of 52 patients with idiopathic aortitis from a cohort of 1204 surgical cases. Arthritis Rheum 2000;43:901–7

Rucker JC, Biousse V, Newman NJ. Ischemic optic neuropathies. Curr Opin Neurol 2004;17(1):27–35

Ruiz-Masera JJ, Alamillos-Granados FJ, Dean-Ferrer A, et al Submandibular swelling as the first manifestation of giant cell arteritis. Report of a case. J Craniomaxillofac Surg 1995;23(2):119–21

Salvarani C, Cantini F, Boiardi L, Hunder GG. Polymyalgia rheumatica and giant-cell arteritis. N Engl J Med 2002a;347(4):261–71

Salvarani C, Giannini C, Miller DV, et al Giant cell arteritis: involvement of intracranial arteries. Arthritis Rheum 2006;55:985–9

Salvarani C, Hunder GG. Giant cell arteritis with a low erythrocyte sedimentation rate: Frequency of occurence in a population-based study. Arthritis Rheum 2001;45:140–5

Salvarani C, Silingardi M, Ghirarduzzi A, et al Is duplex ultrasonography useful for the diagnosis of giant-cell arteritis? Ann Intern Med 2002b;137:232

Schmidt WA, Kraft HE, Vorpahl K, Volker L, Gromnica-Ihle EJ. Color duplex ultrasonography in the diagnosis of temporal arteritis. N Engl J Med 1997;337(19):1336–42

Seo P, Stone JH. Large-vessel vasculitis. Arthritis Care Res 2002;51: 128–39

Small P, Brisson M-L. Wegener's granulomatosis presenting as temporal arteritis. Arthritis Rheum 1991;34:220–3

Smetana GW, Shmerling RH. Does this patient have temporal arteritis? JAMA 2002;287:92–101

Spiera RF, Mitnick HJ, Kupersmith M, et al A prospective, double-blind, randomized, placebo controlled trial of methotrexate in the treatment of giant cell arteritis (GCA). Clin Exp Rheumatol 2001; 19(5):495–501

Stone JH. Hearing voices. Pharos 2006;69:31–2

Stone JH. Antiplatelet versus anticoagulant therapy in patients with giant cell arteritis: which is best? Nat Clin Pract Rheumatol 2007;3: 136–7

Stone JH, Francis HW. Immune-mediated inner ear disease. Curr Opin Rheumatol 2000;12(1):32–40

Tso E, Flamm SD, White RD, et al Takayasu arteritis: utility and limitations of magnetic resonance imaging in diagnosis and treatment. Arthritis Rheum 2002;46(6):1634–42

Wilkinson IM, Russell RW. Arteries of the head and neck in giant cell arteritis: a pathological study to show the pattern of arterial involvement. Arch Neurol 1972;27:378

Takayasu's Arteritis

28

Eamonn S. Molloy, John H. Stone, Carol A. Langford

Overview of Takayasu's Arteritis

> The aorta and its major branches are the prime disease targets in Takayasu's arteritis (TA).

> Clinical symptoms of vascular inflammation and vascular insufficiency are usually accompanied or preceded by a systemic inflammatory process.

> TA disease tends to affect women much more often than men (female:male ratio 9:1), and has a predilection for Asian women. However, the disease has been described in individuals of all racial and ethnic backgrounds.

> TA is associated with granulomatous inflammation within the blood vessel wall. The histopathologic features of the disease closely resemble those of giant cell arteritis.

> TA leads to vascular narrowing in most of the blood vessels it affects. However, in the aorta, the disease can cause aneurysms. These often lead to aortic regurgitation of the ascending aorta.

> A lesion of great concern in TA is renal artery stenosis, which can lead to a rennin-mediated hypertension. If the patient has narrowings in all of the blood vessels to the four extremities, then peripheral blood pressure measurements may not be accurate assessments of the true central aortic pressures. Catheterization may be required to determine the patient's blood pressure accurately.

> Eye lesions in TA are of two major types: hypertensive retinopathy (particularly in the setting of renal artery stenosis) and proliferative retinopathy (caused by extreme narrowing of the blood vessels supplying the head, which leads to neovascularization of the retinal vascular supply). Anterior ischemic optic neuropathy, the most common ocular lesion of giant cell arteritis, occurs very rarely in TA.

Pearl: Both upper back pain or neck pain and tenderness in a young woman both suggest TA.

Comment: Just as tearing of the aorta in aortic dissection can result in thoracic back pain, inflammation within the aortic wall can lead to similar, though generally less severe, symptoms. In some TA patients, thoracic back pain is the chief complaint. Pain and tenderness may also be noted over peripheral arteries, especially the carotid artery (carotidynia). Most patients also have other, more common manifestations of the disease (such as fever of unknown origin, loss of a pulse, new onset hypertension, aortic regurgitation, or claudication in an arm or leg). Still, unfamiliarity with thoracic back pain or carotidynia as a manifestation of TA can lead to delays in the diagnosis.

Pearl: Digital gangrene is not an expected feature of TA.

Comment: Pulseless limbs are common in TA, hence the name "pulseless disease," which was bestowed by Japanese clinicians. The pulselessness of TA classically develops in a "reverse coarctation" form: the upper extremity pulses are absent, while the lower extremity pulses are present (and even bounding, if the disease has led to aortic regurgitation). Coarctation, in contrast, because it usually involves the descending aorta, is associated with diminished pulses in the feet. The contrast between these two diseases is not always so stark, though: TA also frequently involves the large vessels to the lower extremities, leading to absent pedal pulses, as well (Fig. 28.1).

In any event, despite the frequent occurrence of proximal limb arterial occlusion in TA, distal gangrene is extremely uncommon. The development of this complication should prompt an evaluation for contributing cofactors, e.g., thromboembolism and hypercoagulable states. The relative immunity from distal gangrene in TA relates to the fact that vascular occlusions in this disorder develop insidiously, thereby allowing the development of dramatic collateral circulation. The spiderweb of collateral vessels in Takayasu's is generally not associated with a palpable pulse, yet provides sufficient blood flow to the extremities.

J. H. Stone (ed.), *A Clinician's Pearls and Myths in Rheumatology,*
DOI:10.1007/978-1-84800-934-9_28, © Springer Science + Business Media B.V. 2009

Fig. 28.1 Involvement of the femoral artery by Takayasu's arteritis (TA). The Figure shows a long, smooth tapering of the femoral artery of a 19-year-old woman with TA. The lesion was not amenable to angioplasty or stent placement because of its length, but responded with the resolution of leg claudication when the patient was treated with glucocorticoids and an exercise regimen of walking for 1 h each day. The development of collateral circulation is assumed to have mediated the symptomatic improvement. (Figure courtesy of Dr. John Stone)

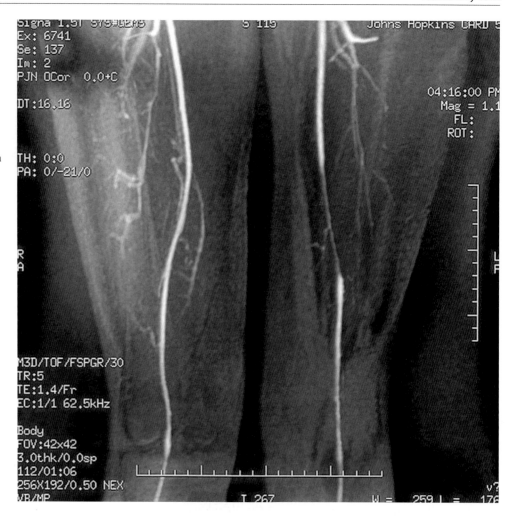

Pearl: TA is in the differential diagnosis of a young woman presenting with cardiomyopathy.

Comment: Although best known for its large vessel involvement, TA can also involve the myocardium with histological features of an inflammatory myocarditis. Patients with TA can present with variable degrees of dilated cardiomyopathy and congestive heart failure. Heart failure may also occur in TA patients as a consequence of uncontrolled hypertension, severe aortic regurgitation, or coronary artery disease.

Myth: TA is a monophasic illness in the majority of patients.

Reality: Large series emphasize that TA is a monophasic illness in only a minority of patients (less than 20%) (Maksimowicz-McKinnon et al. 2007; Kerr et al. 1994). The large majority of patients follow a chronic, relapsing course over time, with significant accrual of disease- and medication-related morbidity.

Pearl: Large-vessel vasculitis is associated with a number of systemic inflammatory diseases besides TA.

Comment: TA is the prototypical large-vessel vasculitis, and inflammation within the great vessels is the cardinal mani-

festation of that condition. However, a variety of other systemic inflammatory disorders may be associated with large-vessel vasculitis. These include giant cell arteritis, Behçet's disease, Cogan's syndrome, relapsing polychondritis, and sarcoidosis (See appropriate chapters). Aortitis may also be associated with systemic autoimmune diseases such as systemic lupus erythematosus, rheumatoid arthritis, and spondyloarthropathies.

Up to 20% of patients with giant cell arteritis have large artery disease detectable by careful auscultation. Moreover, the majority of giant cell arteritis patients have subclinical large artery involvement. Behçet's disease may involve blood vessels of all types and sizes, and large artery lesions may lead to bruits in the chest or abdomen; it is associated with inflammatory venous thromboses and large artery aneurysms. Behçet's disease should particularly be suspected in young males with features of large-vessel vasculitis. These differential diagnoses can usually be distinguished from TA on the basis of a thorough history and physical examination. Infectious etiologies such as syphilis, tuberculosis, and mycotic aneurysms must also be considered in the differential diagnosis of large-vessel vasculitis.

Finally, aortitis that is not related to any known infection may occur in the absence of disease of the primary aortic branches and other large vessels. This entity is termed "idiopathic aortitis."

Myth: TA can be distinguished from giant cell arteritis by its greater tendency to involve the primary branches of the aorta.

Reality: There is much overlap between TA and giant cell arteritis with regard to vascular distribution. This overlap renders any conclusions about diagnosis that are based on the distribution of vascular involvement unreliable. Both TA and giant cell arteritis can involve the proximal aorta, leading to dilatation of the aortic root and aortic regurgitation. In addition, both disorders can involve vessels supplying the upper extremity involving regions as distal as (and perhaps even beyond) the axillary-brachial junction.

The same is true with regard to lower extremity vessels. Both TA and giant cell arteritis can be associated with large-vessel inflammation and vascular narrowing that extends to the knee and possibly beyond.

Pearl: A number of noninflammatory conditions may mimic large-vessel vasculitis.

Comment: Aneurysms of large arteries can occur with genetic disorders such as Marfan's syndrome, Ehlers–Danlos syndrome (type IV), and Loeys–Dietz syndrome. Stenotic lesions are also evident in some patients with neurofibromatosis, Grange syndrome, and congenital disorders such as aortic coarctation and congenital mid-aortic syndrome. Congenital aortic coarctation may be associated with Turner's syndrome and Williams' syndrome.

Fibromuscular dysplasia may cause stenotic and/or aneurysmal lesions, but is distinguished generally by the typical "stack of coins" appearance on angiography (Fig. 28.2. In some cases, there may be other clinical features to point toward the diagnoses listed earlier. The presence of constitutional symptoms, abnormal acute phase reactants, or evidence of arteritis on pathologic examination of surgical specimens distinguishes TA from these genetic and congenital disorders. However, these features are absent in a significant proportion of patients with TA. In such cases, consultation with a medical geneticist may help resolve the underlying diagnosis.

Myth: TA does not involve the skin.

Reality: This Myth illustrates the fallacy of placing too much emphasis on classification schemes that focus on the size of the blood vessels typically affected by a given disorder. Although such systems are useful, they must be regarded as guidelines rather than rules.

TA is the prototypical large vessel vasculitis, and the cutaneous blood supply is generally confined to vessels smaller than 150 μm. Nevertheless, nodular and ulcerative skin lesions can occur in patients with TA and may be the presenting

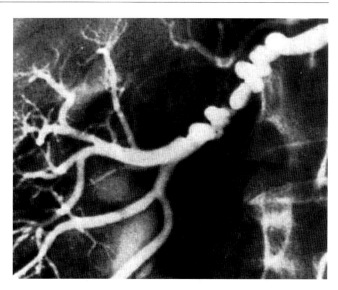

Fig. 28.2 Fibromuscular dysplasia. This disorder is frequently confused clinically with Takayasu's arteritis, but the "stack of coins" lesion evident in this figure is classic for fibromuscular dysplasia. (Figure courtesy of Dr. John Stone)

features of the disease (Pernicario et al. 1987). Failure to include TA in the differential diagnosis may lead to serious delays in diagnosis. However, given the rarity of this association, other disorders associated with large-vessel vasculitis that have prominent skin manifestations, including Behcet's disease and sarcoidosis, also warrant careful consideration in this setting.

Pearl: Peripheral blood pressure readings should be interpreted with caution in patients with TA.

Comment: TA frequently causes bilateral subclavian artery stenoses and may also lead to stenosis of the infra-renal aorta or narrowing of the large vessels to both lower extremities. Unfortunately, it can also cause renal artery stenosis, leading to renin-mediated hypertension. The combined effects of these various stenoses over time are that blood pressure measurements in the arms and even the legs do not accurately reflect the central aortic pressure, which may become dangerously elevated.

Patients with TA and symptoms or signs referable to severe hypertension (e.g., intractable headaches) require a serum renin measurement, a thorough investigation of the circulation to all extremities, precise imaging of the renal arteries, and an accurate determination of the central aortic pressure. This usually means a catheter-directed angiogram and measurement of central aortic pressures directly.

Myth: Normal acute phase reactants effectively exclude the diagnosis of TA.

Reality: Up to 11% of TA patients have normal acute phase reactants at their initial diagnosis (Maksimowicz-McKinnon et al. 2007; Kerr et al. 1994). Furthermore, approximately 25% of patients have normal acute phase reactants during periods of overtly active disease. Therefore, the erythrocyte sedimentation rate and C-reactive protein level cannot be relied upon to exclude the diagnosis of TA.

Pearl: TA can be associated with a markedly abnormal acute phase response.

Comment: A young woman with a markedly abnormal acute phase response, for example, thrombocytosis, a hematocrit compatible with anemia of chronic disease, and a bone marrow examination that shows "reactive hyperplasia," should be evaluated for TA. Platelet counts greater than 1 million/mm^3 have been observed in TA, and the erythrocyte sedimentation rate may exceed 100 mm/h.

Myth: The ESR and CRP are accurate gauges of disease activity in TA.

Reality: Assessing disease activity is one of the greatest challenges in caring for patients with TA. Acute phase reactants correlate with disease activity in only 70% of patients (Maksimowicz-McKinnon et al. 2007; Kerr et al. 1994). Furthermore, longitudinal series of treated TA patients undergoing vascular surgery indicate that active arteritis is found in up to 44% of patients, often in the absence of systemic symptoms or elevations of acute phase reactants and, in some cases, without abnormal findings on vascular imaging studies (Hoffman 1997; Kerr et al. 1994; Lagneau et al. 1987).

Myth: The angiogram is always abnormal in TA.

Reality: Catheter-directed angiography has been a key tool for diagnosis of TA and assessment of disease activity. However, because angiography only detects luminal abnormalities (stenoses, dilatations), which may be absent in the early stages of disease, patients with TA may have a normal angiogram. Although not invariably abnormal in TA, catheter-directed angiography remains important for certain patients even if the diagnosis has been established by magnetic resonance angiography or computed tomography angiography, as it offers the opportunity to measure directly the central aortic pressures.

Pearl: Noninvasive imaging techniques can detect evidence of large vessel vasculitis, but their role in monitoring disease activity remains poorly defined.

Comment: While catheter-directed angiography has traditionally been the gold standard for vessel imaging in TA patients, it is impractical for repeated monitoring because of the associated risks, including hemorrhage, arterial injury, infection, contrast-induced nephropathy, and radiation exposure. Consequently, it is increasingly being supplanted by noninvasive modalities, particularly magnetic resonance angiography (MRA) (Atalay and Bluemky 2001; Flamm et al. 1998) and computed tomography angiography (CTA).

MRA can detect anatomic abnormalities such as luminal stenosis, aneurysm formation, vessel wall thickening, and collateral vessel formation (Tso et al. 2002). MRA can also detect signal changes or brightness in the vessel wall, which is purported to represent neovascularization of the vasa vasorum, edema, or inflammation. The precise significance of these findings in the vessel wall and their correlation with disease activity in TA patients has yet to be defined.

Positron emission tomography (PET) scanning is a promising modality for the assessment of disease activity in TA (Gotway et al. 2005; Moreno et al. 2005). However, the performance characteristics of this technique in TA are still being defined. PET also requires concomitant performance of computed tomography imaging to detect vascular stenoses and aneurysms.

In short, although imaging modalities such as MRA, CTA, and PET now play a major role in establishing the diagnosis of large-vessel vasculitis, much remains to be learned about the utility and pitfalls of these techniques in gauging disease activity.

Pearl: The finding of one vascular lesion in a patient with suspected large vessel vasculitis mandates screening for additional asymptomatic lesions.

Comment: Lesions in TA may be asymptomatic, especially when not associated with hemodynamically significant stenosis or occlusion of the vessel or when associated with aneurysm. Imaging of the entire aorta and major branch vessels should be performed in all patients with suspected large vessel vasculitis. Identification of additional vascular lesions upon the initial assessment of patients with suspected large vessel vasculitis may help establish the diagnosis of TA. A comprehensive noninvasive imaging evaluation is a key component of the baseline patient evaluation. Without a full assessment of the extent of disease at baseline, any abnormality discovered subsequently may be difficult to interpret.

Myth: Radiographic worsening of a preexisting stenotic or aneurysmal lesion in TA indicates active disease and warrants intensification of immunosuppressive therapy.

Reality: Preexisting stenotic or aneurysmal lesions are not generally considered to be reversible, even if immunosuppression is effective. Moreover, such lesions may worsen because of hemodynamic factors even if the disease is controlled effectively. Turbulent flow due to preexisting stenosis may lead to a greater degree of stenosis or occlusion as a result of secondary atherosclerosis, especially in the presence of cofactors such as hypertension, dyslipidemia, and smoking. Worsening stenosis may also occur as a result of tightening of scar tissue within the vessel wall over time. Aneurysms may enlarge or rupture because of mechanical factors, particularly hypertension. Therefore, only a new lesion in a previously unaffected vascular territory should be interpreted as unequivocal evidence of active arteritis.

Myth: Prednisone monotherapy is sufficient for the treatment of TA in the large majority of patients throughout the course of their illness.

Reality: Prednisone remains the foundation of treatment for TA. Although other therapies are often used to treat this disease, no randomized clinical trial of any TA treatment has ever been published.

Prednisone monotherapy is usually the initial treatment of choice for TA patients who do not exhibit severe manifestations. However, most patients are unable to taper glucocorticoids entirely without suffering disease relapses. Consequently, additional therapies must be considered in order to spare excessive toxicity from high-dose glucocorticoids.

Open-label studies have suggested potential benefit with methotrexate, anti-TNF therapy, and a handful of other immunosuppressive agents (Kerr et al 1994; Hoffman et al. 1994; Liang and Hoffman 2005; Maksimowicz-McKinnon et al. 2007; Molloy et al. 2008). It must be emphasized that all these studies involve small numbers of patients, and none have been randomized, controlled trials. As a general rule, cyclophosphamide should be avoided in TA unless there are critical lesions that affect the coronary arteries or multiple cerebral blood vessels. A randomized controlled trial of abatacept for the treatment of TA began its enrollment in the late 2008.

Pearl: Many attempts at revascularization in large-vessel vasculitis are unnecessary or even ill-advised.

Comment: In TA, everything narrowed does not need to be "fixed." The risks and benefits of potential interventions should be considered carefully and with the full knowledge of the extensive collateral blood vessel involvement that characterizes this disease.

Stenotic lesions in large blood vessels such as the subclavian artery require many months or years to form. The slow development of these lesions permits dramatic neovascularization to occur naturally. The network of collateral blood vessels that form in large-vessel vasculitis are not usually associated with palpable pulses at the brachial or radial sites; hence, the term "pulseless disease." However, this collateral circulation is sufficient to provide blood flow to the extremities that prevents ischemia quite effectively.

Critical stenoses to vital organs in which the collateral circulation is poor may be candidates for revascularization with bypass surgery, angioplasty, or stent placement. The limited outcomes data available for these procedures suggest that the failure rates are high.

Pearl: In TA, carotid bypass grafts for central nervous system symptoms should originate from the aortic root or arch.

Comment: Stenoses of the carotid or vertebral artery occur in about 60% of all patients with TA. Depending on the severity of symptoms and anatomic abnormalities, these patients may be candidates for bypass procedures. In such cases, the subclavian or innominate arteries should not serve as the origin of these grafts because of the high frequency with which these vessels are affected in TA.

The subclavian and innominate vessels become stenotic in more than 90% of patients over time, threatening the utility of the bypasses that originate from these vessels. In contrast, even if the aortic arch were involved in TA, occlusive disease at that site is almost unknown (Giordano et al. 1991; Kerr et al. 1994). In addition, there is a much higher flow rate in the aorta, which also lessens the risk of occlusion.

Myth: Patients with the unexpected finding of an inflammatory infiltrate within the aortic root at surgery require treatment with large doses of glucocorticoids.

Reality: The unexpected histologic finding of aortic root inflammation at the time of aortic surgery is more common than generally appreciated. In one study of 1,204 patients who underwent aortic surgery at one institution, 52 of the patients (4%) were found to have idiopathic aortitis (Rojo-Leyva et al. 2000). Among those 52 patients, 51 did not have current features of a systemic illness at the time of their surgery. Despite the absence of systemic symptoms and signs in patients with idiopathic aortitis, the degree of inflammatory change within the aortic wall is often striking. In 16 of the 52 patients (31%), aortitis was associated with a remote history of vasculitis or other systemic disorder that was not considered to be active at the time of surgery.

This observation has profound implications on our perception and assessment of apparent "remission" in patients with large-vessel vasculitis. Among the 52 patients with idiopathic aortitis, 36 were followed for a mean period of 41 months, over which time new aneurysms were identified in only 6 patients (16% of those followed longitudinally). This experience suggests that most patients with isolated focal aortitis identified at aortic surgery have no indication for immunosuppressive therapy. However, such patients require careful imaging of the entire aorta and its primary branches to ensure that disease was unifocal, and careful follow-up to detect the development of other features of large vessel vasculitis.

Pearl: IgG4-related systemic disease can involve the aorta.

Comment: IgG4-related systemic disease is an emerging disorder associated with lymphoplasmacytic infiltration into a variety of organs, plasma cells that stain intensely for IgG4, and elevated serum IgG4 levels (Terumi and Atsutake; Stone et al., 2009) (See Chap. 12). IgG4-related systemic disease, first described in the pancreas and termed "autoimmune pancreatitis" (Yoshida et al. 1995), is now known to involve the biliary tree, salivary glands, kidneys, lungs, and other organs. Cases of aortitis caused by IgG4-related systemic disease have been reported (Fig. 28.3) (Satomi et al. 2008). The measurement of serum IgG4 levels is an appropriate screening test if this condition is suspected.

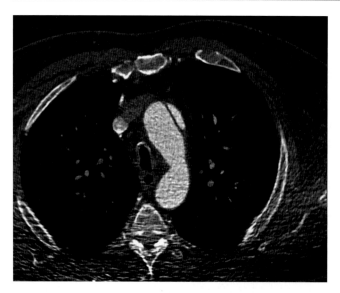

Fig. 28.3 IgG4-related systemic disease involving the aorta. This patient suffered an aortic dissection, and the diagnosis of IgG4-related systemic disease was made upon histopathological examination of the replaced aorta. (Figure courtesy of Dr. Arezou Khosroshahi)

Myth: Pregnancy is contraindicated in patients with TA.

Reality: The striking (9:1) female predominance in TA and the inference that the increased estrogen concentrations of pregnancy are likely to aggravate the illness have raised concerns about the safety of pregnancy in such patients. However, the data available to address this question do not suggest that pregnancy exacerbates TA.

If complications of TA already include uncontrolled hypertension, renal insufficiency, or aortic regurgitation, pregnancy-associated increases in intravascular volume may make pregnancy risky and unadvised. Several small series have demonstrated that in the absence of these risk factors, however, patients with TA may have successful pregnancies, uncomplicated deliveries, and healthy children (Matsumura et al. 1992; Aso et al. 1992; Sharma et al. 2000).

References

Aso T, Abe S, Yaguchi T. Clinical gynecologic features of pregnancy in Takayasu's arteritis. Heart Vessels. 1992;7:S125–132

Atalay M, Bluemke D. Magnetic resonance imaging of large vessel vasculitis. Curr Opin Rheum. 2001;13:41–47

Flamm S, White R, Hoffman G. The clinical application of "edema-weighted" magnetic resonance imaging in Takayasu's arteritis. Int J Cardiol. 1998;66:151–9

Gotway MB, Araoz PA, Macedo TA, et al Imaging findings in Takayasu's arteritis. Am J Roentgenol. 2005;184:1945–50

Giordano J, Leavitt R, Hoffman G, et al Experience with surgical treatment for Takayasu's disease. Surgery 1991;109:252–8

Hoffman G. Takayasu's arteritis: lessons from the American National Institutes of Health experience. Int J Cardiol. 1997;54:S99–102

Hoffman GS, Leavitt RY, Kerr GS, et al Treatment of glucocorticoid-resistant or relapsing Takayasu arteritis with methotrexate. Arthritis Rheum. 1994;37:578–82

Hoffman GS, Merkel PA, Brasington RD, et al Anti-tumor necrosis factor therapy in patients with difficult to treat Takayasu arteritis. Arthritis Rheum. 2004b;50:2296–304

Kerr GS, Hallahan CW, Giordano J, et al Takayasu arteritis. Ann Intern Med. 1994;20:919–29

Lagneau P, Michel J-B, Vuong P. Surgical treatment of Takayasu's disease. Ann Surg. 1987;205:157–66

Liang P, Hoffman GS. Advances in the medical and surgical treatment of Takayasu's arteritis. Curr Opin Rheumatol. 2005;17:16–24

Maksimowicz-McKinnon K, Clark TM, Hoffman GS. Takayasu's arteritis: limitations of therapy and guarded prognosis in an American cohort. Arthritis Rheum. 2007;56:1000–9

Matsumura A, Moriwaki R, Numano F. Pregnancy in Takayasu arteritis from the view of internal medicine. Heart Vessels. 1992;7(S):120–4

Molloy ES, Langford CA, Clark TM, et al Durable remission in patients with refractory Takayasu's arteritis treated with infliximab and etanercept. Ann Rheum Dis. 2008;67:1567–9

Moreno D, Yuste JR, Rodriguez M, et al Positron emission tomography use in the diagnosis and follow up of Takayasu's arteritis. Ann Rheum Dis. 2005;64:1091–3

Pernicario CV, Winkelmann RK, Hunder GG. Cutaneous manifestations of Takayasu's arteritis. J Am Acad Dermatol. 1987;17:998–1005

Rojo-Leyva F, Ratliff N, Cosgrove D, et al Study of 52 patients with idiopathic aortitis from a cohort of 1,204 surgical cases. Arthritis Rheum. 2000;43:901–7

Satomi K, Yoh Z, Atsuhiro K, et al Inflammatory abdominal aortic aneurysm: close relationship to IgG4-related periaortitis. Am J Surg Pathol. 2008;32:197–204

Sharma B, Jain S, Vasishta K. Outcome of pregnancy in Takayasu arteritis. Int J Cardiol. 2000;75:S159–62

Stone JH, Khosroshahi A, Hilgenberg AD et al IgG4-related systemic disease and lymphoplasmacytic aortitis. Arthritis Rheum 2009 (in press)

Terumi K, Atsutake O. IgG4-related sclerosing disease. World J Gastroenterol. 2008;14:3948–55

Tso E, Flamm SD, White RD, et al Takayasu arteritis: utility and limitations of magnetic resonance imaging in diagnosis and treatment. Arthritis Rheum. 2002;46:1634–42

Yoshida K, Toki F, Takeuchi T, et al Chronic pancreatitis caused by an autoimmune abnormality. Proposal of the concept of autoimmune pancreatitis. Dig Dis Sci. 1995;40:1561–8

Primary Angiitis of the Central Nervous System and Reversible Cerebral Vasoconstriction Syndromes

29

Leonard H. Calabrese and Aneesh B. Singhal

29.1 Overview of Primary Angiitis of the Central Nervous System

> Vasculitis that exclusively involves the central nervous system (CNS) is among the most complex and poorly understood forms of vascular inflammatory disease.

> The variable terminology for CNS vasculitis continues to pose significant challenges. CNS vasculitis that is not associated with a known underlying cause or some form of systemic vasculitis is termed primary angiitis of the CNS (PACNS).

> Some cases of PACNS confirmed by histopathology have granulomatous features of inflammation. The term "granulomatous inflammation of the nervous system" has been used for such cases. For practical purposes, now GANS and PACNS are considered to be largely synonymous terms.

> PACNS presents in a subacute manner, with an elapse of many months between the time of first symptom onset and diagnostic confirmation.

> The clinical hallmarks of PACNS are headache, slowly-evolving encephalopathy, and multi-focal strokes. Fever, other constitutional symptoms, and extra-CNS manifestations are absent.

> Acute phase reactants tend to be normal in PACNS.

> Lumbar puncture typically reveals a lymphocytic pleocytosis.

> Magnetic resonance imaging (MRI) usually reveals multiple foci of strokes, some of which may be asymptomatic. Imaging findings typical of PACNS are shown in Fig. 29.1. CNS angiography is normal in many patients with PACNS, but when abnormal, can reveal arterial beading (see Fig. 29.1d, e), focal narrowing, apparent vascular cutoffs, and even microaneurysms.

Pearl: A thorough evaluation of a patient for possible PACNS always must include a lumbar puncture.

Comment: A lumbar puncture is essential for the diagnostic evaluation of patients with potential PACNS. The cerebrospinal fluid (CSF) must be examined for signs of inflammation, infection, and malignancy.

The CSF is abnormal in more than 95% of cases of granulomatous angiitis of the CNS (GACNS). Thus, a normal CSF analysis has a high negative predictive value for this condition. The mean CSF protein in patients with PACNS is 177 mg/dL, and the mean cell count is 77/mm^3 (Calabrese et al. 1997). An equally compelling reason to analyze CSF is to exclude mimics such as infection and malignancy, which can yield angiographic findings identical to those of PACNS.

Pearl: PACNS almost never presents as a simple stroke.

Comment: Although CNS vasculitis remains in the differential diagnosis of an unexplained ischemic event, patients with this rare disorder almost never present with a simple stroke. In patients with GACNS as well as other pathologically documented cases, the usual clinical manifestations include headaches, mental changes, and multiple small-vessel strokes that occur over weeks to many months (Moore 1998). Additional clinical settings that raise the likelihood of PACNS include chronic meningitis and multifocal strokes that occur in a subacute fashion (see Fig. 29.1a–c).

Pearl: PACNS can present as a mass lesion.

Comment: Patients presenting with a mass lesion on a neuroimaging study, regardless of the associated signs or symptoms, must be considered to have a malignancy or an infection until proven otherwise. However, approximately 5% of patients with PACNS also present with mass lesions (see Fig. 29.1f). Biopsy confirmation is always required.

The optimal management of this disorder has not been defined clearly, but CNS vasculitis that presents as a mass lesion occasionally appears to have been cured by surgical resection. Other cases have proved to require immunosuppressive therapy (Molloy et al. 2008).

Pearl: PACNS is usually not associated with constitutional symptoms or signs of systemic inflammation.

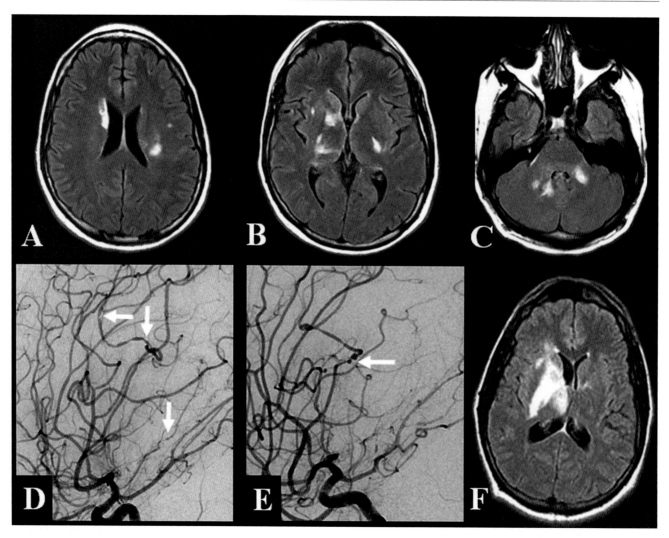

Fig. 29.1 Brain imaging in primary angiitis of the CNS (PACNS). Brain MRI, axial FLAIR images (**a–c**) from a 21-year man with PACNS show hyperintense lesions (subacute and chronic ischemic strokes) in multiple deep locations. Digital subtraction angiographic images from the same patient show areas of irregularity, "beading," and ectasia in branches of the left (**d**) and right (**e**) middle cerebral arteries. Brain MRI, axial FLAIR image (**f**) from a 26-year man shows a mass lesion that proved to be PACNS on brain biopsy

Comment: This concept flies in the face of most clinicians' preconceived notions of vasculitis and frequently confounds the diagnostic evaluation of PACNS. However, it is quite true. The complete blood count is usually normal in PACNS, as are acute phase reactants such as the erythrocyte sedimentation rate and C-reactive protein. When the diagnosis is suspected on clinical neurologic grounds, the clinician should not be dissuaded by the absence of features normally associated with systemic vasculitis. The lack of symptoms and signs to suggest an inflammatory process is actually a point in favor of PACNS.

Myth: Biopsy of the CNS or brain biopsy is not worth the risk.

Reality: This is probably one of the greatest myths and pitfalls in the diagnosis of PACNS. Pathologically-documented PACNS has serious prognostic implications and requires intensive immunosuppression. For these reasons, diagnostic certainty is invaluable whenever it can be established. Furthermore, numerous PACNS mimickers, including infections and malignancies, can be diagnosed only by obtaining histopathology. Although the sensitivity of tissue biopsy is only in the range of 75–80%, the morbidity of brain biopsy is less than 2% when biopsies are performed under appropriate circumstances in the setting of nonmalignant conditions (Parisi and Moore 1994). The optimal approach to brain biopsy is to go directly to accessible lesions by a stereotactic technique. In the absence of a focal lesion, an open biopsy of the tip of the nondominant temporal lobe with overlying leptomeningies is reasonable.

Myth: The high rate of false-negative results on brain biopsy even in patients who really have PACNS makes the procedure relatively useless.

Reality: The most reliable data available suggest that the sensitivity of brain biopsy in PACNS is as low as 75%. Thus, in the presence of PACNS, the procedure will miss the pathological area of tissue in up to a quarter of cases. It is regrettable that this fact often discourages clinicians from performing brain biopsies in cases in which PACNS is suspected. However, an equally important justification for the performance of brain biopsy is the efficiency of this procedure in excluding nonvasculitic conditions.

In a series of 30 consecutive brain biopsies from the Duke University Medical Center, the predictive value of brain biopsy was greater than 90% in patients suspected of PACNS (Chu et al. 1998). In a series of 61 consecutive patients from the University of Michigan, brain biopsy suggested alternative diagnoses in 22 cases (36%) (Alrawi et al. 1999). In our estimation, brain biopsy is underutilized in patients for whom PACNS is a true possibility.

29.2 Overview of Reversible Cerebral Vasoconstriction Syndromes

- Reversible cerebral vasoconstriction syndromes (RCVS) include a diverse array of conditions, such as eclampsia, the postpartum state, hypertensive encephalopathy, migraine, and exposure to vasoconstrictive drugs.
- The angiographic phenomenon of reversible "beading" has been reported using a variety of terms, each reflecting a presumed mechanism or associated underlying condition: migrainous vasospasm, migraine angiitis, thunderclap headache with reversible vasospasm, drug-induced vasospasm, drug-induced arteritis, eclamptic vasospasm, postpartum angiopathy, benign angiopathy (Hajj-Ali et al., 2002), cerebral pseudovasculitis, and Call's syndrome.
- Patients with reversible cerebral arterial narrowing appear to have similar clinical, laboratory, imaging, and prognostic features, regardless of the associated underlying condition.
- Provisional diagnostic criteria for RCVS have been proposed (Table 29.1) (Calabrese et al. 2007).
- Patients with RCVS are typically young (age 20–60 years). More than 80% of patients present with "thunderclap" headaches, which occur suddenly, have great intensity, and can recur over the next few days (Chen et al. 2006).
- Imaging features typical of RCVS are shown in Fig. 29.2. with RCVS, by definition, have segmental cerebral arterial vasoconstriction that resolves over a period of weeks.
- RCVS has many features that overlap with PACNS: headache, potential for strokes and seizures, and "beading" of the cerebral arteries on angiographic studies.
- Despite the ominous presentation and impressive angiographic and imaging abnormalities, the prognosis of

Table 29.1 RCVS: key elements for diagnosis

Digital subtraction angiography or a CT or MR angiogram that documents multifocal cerebral artery vasoconstriction
No evidence for ruptured brain aneurysm or ruptured cerebral vascular malformation
Normal or near-normal cerebrospinal fluid analysis (protein < 80 mg/dL, white blood cells < 10/mm^3)
Onset with severe headache, with or without additional neurologic signs or symptoms
The diagnosis cannot be confirmed until (a) reversibility of the angiographic abnormalities is documented, usually within 12 weeks after onset; or (b) if death occurs before the follow-up neurovascular imaging is obtained, autopsy rules out conditions such as cerebral vasculitis, intracranial atherosclerosis, and aneurysmal subarachnoid hemorrhage that can also manifest with headache, stroke, and cerebral angiographic abnormalities.

Adapted from Calabrese et al. (2007)

RCVS is usually benign. Nearly 90% of patients have few or no residual neurological deficits (Hajj-Ali et al., 2002).

Pearl: Specific clinical features can distinguish RCVS from PACNS.

Comment: The confusion between RCVS and PACNS is attributable to overlapping clinical-angiographic features, low specificity of diagnostic tests, and lack of validated diagnostic criteria for either condition. Nevertheless, these disorders have major differences in their clinical presentations, and clinicians ignore them at their peril.

Patients with PACNS usually come to medical attention because of smoldering, low-grade headaches, subacute encephalopathy, or progressive neurological deficits. In contrast, the onset of RCVS is typically dramatic. RCVS patients report the explosive onset of the worst headache of their lives. Most patients have three to five headaches over a period of days to a couple of weeks. These headaches are exacerbated by the Valsalva maneuver (Ducros et al. 2007). A significant minority of patients develop generalized seizures or focal neurological deficits.

Cortical blindness (Balint syndrome) and visual scotomas occur in approximately 30% of patients. Bilateral hyperreflexia is common. The headaches resolve spontaneously over days to weeks, and unlike PACNS, most patients recover completely within weeks.

Two critical clues in the presentation distinguish RCVS from PACNS with great reliability. First, RCVS begin quickly (explosively) with the onset of a thunderclap headache, in contrast to the subacute development characteristic of PACNS. Second, the clinical setting of RCVS is highly typical: onset after childbirth or after exposure to vasoconstrictive drugs such as sumatriptan, nasal decongestants, certain antidepressants, and illicit drugs of abuse such as cocaine or ecstasy favors the diagnosis of RCVS.

Pearl: Cross-sectional neuroimaging studies help distinguish RCVS from PACNS.

Comment: Computed tomography (CT) or MRI of the brain should be performed immediately in all patients with "thunderclap" headaches. These studies are essential for the exclusion of explanations such as cerebral venous sinus thrombosis, pituitary apoplexy, carotid or vertebral artery dissection, and CNS hemorrhage (Schwedt et al. 2006). Once these conditions have been excluded, consideration can be given to RCVS and PACNS as potential diagnoses.

Analysis of the type and distribution of brain lesions on neuroimaging studies is helpful. Patients with PACNS virtually always have small, disseminated, punctuate infarcts that are of variable age (acute, subacute, and even chronic). Diffused white matter lesions are also often present, suggesting a chronic microangiopathy. Brain hemorrhages seldom occur in bona fide cases of PACNS.

On the other hand, approximately 70% of patients with RCVS have no parenchymal brain lesions on CNS imaging.

RCVS patients who do have brain imaging abnormalities usually have a combination of parenchymal hemorrhage (see Fig. 29.2b), small subarachnoid hemorrhages on the cortical surface (see Fig. 29.2d), brain infarctions, and transient vasogenic brain edema. RCVS-associated brain infarctions tend to be bilateral, symmetric, and located in cortical-subcortical regions. They are surrounded by areas of cerebral hypoperfusion. Brain edema (see Fig. 29.2c) is similarly bilateral, symmetric, and located in the cerebral or cerebellar hemispheres. The edema associated with RCVS is similar to that of the edematous brain lesions found in the reversible posterior leukoencephalopathy syndrome (RPLS), also known as the posterior reversible encephalopathy syndrome (PRES) (Singhal 2004).

Myth: RCVS and PACNS can be differentiated by their angiographic features if classic findings of PACNS are present.

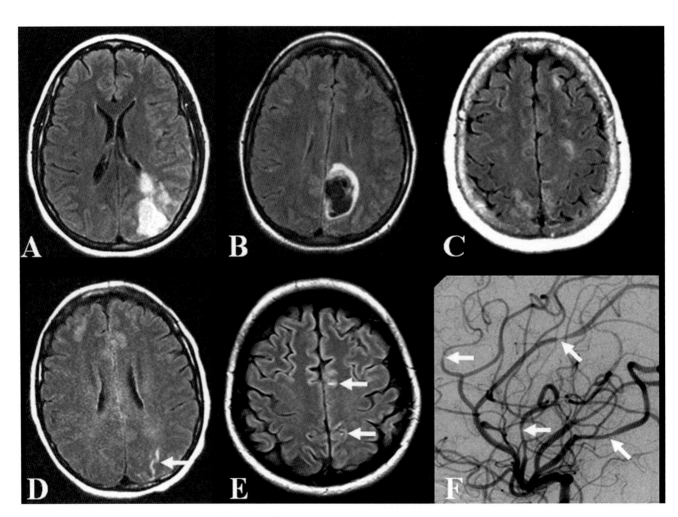

Fig. 29.2 Brain imaging in the reversible cerebral vasoconstriction syndrome (RCVS). Brain MRI, axial FLAIR images (**a–e**) show the typical brain imaging abnormalities in RCVS, including an ischemic stroke in the watershed distribution of the left middle and posterior cerebral artery (**a**), parenchymal brain hemorrhage (**b**), reversible hyperintense lesions (brain edema) in subcortical regions (**c**), non-aneurysmal cortical surface subarachnoid hemorrhage (*arrow*) overlying the left hemisphere (**d**), and dilated cortical surface vessels (*arrows*) overlying the left hemisphere (**e**). However, it is important to note that most patients with RCVS have no parenchymal lesion on brain MRI. Digital subtraction angiogram (**f**) from a patient with RCVS shows the typical segmental narrowing ("sausaging") of multiple cerebral arteries that usually reverse within weeks

Reality: The single greatest pitfall in evaluating patients with possible CNS vasculitis is over-reliance upon cerebral arteriography as a diagnostic test. There is not a single angiographic feature that is pathognomonic for PACNS; RCVS can mimic every last one. Thus, a CNS angiogram read as "consistent with vasculitis" (see Fig. 29.2f) merely indicates that insightful clinical correlation is required and additional work-up (e.g., lumbar puncture and an MRI) are probably necessary.

Although the cerebral angiographic abnormalities can be identical in RCVS and PACNS, the evolution over time of angiographic lesions is very helpful in distinguishing these two entities. Cerebral angiography is abnormal by definition in RCVS, but shows reversibility within 10–12 weeks in nearly all cases. It must be acknowledged that in a minority of RCVS cases, the intense vasoconstriction characteristic of RCVS invokes a secondary inflammatory response that leads to some permanent changes on angiography.

Clinicians must bear in mind that PACNS patients can have normal cerebral angiograms. This is because the caliber of the arteries affected is sometimes below the resolution of angiography. Arterial irregularities, if present, seldom get reversed in PACNS without chronic immunosuppressive treatment.

Myth: Blood and CSF test results generally distinguish RCVS from PACNS quite reliably.

Reality: Neither RCVS nor PACNS has a characteristic serologic marker of the disease. Peripheral blood markers of inflammation such as the erythrocyte sedimentation rate and C-reactive protein are usually normal in both conditions, but are helpful (if markedly abnormal) in suggesting diagnoses other than RCVS or PACNS. Perhaps, the only clue to a cause of RCVS is the finding of elevated norepinephrine metabolites in the blood and urine of patients with cerebral vasoconstriction associated with a pheochromocytoma.

CSF analysis is more helpful but remains imperfect. A "benign" CSF favors the diagnosis of RCVS. However, the CSF is normal in at least 20% of patients with PACNS and also has mild abnormalities in up to 20% of those with RCVS.

Myth: Angiographic "beading" in RCVS results from subarachnoid blood or transient inflammation.

Reality: The precise mechanism of vasoconstriction in RCVS remains unknown. At the molecular level, the pathophysiology may be related to the immunological and biochemical factors such as endothelin-1, serotonin, nitric oxide, and prostaglandins that are known to be involved in subarachnoid hemorrhage-related vasospasm. One-third of patients with RCVS have minor subarachnoid hemorrhages localized to the cortical surface, raising the question of hemorrhage-induced cerebral vasospasm, similar to that which occurs in patients following the rupture of berry aneurysms. However, the widespread distribution of vasoconstriction in RCVS cannot be explained by the small surface hemorrhages.

Moreover, the presence of vasoconstriction at the onset of RCVS is contrary to what is observed normally in subarachnoid hemorrhage, a setting in which vasospasm ensues after a period of 5–10 days.

Despite the important differences between the vasoconstriction of RCVS and subarachnoid hemorrhage, many patients with RCVS are subjected to serial angiograms designed to detect occult sources of CNS bleeding or exclude unruptured aneurysms as the cause of their recurrent thunderclap headaches. Such serial studies are unnecessary. The role of follow-up angiography in RCVS is to confirm the diagnosis by documenting the resolution of vasospasm 4–6 weeks after the initial study. In practice, few patients undergo such second studies.

Myth: RCVS is simply a bad migraine attack.

Reality: Patients with RCVS present with headaches and 25% have histories of migraine headaches. A significant proportion of RCVS patients develop "migraine-like strokes" in watershed arterial territories (see Fig. 29.2a). These features, combined with the rare observation of angiographic vasoconstriction during acute migraine attacks, have made some authors question whether RCVS is simply a severe migraine attack.

A true relationship between RCVS and migraines is unlikely, for several reasons. The character of thunderclap headache is quite different from migraines. In addition, RCVS rarely recur, in contrast to migraines. However, the spectrum of RCVS probably does include primary headache disorders such as benign sexual, cough, and exertional headaches, all of which have been associated with cerebral vasoconstriction. In a prospective study, MR angiography showed beading of the cerebral arteries in 39% of patients with unexplained thunderclap headache. The clinical features of those with and without vasoconstriction were similar (chen et al., 2006).

Pearl: Transcranial Doppler studies are useful in RCVS.

Comment: Conventional angiography is the modality of choice for making the diagnosis of RCVS. MR and CT angiographic studies are also helpful if the blood vessels involved are not below the resolution of these instruments (Remember, even conventional angiography is not sufficiently sensitive to detect disease in the smallest blood vessels). Transcranial Doppler studies, noninvasive investigations that measure blood flow velocities in multiple intracranial arteries, can also provide support for the diagnosis of RCVS.

Transcranial Doppler studies have potential shortcomings. Hyperemia and other factors can raise blood flow velocities, leading to false impressions of vessel narrowing. In addition, some patients with vasoconstriction demonstrated on angiography have normal blood flow velocities. Transcranial Doppler studies are probably most useful when employed in a serial fashion in individual patients. These procedures permit simple, noninvasive, contrast-free, bedside monitoring of the progression and resolution of vasoconstriction (Chen et al. 2008).

Pearl: Vasoconstrictive medications should be avoided in patients with RCVS.

Comment: Numerous vasoconstrictive drugs and medications such as amphetamine derivatives, sumatriptan, ergot derivatives, diet pills, nasal decongestants, serotonergic antidepressants, cocaine, ecstasy, and marijuana have been identified as triggers of RCVS (Ducros et al. 2007; Singhal 2002; Singhal et al. 2002). These data are anecdotal. Confirmatory prospective studies are warranted, but avoidance of further exposure to such agents in patients with evidence for cerebral vasoconstriction is reasonable.

This issue is particularly relevant because the majority of patients present with the sudden onset of intense headaches and often receive medications such as sumatriptan before undergoing neurovascular imaging tests.

Pearl: Pharmacological blood pressure modulation should be avoided in patients with RCVS. Simple observation is an appropriate management option.

Comment: It is tempting to use pharmacological maneuvers to raise blood pressure so as to improve cerebral perfusion, or to lower the blood pressure in hypertension in the interest of minimizing brain hemorrhage. Clinicians should understand, however, that blood pressure fluctuations in RCVS may represent autoregulatory phenomena. Therefore, blood pressure modulation should be avoided. Drug-induced hypertension can exacerbate vasoconstriction, and relative hypotension carries the risk of precipitating infarction within hypoperfused brain tissue.

Angioplasty and direct infusion of vasodilators have been attempted as measures to relieve severe arterial narrowing. These intra-arterial strategies carry the risk of reperfusion injury (edema and hemorrhage). They should be reserved for patients who have declined clearly as a result of progressive vasoconstriction. Calcium-channel blockers such as verapamil and nimodipine may be useful in mitigating headaches, but to date, have not been found to influence the course of vasoconstriction (Chen et al. 2008; Ducros et al. 2007). They may also lead to vascular steal phenomena in which vasoconstricted vessels are further deprived of blood.

Myth: RCVS is an extremely rare condition.

Reality: Reports of RCVS have increased steadily since the turn of the current century. Our two centers have encountered more than 140 RCVS cases, and a single-center prospective study reported 67 cases occurring over a period of only 5 years (Ducros et al. 2007). Several factors account for this – the advent of CT and MR technologies for the assessments of the cerebral vasculature, the widespread use and abuse of vasoconstrictive drugs and medications, and use of the term "RCVS," which has brought together a group of related conditions that previously seemed disparate.

The recognition that cerebral vasoconstriction is often present in isolated thunderclap headache and RPLS has increased the use of neurovascular testing in these conditions. It is likely that primary care physicians, rheumatologists, obstetricians, neurologists, neurosurgeons, intensivists, emergency department physicians, and other specialists will encounter and report more cases of RCVS in the years ahead.

References

Alrawi A, Trobe JD, Blaivas M, Musch DC. Brain biopsy in primary angiitis of the central nervous system. Neurology 1999;53:858–60

Calabrese LH, Dodick DW, Schwedt TJ, Singhal AB. Narrative review: reversible cerebral vasoconstriction syndromes. Ann Intern Med. 2007;146:34–44

Calabrese LH, Duna GF, Lie JT. Vasculitis in the central nervous system. Arthritis Rheum. 1997;40:1189–201

Chen SP, Fuh JL, Chang FC, Lirng JF, Shia BC, Wang SJ. Transcranial color Doppler study for reversible cerebral vasoconstriction syndromes. Ann Neurol. 2008;63:751–7

Chen SP, Fuh JL, Lirng JF, Chang FC, Wang SJ. Recurrent primary thunderclap headache and benign CNS angiopathy: spectra of the same disorder? Neurology 2006;67:2164–9

Chu CT, Gray L, Goldstein LB, Hulette CM. Diagnosis of intracranial vasculitis: a multi-disciplinary approach. J Neuropathol Exp Neurol. 1998;57:30–8

Ducros A, Boukobza M, Porcher R, Sarov M, Valade D, Bousser MG. The clinical and radiological spectrum of reversible cerebral vasoconstriction syndrome. A prospective series of 67 patients. Brain 2007;130:3091–101

Hajj-Ali RA, Furlan A, Abou-Chebel A, Calabrese LH. Benign angiopathy of the central nervous system: cohort of 16 patients with clinical course and long-term followup. Arthritis Rheum. 2002;47: 662–9

Molloy ES, Singhal AB, Calabrese LH. Tumor-like mass lesion – an under-recognized presentation of primary angiitis of the central nervous system. Ann Rheum Dis. 2008;67:1732–5

Moore PM. Central nervous system vasculitis. Curr Opin Neurol. 1998;11:241–6

Parisi JE, Moore PM. The role of biopsy in vasculitis of the central nervous system. Semin Neurol. 1994;14:341–8

Schwedt TJ, Matharu MS, Dodick DW. Thunderclap headache. Lancet Neurol. 2006;5:621–31

Singhal AB. Cerebral vasoconstriction without subarachnoid blood: associated conditions, clinical and neuroimaging characteristics. Ann Neurol. 2002;S:59–60

Singhal AB. Postpartum angiopathy with reversible posterior leukoencephalopathy. Arch Neurol. 2004;61:411–16

Singhal AB, Caviness VS, Begleiter AF, Mark EJ, Rordorf G, Koroshetz WJ. Cerebral vasoconstriction and stroke after use of serotonergic drugs. Neurology 2002;58:130–3

Eric L. Matteson and John H. Stone

30.1 Overview of Thromboangiitis Obliterans (Buerger's Disease)

> A form of vasculitis associated with a highly inflammatory clot within the lumen as well as inflammation within the vascular wall.
> Associated with active cigarette smoking, typically moderate to heavy.
> Tends to involve medium-sized arteries and veins, with the most striking clinical pathology related to arterial disease.
> Digital ischemia in all four extremities is a hallmark of the disorder, with the involvement of some extremities more characteristic than others.
> Severe digital ischemia without the evidence of internal organ involvement.
> Angiography reveals segmental involvement of medium-sized arteries, with abrupt vascular cut-offs and corkscrew collaterals. The major vessel involvement occurs at the levels of the ankle and wrist, with major consequences to the distal extremities.
> Smoking cessation is the only therapy known to be effective for Buerger's disease.

Myth: Patients with thromboangiitis obliterans are more addicted to nicotine than are those with atherosclerotic coronary artery disease.

Reality: The "classic" patient with thromboangiitis obliterans is a young male who smokes heavily. As discussed in this chapter, several parts of this stereotype are misleading. For example, in a prospective study, patients with thromboangiitis obliterans actually smoked significantly fewer cigarettes per day than did patients with coronary atherosclerosis (Cooper et al. 2006). Patients with thromboangiitis obliterans are also more likely to have made serious attempts to quit smoking. Their degree of tobacco dependence was judged to be comparable to that of patients with atherosclerotic coronary artery disease, not greater.

Myth: The risk of amputation in patients with thromboangiitis obliterans is low in the first years of disease but increases markedly over time.

Comment: This statement is too optimistic. It boils down to this: the risk of amputation in patients with thromboangiitis obliterans is high in the first years of disease and even higher in the long run, particularly among patients who continue to smoke.

The probability of having an amputation of either a terminal digit or a larger part of a limb is 50% at 15 years of disease (Fig. 30.1) (Cooper et al. 2004). As shown in Fig. 30.1, the risk of amputation is already high in the first 5 years of disease. The risk of amputation persists up to at least 18 years following the diagnosis in thromboangiitis obliterans patients.

Pearl: Thromboangiitis obliterans never involves only one limb.

Comment: Thromboangiitis obliterans is always present in more than arm or leg, and often in both arms and both legs, even if clinical evidence of multi-limb involvement is not

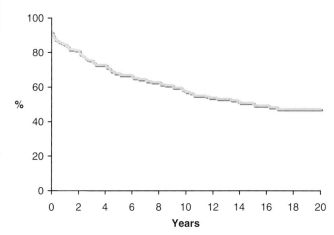

Fig. 30.1 Survival free of amputation in patients with thromboangiitis obliterans. The risk of major or minor amputation at 20 years was 56%. From Dr. Leslie T. Cooper, Mayo Clinic. Reprinted with kind permission from Elsevier Limited

J. H. Stone (ed.), *A Clinician's Pearls and Myths in Rheumatology,*
DOI:10.1007/978-1-84800-934-9_30, © Springer Science + Business Media B.V. 2009

Fig. 30.2 Clinical and angiographic findings in thromboangiitis obliterans. (**a**) Left foot of a patient with thromboangiitis obliterans and critical limb ischemia, illustrating dependent rubor and hair loss. (**b**) The contrast angiogram of the same foot illustrates diffuse thrombosis of the distal pedal arteries. Numerous small collateral blood vessels, including adventitial "corkscrew"-type vessels, can be seen in the region of the occluded distal peroneal and dorsalis pedis arteries. (Courtesy of Cooper, Mayo Clinic.)

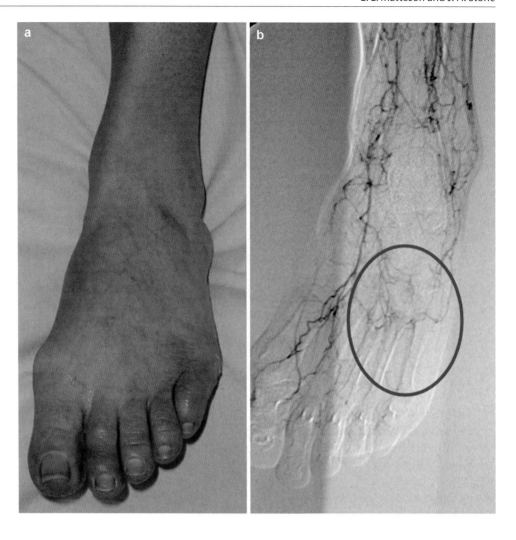

apparent immediately (Hirai and Shionoya 1979) (Fig. 30.2a, b). If called to see a patient who has intense ischemia in only one limb and no angiographic evidence of disease in other extremities, thromboangiitis obliterans is not the diagnosis (Fig. 30.3).

Myth: Thromboangiitis obliterans is a systemic vasculitis.

Reality: Although often classified as a systemic vasculitis, there are several important distinctions between thromboangiitis obliterans and other forms of vasculitis (Puechal and Fiessinger 2007). Thromboangiitis obliterans is characterized pathologically by a highly cellular thrombus with relative sparing of the blood vessel walls (Fig. 30.4). Multinucleated giant cells can even be observed within the clot in thromboangiitis obliterans. The architecture of the vascular wall is preserved, and fibrinoid necrosis is absent.

The occlusive clot found within the lumen of blood vessels involved by thromboangiitis obliterans explains why immunosuppressive therapy is ineffective in this disorder. Unfortunately,

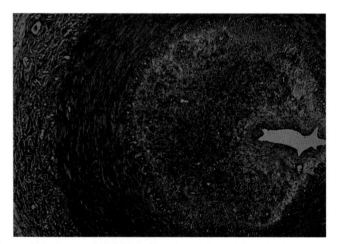

Fig. 30.3 Early lesions in thromboangiitis obliterans (hematoxylin and eosin staining). Thrombosed artery with highly cellular thrombus and intact internal elastic lamina, illustrating the typical early lesion of thromboangiitis obliterans (hematoxylin and eosin, medium power). (Courtesy of William Edwards, Mayo Clinic.)

anticoagulation and thrombolytic treatment approaches are also either unhelpful or unproven. Smoking cessation is the critical component of thromboangiitis obliterans therapy.

Myth: Thromboangiitis obliterans is a disease of young men.

Reality: In a Mayo Clinic series from the 1930s, less than 1% of the patients were women (Horton 1938). As the proportion of smokers who are women has grown, the percentage of thromboangiitis obliterans patients who are women has expanded proportionally. More recent estimates of the percentage of thromboangiitis obliterans patients who are women are as high

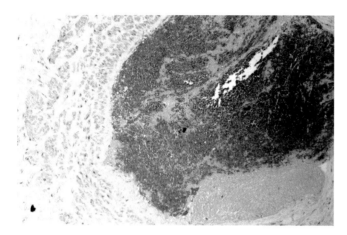

Fig. 30.4 Highly cellular thrombus with relative sparing of the blood vessel walls (Courtesy of Dr. John Stone)

as 23% (Lie 1987; Olin 2000). Thromboangiitis obliterans has a lot more to do with whether or not one smokes than whether or not a Y chromosome is present.

Myth: Smoking marijuana can cause a disease identical to Buerger's disease.

Reality: Digital ischemia has been reported as a result of marijuana use (Fig. 30.5) (Sterne and Ducastaing 1960). Scrutiny of these results indicates that "cannabis arteritis" bears a remarkable resemblance to thromboangiitis obliterans clinically, that most of the patients reported smoked cigarettes as well as marijuana, and that the reported pathological differences between these allegedly separate entities are unconvincing (Combemale et al. 2005; Disdier et al. 1999). Cannabis arteritis is probably really just thromboangiitis obliterans.

Pearl: Superficial thrombophlebitis may be the first manifestation of thromboangiitis obliterans.

Comment: Buerger himself noted that fleeting, painful, erythematous lesions—symptomatic of a superficial thrombophlebitis—are frequently the initial manifestation of this disorder (Buerger 1908). Buerger called attention to two distinct disease phases: (1) a migratory thrombophlebitis; (2) an occlusive disease of deeper vessels. Describing the first phase, Buerger wrote: "Most interesting is the acute stage or earliest lesion, which occurs simultaneously with or shortly after the onset of thrombosis." Histologic examination of these lesions reveals an acute thrombophlebitis with marked perivascular infiltration.

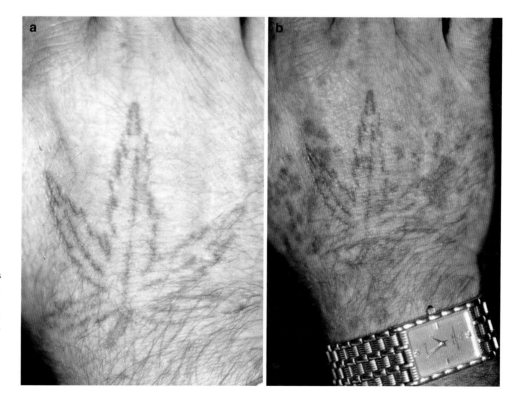

Fig. 30.5 (**a, b**) "Cannabis arteritis" is probably caused by concomitant cigarette smoking and consequent thromboangiitis obliterans and is therefore not a true vasculitic entity itself. However, this cannabis user did develop a vasculitis: cryoglobulinemia secondary to hepatitis C, acquired through injection drug use (Courtesy of Dr. John Stone)

The superficial thrombophlebitis of thromboangiitis obliterans is migratory, recurrent, and may affect the arms and legs. Migrating phlebitis (phlebitis saltans) in a young smoker is therefore highly suggestive of thromboangiitis obliterans. Biopsy of a subcutaneous nodule can be used to confirm the presence of superficial thrombophlebitis at an early phase of thromboangiitis obliterans, before the onset of larger vessel thrombosis (Hill 1974).

Patients rarely consult physicians at the time of this early complaint, and therefore these lesions are usually overlooked or disregarded. This "herald lesion," however, is generally followed by progressive occlusive disease in the deeper arteries and veins, leading the patient to medical attention.

Pearl: Thromboangiitis obliterans targets medium-sized vessels at the level of the wrists and ankles.

Comment: Again, Buerger's elegant description: *"The beginnings of the obliteration are not to be sought in the capillaries nor in the finest branches. If we follow the vessels upward, we frequently see a sudden cessation of the process, and in a number of instances we find that some 5 or 10 cm of a vessel's length is closed, and that the portions above and below are apparently normal"* (Buerger 1908).

Radiologic findings often correlate well with this pathologic observation (Fig. 30.6). An angiogram of the extremities often demonstrates areas of flagrantly abnormal arteries, followed by stretches of radiographically normal blood vessels.

Pearl: Thromboangiitis obliterans may begin with joint manifestations.

Comment: Recurrent episodes of large-joint arthritis and transient, migratory single joint episodes accompanied by local signs of inflammation have been described in thromboangiitis obliterans (Puechal et al. 1999). When present, joint symptoms usually precede the onset of digital ischemia. In this way, thromboangiitis obliterans resembles many other forms of vasculitis, which are often heralded by nonspecific musculoskeletal complaints, including a migratory oligoarthritis.

In thromboangiitis obliterans, the arthritis disappears with the appearance of ischemic signs, much as asthma disappears once the vasculitic phase of the Churg–Strauss syndrome begins.

Myth: Thromboangiitis obliterans may present with Raynaud's phenomenon.

Reality: A century and a half after Maurice Raynaud (1862) first described *De l'asphyxie locale et de la gangrène symétrique des extrémités* (On the local asphyxia and symmetric gangrene of the digits), there remains a tendency to lump many forms of digital ischemia under the rubric of "Raynaud's disease." Thromboangiitis obliterans causes digital ischemia equaled by few other disorders, but it is not because of Raynaud's phenomenon.

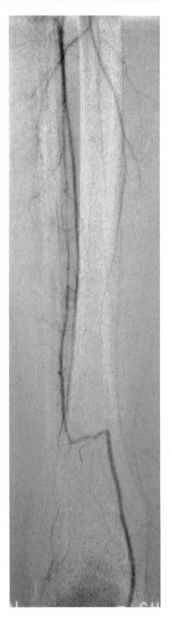

Fig. 30.6 Angiogram in thromboangiitis obliterans showing an area of normal-appearing artery distal to severely diseases vessels (Courtesy of Dr. John Stone)

Raynaud's phenomenon, so typical of "true" connective tissue disorders (i.e., systemic sclerosis, systemic lupus erythematosus, and dermatomyositis), is caused by vasospasm. This is usually induced by cold, emotional upset, and other stimuli recognized by the patient. Conversely, thromboangiitis obliterans is not the result of vasospasm but rather a highly inflammatory clot in the medium-sized arteries at the level of the wrists and ankles. The term "Raynaud's phenomenon" should not be applied to patients who have thromboangiitis obliterans, nor to any other form of vasculitis that causes digital ischemia.

Pearl: Patients who continue to smoke are the ones who lose limbs.

Comment: An analysis of 850 patients identified by a national study in Japan showed that the risk for amputation was 2.7

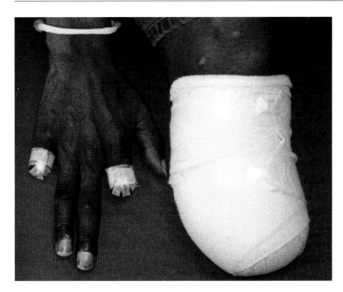

Fig. 30.7 Patients who have thromboangiitis obliterans who continue to smoke continue to lose digits and other portions of their extremities. This patient lost every finger on both hands and had bilateral below-the-knee amputations (Courtesy of Dr. John Stone)

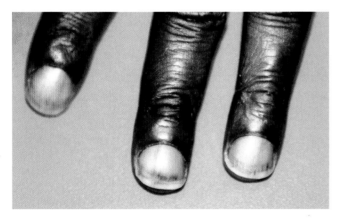

Fig. 30.8 Splinter hemorrhages at presentation in a patient who had thromboangiitis obliterans (Courtesy of Dr. John Stone)

times higher (95% confidence interval: 1.9–4.0) in patients who continued to smoke (Sasaki et al. 2000). Patients who have thromboangiitis obliterans must choose between their cigarettes and their fingers (Fig. 30.7).

Pearl: Thromboangiitis obliterans may present with splinter hemorrhages.

Comment: Endocarditis is not the only disorder that causes splinter hemorrhages. A variety of systemic vasculitides, including thromboangiitis obliterans, also cause this physical finding (Fig. 30.8) (Quenneville et al. 1981). Other vasculitides known to cause these subungual lesions are the ANCA-associated vasculitides and cryoglobulinemia.

Pearl: Extra-extremity disease occurs in thromboangiitis obliterans very rarely.

Comment: Cases of extra-extremity involvement are sufficiently rare as to constitute exceptions to the rule that parenchymal organ involvement by this disorder does not happen. Only a handful of well-documented cases of exist in which thromboangiitis obliterans has involved the vessels of the mesentery or central nervous system (Puechal and Fiessinger 2007). If a patient presents with intense digital ischemia to the virtual exclusion of ischemia in other vascular beds, think of thromboangiitis obliterans.

Pearl: The three forms of vasculitis most likely to lead to the loss of a pulse are Takayasu's arteritis, giant cell arteritis, and thromboangiitis obliterans.

Comment: Takayasu's arteritis has been termed "pulseless disease" because of the frequency with which it causes the extinction of pulses in the arms (and less often the legs) (Fig. 30.9a). Subclavian and axillary artery disease in giant cell arteritis also leads to the loss of pulses in the upper extremity. In comparison to thromboangiitis obliterans, the vascular occlusions are more proximal in Takayasu's arteritis and giant cell arteritis. Thus, the entire arm or leg is affected, and extremity claudication is a common symptom. Because of the effectiveness of collateral circulation in Takayasu's and giant cell arteritis, ischemia sufficient to cause gangrene of the extremities is seldom seen in those disorders today.

Through its involvement of medium-sized arteries at the levels of the wrist and ankles, thromboangiitis obliterans also obliterates pulses in the upper and lower extremities (Fig. 30.9b). In thromboangiitis obliterans, severe ischemic changes tend to develop in the distal extremities, usually in one or more digits of the hands or feet, often accompanied by gangrene.

Myth: Smoking must be heavy for thromboangiitis obliterans to occur.

Comment: The definitions of "heavy" vary among patients and between physicians and patients, but thromboangiitis obliterans has been reported in patients who smoke less than a pack of cigarettes a day (Fig. 30.10). Furthermore, even second-hand smoke has been implicated in thromboangiitis obliterans. Although a compelling case for thromboangiitis obliterans cannot be made without a history of cigarette exposure, there is no two-pack per day minimum requirement.

Myth: Necrotic fingertips should be amputated for pain relief and avoidance of other complications, such as infection.

Reality: Although there is nothing like timely surgical intervention for many conditions, it is usually a mistake to have a patient with digital ischemia due to thromboangiitis obliterans (or any form of vasculitis) evaluated first by a surgeon. Such patients often wind up having amputations prematurely and lose more tissue than they would have had Nature been allowed to take its course—partly redirected by smoking

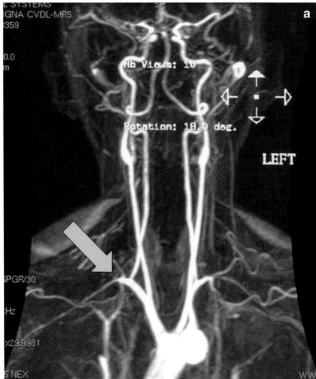

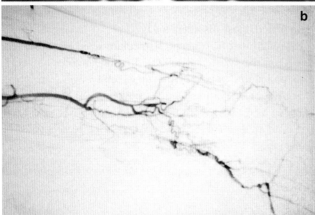

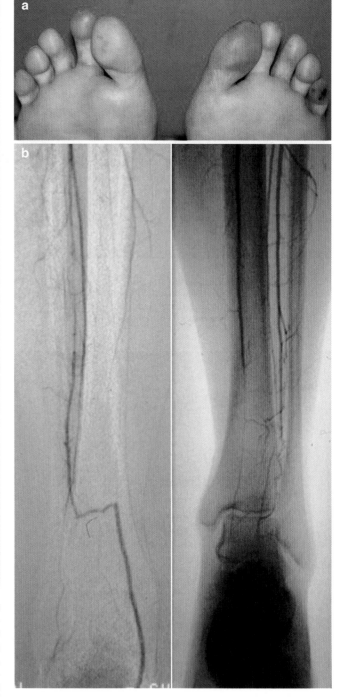

Fig. 30.9 Imaging findings in Takayasu's arteritis (**a**) as opposed to Buerger's disease (thromboangiitis obliterans) (**b**). (**a**) Magnetic resonance angiogram in Takayasu's arteritis. There is an abrupt vascular narrowing right at the take-off of the right subclavian artery, the branch of the aorta most commonly involved in Takayasu's arteritis (*arrow*). (**b**) Conventional angiogram in a patient with Buerger's disease (thromboangiitis obliterans). The image shows the radial and ulnar arteries near the level of the patient's wrist, far more distal that the typical involvement in Takayasu's. The findings include "corkscrew" collaterals and obliteration of the distal vessels. The proximal arteries (e.g., the subclavians) were normal in this patient (Courtesy of Dr. John Stone)

Fig. 30.10 Clinical picture and angiogram of thromboangiitis obliterans in an 18-year-old woman who smoked only one pack of cigarettes a day. Women can get thromboangiitis obliterans, too, and their smoking does not have to be "heavy." (**a**) Bilateral ischemia with small areas of skin necrosis in the toes. (**b**) Angiography of both lower extremities revealing dramatically damaged blood vessels, with an extent of lesions far more proximal and far worse than one would suspect from the clinical picture of the toes alone. Clinical picture and angiogram of thromboangiitis obliterans in an 18-year-old woman who smoked only one pack of cigarettes a day. Women can get thromboangiitis obliterans, too, and their smoking does not have to be "heavy" (Courtesy of Dr. John Stone)

cessation (in thromboangiitis obliterans) or immunosuppression (in other vasculitides).

Despite the sometimes hopeless appearance of digital gangrene, fingers and toes can make astonishing recoveries if the underlying inflammatory process is arrested. After a period of some months, traces of vasculitis can be difficult to find even in patients who had gangrene. Patients usually require ample support with pain medications during the resolution of these events.

References

Buerger L. Thromboangiitis obliterans: a study of the vascular lesions leading to presenile spontaneous gangrene. Am J Med Sci 1908; 136:567–80

Combemale P, Consort T, Denis-Thelis L, et al Cannabis arteritis. Br J Dermatol 2005;152:166–9

Cooper LT, Henderson SS, Ballman KV, et al A prospective, case control study of tobacco dependence in thromboangiitis obliterans (thromboangiitis obliterans). Angiology 2006;57:73–8

Cooper LT, Tse PS, Mikhail MA, et al Long-term survival and amputation risk in thromboangiitis obliterans (thromboangiitis obliterans). J Am Coll Cardiol 2004;44:2410–11

Disdier P, Swiader L, Jouglard J, et al Arterite du cannabis versus maladie de leo buerger. Discussion nosologique a propos de deux nouveaux cas. Presse Med 1999;28:71–4

Hill GL. A rational basis for management of patients with the Buerger syndrome. Br J Surg 1974;61:476–81

Hirai M, Shionoya S. Arterial obstruction of the upper limb in thromboangiitis obliterans: its incidence and primary lesion. Br J Surg 1979;66:124–8

Horton BT. The outlook in thromboangiitis obliterans. JAMA 1938; 111:2184–9

Lie JT. Thromboangiitis obliterans (Buerger's disease) in women. Medicine (Baltimore) 1987;66:65–72

O'Dell J, Linder R, Markin RS, Moore GF. Thromboangiitis obliterans (Buerger's disease) and smokeless tobacco. Arthritis Rheum 1987; 30(9):1054–6

Olin J. Thromboangiitis obliterans (Buerger's disease). N Eng J Med 2000;343:864–70

Puechal X, Fiessinger JN, Kahan A, et al Rheumatic manifestations in patients with Thromboangiitis obliterans (Buerger's disease). J Rheumatol 1999;26:1764–8

Puechal X, Fiessinger JN. Thromboangiitis obliterans or Buerger's disease: challenges for the rheumatologist. Rheumatology 2007;46:192–9

Quenneville JG, Prat A, Gossard D. Subungual-splinter hemorrhage: an early sign of thromboangiitis obliterans. Angiology 1981;32:424–32

Sasaki S, Sakuma M, Yasuda K. Current status of thromboangiitis obliterans (Buerger's disease) in Japan. Int J Cardiol 2000;75 Suppl 1:S175–81

Sterne J, Ducastaing C. [Arteritis caused by *Cannabis indica*]. Arch Mal Coeur Vaiss 1960;53:143–7

Less Common Forms of Vasculitis

31

Eric L. Matteson and John H. Stone

31.1 Cogan's Syndrome

31.1.1 Overview of Cogan's Syndrome

> The hallmark of Cogan's syndrome is the presence of ocular inflammation and audiovestibular dysfunction. These findings may be accompanied by the evidence of a systemic vasculitis that involves large blood vessels.
> Interstitial keratitis is the most common form of ocular involvement.
> Audiovestibular dysfunction may lead to the acute onset of vertigo, tinnitus, nausea, and vomiting.
> Vasculitis in Cogan's syndrome may take the form of aortitis, renal artery stenosis, or occlusion of the great vessels.

Myth: Hearing loss in Cogan's syndrome is preventable by aggressive use of glucocorticoid therapy and additional immunosuppressive agents.

Reality: It is important to recognize the limitations of current therapies for the auditory component of Cogan's syndrome. Prompt implementation of high-dose glucocorticoid treatment (1 mg/kg/day) initially results in the improvement in hearing for many patients, but severe hearing loss and deafness eventually occur in at least 50% of patients with Cogan's syndrome (Gluth et al. 2006; Mazlumzadeh and Matteson 2007). The deafness often occurs gradually, through incremental hearing losses resulting from disease "flares." Patients often recover some but not all of the hearing they possessed before an individual disease exacerbation.

After an initial 2 weeks of 1 mg/kg prednisone, it is important to taper in decrements of 5–10 mg every 1–2 weeks. In the absence of other systemic manifestations, prednisone should be reduced even more quickly (e.g., 5–10 mg/day) to avoid excessive morbidity from glucocorticoids (Fig. 31.1a, b).

There is little evidence that protracted use of high-dose glucocorticoids is effective in preserving hearing over the long term (Gluth et al. 2006; Mazlumzadeh and Matteson 2007).

A variety of adjunct therapies have been employed, including azathioprine, cyclophosphamide, methotrexate, and tumor necrosis factor (TNF) inhibitors, in efforts to improve outcomes and reduce glucocorticoid-related side effects.

Cogan's syndrome patients who suffer profound hearing loss are good candidates for cochlear implantation (Pafanisi et al. 2003). Hence, a protracted course of immunosuppressive and glucocorticoids should not be pursued, especially if there is only marginal response to treatment, and hearing loss is the major disease manifestation. Unfortunately, in some patients, refractory eye disease necessitates ongoing immunosuppression.

Pearl: If disease remission is achieved in Cogan's syndrome, treatment should never be stopped completely.

Comment: Clinicians' efforts to control most forms ocular inflammation with immunosuppression are usually rewarded. In contrast, the challenge of preventing deafness in Cogan's syndrome can be humbling (Mazlumzadeh and Matteson 2007; Riente et al. 1996). The two largest series of Cogan's syndrome patients reported to date paint discouraging pictures of the likelihood of retaining useful hearing over time. In a study from the Mayo Clinic, 42 of 60 patients became deaf in at least one ear, and 31 of 60 became completely deaf over time (Gluth 2006). In a study from France, 30 of 32 patients developed significant auditory dysfunction; 11 became completely deaf (Grasland et al. 2004).

These reports and anecdotal experiences inform the bias that patients who achieve disease control should never discontinue their treatment entirely. Useful hearing loss is usually not restored entirely by treatment. The optimal remission maintenance regimen is far from clear (to be more precise, it is entirely empirical). Remission maintenance regimens may include immunomodulating agents such as methotrexate, azathioprine, or mycophenolate mofetil, as well as low-dose glucocorticoids.

Myth: Cogan's syndrome has a specific autoantibody profile.

Reality: To date, no immune abnormality unique to Cogan's syndrome has been identified. Autoantibody testing may be performed to rule out other causes of sensorineural hearing

Fig. 31.1 Audiograms of a patient with Cogan's syndrome before and after therapy. There is typical bilateral hearing loss (**a**), and some improvement on glucocorticoid therapy 2 months later (**b**). *HL* hearing level (this is the decibel (dB) level that corresponds to the numbers on the ordinate of the audiogram); masked AC: masked air conduction threshold; masked BC: masked bone conduction threshold; *SL* sensation level (this is the dB level above the SRT, usually 25 or 40dB SL); speech reception threshold is the lowest dB level at which a patient accurately repeats common two-syllable words, such as "bottle" or "marriage" 50% of the time (Courtesy of Dr. Eric Matteson)

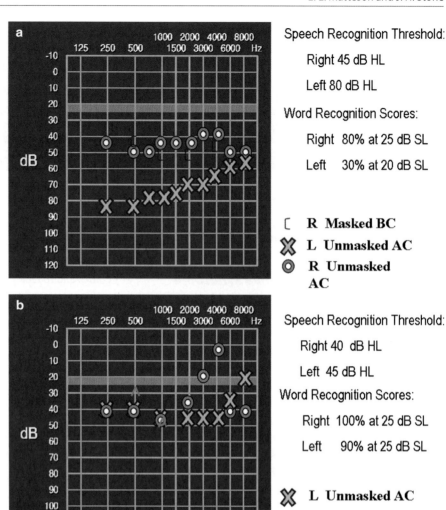

Speech Recognition Threshold:

Right 45 dB HL

Left 80 dB HL

Word Recognition Scores:

Right 80% at 25 dB SL

Left 30% at 20 dB SL

[**R Masked BC**

✕ **L Unmasked AC**

◎ **R Unmasked AC**

Speech Recognition Threshold:

Right 40 dB HL

Left 45 dB HL

Word Recognition Scores:

Right 100% at 25 dB SL

Left 90% at 25 dB SL

✕ **L Unmasked AC**

◎ **R Unmasked AC**

loss, dizziness, and eye disease in patients with suspected Cogan's syndrome, but there are no specific autoantibody tests which are present in patients with Cogan's syndrome (Mazlumzadeh and Matteson 2007). Antibodies to heat shock protein-70 have been posited as a marker of active inflammation in various forms of autoimmune inner ear disease, but the experience with this antibody testing has been disappointing.

The work-up for patients with clinical presentations compatible with Cogan's syndrome includes a slit-lamp examination, audiogram, vestibular studies, chest radiography, and a magnetic resonance imaging study to exclude acoustic neuroma and other intracranial pathology (Mazlumzadeh and Matteson 2007).

Pearl: Interstitial keratitis is the most common ocular manifestation of Cogan's syndrome.

Comment: In most cases, interstitial keratitis occurs early in the disease course and responds well to glucocorticoid eyedrops. In some cases, atropine or cyclosporine eyedrops are required (Mazlumzadeh and Matteson 2007) (Fig. 31.2a, b).

Pearl: Any kind of ocular inflammation can occur in Cogan's syndrome.

Comment: Nonsyphilitic interstitial keratitis is the classic ocular manifestation of Cogan's syndrome, but just about any type of ocular inflammation can occur in this disorder. In addition to interstitial keratitis and scleritis, other ocular lesions in Cogan's syndrome include conjunctivitis, episcleritis, uveitis, retinal vasculitis, orbital pseudotumor, and a pan-ophthalmitis that resembles orbital pseudotumor (Vollertsen et al. 1986).

Patients who do not have the classic interstitial keratitis at diagnosis are sometimes referred to as having "atypical" Cogan's syndrome, but it is not clear that the courses of such patients differ significantly from those of patients who have textbook presentations. If an atypical eye lesion develops before the onset of sensorineural hearing loss, the diagnosis of Cogan's syndrome is impossible to make until both ocular and auditory findings are present.

In some patients, the diagnosis of Cogan's syndrome becomes clear only when interstitial keratitis occurs following

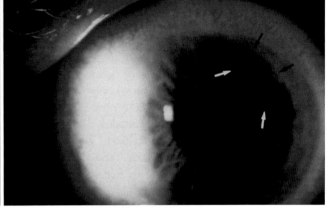

Fig. 31.2 (a, b) The eye in Cogan's syndrome. A 54-year-old man with Cogan's syndrome. There is interstitial keratitis that appears as an area of oval-shaped haziness in the upper inner quadrant of the cornea

(*arrows*). The lesion responded to glucocorticoid therapy, but the patient suffered hearing loss and eventually required cochlear implantation (note cochlear wire behind patient's left ear)

the treatment of another ocular manifestation of this disorder such as scleritis.

Pearl: Cogan's syndrome can cause meningitis.

Comment: Cogan's syndrome can be complicated by intense headaches, photophobia, and neck stiffness. Lumbar puncture in such cases often reveals a lymphocytic pleocytosis. The presentation raises obvious concerns about infections (opportunistic or otherwise), but following the appropriate exclusion of microbial pathogens the meningitis responds promptly to glucocorticoids.

31.2 Erythema Elevatum Diutinum

31.2.1 Overview of Erythema Elevatum Diutinum

- Erythema elevatum diutinum (EED) is an extremely rare form of small-vessel vasculitis that leads to the formation of distinctive nodules or papules, usually over the extensor surfaces of joints.
- New lesions come in the form of tender papules that are associated with pruritus or a burning sensation.
- Lesions develop into red, reddish-brown, or purple papules or nodules, and may coalesce to form large plaques.

Pearl: The skin lesions of EED usually appear on the extensor surfaces, especially near joints of the hands, elbows, knees, and ankles.

Comment: EED lesions are usually symptomatic at onset, with itching and burning in affected areas (Gibson and El-Azhary 2000). They are initially tender to touch in many

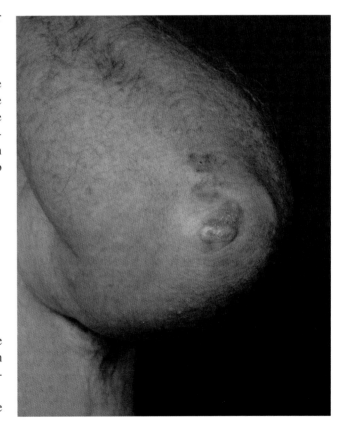

Fig. 31.3 Erythematous, firm, papular, and nodular lesions over the elbow of a 54-year-old male with EED. (Courtesy of Dr. L.E. Gibson, Mayo Clinic)

patients. The skin lesions of EED can be reddish, purplish, and yellowish cutaneous papules, plaques, and nonblanching nodules, occurring preferentially over the extensor surfaces, especially near joints of the hands, elbows, knees, and ankles (Fig. 31.3). They may also occur on the trunk and scalp.

Myth: EED is a systemic vasculitis.

Reality: EED is a rare form of chronic, recurring cutaneous leukocytoclastic vasculitis. It is frequently associated with a variety of underlying infectious, malignant, autoimmune conditions, but it is not a systemic vasculitis *sui generis*. EED is believed to be secondary to immune complex deposition, which can occur in the context of a number of underlying disorders (Gibson and El-Azhary 2000; Wahl et al. 2005).

Pathogens associated with EED include the human immunodeficiency virus (HIV), hepatitis B and C, *Treponema pallidum*, *Mycobacterium tuberculosis*, and *Streptococcus* species. EED had also been reported in hematopoietic malignancies such as lymphoma, myelodysplasia, and the POEMS syndrome (polyneuropathy, organomegaly, endocrinopathy, monoclonal gammopathy, and skin changes). Autoimmune conditions with which EED is associated include Crohn's disease, celiac disease, relapsing polychondritis, Wegener's granulomatosis, rheumatoid arthritis, pyoderma gangrenosum, and type 1 diabetes mellitus.

Pearl: The optimal therapy for EED is treatment of the underlying condition.

Comment: Amelioration of the underlying condition improves EED (presumably) by decreasing the formation of immune complexes related to the underlying disease (Gibson and El-Azhary 2000; Wahl et al. 2005). This explanation is compatible with the best current hypothesis about disease pathogenesis, but is likely incomplete.

Dapsone is also effective in treating many cases of EED. Other therapies have included antibiotics, colchicine, glucocorticoids (intralesional, topical, or oral), niacinamide, and chloroquine. In patients who have advanced fibrotic skin disease, these interventions are less effective than when used in patients with early skin lesions.

Pearl: EED lesions are most likely to respond to therapy if they are treated early.

Comment: EED is a chronic disease that can present as an acute leukocytoclastic vasculitis. The histopathologic features are a diffuse, mixed cellular infiltrate with polymorphonuclear cell infiltration of the vessel wall, nuclear dust, and spindle cells (histiocytes, fibroblasts, and myofibroblasts) (Figs. 31.4 and 31.5) (Gibson and El-Azhary 2000). In the later stages of disease evolution, the lesions become fibrotic and contain lipid deposits (Fig. 31.6a, b). At this advanced stage, the skin lesions respond poorly to treatment.

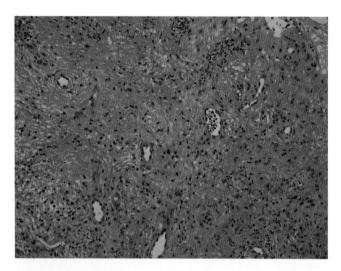

Fig. 31.4 Photomicrograph (hematotoxin and eosin staining) demonstrating leukocytoclastic vasculitis with a diffuse dermal mixed cellular infiltrate in EED. (Courtesy of Dr. L.E. Gibson, Mayo Clinic)

31.3 Urticarial Vasculitis

31.3.1 Overview of Urticarial Vasculitis

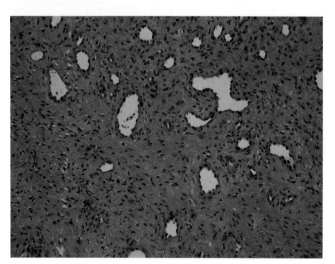

Fig. 31.5 Photomicrograph (hematotoxin and eosin staining) demonstrating more mature changes as vascular damage and polymorphonuclear cell infiltrate is replaced by a fibrosing response in EED. (Courtesy of Dr. L.E. Gibson, Mayo Clinic)

- Urticarial vasculitis can be divided into a form associated with normal complement levels and a form associated with hypocomplementemia.
- Normocomplementemic patients are likely to have a self-limited course that resembles hypersensitivity vasculitis. In contrast, hypocomplementemic patients are more likely to have chronic disease.
- The lesions of urticarial vasculitis are frequently associated with burning or pain rather than pruritus and require more than 24 h to resolve.
- Hypocomplementemic urticarial vasculitis has many similarities to systemic lupus erythematosus (SLE), and is considered by some to be part of the SLE spectrum.

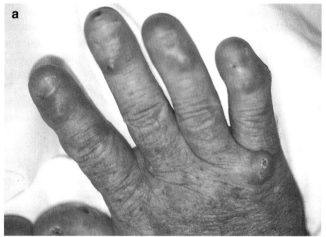

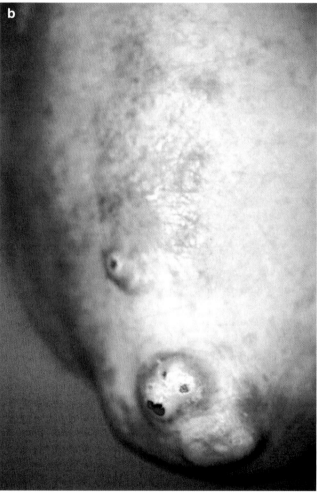

Fig. 31.6 Advanced lesions of EED over the knuckles (**a**) and elbow (**b**). Lesions that have become indurated are typically refractory to therapy (Courtesy of Dr. John Stone)

- Patients with hypocomplementemic urticarial vasculitis can develop a number of features that are atypical of SLE, including scleritis and chronic obstructive pulmonary disease.

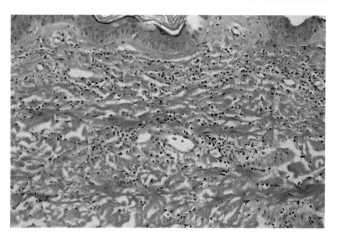

Fig. 31.7 Photomicrograph (hematoxylin and eosin staining) demonstrating leukocytoclastic vasculitis in a skin biopsy from a patient with normocomplementemic urticarial vasculitis. Red blood cell extravasation, leukocyte fragmentation, and perivascular infiltrate composed mostly of neutrophils in the background of dermal edema are seen. These findings can be present in any type of leukocytoclastic vasculitis that involves small blood vessels. (Courtesy of Dr. L.E. Gibson, Mayo Clinic)

- Hypocomplementemic urticarial vasculitis is associated with heritable deficiencies of complement in some patients.
- Direct immunofluorescence of a skin biopsy specimen is the critical test. Intense staining for immunoreactants (i.e., IgG, IgM, C3, C4, and C1q) is found not only in and around small blood vessel walls but also in a ribbon along the dermal/epidermal junction. In the proper clinical setting, these findings are diagnostic of hypocomplementemic urticarial vasculitis.

Myth: All forms of urticarial vasculitis are alike.

Reality: The critical distinction between the two major forms of urticarial vasculitis is whether or not the patient is hypocomplementemic, based on the measurements of C3, C4, and total complement (CH50). Normocomplementemic urticarial vasculitis is viewed most appropriately as a subset of cutaneous leukocytoclastic angiitis (hypersensitivity vasculitis) in which the skin manifestation of small-vessel vasculitis takes the form of urticaria rather than the more familiar palpable purpura. The histopathologic features of normocomplementemic urticarial vasculitis are shown in Fig. 31.7.

Normocomplementemic urticarial vasculitis normally as a self-limited course whether or not the underlying stimulus – often a medication – can be identified and removed. In chronic cases, normocomplementemic ultraviolet must be distinguished carefully from neutrophilic urticaria, a persistent form of urticaria not associated with vasculitis (Mehregan et al. 1992; Davis et al. 1998; Davis and Brewer 2004; Toppe et al. 1998).

In contrast to the normocomplementemic variant, hypocomplementemic urticarial vasculitis represents a unique form of small-vessel vasculitis that is characterized by a high likelihood of extracutaneous manifestations. Hypocomplementemic urticarial vasculitis often occurs with other disease features that suggest an SLE-like illness. In such cases, the term *hypocomplementemic urticarial vasculitis syndrome* is sometimes used (Wisnieski et al. 1995).

Myth: Patients with urticarial vasculitis must be treated with prednisone.

Reality: Urticarial vasculitis patients have urticarial lesions that usually persist more than 24 h can be painful, and frequently resolve with residual pigmentation in the skin. The infiltrate is neutrophilic, as opposed to the lymphocytes seen in most patients with cutaneous lupus. Patients who have low complement levels frequently have SLE as the underlying disease. For patients with skin-predominant disease, colchicine and dapsone can be an effective therapy and patients may not always need treatment with prednisone (Sunderkötter et al. 2005).

A G6PD should be checked before starting dapsone to make sure that the patient can metabolize the drug. Dapsone is usually begun at a dose of 50 mg/day if baseline blood count and liver function tests are normal. The dose is titrated up by 25 mg/day each week, as long as the weekly hemoglobin and liver functions tests are fine. A target dose is normally 150 mg/day, but may be less if control is achieved at a lower dose. After attaining the maximum stable dose, laboratories are checked monthly for 3 months, and thereafter every 3 months.

Pearl: Patients with urticarial vasculitis who have low complements are more likely to have severe, systemic, and treatment-resistant disease.

Comment: Patients with normal complementemic urticarial vasculitis have good prognoses with waxing and waning disease courses that usually resolve within 1–4 years. Patients with hypocomplementemic urticarial vasculitis are more likely to have a systemic underlying disease and to have clinical manifestations that require ongoing therapy.

Pearl: Many patients with urticarial vasculitis (with or without hypocomplementemia) experience tenderness, burning, and pruritus. This contrasts with common urticaria that is neither tender nor painful.

Comment: Common chronic urticaria is associated with itching but not pain (Mehregan et al. 1992; Davis et al. 1998). On physical examination, the lesions of urticarial vasculitis can be differentiated from chronic urticaria by applying a magnifying glass or glass slide to the skin (diascopy). Diascopy reveals a central, dark brown or red macule, indicative of the purpuric nature of urticaria. This finding is absent in chronic urticaria.

The lesions of urticarial vasculitis typically last for 1–3 days. In contrast, the lesions of chronic urticaria generally resolve within 24 h of their first appearance. Whereas chronic urticarial lesions resolve without skin discoloration, hyperpigmentation is often observed following the resolution of the lesions of urticarial vasculitis, particularly if the lesions recur multiple times (more likely among patients with hypocomplementemia) (Fig. 31.8a–c).

Pearl: Urticarial lesions persisting for more than 48 h are more likely to be related to an underlying vasculitis than such lesions of shorter duration.

Comment: Common urticaria is encountered far more commonly in clinical practice than urticarial vasculitis. Urticaria can be troubling and even disabling, but does not require (or respond to) the type of therapy used in urticarial vasculitis. Thus, it is critical to distinguish these two conditions. Aside from the duration of skin lesions, indications that urticaria may be associated with vasculitis include a stinging or burning component to the symptoms, rather than mere pruritus. In addition, visual inspection or diascopy reveals a purpuric component to the urticarial lesions in vasculitis (Fig. 31.9), and laboratory studies may reveal hypocomplementemia.

One other word of caution with regard to urticarial vasculitis is in order. Neutrophilic urticaria, a nonvasculitic condition, is readily confused histopathologically with the leukocytoclastic vasculitis associated with urticarial vasculitis. Having the skin biopsy reviewed by an experienced dermatopathologist is usually worthwhile.

Pearl: To establish the diagnosis of urticarial vasculitis, skin biopsy should be performed of a recent lesion.

Comment: It is helpful to obtain two punch biopsies (Davis et al. 1998). Because the lesions of urticarial vasculitis are in the superficial dermis, punch biopsies usually suffice for diagnosis. Each punch biopsy should be cut in half. One half should be sent for formalin fixation and for hematoxylin and eosin staining. The second half should be placed into liquid nitrogen without formalin fixation and sent for direct immunofluorescence. The immunoreactants worth testing for on DIF are C3, C4, C1q, IgG, IgA, and IgM.

Repeat biopsies of new lesions are occasionally required to confirm the diagnosis of urticarial vasculitis.

Pearl: The major entities from which hypocomplementemic urticarial vasculitis must be distinguished are Henoch–Schönlein purpura, cryoglobulinemia, and hypersensitivity vasculitis.

Comment: The legs in Fig. 31.10a, b could belong to a patient with any of those other three disorders. These are the legs of a 77-year-old man who had extensive palpable purpura on the lower extremities, trunk, and upper extremities. A direct immunofluorescence study of his skin biopsy showed granular deposition of C3, C4, IgG, and IgM along the dermal–epidermal junction and around small blood vessels in the superficial dermis.

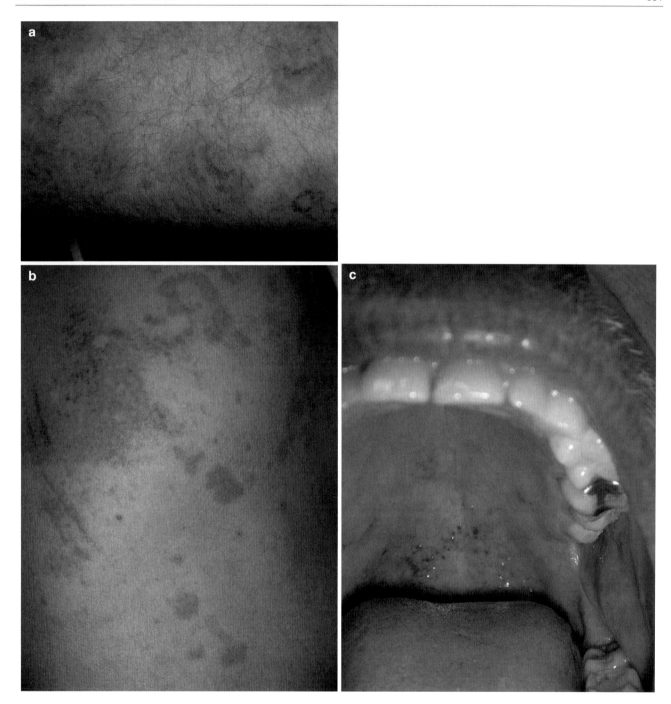

Fig. 31.8 Urticarial vasculitic lesions of 3 days' duration in a 52-year-old male with an 8-year history of rheumatoid arthritis. (**a**) The lesions on the leg are moderately pruritic and painful, raised, erythematous, and develop central clearing with resolution. Where red blood cell extrava-sation has occurred, they are nonblanching. (**b**) Trunk of same patient with scratch efflorescences. (**c**) Purpuric lesions on the soft palate. (Courtesy of Dr. Eric Matteson)

Pearl: The level of complement C1q is low in most patients with hypocomplementemic urticarial vasculitis.

Comment: In hypocomplementemic urticarial vasculitis, any one or all of the complements involved in the classic complement pathway may be reduced (Davis et al. 1998; Davis and Brewer 2004). This includes total complement, C1, C1q, C2, C3, and C4.

Myth: Hypocomplementemic urticarial vasculitis is almost always associated with a systemic underlying disease.

Reality: Most cases of hypocomplementemic urticarial vasculitis are idiopathic, just as SLE is idiopathic (Mehregan et al. 1992; Davis et al. 1998). Thorough histories, physical examinations, and extensive laboratory evaluations are conducted in most patients with this disorder, but at the end of it

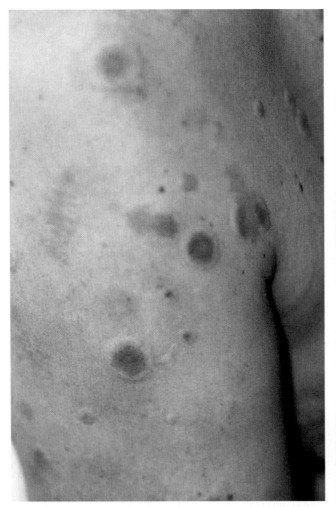

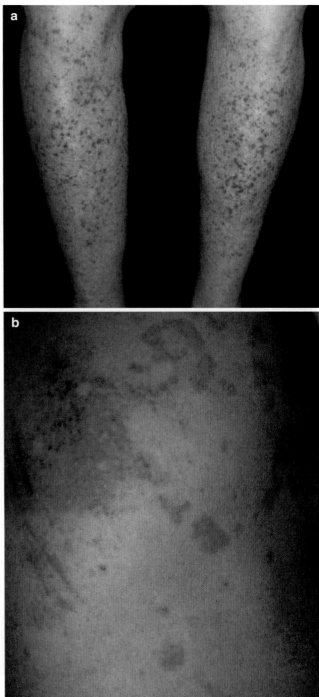

Fig. 31.9 This urticarial lesion has a central purpuric component, suggestive of an underlying vasculitic nature (Courtesy of Dr. John Stone)

all the proper conclusion in most patients is that an independent disorder is present and there lurks no occult malignancy, infection, or other idiopathic inflammatory disorder as a rational explanation.

In contrast, normocomplementemic urticarial vasculitis has multiple potential causes: the lengthy list of disorders that can cause hypersensitivity vasculitis.

Pearl: Eye findings can help distinguish between hypocomplementemic urticarial vasculitis and SLE.

Comment: Scleritis is a common ocular complication of hypocomplementemic urticarial vasculitis (Fig. 31.11). This complication is highly atypical of lupus.

Fig. 31.10 Palpable purpura in a patient with hypocomplementemic urticarial vasculitis involving (**a**) the lower extremities, (**b**) trunk, and upper extremities (not shown) (Courtesy of Dr. John Stone)

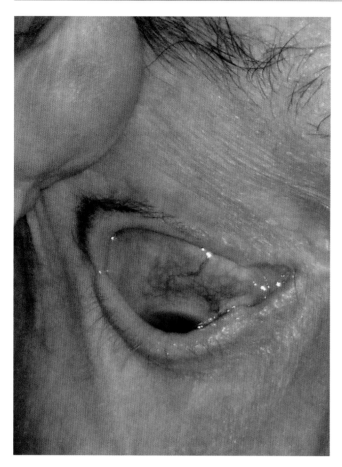

Fig. 31.11 Scleritis in a patient with hypocomplementemic urticarial vasculitis. (Courtesy of Dr. John Stone.)

References

Davis MD, Brewer JD. Urticarial vasculitis and hypocomplementemic urticarial vasculitis syndrome. Immunol Allergy Clin North Am 2004;24:183

Davis MDP, Daoud MS, Kirby B, et al Clinicopathologic correlation of hypocomplementemic and normocomplementemic urticarial vasculitis. J Am Acad Dermatol 1998;38:899

Gibson LE, El-Azhary RA. Erythema elevatum diutinum. Clin Dermatol 2000;18:295–99

Gluth MB, Baratz KH, Matteson EL, et al Cogan's syndrome: a retrospective review of 60 patients throughout a half-century. Mayo Clin Proc 2006;81:483–8

Grasland A, Pouchot P, Hachulla E, et al Typical and atypical Cogan's syndrome: 32 cases and review of the literature. Rheumatology 2004;43:1007–15

Mazlumzadeh M, Matteson EL. Cogan's syndrome: an audiovestibular, ocular, and systemic autoimmune disease. Rheum Dis Clin North Am 2007;33:855–74

Mehregan DR, Hall MJ, Gibson LE. Urticarial vasculitis: a histopathologic and clinical review of 72 cases. J Am Acad Dermatol 1992;26(3 Pt 2):441–8

Pafanisi, Pafanisi E, Vincenti V, et al Cochlear implantation and Cogan's syndrome. Otol Neurotol 2003;24:601–4

Riente L, Taglione E, Berrettini S. Efficacy of methotrexate in Cogan's syndrome. J Rheumatol 1996;23:1830–1

Sunderkötter C, Bonsmann G, Sindrilaru A, et al Management of leukocytoclasticvasculitis. J Dermatol Treat 2005;16:193–206

Toppe E, Haas N, Henz BM. Neutrophilic urticaria: clinical features, histologic changes, and possible mechanisms. Br J Dermatol 1998;138:248–53

Vollertsen R, McDonald T, Younge B, et al Cogan's syndrome: 18 cases and a review of the literature. Mayo Clin Proc 1986;61: 344–61

Wahl CE, Bouldin MB, Gibson LE. Erythema elevatum diutinum: clinical, histopathologic, and immunohistochemical characteristics of six patients. Am J Dermatopathol 2005;27:397–400

Wisnieski JJ, Baer AN, Christensen J, et al Hypocomplementemic urticarial vasculitis syndrome: clinical and serologic findings in 18 patients. Medicine 1995;74:24–41

Relapsing Polychondritis

32

Harvinder S. Luthra

32.1 Overview of Relapsing Polychondritis

> Relapsing polychondritis (RP) is a multisystem inflammatory disease of unknown etiology in which the cartilaginous structures of the ears, nose, trachea, and joints are the main sites of damage.
> A variety of other organs and tissues, including the eyes, heart, and blood vessels, can also be affected by RP.
> Clues from human and animal studies suggest that cartilage components may be the antigens driving the immune response, leading to damage from the resulting inflammation.
> First described by Jaksch–Wartenhorst (1923), more than 500 patients with RP have been reported in the medical literature.
> RP has a worldwide distribution.
> Some RP cases are associated with other conditions, particularly myelodysplastic syndromes and connective tissue disorders such as rheumatoid arthritis or systemic lupus erythematosus.

32.2 Ear Involvement

Pearl: Inflammatory changes in RP are localized to the cartilaginous part of the external ear, the pinna, and do not involve the noncartilaginous area: the lobule (Fig. 32.1a).

Comment: The ear is the most common site of inflammation in RP. Inflammation can involve the outer, middle, and inner ear. The pinna is the most commonly involved part of the ear; the inflammation in RP localizes to the cartilagenous portion of the ear, sparing the lobule. If the lobule is inflamed, one should consider other diagnosis such as cellulitis. The acutely inflamed pinna is warm to touch, exquisitely tender, and painful to move in any direction.

The pinna may return to its normal shape between attacks or remain thick because of the fibrosis that has occurred during the period of acute inflammation. In some cases, one may find in the pinna bony hard changes that are a reflection of previously active disease, some of which may have been subclinical (Fig. 32.1b) (Kent et al. 2004).

Myth: Hearing loss in RP is irreversible.

Reality: The auditory canal comprises the cartilaginous structure in the outer third of the ear. This portion can become inflamed in RP (see Fig. 32.1a). Similarly, the Eustachian tube is cartilaginous in its medial two-thirds of the canal. Inflammation in the auditory canal or in the Eustachian tube can lead to conductive hearing loss. Nerve deafness caused by dysfunction of the auditory nerve has been described in RP and is presumed to be secondary to "vasculitis" of the internal auditory artery. Histologic proof of vasculitis in such cases is lacking because of the general inaccessibility of the inner ear (see Chap. 39).

Both conductive and sensorineural hearing loss in RP generally responds well to therapy, particularly if treatment is initiated early.

Pearl: Occasionally, patients with RP develop hearing difficulties along with vertigo.

Comment: This combination of symptoms usually reflects inner ear disease. These symptoms may be mild and may be ignored by the patient. On the other hand, these may be severe enough to cause nausea, vomiting, difficulty sitting up in a chair or bed, standing, and walking. As noted above, the occurrence of inner ear symptoms in RP is presumed to be related to a vasculopathy (and possibly vasculitis) of the cochlear and/or vestibular branch of the internal auditory artery. Endolymphatic hydrops may occur in this setting (Murata et al. 2006).

Such complications require urgent intervention with immunosuppressive therapy, typically high doses of glucocorticoids.

Myth: Nasal bridge collapse cannot be surgically repaired because of the inherently fragile tissue and the risk of inducing a disease flare.

Reality: Nasal involvement in RP is very common and may affect as many as 54% of patients. Nasal disease can present in a subacute manner as mild tenderness or redness of the nasal

J. H. Stone (ed.), *A Clinician's Pearls and Myths in Rheumatology*,
DOI:10.1007/978-1-84800-934-9_32, © Springer Science + Business Media B.V. 2009

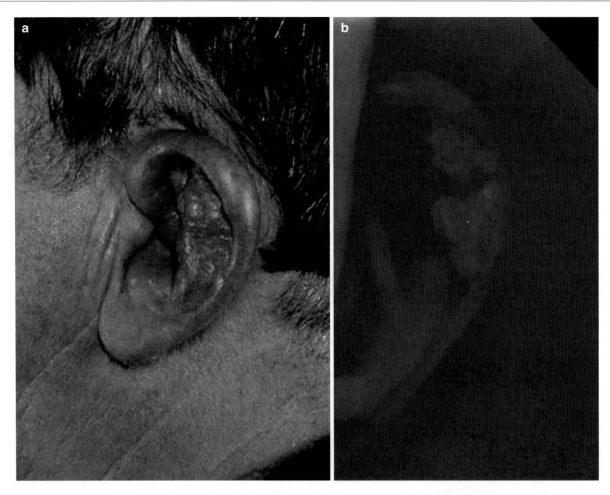

Fig. 32.1 (**a**) Involvement of the pinna is the most common manifestation of RP. Note involvement of the cartilagenous portions of the pinna and the external auditory canal while sparing of the lobule. (**b**) Ossification of the cartilage in a patient with recurrent attacks of RP

bridge and tip of the nose. Alternatively, it may appear rapidly in a day or so. In many patients with RP, nasal disease resolves either spontaneously or with modest degrees of treatment, with no residual damage. In others, however, nasal disease leads to collapse of the nasal bridge due to inflammatory changes in the cartilage, resulting in a saddle nose deformity (Fig. 32.2a>).

Because of its cosmetic implications, there is generally a strong desire on the part of the patient to have a surgical repair of the nose. Surgery should be undertaken only when the disease is under excellent control and the patient is maintained on minimal immunosuppression (Fig. 32.2b, c) (Cody and Sones 1971).

Pearl: Respiratory symptoms should always be taken seriously.

Comment: Patients with RP often develop hoarseness, nonproductive cough, wheezing, dyspnea, or stridor. There is frequently little correlation between the severity of symptoms and the extent of laryngotrachael involvement. Most of these patients have inflammation of the cartilaginous structures and the soft tissues surrounding them.

A routine chest radiograph can show narrowing of the tracheal outline (Fig. 32.3a). Appreciation of this abnormality can be accentuated if a tomogram (i.e., computed tomography (CT)) is performed (Fig. 32.3b). All RP patients should have flow-volume loops performed on their first visit, with follow-up comparisons every 6–12 months. Flow-volume loops help determine if the patient has an obstructive pattern to the air flow, consistent with the presence of a stricture or fixed narrowing.

In every patient who has an abnormal flow-volume loop study, in patients in whom the flow-volume loop study worsens on follow-up, and in all patients who have respiratory symptoms, further investigations of the airway are very important. CT scans of the airway can show thickening of the airway wall, which leads eventually to airway narrowing. The thickening is considered a reflection of the inflammatory process (Fig. 32.4a).

Cartilage calcification, if present, reflects sequelae of old inflammation. Dynamic CT scanning at end-inspiration and end-expiration can help evaluate the collapsibility of the airway. Direct laryngoscopy (Fig. 32.4b) can be helpful in the

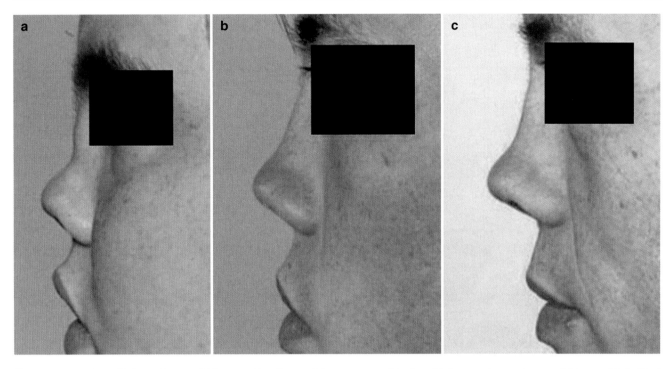

Fig. 32.2 (**a**) Patient with RP at the age of 16 years with collapse of the bridge of the nose due to destruction of the cartilage. (**b**) Same patient at the age of 19 years, after plastic repair. He was off all therapy for over a year at this time. (**c**) Same patient at the age of 47 years. He had had no further attacks of nasal chondritis

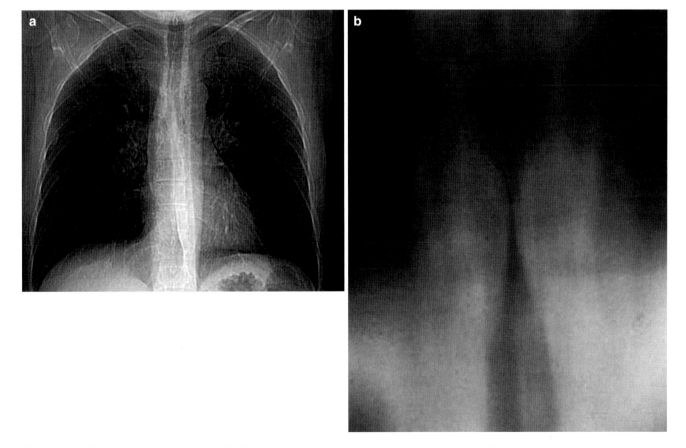

Fig. 32.3 (**a**) Chest radiograph of a patient with RP. Note the narrowing of the trachea and main bronchi. (**b**) Tomogram of a patient with subglottic stenosis

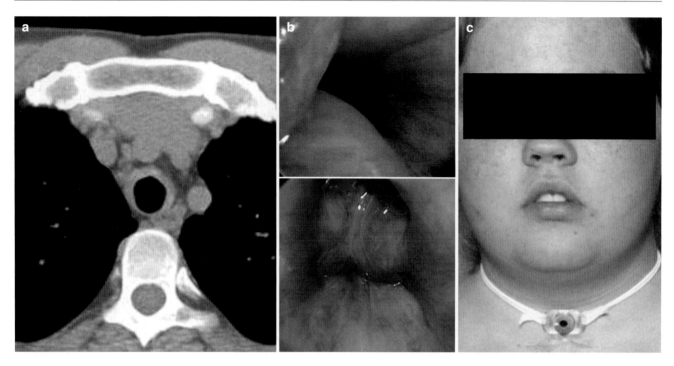

Fig. 32.4 (**a**) CT scan of a patient with tracheal involvement in RP. Note the thickness of the tracheal wall from inflammation. (**b**) Direct laryngoscopy of a patient with RP showing subglottic stenosis. (**c**) Patient with RP with traschestomy in place

assessment of the upper airway, but bronchoscopy is used for more detailed examination. Bronchoscopy should be performed with great caution in patients with airway narrowing. Both the patient and family must be prepared for the possibility of tracheostomy in the event of a complicated procedure, because complete or near-complete obstruction of the airway can occur very rapidly. (Fig. 32.4c) (Staats et al. 2002; Ernst et al. 2009).

Pearl: Recurrent pneumonias or bronchiectasis may reflect a narrowed or collapsed bronchus.

Comment: In RP, the pulmonary parenchyma is spared and does not become involved by the disease process. However, there are circumstances in which a patient may experience recurrent episodes of pneumonias or give a history of a chronic, productive cough. In such circumstances, one should suspect the presence of a stenotic or collapsed bronchus (Fig. 32.5). In such circumstances a balloon dilation, stenting, or even resection of that segment need to be considered.

Significant respiratory involvement should be managed by the rheumatologist in partnership with a pulmonologist.

Pearl: Any surgical repairs of cardiovascular lesions should be undertaken when disease is under control.

Comment: RP can involve the heart and great vessels. In the heart, the aortic root dilation resulting in aortic regurgitation is the most common manifestation. Other manifestations of the heart include conduction abnormalities and mitral valve regurgitation due to mitral valve prolapse. This occurs

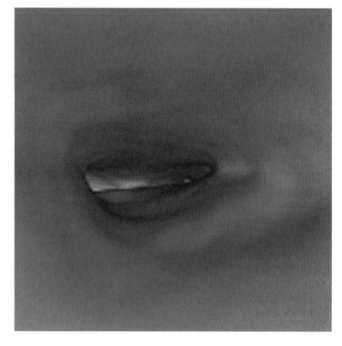

Fig. 32.5 3D reconstructed image of the bronchus showing the severity of narrowing

because of the inflammatory process that involves the media, leading to vascular destruction.

In cases of significant cardiac valve disease (or dilation of the aorta leading to secondary valvular dysfunction), many patients require valve replacements as well as vascular grafts. Valve-sparing surgeries can be performed in some patients if the process is diagnosed in sufficient time, before valvular damage ensues. Whenever possible, surgical therapy should be deferred until such time that the vascular inflammation is controlled, usually with glucocorticoids and often with other immunosuppressive medications (Esdaile et al. 1977; Dib et al. 2006; Barretto et al. 2002).

References

Barretto S, Oliveira GH, Michet CJ, Nyman M, Edwards WD, Kullo IJ. Multiple cardiovascular complications in a patient with relapsing polychondritis. Mayo Clin Proc. 2002;77:971–4

Cody DTR, Sones DA. Relapsing polychondritis: audiovestibular manifestations. Laryngoscope. 1971;81:1208–22

Dib C, Moustafa SE, Mookadam M, Zehr K, Michet CJ, Mookadam F. Surgical treatment of the cardiac manifestations of relapsing polychondritis. Mayo Clin Proc. 2006;81:772–6

Ernst A, Rafeq S, Boiselle P, Sung A, Reddy C, et al Relapsing polychondritis and airway involvement. Chest 2009;135:1024–30

Esdaile J, Hawkins D, Gold P, Freedman SO, Duguid WP. Vascular involvement in relapsing polychondritis. Can Med Assoc J. 1977;1019–22

Jaksch-Wartenhorst R. Polychondropathia. Wien Arch F Inn Med. 1923;6:93–100

Kent PD, Michet CJ, Luthra HS. Relapsing polychondritis. Curr Opin Rheumatol. 2004;16:56–61

Murata J, Horii A, Tamura M, et al Endolymphatic hydrops as a cause of audio-vestibular manifestations of relapsing polychondritis. Acta Otolaryngol. 2006;126:548–52

Staats BA, Utz JP, Michet CJ. Relapsing polychondritis. Sem Resp Crit Care Med. 2002;23:145–54

Fibromyalgia

33

Daniel Clauw and Don L. Goldenberg

33.1 Overview of Fibromyalgia

> Fibromyalgia (FM) is a soft tissue pain syndrome that has been estimated to affect 4% of the U.S. population.

> Precursor terms such as "neurasthenia" and "fibrositis" were used as early as the nineteenth century. The controversy about whether FM is a disorder of the mind or of the body still rages.

> The American College of Rheumatology (ACR) criteria for the classification of FM include a history of chronic, widespread body pain and at least 11 of 18 designated tender points on physical examination.

> Patients with FM often have a variety of nonspecific complaints. As examples, fatigue, paresthesias, irritable bowel complaints, subjective swelling of the hands and feet, sleep disturbances, migraine headaches, and deficits of attention and memory are reported commonly in FM.

> Exercise is a critical part of therapy for FM.

Myth: FM is a psychiatric disorder.

Reality: There is a higher rate of psychiatric disorders in FM patients compared with the general population. Depression and anxiety are the disorders most commonly associated with FM. However, FM 0is not a psychiatric illness. At the time of the diagnosis of FM, mood disturbances are present in 30–50% of patients with FM (Table 33.1) (Arnold et al. 2004a, b).

Estimates of the prevalence of psychiatric disturbances among patients with FM are probably elevated artifactually because of the fact that most studies of the disorder have been performed in tertiary care centers. Community-dwelling individuals who fulfill the ACR criteria for the classification of FM have a much lower rate of identifiable psychiatric conditions (White et al. 2002).

In short, rheumatologists should not get off the hook simply by regarding FM as a psychiatric disorder (Fig. 33.1).

Table 33.1 FM and mood disorders

- At the time of FM diagnosis, mood disorders (primarily depression) are present in 30–50% of cases.
- The increased prevalence of mood disorders is observed primarily in tertiary-referral patients.
- There is an increased lifetime risk or family history of mood disorders in FM compared with rheumatoid arthritis (odds ratio = 2.0).
- FM co-aggregates with major mood disorders in families (odds ratio = 1.8).

Adapted from Arnold et al. (2004b)

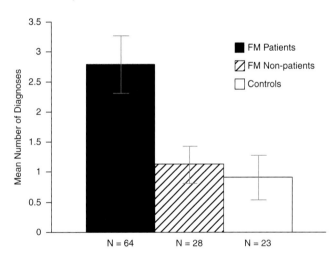

Fig. 33.1 Psychiatric disorders in FM, non-FM patients, controls. From Aaron et al. (1996)

Pearl: Dividing chronic illnesses such as FM into mutually exclusive mind or body disorders is harmful to patients and unproductive for clinicians.

Comment: There is ample evidence to suspect shared biologic and genetic factors in FM and depression. Furthermore, FM and mood disturbances often occur together. Higher rates of psychiatric disorders are reported in all chronic pain conditions, including headaches and idiopathic low back pain. The nature of the cause and effect relationship between chronic pain psychiatric disorders, especially depression, is

J. H. Stone (ed.), *A Clinician's Pearls and Myths in Rheumatology*,
DOI:10.1007/978-1-84800-934-9_33, © Springer Science + Business Media B.V. 2009

not clear. FM patients often become defensive if they believe that another doctor is "telling me it's all in my head."

Myth: FM is not the legitimate cause of chronic pain, in contradistinction to diseases such as rheumatoid arthritis. Patients with FM exaggerate their symptoms.

Reality: Such statements, often muttered in frustration even by rheumatologists, arise from the notion that illnesses are not real if they have no defined organ pathology. In such a scenario, objective findings are considered to be hard, scientific proof of a person's suffering. In contrast, subjective symptoms are regarded as "soft" and prone to "interpretation" by the patient and physician. Assigning such a disease hierarchy creates a second-class status for many common chronic illnesses, including FM, but also for headaches, low back pain, chronic neck and shoulder pain, chronic fatigue, and mood disorders (Table 33.1).

Pearl: Physicians should accept FM symptoms as real.

Comment: Health care professionals no longer question the legitimacy of conditions such as depression or headaches, even though they cannot see evidence that these conditions are "real." FM should be regarded in the same context as these conditions. A biopsychologic framework fits current concepts of FM and lends itself to a comprehensive, multidisciplinary treatment program. This model takes into account the complex interaction of pain and stress. When pain causes distress, individuals function less well in their various roles. They may have difficulties with spouses, children, and work inside or outside the home. These stressors exacerbate symptoms and lead to maladaptive illness behaviors such as social isolation, cessation of pleasurable activities, and reductions in physical activity and exercise.

In the worst-case scenario, the patient becomes entangled with disability and compensation systems. These programs almost guarantee that the patient will not improve (Hadler 1996). If a patient senses that his/her doctor or family "does not believe" him/her – a common complaint among patients with FM – he/she may unconsciously exaggerate his/her illness behavior. However, there is no evidence that malingering is any more common in FM than in other chronic medical disorders.

Myth: FM occurs more commonly in industrialized countries and Western cultures.

Reality: The prevalence of FM is just as high in rural or non-industrialized societies as is in "developed" countries (Raspe 1992; Peleg et al. 2008; White and Thompson 2003). Individuals who have greater access to health care are more likely to present for care with symptoms of FM than are those whose access in inferior, but FM occurs as commonly in Amish communities and Bedouin tribes as it does in the general US population. In fact, the prevalence of FM is remarkably consistent in different countries and cultures, about 2–4% of most populations.

Myth: FM only occurs in women.

Reality: Gender differences in pain sensitivity and tolerance extend across the human species (Kim et al. 2004). These gender differences influence tender point counts. Women are only 1.5 times more likely than men to experience chronic widespread pain, but are 10 times more likely than men to have 11 or more tender points (Wolfe et al. 1995). Because of this, women are about 10 times more likely to meet ACR criteria for FM than are men.

Most men who have chronic widespread pain but are not tender enough to meet criteria for FM probably have the same underlying problem as the women who do. Such male FM patients are often misdiagnosed as having regional musculoskeletal disorders (e.g., chronic low back pain or cervical osteoarthritis) and therefore are treated with inappropriate medications, injections, or surgical procedures. Although men are less likely to be diagnosed with FM, the clinical features and disease outcomes do not differ significantly between the sexes (Yunus et al. 2000).

Myth: A patient must have at least 11 tender points to be diagnosed with FM.

Reality: The ACR criteria for FM were intended for use in patient classification for research studies, not clinical diagnosis. Tender points are representative of heightened pain perception rather than anatomic sites of true inflammation or tissue pathology. Thus, they are proxies for abnormal pain processing. This number of 11 tender points that is required to fulfill research diagnostic criteria is totally arbitrary.

At the time the ACR criteria were formulated, it was thought that the location of tender points might have diagnostic significance. In fact, the concept of "control points" was coined to describe areas of the body that should not be tender, even in patients with FM. Individuals who were tender at such control points were assumed to have a psychologic cause of their pain. Since the ACR criteria were published, it has become clear that tenderness in FM patients extends throughout the entire body and is not confined inevitably to specific body regions (albeit tenderness is more common in some areas than in others). We now know that, relative to a non-FM patient, these regions such as the thumb nail and the forehead are just as tender as areas of tender points – it is just that everyone is more tender at tender point regions (Petzke et al. 2001; Granges and Littlejohn 1993; Cohen and Quintner 1993).

Pearl: The laying on of hands is important. Formal tender point examinations are not.

Comment: The recognition that an individual has tenderness that is diffuse and not confined to the joints is helpful in diagnosing FM. Clinicians should incorporate this approach into

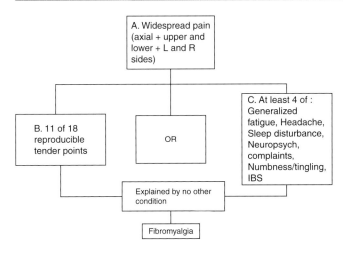

Fig. 33.2 Structured interview with or without a tender point examination for FM

Table 33.2 Laboratory evaluation in FM

In most patients:
Erythrocyte sedimentation rate or C-reactive protein
Complete blood count
Thyroid function tests
In some patients: serum hepatic aminotransferases, creatine kinase
Avoid:
Serologic screening tests (e.g., antinuclear antibodies and rheumatoid factor) clinical suspicion for a systemic connective tissue disease exists
Extensive neurologic testing, radiographs, or other imaging unless clinical picture warrants

their physical examination routines, using the same degree of pressure on all patients to get a sense of any individual patient's pain threshold. This combines a general assessment of a patient's pain threshold with a specific examination of the joints affected in inflammatory or noninflammatory arthritis.

Some investigators have suggested guidelines to diagnose FM using a structured interview, without performing a tender point examination (Fig. 33.2) (Pope et al. 1991). Even if no formal tender point examination is performed, in our experience, patients find "the laying on of hands" an essential part of the evaluation process.

Pearl: The most critical parts of the FM evaluation are the history and physical examination.

Comment: Diagnosing FM efficiently and confidently requires considerable clinical acumen and breadth of experience. FM patients often have symptoms that mimic those of inflammatory disease. These include fatigue, arthralgias, myalgias, stiffness, and the subjective swelling of the hands and feet. Certain dermatologic features commonly seen among patients with FM (e.g., flushing over the malar region, livedo reticularis, and erythema over the digits) are reminiscent of a malar rash or Raynaud's phenomenon.

Endocrine disorders that cause unexplained fatigue and muscles aches, most notably hypothyroidism, may mimic FM. It is reasonable to obtain thyroid function tests in the work-up for possible FM. Tests such as electromyography and nerve conduction velocities should be limited to patients with abnormal neurologic findings.

Pearl: Acute phase reactants should be ordered in patients suspected of FM.

Comment: The only screening tests generally recommended for FM are erythrocyte sedimentation rate, C-reactive protein, and thyroid-stimulating hormone (TSH) (Table 33.2).

Because FM is not an inflammatory condition, normal acute phase reactants immediately provide confidence that an occult inflammatory disorder is unlikely.

Myth: All patients should have routine autoantibody testing before the diagnosis of FM is considered "final" or "confirmed."

Reality: Serologic studies such as antinuclear antibody (ANA) and rheumatoid factor assays should generally be avoided, unless there are historic features or findings on physical examination that suggest diagnoses other than FM (see Table 33.2). The promiscuous use of autoantibody testing poses a major problem in clinical practice because of the high sensitivity of many autoantibody assays. "False-positive" results lead to incorrect diagnostic labels ("lupus," "rheumatoid arthritis," and "undifferentiated connective tissue disease"), further unnecessary testing and, perhaps most damaging, heightened patient anxiety (Tan et al. 1997).

The scope of the diagnostic evaluation for patients with possible FM depends upon the duration of pain and other somatic complaints, as well as the presence or the absence of specific symptoms that suggest alternative diagnoses. The only patients who require serologic studies are those with symptoms of relatively short duration (e.g., <1 year) who also have symptoms or signs that suggest an inflammatory or autoimmune disorder.

Myth: FM is due to a sleep disturbance.

Reality: One of the first biologic findings in FM was that selective sleep deprivation leads to symptoms of FM in healthy individuals (Moldofsky et al. 1975). These findings have been replicated by several groups (Older et al. 1998). However, the EEG abnormalities that were noted in this first study and initially thought to be a marker for FM, the so-called "alpha intrusions," have subsequently been found to occur in normal individuals and among patients with other conditions (Branco et al. 1994; Drewes and Svendsen 1994).

Polysomnography evaluations in FM do find a variety of nonspecific findings including fewer sleep "spindles," an increase in cyclic alternating pattern rate, upper airway resistance syndrome, and poor sleep efficiency. However, it is not clear that correction of any sleep problems identified (e.g., obstructive sleep apnea, upper airway resistance, and restless leg or periodic limb movement syndromes) result in the improvement of patients' core FM symptoms.

Myth: Patients given the "label" of FM begin to think they have an illness. This will only make them worse.

Reality: "Labeling" an individual with an illness always has the potential to increase illness behavior. Some physicians contend that the diagnosis of FM "medicalizes" everyday symptoms. However, this scenario is unlikely if the FM diagnosis is coupled with appropriate patient education, and a treatment plan that emphasizes the patient's role in improving

their symptoms. Furthermore, studies to date in FM do not suggest that health care utilization is increased following the diagnosis of FM (White et al. 2002). On the contrary, a recent study in the U.K. showed significantly *reduced* health care costs in the year following the diagnosis of FM, most likely because individuals stopped going from doctor to doctor and from test to test (Annemans et al. 2008) (Fig. 33.3).

Management of any illness begins with an accurate diagnosis. Most FM patients report that a diagnosis, even if based upon "soft" findings such as the history and physical examination, reassures them that a degenerative structural disease is not present. It also validates their sense that the problem is not in their head.

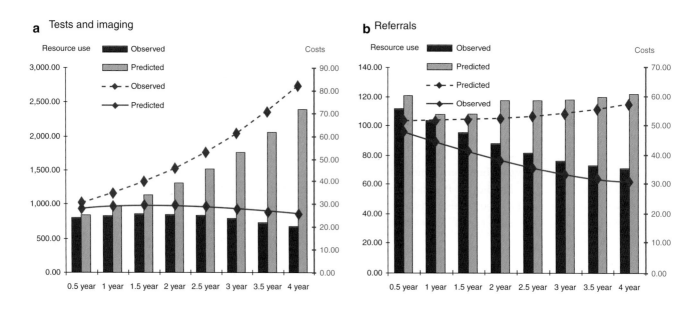

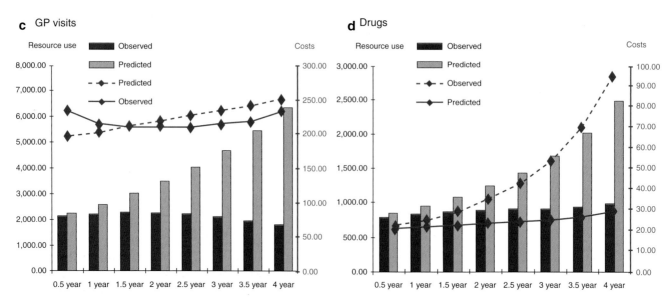

Fig. 33.3 Impact on National Health Service resources and expenses (in British pounds) of making a diagnosis of FM syndrome. (a) Tests and imaging. (b) Referrals. (c) General practitioner (GP) visits. (d) Drugs. From Annemans et al. (2008)

Pearl: Attempting to establish links between the diagnosis of FM and possible "etiologies" can be counterproductive.

Comment: Clinicians should avoid linking the diagnosis of FM to putative causes, such as an injury or exposure to an environmental toxin. In the overwhelming majority of cases, causal associations are speculative. All too often, the affirmation of such an association leads to blame, inactivity, and a sense of being victimized and litigation.

Patients establish tentative (or firm) links in their own minds about previous exposures and the development of FM, usually long before they see a rheumatologist.

Myth: Patients with FM require specialist care.

Reality: The diagnosis and management of FM should be approached like that of chronic headaches or chronic mood disturbances. FM is a chronic illness and needs to be managed as such. As with any chronic illness, management requires the imparting of appropriate information about the diagnosis to the patient, as well as both medications and non-drug therapies. Patients must exercise, follow a good diet, and become educated about self-management techniques, just as they would for the management of other disorders such as diabetes or high blood pressure. These illnesses are largely diagnosed and treated by primary care physicians. Specialists should be consulted when the diagnosis is uncertain or when the initial management has been unsuccessful.

More than half of all patient visits for FM are to primary care physicians. Specialists are involved in about 25% of cases, and 16% of FM visits are to rheumatologists. The ACR suggests that the role of rheumatologists should be primarily as consultants to primary care physicians. With an estimated 6–10 million FM patients in the U.S., rheumatologists cannot possibly accommodate the longitudinal care of all such patients. Rheumatologists should advise primary care physicians with regard to team management, which often will include other specialists such as mental health professionals, physiatrists, and pain management experts.

The close association of FM with mood disturbances mandates that every new FM patient be carefully evaluated for comorbidity of psychiatric illness. Even in patients with no psychiatric diagnosis, levels of psychosocial stressors, coping ability, and locus of control should be ascertained. Often this requires formal referral to a mental health professional.

Myth: There is no reasonable pathophysiologic explanation that accounts for the multitude of symptoms in FM.

Reality: There is substantial evidence that FM is associated with abnormalities in neural pain regulation. These data are consistent with the notion that FM and related syndromes represent biologic amplification of all sensory stimuli (Gracely et al. 2002). Functional imaging studies indicate that the insula is the most consistently hyperactive brain

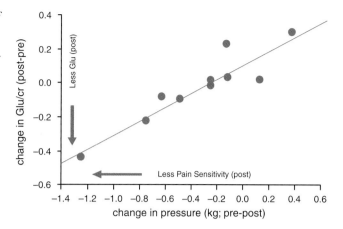

Fig. 33.4 Higher glutamate levels associated with increased FM pain. From Harris et al. (2008)

region in patients with FM (Fig. 33.4) (Harris 2008). The insula plays a critical role in sensory integration. The anterior insula is linked with the emotional processing of sensations (Tracey and Mantyh 2007). The posterior insula has a more purely sensory role.

FM should be thought of as part of functional pain disorders such as chronic fatigue syndrome, irritable bowel syndrome, chronic headaches, and chronic pelvic and bladder pain. Research indicates a strong familial component to the development of FM. First-degree relatives of individuals with FM display an eightfold greater risk of developing this condition compared with the general population (Arnold et al. 2004b). Family members of individuals with FM are also much more likely to complain of tenderness on examination than are the family members of healthy controls, regardless of whether they have pain. Family members of FM patients are also much more likely to have irritable bowel syndrome, temporomandibular dysfunction, headaches, and a host of other regional pain syndromes (Buskila et al. 1996; Hudson et al. 1985; Kato et al. 2006a, b).

This familial and personal co-aggregation of painful conditions was originally termed *affective spectrum disorder* (Hudson et al. 1993). More recently, the term *central sensitivity syndromes* and *chronic multisymptom illnesses* have been employed (Yunus, 2008; Fukuda et al. 1998). In population-based studies, the key symptoms (in addition to pain) that often co-aggregate are fatigue, memory difficulties, and mood disturbances (Fukuda et al. 1997, 1998). Twin studies suggest that about half of the risk of developing chronic widespread pain can be attributed to genetic factors, and the other half to environmental influences (Kato et al. 2006b).

Certain genetic polymorphisms are associated with a higher risk of developing FM. To date, the serotonin 5-HT2A receptor polymorphism T/T phenotype, serotonin transporter, dopamine 4 receptor, and catecholamine *o*-methyl transferase (COMT) polymorphisms have all been detected in a higher frequency among patients with FM (Bondy et al. 1999; Offenbaecher et al. 1999; Buskila et al. 2004; Buskila, 2007). All of the polymorphisms identified to date involve the metabolism or transport of monoamines, compounds that play a critical role in activity of the human stress response. Multiple genetic polymorphisms probably help determine individuals' "set point" for pain and sensory processing.

Pearl: When considering the diagnosis of FM, ask patients if they are sensitive to noises, odors, and other sensory stimuli.

Comment: FM might be related to a generalized disturbance in the processing of sensory information. FM patients are hyperresponsive not only to painful stimuli, but also to other sensory stimuli. For example, FM patients display a low noxious threshold to auditory tones (Gerster and Hadj-Djilani 1984; McDermid et al. 1996). Yunus coined the term "central sensitivity syndrome" to describe illnesses such as FM, irritable bowel syndrome, tension headache, and other disorders than tend to cluster in the same patients (Yunus 2008).

One study used an identical random staircase paradigm to test FM patients' thresholds to the loudness of auditory tones and to pressure (Geisser et al. 2007). In that study, FM patients displayed low thresholds to both types of stimuli. Moreover, the correlation between the results of auditory and pressure pain threshold testing suggested that some of these differences were due to shared variance to the different stimuli and that other portions were unique to one stimulus or the other.

Pearl: Patients with FM can understand their disorder as one of "increased volume control" in which their central nervous system processes pain and other sensory stimuli in an altered (do not say aberrant!) manner.

Comment: Pain and sensory processing are physiologic processes in which large differences exist among individuals across the population. In this way, pain and sensory processing are similar to blood pressure, glucose metabolism, or any other physiologic process. Ample data suggest that the fundamental neurobiologic problem in FM and related syndromes is that patients perceive more pain from a certain amount of pressure or heat applied to their skin than do individuals without FM. As noted above, this sensitivity extends to other sensory processes. Patients should be informed that pain and other sensory symptoms do not relate necessarily to something "wrong" with the symptomatic part of their body, but rather to their underlying sensitivity.

Myth: FM is an intractable illness and a carries a poor prognosis. There is no effective therapy.

Reality: The medical literature (especially older literature) often depicts FM as an intractable illness for which very limited therapeutic options exist. On the contrary, patients

Table 33.3 Typical outcome in FM

FM does not herald the onset of a systemic disease
There is no progressive, structural or organ damage
Most patients in specialty practice have chronic, persistent symptoms (Felson)
Primary care patients more commonly report complete remission of symptoms and 50% no longer had FM after 1 year (Granges)
Most patients continue to work, but 10–15% are disabled (Felson)
There is often adverse impact on work and leisure activities
Most patients' quality of life improves with medical management

Summarized from Felson and Goldenberg (1986); Granges et al. (1994)

diagnosed with FM in the community often have spontaneous remission of their symptoms (Table 33.3). Nearly 50% of FM patients in primary care no longer had symptoms of FM 1 year after the initial diagnosis (Granges et al. 1994). Even in tertiary referral clinics dedicated to FM, most patients continue to work full time and nearly two-thirds report feeling well or very well (Felson 1986). The notion that FM carries a poor prognosis whether diagnosed in the community or in specialty clinics contributes to pessimism on the part of both patients and clinicians. In the majority of patients, FM responds favorably to a combination of pharmacologic and nonpharmacologic therapy (Table 33.3).

Pearl: Emphasize a "disease management" approach to FM.

Comment: Optimal management of FM requires multidisciplinary health care team. It is useful in discussions with patients to compare their problem with diabetes. If they had been diagnosed with diabetes rather than FM, they would understand that they would not simply be given a prescription for insulin and syringes and expect that this would manage their illness. Rather, they would receive education about their diagnosis, they would learn of the importance of exercise and following a diet, and other information. In FM, the patient must also take an active role in their overall disease management. The patient and primary care provider should be at the helm of that team. Specialists, including rheumatologists, physiatrists, mental health professionals, pain management specialists, physical therapists, and occupational therapists also often participate in the care of these patients.

Specialists can provide important education to FM patients. This teaching can be accomplished in either small or large group settings. Rheumatologists or physiatrists are ideal specialists to develop such educational sessions, either as part of office practice or as a stand-alone education program. The patient's spouse and immediate family members should be encouraged to attend.

Myth: Antidepressants work in FM because most FM patients are depressed.

Reality: Two new serotonin-norepinephrine reuptake inhibitors (SNRIs), milnacipran and duloxetine, have undergone recent multicenter trials and were shown to be effective in a number of outcome variables (Vitton et al. 2004; Arnold et al. 2004a). In these trials, significant differences were reported in such parameters as overall improvement, physical functioning, fatigue levels, degree of reported physical impairment, self-reported pain and stiffness, and the number of tender points. With both of these drugs and more broadly in the pain field, the analgesic and other benefits of the drugs were equal in depressed and nondepressed patients. These findings suggest that the analgesic and other positive effects of tricyclics and SNRIs in FM are not simply due to their antidepressant effects.

Pearl: Cognitive behavioral therapy is effective in the treatment of FM.

Comment: The two forms of nonpharmacologic therapy studies most thoroughly to date are cognitive behavioral therapy and exercise. Both of these therapies are efficacious in the treatment of FM, as well as a plethora of other medical conditions (Williams et al. 2000; Goldenberg et al. 2004). Both of these treatments can lead to sustained improvements when an individual complies with therapy.

Pearl: Start low, go slow when initiating new therapy for FM.

Comment: Perhaps because of their generalized sensory hypersensitivity, patients with FM are much more likely to experience adverse effects of drugs than patients without FM. Thus, it is often quite helpful to begin at very low doses of drugs, and to escalate the dose very slowly.

Pearl: Patients on selective serotonin reuptake inhibitors may require higher doses than those necessary to treat depression.

Comment: Studies that have demonstrated the efficacy of SSRIs in FM have either combined the drug with a low dose of a tricyclic medication (e.g., amitriptyline) or used much higher doses of the SSRI than is often used for depression (Goldenberg et al. 1996; Arnold et al. 2002). For example, the dose of fluoxetine necessary to treat FM in one of the above studies was 45 mg/day, much higher than the average dose used as an antidepressant. These higher doses of SSRIs might achieve their outcomes through the recruitment of noradrenergic effects.

Thus, although there is some evidence that SNRIs may be preferable to SSRIs in the treatment of FM, if SSRIs are used they may need to be used at higher doses.

Myth: Exercise makes people with FM worse, such that they are never able to comply.

Reality: Several studies have demonstrated that cardiovascular exercise is helpful in FM (Fig. 33.5). A large meta-analysis of about 40 clinical trials demonstrated that exercise improves physical status, daily function, and FM symptoms (Busch et al. 2007).

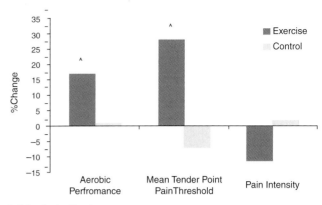

statistically significant

Fig. 33.5 Improvements in aerobic exercise vs. nonexercise controls

Women with FM gain the same physiologic benefits from exercise, including cardiovascular fitness and strength, as do healthy women. In most patients, it is best to initiate exercise a few months after the start of drug therapy so that the patient is less symptomatic and able to tolerate the exercise program better. Any cardiovascular exercise should be initiated slowly and incrementally, with a target goal of 30–40 min of aerobic cardiovascular fitness training 3 or 4 times weekly. Exercise programs of moderate intensity (55–75% of age-adjusted maximal heart rate) are usually tolerated well, but high-intensity (heart rate >150/min) aerobic exercise is not.

Pearl: Describe exercise as a "drug" to patients.

Comment: Exercise likely works in part in FM by raising levels of serotonin and norepinephrine. This intervention is most effective if administered in low, frequent doses several times a week rather than high doses taken intermittently. Clinicians caring for patients with FM need to mount the exercise soapbox and ask patients continually how much activity and exercise they undertake. Patients often resist beginning exercise programs for years, but perseverance on the part of the clinician pays off. Once patients become "sick and tired of being sick and tired" and begin to exercise, they usually continue this as part of their treatment program.

Exercise should be considered similar to any medication and explained to the patient in detail. Make a show of writing the patient a prescription for exercise. Referral of the patient to a physical therapist can be helpful, especially for patients who are reluctant to begin an exercise program.

Pearl: Ask patients if they had been were active before developing FM.

Comment: Several studies suggest that FM patients have higher levels of premorbid activity and exercise than do controls. These data suggest that individuals learned early in life that regular exercise made them feel better. Pointing this out to patients often assists in getting individuals to begin an exercise program. Exercise has a salutatory effect on pain, fatigue, and other symptoms, even in healthy individuals.

Myth: When patients experience a flare of their FM symptoms, switch them to a new therapy.

Reality: FM flares occur most often because of stressors such as psychologic pressure, infections, trauma, and other events. In these settings, the discontinuation of current therapy can be counterproductive. However, when patients are consistently doing poorly, it is reasonable to consider switching medications or adding a different drug. Whatever initial drug is chosen should be titrated to an adequate therapeutic dosage for an adequate duration before deciding on response. If no response occurs consider switching to a different antidepressant or using combinations, such as an antidepressant in the morning with either gabapentin or pregabalin at night.

References

Aaron LA, et al Psychiatric diagnoses in patients with fibromyalgia are related to health care-seeking behavior rather than to illness [see comments]. Arthritis Rheum. 1996;39:436–45

Annemans L, Wessely S, Spaepen E, et al Health economic consequences related to the diagnosis of fibromyalgia syndrome. Arthritis Rheum. 2008;58:895–902

Arnold LM, et al A double-blind, multicenter trial comparing duloxetine with placebo in the treatment of fibromyalgia patients with or without major depressive disorder. Arthritis Rheum. 2004a;50: 2974–84

Arnold LM, et al A randomized, placebo-controlled, double-blind, flexible-dose study of fluoxetine in the treatment of women with fibromyalgia. Am J Med. 2002;112:191–7

Arnold LM, et al Family study of fibromyalgia. Arthritis Rheum. 2004b;50:944–52

Bondy B, et al The T102C polymorphism of the 5-HT2A-receptor gene in fibromyalgia. Neurobiol Dis 1999; 6: 433–439

Branco J, Atalaia A, Paiva T. Sleep cycles and alpha-delta sleep in fibromyalgia syndrome. J Rheumatol. 1994;21:1113–7

Busch AJ, Barber KA, Overend TJ, et al Exercise for treating fibromyalgia syndrome. Cochrane Database Syst Rev. 2007;4

Buskila D, Neumann L, Hazanov I, Carmi R. Familial aggregation in the fibromyalgia syndrome. Semin Arthr Rheum. 1996;26: 605–11

Buskila D, Cohen H, Neumann L, Ebstein RP. An association between fibromyalgia and the dopamine D4 receptor exon III repeat polymorphism and relationship to novelty seeking personality traits. Mol Psychiatry. 2004;9:730–1

Buskila D. Genetics of chronic pain states. Best Pract Res Clin Rheumatol. 2007;21:535–47

Cohen ML, Quintner J. Fibromyalgia syndrome: a problem of tautology. Lancet 1993;342:906–9

Drewes AM, Svendsen L. Quantification of alpha-EEG activity during sleep in fibromyalgia: a study based on ambulatory sleep monitoring. J Musculoskel Pain. 1994;2:33–53

Felson DT, Goldenberg DL. The natural history of fibromyalgia. Arthritis Rheum. 1986;29:1522–6

Fukuda K, et al Chronic multisymptom illness affecting Air Force veterans of the Gulf War. JAMA 1998;280:981–8

Fukuda K, et al An epidemiologic study of fatigue with relevance for the chronic fatigue syndrome. J Psychiatr Res. 1997;31:19–29

Geisser ME, et al The association between experimental and clinical pain measures among persons with fibromyalgia and chronic fatigue syndrome. Eur J Pain. 2007;11:202–07

Gerster JC, Hadj-Djilani A. Hearing and vestibular abnormalities in primary fibrositis syndrome. J Rheumatol. 1984;11:678–80

Goldenberg DL, Burckhardt C, Crofford L. Management of fibromyalgia syndrome. JAMA 2004;292:2388–95

Goldenberg D, Mayskiy M, Mossey C, et al A randomized, double-blind crossover trial of fluoxetine and amitriptyline in the treatment of fibromyalgia. Arthritis Rheum. 1996;39:1852–59

Gracely RH, Petzke F, Wolf JM, Clauw DJ. Functional magnetic resonance imaging evidence of augmented pain processing in fibromyalgia. Arthritis Rheum. 2002;46:1333–43

Granges G, Littlejohn G. Pressure pain threshold in pain-free subjects, in patients with chronic regional pain syndromes, and in patients with fibromyalgia syndrome. Arthritis Rheum. 1993;36:642–6

Granges G, Zilko P, Littlejohn GO. Fibromyalgia syndrome: assessment of the severity of the condition 2 years after diagnosis. J Rheumatol. 1994;21:523–29

Hadler NM. If you have to prove you are ill, you can't get well. The object lesson of fibromyalgia. Spine 1996;21:2397–400

Harris R, Sundgren P, Pang Y, et al Dynamic levels of glutamate within the insula are associated with improvements in multiple pain domains in fibromyalgia. Arthritis Rheum. 2008;58:903–7

Hudson JI, Hudson MS, Pliner LF, et al Fibromyalgia and major affective disorder: a controlled phenomenology and family history study. Am J Psychiatr. 1985;142:441–6

Hudson JI, Goldenberg DL, Pope HGJ, et al Comorbidity of fibromyalgia with medical and psychiatric disorders. Am J Med. 1993;92: 363–7

Kato K, Sullivan PF, Evengard B, Pedersen NL. Chronic widespread pain and its comorbidities: a population-based study. Arch Intern Med. 2006a;166:1649–54

Kato K, Sullivan PF, Evengard B, Pedersen NL. Importance of genetic influences on chronic widespread pain. Arthritis Rheum. 2006b; 54:1682–6

Kim H, Neubert JK, San Miguel A, et al Genetic influence on variability in human experimental pain sensitivity associated with gender, ethnicity and psychological temperament. Pain 2004;109:488–96

McDermid AJ, Rollman GB, McCain GA. Generalized hypervigilance in fibromyalgia: evidence of perceptual amplification. Pain 1996;66: 133–44

Moldofsky H, Scarisbrick P, England R, Smythe H. Musculoskeletal symptoms and non-REM sleep disturbance in patients with "fibrositis syndrome" and healthy subjects. Psychosomatic Med. 1975; 37:341–51

Offenbaecher M, et al Possible association of fibromyalgia with a polymorphism in the serotonin transporter gene regulatory region. Arthritis Rheum. 1999;42:2482–8

Older SA, et al The effects of delta wave sleep interruption on pain thresholds and fibromyalgia-like symptoms in healthy subjects; correlations with insulin-like growth factor I. J Rheumatol 1998;25: 1180–6

Peleg R, et al Characteristics of fibromyalgia in Muslim Bedouin women in a primary care clinic. Semin Arthritis Rheum. 2008;37(6): 398–402

Petzke F, et al Dolorimetry performed at 3 paired tender points highly predicts overall tenderness. J Rheumatol 2001;28:2568–69

Pope HGJ, Hudson JI. A Supplemental interview for forms of "affective spectrum disorder". International Journal of Psychiatry in Medicine 1991; 21(3): 205–32

Raspe H. [Rheumatism epidemiology in Europe]. Soz Praventivmed. 1992;37:168–78

Tan EM, et al Range of antinuclear antibodies in "healthy" individuals. Arthritis Rheum. 1997;40:1601–11

Tracey I, Mantyh PW. The cerebral signature for pain perception and its modulation. Neuron. 2007;55:377–91

Vitton O, Gendreau M, Gendreau J, et al A double-blind placebo-controlled trial of milnacipran in the treatment of fibromyalgia. Hum Psychopharmacol. 2004;19(Suppl 1):S27–35

White KP, Nielson WR, Harth M, et al Does the label "fibromyalgia" alter health status, function, and health service utilization? A prospective, within-group comparison in a community cohort of adults with chronic widespread pain. Arthritis Rheum. 2002;47:260–5

White KP, Thompson J. Fibromyalgia syndrome in an Amish community: a controlled study to determine disease and symptom prevalence. J Rheumatol. 2003;30:1835–40

Williams DA, Cary MA, Glazer LJ, et al Randomized controlled trial of CBT to improve functional status in fibromyalgia. Arthritis Rheum. 2000;43:S210

Wolfe F, Ross K, Anderson J, et al Aspects of fibromyalgia in the general population: sex, pain threshold, and fibromyalgia symptoms. J Rheumatol. 1995;22:151–6

Yunus MB Central sensitivity syndromes: a new paradigm and group nosology for fibromyalgia and overlapping conditions, and the related issue of disease versus illness. Semin Arthritis Rheum. 2008;37(6):339–52

Yunus MB, Inanici F, Aldag JC, et al Fibromyalgia in men: comparison of clinical features with women. J Rheumatol. 2000;27:485–90

The Clinical Features of Gout

34

Bruce N. Cronstein and Michael H. Pillinger

34.1 Overview of the Clinical Features of Gout

> Gout is caused by the crystal deposition of monosodium urate in and around joint tissues.
> The first joint affected in the majority of cases is the first metatarsophalangeal joint, a condition known as podagra.
> Acute gout is characterized by the rapid development of warmth, swelling, erythema, and pain in the affected joint.
> The natural history of gout is to worsen with time, progressing through the stages of asymptomatic hyperuricemia and acute intermittent gouty attacks to tophaceous gout.
> The time period between the first development of acute intermittent gouty attacks and the appearance of chronic tophaceous gout is approximately a decade in most cases.
> The development of tophaceous deposits of monosodium urate is a function of the degree and duration of hyperuricemia.
> However, most people with hyperuricemia never develop clinical gout.

Myth: The presence of polymorphonuclear neutrophils (PMNs) and EXTRACELLULAR urate crystals in a synovial fluid aspirate is pathognomonic of acute gout.

Reality: The *sine qua non* of an acute gouty attack is the presence in synovial fluid of PMNs whose response is directed against urate crystals. Examination of the joint fluid in a true gout attack usually demonstrates urate crystals both within PMNs and in the extracellular fluid. Only the presence of intracellular crystals provides unequivocal evidence that the PMN attack is directed toward the crystals.

Individuals with a history of gout can have "residual" extracellular crystals in the joint between gouty attacks. These "old"

crystals do not induce inflammatory responses, for reasons that are not fully understood (Bomalaski et al. 1986). Thus, the finding of only extracellular crystals in a joint aspirate raises the possibility that extracellular crystals are not the "primum mobile" of the inflammatory response. Other potential etiologies for the presence of PMNs (e.g., infection) must be excluded.

Myth: A therapeutic response to colchicine confirms that the cause of acute monoarticular arthritis was gout.

Reality: The major mechanism of action of colchicine is the disruption of microtubules. The consequence of this is the impairment of the ability of PMNs to infiltrate into joints. Other potential mechanisms of action for colchicine include effects on adhesion molecules and interleukin-I (Molad et al. 1998; Cronstein and Terkeltaub 2006). These effects make colchicine a useful drug for acute gouty attacks. In the setting of a high suspicion of acute gout, a response to colchicine supports the diagnosis.

However, colchicine also inhibits inflammatory responses in other conditions, including pseudogout, familial Mediterranean fever, and leukocytoclastic vasculitis (Famaey 1988; Ben-Chetrit and Levy 1998; Chen and Carlson 2008). Pseudogout is the disorder most likely to mimic gout, and the two cannot be rigorously distinguished by a therapeutic response to colchicine. Because the long-term management strategies of these two crystal diseases differ, establishing the definitive diagnosis of one or the other by joint aspiration and crystal examination is important.

Myth: A normal serum uric acid level at the time of acute monoarticular arthritis excludes the possibility of gout.

Reality: Hyperuricemia, defined as chronic elevation of the serum uric acid level above 6.8 mg/dL, is the *sine qua non* for the development of the condition of gout. However, serum uric acid levels fluctuate over time and are not always elevated at the time of an acute attack. Acute attacks of gout can be caused by the liberation of preformed urate crystals from tophaceous or microtophaceous deposits within joints, bursae, skin, and other organs. In such cases, an elevated uric acid is not required at the time of the attack.

J. H. Stone (ed.), *A Clinician's Pearls and Myths in Rheumatology*,
DOI:10.1007/978-1-84800-934-9_34, © Springer Science + Business Media B.V. 2009

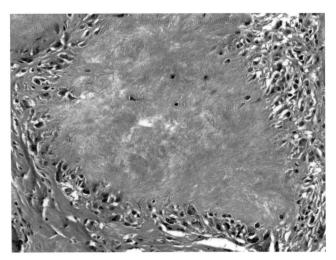

Fig. 34.1 Tophaceous deposits within synovial tissue. This patient had a clinical course complicated by both fungal arthritis (*Candida tropicalis*) and chronic gouty arthropathy in the knee. He underwent an orthopedic procedure to help eradicate the fungal infection. The synovial pathology revealed extensive tophaceous deposits. The patient's fungal infection was believed to have led to continuous "crystal stripping" from the synovium (Figure courtesy of Dr. John Stone)

A common scenario on the Inpatient Rheumatology Consult Service is as follows: (1) Elderly patient with or without a recognized history of gout is admitted for elective surgery; (2) The patient is made NPO in anticipation of surgery; (3) The serum uric acid level declines acutely; and (4) Uric acid crystals are leeched from tophaceous deposits within joint synovium, triggering an acute attack of gout (Fig. 34.1).

Individuals who begin a xanthine oxidase inhibitor (e.g., allopurinol) or uricosuric agent (e.g., probenicid) are actually at higher risk of an acute gout flare during the first 6 months of therapy (Becker et al. 2005) (for this reason, colchicine should be administered along with the urate-lowering agent for the first 6 months). In addition, some data suggest that the inflammatory response that accompanies acute gout induces a urate diuresis, transiently leading to a lowering of the serum urate level (Urano et al. 2002). Thus, a normal serum urate level during a flare of acute joint disease does not exclude gout as the cause.

Myth: A negative Gram stain excludes a joint infection and implicates a microcrystalline disorder as the cause of joint inflammation.

Reality: Gram stain should be performed on any joint fluid in which infection is considered as an alternative to acute gout or another microcrystalline disorder (this, of course, includes essentially all cases). A positive Gram stain strongly supports the diagnosis of infection and frequently provides important clues to the nature of the offending organism. However, the sensitivity of Gram stain is limited. As many as 55% of patients with infected joints have negative Gram stains of synovial fluid (Faraj et al. 2002).

A patient with a negative Gram stain should not be presumed to be infection-free based on that result alone. Indeed, in patients whose joint fluid cell count approaches or exceeds 100,000 cells/mm^3, it is often wise to assume the patient has an infection until the results of synovial fluid cultures are available.

Pearl: A 24-h urine collection for uric acid should not be performed during or immediately after an acute gout attack.

Comment: The quantity of uric acid present in a 24-h collection can provide insight into the etiology of the patient's hyperuricemia:

- In a patient with relatively normal glomerular filtration rate and hyperuricemia, the excretion of more than 800 mg of uric acid in a 24-h period indicates metabolic overproduction of urate. In other words, the excretion of urate is insufficient to keep pace with production. Such a patient is said to be an "overproducer."
- On the other hand, hypoexcretion of uric acid (e.g., less than 600 mg in a 24-h period) suggests a failure of the renal tubular system to excrete a normal load of urate. Such patients are termed "underexcreters."

Classification of a patient as an "overproducer" or "underexcreter" can be useful in selecting the appropriate urate-lowering therapy. In the absence of contraindications to one drug or the other, allopurinol would be an appropriate choice for an overproducer and probenicid a reasonable selection for an underexcreter.

Many aspects of urate handling are in flux around the time of an acute gout attack. Cytokines associated with the attack can increase the degree of urate excretion. Conversely, the presence of acidosis or the recent institution of a diuretic can lead to decreased urate excretion. Under these circumstances, a 24-h collection is unlikely to reflect accurately the patient's baseline urate metabolism and excretion. Clinicians wishing to assess urate excretion should not obtain a 24-h urine collection until the intercritical period is reached, several weeks after an acute gout flare.

Pearl: Subchondral defects with "overhanging edges" are virtually pathognomonic of tophaceous deposits on radiographs of the hands or feet.

Comment: In assessing a patient for the diagnosis of chronic gout, one radiographic finding is highly characteristic: the punched-out lesion with an overhanging edge (Fig. 34.2) (Choi et al. 2006). Subchondral defects with classic overhanging edges confirm the presence of small tophaceous deposits consistent with chronic gout.

These lesions typically are located in a juxta-articular region, at either the distal or proximal ends of bones (e.g., near the metacarpophalangeal or interphalangeal joints). Gouty erosions often have a cystic quality to them and can be

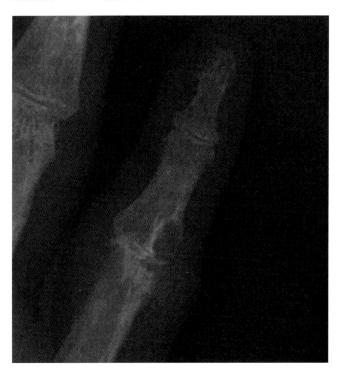

Fig. 34.2 Radiograph of a chronic gouty arthropathy, characterized by joint erosions with overhanging edges (Figure courtesy of Dr. John Stone)

confused with the kind of bone cysts found in osteoarthritis. However, they differ from such cysts in that their cortical "roof" has been broken, leading to the overhanging edge. Gouty lesions therefore often appear to have an open lid.

Many other radiologic features of gout are nonspecific. As examples, gouty erosions may be indistinguishable from those of rheumatoid arthritis or osteomyelitis. In addition, although tophi are not usually radio-opaque, they may become so if they undergo secondary calcification.

Pearl: The diagnosis of gout can often be confirmed in an asymptomatic patient by aspirating a previously involved joint and examining the synovial fluid for uric acid crystals.

Comment: Urate crystals persist in the joint during the intercritical phase in the great majority of patients with gout (perhaps all patients with gout) (Bomalaski et al. 1986; Pascual et al. 1999). For reasons that remain unclear, these "old" crystals are no longer inflammatory.

A common scenario in the rheumatology clinic is the arrival of a patient alleged to have gout who is no longer symptomatic. In the usual situation, the patient has been managed empirically 2 weeks before the clinic appointment during an acute presentation, without the performance of an arthrocentesis to confirm the presence of monosodium urate crystals.

Aspiration of the previously affected but no longer symptomatic joint can be considered in this setting. Moreover, this procedure is strongly indicated if the joint in question (e.g.,

the knee) is easily "tappable," and if the result of the synovial fluid analysis would alter the decision about whether or not to begin longitudinal treatment.

Pearl: The occurrence of acute monoarticular arthritis in a premenopausal woman who is otherwise well is almost never gout.

Comment: Clinicians who are consulted to "rule out gouty attack" in a premenopausal woman with joint pain should recall the wisdom of Hippocrates, who observed that "A woman does not take the gout, unless her menses be stopped" (Hippocrates 1886).

Premenopausal women normally have persistently low serum urate levels because of a high rate of renal excretion. Thus, they lack the conditions necessary to develop gout. Indeed, the prevalence of gout in premenopausal women is on the order of only 2 cases per 10,000 (Centers for Disease Control 1996). Premenopausal women who develop gout almost certainly have one or more well-defined risk factors (e.g., diuretic use or renal failure).

Pearl: Gout is a hereditary disease.

Comment: Most clinicians pay little attention to the family history when evaluating a patient with gout. However, it has been known for at least a century that the risk of gout can be conveyed in families. A family history of gout is identified approximately 40% of patients with this disease. For the purposes of initial diagnosis, the specific gene in question is not important, but a positive family history of gout can provide strong supporting evidence for the diagnosis of gout as the course of an evaluation is underway. The precise genetic bases for the risk of gout are understood only partly. Pertinent known genes include hypoxanthine–guanine phosphoribosyl transferase, phosphoribosyl pyrophosphate synthase, fructose-1-phosphatase aldolase, and the URAT-1 renal transporter, among others.

Pearl: Gout and hyperuricemia are strongly associated with other chronic diseases, including obesity, hypertension, and coronary artery disease.

Comment: Gout or hyperuricemia often occur as part of a constellation of other problems. The high purine intake associated with hyperuricemia in most cases contributes to obesity, a condition common among patients with gout (Annemans et al. 2008). In addition, the prevalence of hypertension among patients with gout may be as high as 40%. Some data from both animal and human studies suggest that hyperuricemia is a direct cause of high blood pressure (Edwards 2008). Finally, myocardial infarction is a common cause of morbidity in patients with gout.

The true relationship between hyperuricemia and clinical entities that are associated clearly with the metabolic syndrome requires further study. However, from the clinical standpoint, the diagnosis of gout is a marker for a patient who may benefit from a number of interventions in addition to the direct treatment of hyperuricemia complications. Weight loss, blood pressure treatment, and other strategies designed to reduce the risk of cardiovascular disease may be appropriate.

Pearl: Gout often complicates a joint that is infected, and vice versa.

Comment: Gout is often a sufficient explanation for inflammation in a joint, particularly if intracellular urate crystals are demonstrated within synovial fluid neutrophils. However, the positive finding of crystals does not exclude a concurrent problem. Gout probably leads to an increased risk of joint infections in the same way that rheumatoid arthritis does: the existence of baseline structural damage, the presence of an effusion, and alterations in the local immune response.

Conversely, joint infections are proposed to result in the liberation of monosodium urate crystals sites of synovial deposition – a phenomenon known as "crystal stripping" – and secondary gout attacks. One study revealed the prevalence of infection to be low in the setting of known crystal disease, but reported a substantial increase (from 1.5% to 22%) when only joints with synovial fluid counts $\geq 100,000/mm^3$ were considered (Shah et al. 2007). Given the potentially disastrous consequences of an untreated septic joint, even the lower value is concerning. Thus, the diagnosis of acute gout attack should not cause the clinician to disregard the possibility of infection.

References

Annemans L, Spaepen E, Gaskin M, Bonnemaire M, Malier V, Gilbert T, Nuki G. Gout in the UK and Germany: prevalence, comorbidities and management in general practice 2000–2005. Ann Rheum Dis. 2008;67:960–6

Becker MA, Schumacher HR Jr, Wortmann RL, MacDonald PA, Eustace D, Palo WA, Streit J, Joseph-Ridge N. Febuxostat compared with allopurinol in patients with hyperuricemia and gout. N Engl J Med. 2005;353:2450–61

Ben-Chetrit E, Levy M. Colchicine: 1998 update. Semin Arthritis Rheum. 1998;28(1):48–59

Bomalaski JS, Lluberas GR, Schumacher HR Jr. Monosodium urate crystals in the knee joints of patients with asymptomatic nontophaceous gout. Arthritis Rheum. 1986;29(12):1480–4

Centers for Disease Control and Prevention, national Center for Health Statistics. Vital and health statistics: current estimates from the national Health Interview Survey, 1996. Series 10, No. 200. Atlanta: Department of Health and Human Services (US). Available at http://www.cdc.gov/nchs/data/series/sr_10/sr10_200.pdf

Chen KR, Carlson JA. Clinical approach to cutaneous vasculitis. Am J Clin Dermatol. 2008;9(2):71–92

Choi MH, MacKenzie JD, Dalinka MK. Imaging features of crystal-induced arthropathy. Rheum Dis Clin N Am. 2006;32:427–46

Cronstein BN, Terkeltaub R. The inflammatory process of gout and its treatment. Arthritis Res Ther. 2006;8(Suppl 1):S3

Edwards NL. The role of hyperuricemia and gout in kidney and cardiovascular disease. Cleve Clin J Med. 2008;75(Suppl 5):S13–6

Famaey JP. Colchicine in therapy. State of the art and new perspectives for an old drug. Clin Exp Rheum. 1988;6(3):305–17

Faraj AA, Omonbude OD, Godwin P. Gram staining in the diagnosis of acute septic arthritis. Acta orthop Belg. 2002;68(4):388–91

Hippocrates. The genuine works of Hippocrates, volumes 1 and 2. Translated and edited by Adams F. New York: Wood; 1886

Molad Y, Cronstein BN, Malawista SE. Colchicine. In: Smyth CJ, Holers VM, editors. Gout, hyperuricemia, and other crystal-associated arthropathies. New York: Marcel Dekker; 1998. p. 193–204

Pascual E, Batlle-Gualda E, Martinez A, Rosas J, Vela P. Synovial fluid analysis for diagnosis of intercritical gout. Ann Intern Med. 1999;131:756–9

Shah K, Spear J, Nathanson LA, McCauley J, Edlow JA. J Emerg Med. 2007;32(1):23–26

Urano W, Yamanaka H, Tsutani H, Nakajima H, Matsuda Y, Taniguchi A, Hara M, Kamatani N. The inflammatory process in the mechanism of decreased serum uric acid concentrations during acute gouty arthritis. J Rheumatol. 2002;29:1950–3

Gout Epidemiology

35

Hyon K. Choi

35.1 Overview of Gout Epidemiology

> The prevalence of gout rises with advancing age. Among men and women older than 80 years of age, the prevalence of the disorder is 9% and 6%, respectively.

> Gout is more common among individuals with lower family income levels. This is probably attributable to a disproportionate occurrence within those income strata of other risk factors for gout, including hypertension, obesity, and dietary patterns.

> Ethanol or fructose consumption increases uric acid production by net adenosine triphosphate (ATP) degradation to adenosine monophosphate (AMP). AMP is degraded rapidly to uric acid.

> Two major genetic mutations lead to gout, urolithiasis, and related problems:

> Mutations in the gene that encodes hypoxanthine-guanine phosphoribosyl transferase are associated with a spectrum of diseases in children, which ranges from the Lesch–Nyhan syndrome at the severe end of the spectrum to simple hyperuricemia at the mild end.

> Mutations in the 5'-phosphoribosyl-1-pyrophosphate (PRPP) synthetase genes can result in overactivity of the pathway, leading ultimately to increased urate production.

Myth: Gout is common among men but rare among women.

Reality: Both the prevalence and incidence of gout are considerably higher in men than in women before the age of menopause, but the burden of gout in women increases substantially after menopause and rises with age. In the National Health and Nutrition Examination Survey (NHANES), the prevalence of gout among women between the ages 60 and 69 years was 3.5%, but increased to 4.6% and 5.6% among those aged 70–79 and 80 years or older, respectively (Kramer and Curhan 2002).

NHANES data may overestimate the prevalence of some disorders, as the survey is based upon individuals' self-reports of physician-diagnosed gout. However, even if the true age-specific prevalence of gout are 50% lower than these estimates, they still rival or exceed that of rheumatoid arthritis among women (2.3% in the NHANES III) (Rasch et al. 2003). Moreover, data from the Rochester Epidemiology project indicate a doubling in the incidence of primary gout among women between the years 1977 and 1996 (Arromdee et al. 2002).

Myth: Gout occurs more often among African-Americans than Caucasians.

Reality: A prospective study of 352 Black men in the Meharry Cohort Study and 571 White men in the Johns Hopkins Precursors Study investigated this issue. Based upon self-reported cases of gout, the study found that the risk of gout was 70% higher among the Black men compared with that among the White men ($p = 0.04$) (Hochberg et al. 1995). However, this excess risk disappeared after adjustment for hypertension (adjusted relative risk = 1.30 (95% CI 0.77–2.19).

These data demonstrate that Black men have a greater incidence of gout than White men. However, this excess risk is explained primarily by a greater incidence of hypertension among Black men.

Myth: Gout is painful but does not affect longevity.

Reality: A large prospective study among men found that those with gout have a higher risk of death from all causes (Choi and Curhan 2007b). Among men without known coronary heart disease at baseline, the increased mortality risk is due primarily to an elevated risk of cardiovascular death. In addition, at least two other major studies confirm the relationship between gout and shortened longevity, primarily through the increased risk of coronary heart disease:

• One study of men with above-average risk for coronary heart disease found that hyperuricemia and a diagnosis of gout were associated with increased long-term all-cause mortality (Krishnan et al. 2008). The excess risk was attributable principally to an increased risk of death from cardiovascular disease.

• Gout also increased the risk of overall mortality among patient with end-stage renal disease by 49%, even after adjustments for gender, race, chronic pulmonary disease, peripheral vascular disease, diabetes, ischemic heart disease, congestive failure, albumin levels, and smoking status (Cohen et al. 2008).

These data suggest that men with gout have a higher risk of death from all causes and that the increased mortality risk is due mainly to an elevated risk of death from cardiovascular disease. These findings indicate that aggressive management of cardiovascular risk factors is appropriate for individuals with gout.

Pearl: The risk of the metabolic syndrome is remarkably high among patients with gout or a high level of hyperuricemia.

Comment: The metabolic syndrome is a constellation of interrelated atherosclerotic risk factors. Abdominal obesity and insulin resistance are two major features. Other metabolic components include atherogenic dyslipidemia, elevated blood pressure, and elevated plasma glucose (Grundy et al. 2005). The metabolic syndrome affects more than 50 million Americans and increases the risk for atherosclerotic cardiovascular disease, type 2 diabetes, and death (Ford et al. 2002; Ford 2005).

Close associations between serum urate levels and individual components of the metabolic syndrome exist (Emmerson 1998; Lee et al. 1995; Rathmann et al. 1998). The prevalence of the metabolic syndrome is high among hospitalized patients with gout (82% in Mexican men (Vazquez-Mellado et al. 2004) and 44% in Korean men) (Rho et al. 2005). These data suggest that hyperuricemia should be regarded as an intrinsic part or surrogate marker for the metabolic syndrome (Emmerson 1998).

The high insulin levels known to be associated with the metabolic syndrome reduce the renal excretion of uric acid (Ter Maaten et al. 1997; Muscelli et al. 1996; Facchini et al. 1991; Dessein et al. 2000). Insulin may enhance renal urate reabsorption via stimulation of urate–anion exchanger URAT1 (Enomoto et al. 2002) and/or the Na^+-dependent anion co-transporter in brush border membranes of the renal proximal tubule (Choi et al. 2005b). The conventional low-purine diet recommended for gout patients that permits unlimited fructose ingestion could also contribute to the high prevalence of the metabolic syndrome among these patients because fructose intake is associated with elevated serum insulin levels, insulin resistance, and adiposity.

A diagnosis of hyperuricemia or gout should trigger a high clinical suspicion for coexistent metabolic syndrome (Ford 2005). Lifestyle interventions in this setting (e.g., enhanced physical activity and dietary modifications) delay or prevent the transition from impaired glucose tolerance to type 2 diabetes (Ford et al. 2002; Eriksson and Lindgarde 1991; Pan et al. 1997; Tuomilehto et al. 2001). Daily exercise and weight control are the foundations of the new healthy eating pyramid and an important recommendation for patients with gout (Choi et al. 2005, b; Willett and Stampfer 2003).

Pearl: Diabetes is associated with lower serum uric acid levels compared to patients with glucose intolerance.

Comment: The relation between serum glucose levels and uric acid levels is not linear. In fact, it is bell shaped, rising to a vertex and then declining. Several studies have shown that a moderate degree of hyperglycemia is associated with higher serum uric acid levels, but marked hyperglycemia is associated with lower serum uric acid levels (Cook et al. 1986; Tuomilehto et al. 1988; Herman and Goldbourt 1982; Whitehead et al. 1992). The biologic explanation for this is the uricosuric effect of glycosuria, which occurs when the blood glucose level is greater than approximately 10 mmol/L (180 mg/dL) (Cook et al. 1986).

Serum uric acid levels rise with moderately increasing levels of serum glucose HbA1c (6–6.9%), but then decrease with further HbA1c elevations (again, a bell-shaped curve). Serum uric acid levels also rise in parallel with increases in the level of fasting C-peptide levels (Choi and Ford 2008).

These data suggest divergent risks for hyperuricemia and gout among prediabetic and diabetic individuals. Individuals with moderately elevated HbA1c levels (i.e., prediabetes) are at higher risk of hyperuricemia and gout. Those with highly elevated HbA1c levels (i.e., diabetes) are at lower risk for these conditions, all other things being equal.

Pearl: With regard to the prevention of gout, Osler got at least part of the equation right: "The sugar should be reduced to a minimum. The sweeter fruits should not be taken."

Comment: A number of foods and beverages are known to affect the risk of hyperuricemia and gout. These are summarized in Table 35.1.

Writing in his *The Principles and Practice of Medicine* (1893), William Osler prescribed a diet low in fructose as a means of preventing gout (Osler and Gout 1893; Nakagawa et al. 2005). Yet conventional dietary recommendations for the prevention of gout have focused on the restriction of purine intake (Fam 2002). Was Osler wrong?

No (Of course not). Both mechanistic data and prospective evidence support Osler's concept that a high intake of fructose poses a substantial risk for gout. Fructose induces uric acid production by increasing ATP degradation to AMP, a uric acid

Table 35.1 Foods and beverages that affect the risk of hyperuricemia and gout

Increase risk	Decrease risk	Risk neutral
Beer	Vitamin C	Vegetables rich in purines: peas, beans, spinach, mushrooms
Whiskey	Low-fat diary products	Wine
Fructose	Coffee (regular or decaffeinated)	Tea
Red meat		Overall protein intake
Seafood		

precursor (Choi et al. 2005b;Gibson et al. 1983; Fox and Kelley 1972; Puig and Fox 1984; Faller and Fox 1982). Fructose phosphorylation in the liver uses ATP, and the accompanying phosphate depletion limits the regeneration of ATP from ADP, which in turn serves as substrate for the catabolic pathway to uric acid formation (Fox et al. 1987). (Ethanol, another known risk factor for gout, acts in the same manner). Thus, diets high in fructose heighten the risk of gout.

Within minutes of a fructose infusion, the plasma uric acid concentrations are increased (Fox and Kelley 1972). In conjunction with purine nucleotide depletion, rates of purine synthesis *de novo* are accelerated, thus potentiating uric acid production (Raivio et al. 1975). In contrast, glucose and other simple sugars do not have the same effect (Nakagawa et al. 2005). Moreover, fructose intake correlates with the levels of serum insulin as well as with insulin resistance (Wu et al. 2004), and therefore could increase indirectly both the serum uric acid level and the risk of gout (Choi et al. 2007; Lee et al. 2004; Vasquez-Mellado et al. 2004). An increase in fructose consumption contributes to a positive energy balance, and therefore to insulin resistance and adiposity (Tordoff and Alleva 1990; Anderson et al. 1989; Gross et al. 2004; Bray et al. 2004; Thorburn et al. 1989).

A prospective study of male professionals confirmed that consumption of sugar-sweetened soft drinks and fructose was associated strongly with an increased risk of gout (Choi and Curhan 2008). The risk of incident gout was 85% higher among men who consumed two or more servings of sugar-sweetened soft drinks per day compared with those who consumed less than one per month. In contrast, diet drinks were not associated with the risk of gout. The consumption of fruit juice or fructose-rich fruits such as apples and oranges is also associated with a modestly increased risk of gout.

Data from the NHANES indicate that serum uric acid concentrations increase in parallel with intake of sugar-sweetened soft drinks (Choi et al. 2008). Diet soft drinks do not demonstrate this same association. In men, added sugar intake was also associated with serum uric acid concentration (Gao et al. 2007).

These findings indicate that consumption of sugar-sweetened soft drinks and fructose is strongly associated with an increased risk of hyperuricemia and gout. Dietary recommendations that emphasize modest consumption of fructose are appropriate in individuals with these conditions.

Pearl: Moderate- to high-level coffee consumption is associated with a lower risk of gout.

Comment: The more coffee one drinks, the lower one's risk of gout (Choi et al. 2007b). People who imbibe four or five cups of java per day have a 40% lower risk of gout compared to those who do not drink coffee. Individuals who consume more than six cups/day have a 61% lower risk. Decaffeinated coffee is associated with a lowering of the risk of gout, albeit the effect

is somewhat lower with that beverage. In contrast, tea intake and total caffeine ingestion from all sources do not alter the risk of gout. Thus, it seems to be something about the coffee.

Serum uric acid levels in the NHANES decreased as coffee intake increased, but tea consumption and total caffeine ingestion were not linked to serum uric acid levels (Choi and Curhan 2007a). These findings are consistent with a cross-sectional study from Japan in which coffee but not tea consumption was associated inversely with serum uric acid levels (Kiyohara et al. 1999).

The effect of coffee on insulin sensitivity may mediate its decreased risk of gout. Higher long-term coffee intake is associated with lower insulin levels (Wu et al. 2005) and improved insulin sensitivity (Arnlov et al. 2004). Greater insulin sensitivity appears to foster lower serum levels of uric acid.

Pearl: Purine-rich foods of vegetable origin do not lead to gout.

Comment: The relationships between purine-rich foods, high protein intake, and incident gout were examined prospectively over a 12-year period in 47,150 male participants with no baseline history of gout (Choi et al. 2004b). The investigators found *no increased risk* associated with the consumption of purine-rich vegetables (e.g., peas, beans, spinach, and mushrooms) or with overall protein intake. In fact, this study found a protective effect from vegetable and dairy proteins. However, the consumption of meat, particularly red meat, increased the risk of gout significantly. Seafood consumption was associated with a still higher risk (Choi et al. 2004b).

Myth: All alcoholic beverages are equally likely to lead to gout.

Reality: Beer consumption showed the strongest independent association with the risk of new gout in the Health Professionals Follow-up Study (Choi et al. 2004a, b). The risk of gout increased by 50% for every 12-ounce serving/day. Liquor consumption also increased the risk of new gout by approximately 15% for each drink. Moderate levels of wine intake did not increase the risk of gout in this study.

In the NHANES III study, the association between beer consumption and serum uric acid level was strong for beer (an increase of 0.46 mg/dL for each additional serving) and for liquor (0.29 mg/dL for each additional serving), but no independent association existed for wine consumption (Choi and Curhan 2004) It remains unclear whether there are offending factors unrelated to alcohol in beer or liquor or perhaps instead protective factors in that wine mitigate the effect of alcohol upon the risk of gout.

Pearl: Moderate- to high-dose vitamin C intake is associated with a lower risk of gout.

Comment: The suspicion for a potential protective effect of vitamin C intake against gout originated from metabolic experiments that examined the impact of short-term loading of high-dose vitamin C on the serum uric acid levels. For example, ingestion of a single dose of 4 g vitamin C doubled the fractional excretion of uric acid, and a daily ingestion of 8 g of vitamin C for 3–7 days reduced serum uric acid by 2.0–3.1 mg/dL as a result of uricosuria (Stein et al. 1976).

A randomized, double-blind, placebo-controlled trial ($n = 184$) showed that dietary supplementation with as little as 500 mg of vitamin C a day for 2 months reduced serum uric acid by 0.5 mg/dL, compared to no change in the placebo group (Huang et al. 2005). A retrospective case–control study (91 gout cases and 91 controls) reported an inverse association between vitamin C intake and the presence of gout (Lyu et al. 2003).

An updated analysis of the Health Professionals Follow-up Study over a 20-year period found that the risk of gout decreased with increasing vitamin C intake (Choi et al. 2009). Individuals who ingested 1,500 mg or more of vitamin C daily had a risk of gout that was 45% lower than those in the lowest category. This finding was independent of all known dietary factors and other risk factors for gout such as body mass index, age, hypertension, diuretic use, alcohol, and chronic renal failure. These data suggest that vitamin C intake may be beneficial in the prevention and management of gout.

Pearl: Low-fat dairy product consumption is associated with a lower risk of gout.

Comment: The potentially protective role of dairy consumption on gout was suggested by several studies that measured uric acid as a surrogate outcome (Loenen et al. 1990; Garrel et al. 1991; Ghadirian et al. 1995). The ingestion of the milk proteins casein and lactalbumin decreases serum uric acid levels in healthy subjects via a uricosuric effect (Garrel et al. 1991). Conversely, a significant increase in uric acid level was induced by a dairy-free diet in a 4-week randomized clinical trial (Ghadirian et al. 1995). Those who consumed milk one or more times per day had a lower serum uric acid level than those who did not drink milk (p for trend <0.0001) (Choi et al. 2005a). Similarly, those who consumed yogurt at least once every other day had a lower serum uric acid level than those who did not consume yogurt (p for trend <0.0001). The actual risk of gout was 44% lower in the highest quintile of dairy consumption as compared with the lowest quintile. This inverse association was evident with low-fat dairy consumption, but not with high-fat dairy consumption (Choi et al. 2004b).

References

Anderson JW, Story LJ, Zettwoch NC, Gustafson NJ, Jefferson BS. Metabolic effects of fructose supplementation in diabetic individuals. Diabetes Care. 1989;12:337–44

Arnlov J, Vessby B, Riserus U. Coffee consumption and insulin sensitivity. JAMA 2004;291:1199–201

Arromdee E, Michet CJ, Crowson CS, O'Fallon WM, Gabriel SE. Epidemiology of gout: is the incidence rising? J Rheumatol. 2002;29:2403–6

Bray GA, Nielsen SJ, Popkin BM. Consumption of high-fructose corn syrup in beverages may play a role in the epidemic of obesity. Am J Clin Nutr. 2004;79:537–43

Choi HK, Atkinson K, Karlson EW, Willett WC, Curhan G. Alcohol intake and risk of incident gout in men – a prospective study. Lancet 2004a;363:1277–81

Choi HK, Atkinson K, Karlson EW, Willett WC, Curhan G. Purine-rich foods, dairy and protein intake, and the risk of gout in men. N Engl J Med. 2004b;350:1093–103

Choi HK, Curhan G. Beer, liquor, wine, and serum uric acid level – the Third National Health and Nutrition Examination Survey. Arthritis Rheum. 2004:1023–9

Choi HK, Curhan G. Coffee, tea, and caffeine consumption and serum uric acid level: the Third National Health and Nutrition Examination Survey. Arthritis Rheum. 2007a;57:816–21

Choi HK, Curhan G. Independent impact of gout on mortality and risk for coronary heart disease. Circulation 2007b;116:894–900

Choi HK, Curhan G. Soft drinks, fructose consumption, and the risk of gout in men: prospective cohort study. BMJ 2008;336:309–12

Choi HK, Ford ES. Haemoglobin A1c, fasting glucose, serum C-peptide and insulin resistance in relation to serum uric acid levels – the Third National Health and Nutrition Examination Survey. Rheumatology (Oxford) 2008;47:713–7

Choi HK, Ford ES, Li C, Curhan G. Prevalence of the metabolic syndrome in patients with gout: the Third National Health and Nutrition Examination Survey. Arthritis Rheum. 2007a;57:109–15

Choi HK, Liu S, Curhan G. Intake of purine-rich foods, protein, dairy products, and serum uric acid level – the Third National Health and Nutrition Examination Survey. Arthritis Rheum. 2005a;52:283–9

Choi HK, Mount DB, Reginato AM. Pathogenesis of gout. Ann Intern Med. 2005b;143:499–516

Choi HK, Willett W, Curhan G. Coffee consumption and risk of incident gout in men: a prospective study. Arthritis Rheum. 2007b;56:2049–55

Choi HK Gao X, Curhan G. Vitamin C intake and the risk of gout in men: a prospective study. Arch Intern Med 2009;169:502–7

Choi JW, Ford ES, Gao X, Choi HK. Sugar-sweetened soft drinks, diet soft drinks, and serum uric acid level: the Third National Health and Nutrition Examination Survey. Arthritis Rheum. 2008;59:109–16

Cohen SD, Kimmel PL, Neff R, Agodoa L, Abbott KC. Association of incident gout and mortality in dialysis patients. J Am Soc Nephrol. 2008;19:2204–10

Cook DG, Shaper AG, Thelle DS, Whitehead TP. Serum uric acid, serum glucose and diabetes: relationships in a population study. Postgrad Med J. 1986;62:1001–6

Dessein PH, Shipton EA, Stanwix AE, Joffe BI, Ramokgadi J. Beneficial effects of weight loss associated with moderate calorie/carbohydrate restriction, and increased proportional intake of protein and unsaturated fat on serum urate and lipoprotein levels in gout: a pilot study. Ann Rheum Dis. 2000;59:539–43

Emmerson B. Hyperlipidaemia in hyperuricaemia and gout. Ann Rheum Dis. 1998;57:509–10

Enomoto A, Kimura H, Chairoungdua A, et al Molecular identification of a renal urate anion exchanger that regulates blood urate levels. Nature 2002;417:447–52

Eriksson KF, Lindgarde F. Prevention of type 2 (non-insulin-dependent) diabetes mellitus by diet and physical exercise. The 6-year Malmo feasibility study. Diabetologia 1991;34:891–8

Facchini F, Chen YD, Hollenbeck CB, Reaven GM. Relationship between resistance to insulin-mediated glucose uptake, urinary uric acid clearance, and plasma uric acid concentration. JAMA 1991;266:3008–11

Faller J, Fox IH. Ethanol-induced hyperuricemia: evidence for increased urate production by activation of adenine nucleotide turnover. N Engl J Med. 1982;307:1598–602

Fam AG. Gout, diet, and the insulin resistance syndrome. J Rheumatol. 2002;29:1350–5

Ford ES. Risks for all-cause mortality, cardiovascular disease, and diabetes associated with the metabolic syndrome: a summary of the evidence. Diabetes Care 2005;28:1769–78

Ford ES, Giles WH, Dietz WH. Prevalence of the metabolic syndrome among US adults: findings from the third National Health and Nutrition Examination Survey. JAMA 2002;287:356–9

Fox IH, Kelley WN. Studies on the mechanism of fructose-induced hyperuricemia in man. Metabolism 1972;21:713–21

Fox IH, Palella TD, Kelley WN. Hyperuricemia: a marker for cell energy crisis. N Engl J Med. 1987;317:111–2

Gao X, Qi L, Qiao N, et al Intake of added sugar and sugar-sweetened drink and serum uric acid concentration in US men and women. Hypertension 2007;50:306–12

Garrel DR, Verdy M, PetitClerc C, Martin C, Brule D, Hamet P. Milk- and soy-protein ingestion: acute effect on serum uric acid concentration. Am J Clin Nutr. 1991;53:665–9

Ghadirian P, Shatenstein B, Verdy M, Hamet P. The influence of dairy products on plasma uric acid in women. Eur J Epidemiol. 1995; 11:275–81

Gibson T, Rodgers AV, Simmonds HA, Court-Brown F, Todd E, Meilton V. A controlled study of diet in patients with gout. Ann Rheum Dis. 1983;42:123–7

Gross LS, Li L, Ford ES, Liu S. Increased consumption of refined carbohydrates and the epidemic of type 2 diabetes in the United States: an ecologic assessment. Am J Clin Nutr. 2004;79:774–9

Grundy SM, Cleeman JI, Daniels SR, et al Diagnosis and management of the metabolic syndrome: an American Heart Association/National Heart, Lung, and Blood Institute Scientific Statement. Circulation 2005;112:2735–52

Herman JB, Goldbourt U. Uric acid and diabetes: observations in a population study. Lancet 1982;2:240–3

Hochberg MC, Thomas J, Thomas DJ, Mead L, Levine DM, Klag MJ. Racial differences in the incidence of gout. The role of hypertension. Arthritis Rheum. 1995;38:628–32

Huang HY, Appel LJ, Choi MJ, et al The effects of vitamin C supplementation on serum concentrations of uric acid: results of a randomized controlled trial. Arthritis Rheum. 2005;52:1843–7

Kiyohara C, Kono S, Honjo S, et al Inverse association between coffee drinking and serum uric acid concentrations in middle-aged Japanese males. Br J Nutr. 1999;82:125–30

Kramer HM, Curhan G. The association between gout and nephrolithiasis: the National Health and Nutrition Examination Survey III, 1988–1994. Am J Kidney Dis. 2002;40:37–42

Krishnan E, Svendsen K, Neaton JD, Grandits G, Kuller LH. Long-term cardiovascular mortality among middle-aged men with gout. Arch Intern Med. 2008;168:1104–10

Lee J, Sparrow D, Vokonas PS, Landsberg L, Weiss ST. Uric acid and coronary heart disease risk: evidence for a role of uric acid in the obesity–insulin resistance syndrome. The Normative Aging Study. Am J Epidemiol. 1995;142:288–94

Lee WY, Park JS, Noh SY, Rhee EJ, Kim SW, Zimmet PZ. Prevalence of the metabolic syndrome among 40,698 Korean metropolitan subjects. Diabetes Res Clin Pract. 2004;65:143–9

Loenen HM, Eshuis H, Lowik MR, et al Serum uric acid correlates in elderly men and women with special reference to body composition and dietary intake (Dutch Nutrition Surveillance System). J Clin Epidemiol. 1990;43:1297–303

Lyu LC, Hsu CY, Yeh CY, Lee MS, Huang SH, Chen CL. A case–control study of the association of diet and obesity with gout in Taiwan. Am J Clin Nutr. 2003;78:690–701

Muscelli E, Natali A, Bianchi S, et al Effect of insulin on renal sodium and uric acid handling in essential hypertension. Am J Hypertens. 1996;9:746–52

Nakagawa T, Tuttle KR, Short RA, Johnson RJ. Hypothesis: fructose-induced hyperuricemia as a causal mechanism for the epidemic of the metabolic syndrome. Nat Clin Pract Nephrol. 2005; 1: 80–6

Osler W, Gout. The principles and practice of medicine. New York: Appleton; 1893. p. 287–95

Pan XR, Li GW, Hu YH, et al Effects of diet and exercise in preventing NIDDM in people with impaired glucose tolerance. The Da Qing IGT and Diabetes Study. Diabetes Care. 1997;20:537–44

Puig JG, Fox IH. Ethanol-induced activation of adenine nucleotide turnover. Evidence for a role of acetate. J Clin Invest. 1984;74: 936–41

Raivio KO, Becker A, Meyer LJ, Greene ML, Nuki G, Seegmiller JE. Stimulation of human purine synthesis de novo by fructose infusion. Metabolism 1975;24:861–9

Rasch EK, Hirsch R, Paulose-Ram R, Hochberg MC. Prevalence of rheumatoid arthritis in persons 60 years of age and older in the United States: effect of different methods of case classification. Arthritis Rheum. 2003;48:917–26

Rathmann W, Funkhouser E, Dyer AR, Roseman JM. Relations of hyperuricemia with the various components of the insulin resistance syndrome in young black and white adults: the CARDIA study. Coronary Artery Risk Development in Young Adults. Ann Epidemiol. 1998;8:250–61

Rho YH, Choi SJ, Lee YH, et al The prevalence of metabolic syndrome in patients with gout: a multicenter study. J Korean Med Sci. 2005; 20:1029–33

Stein HB, Hasan A, Fox IH. Ascorbic acid-induced uricosuria. A consequence of megavitamin therapy. Ann Intern Med. 1976;84:385–8

Ter Maaten JC, Voorburg A, Heine RJ, Ter Wee PM, Donker AJ, Gans RO. Renal handling of urate and sodium during acute physiological hyperinsulinaemia in healthy subjects. Clin Sci (Lond). 1997;92: 51–8

Thorburn AW, Storlien LH, Jenkins AB, Khouri S, Kraegen EW. Fructose-induced in vivo insulin resistance and elevated plasma triglyceride levels in rats. Am J Clin Nutr. 1989;49:1155–63

Tordoff MG, Alleva AM. Effect of drinking soda sweetened with aspartame or high-fructose corn syrup on food intake and body weight. Am J Clin Nutr. 1990;51:963–9

Tuomilehto J, Lindstrom J, Eriksson JG, et al Prevention of type 2 diabetes mellitus by changes in lifestyle among subjects with impaired glucose tolerance. N Engl J Med. 2001;344:1343–50

Tuomilehto J, Zimmet P, Wolf E, Taylor R, Ram P, King H. Plasma uric acid level and its association with diabetes mellitus and some biologic parameters in a biracial population of Fiji. Am J Epidemiol. 1988;127:321–36

Vazquez-Mellado J, Conrado GG, Vazquez SG, et al Metabolic syndrome and ischemic heart disease in gout. J Clin Rheumatol. 2004; 10:105–9

Wallace SL, Robinson H, Masi AT, Decker JL, McCarty DJ, Yu TF. Preliminary criteria for the classification of the acute arthritis of primary gout. Arthritis Rheum. 1977;20:895–900

Whitehead TP, Jungner I, Robinson D, Kolar W, Pearl A, Hale A. Serum urate, serum glucose and diabetes. Ann Clin Biochem. 1992;29 (Pt 2):159–61

Willett WC, Stampfer MJ. Rebuilding the food pyramid. Sci Am. 2003;288:64–71

Wu T, Giovannucci E, Pischon T, et al Fructose, glycemic load, and quantity and quality of carbohydrate in relation to plasma C-peptide concentrations in US women. Am J Clin Nutr. 2004;80:1043–9

Wu T, Willett WC, Hankinson SE, Giovannucci E. Caffeinated coffee, decaffeinated coffee, and caffeine in relation to plasma C-peptide levels, a marker of insulin secretion, in U.S. women. Diabetes Care. 2005;28:1390–6

36.1 Overview of the Treatment of Gout

> Treatment of gouty inflammation, hyperuricemia, and comorbidities are distinct but closely linked core elements of therapeutic strategy for patients with gout.

> All gout patients should be evaluated and treated for comorbid medical problems such as hypertension, metabolic syndrome, and coronary artery disease.

> Lifestyle modifications, including weight loss, are important adjuncts to pharmacologic urate lowering.

> The target serum urate level for urate-lowering therapy in most patients is less than 6.0 mg/dL.

> Serial monitoring of serum uric acid levels is essential, following the initiation of urate-lowering therapy.

> High-dose oral colchicine for the treatment of acute gout has an unacceptable risk:benefit ratio.

> Maintenance colchicine should be continued for at least the first 6 months of urate-lowering therapy.

> Allopurinol should not be initiated or discontinued during an acute gout flare.

> In most cases, allopurinol and other urate-lowering therapies should be continued for life.

Pearl: Oral glucocorticoids are an excellent treatment option for acute gout.

Comment: Prednisone and prednisolone are excellent therapeutic choices for acute gout in clinical settings in which NSAIDs, colchicine, or intraarticular glucocorticoids are contraindicated or have not been adequately effective for treatment of acute gout. A randomized clinical trial that compared prednisolone (35 mg/day for 5 days) to naproxen (500 mg twice daily for 5 days) for the treatment of acute gouty arthritis demonstrated comparable efficacy and tolerance (Janssens et al. 2008).

Acute gouty arthritis (Fig. 36.1) requires moderate-to-high doses of glucocorticoids. A typical initial dosing regimen is equivalent to a minimum of 0.5 mg/kg of prednisone each day. As an example, the clinician might prescribe prednisone

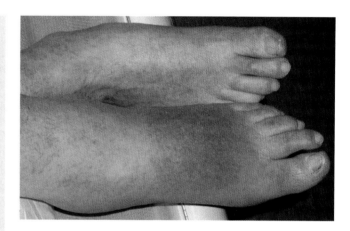

Fig. 36.1 Glucocorticoids are an effective therapy for acute gout flares. The patient whose feet are shown had a known history of gout when he developed intense erythema over the midfoot. Tenderness was most intense over the first metatarsophalangeal joint. Because of existing renal dysfunction (serum creatinine 2.5 mg/dL), he was treated with prednisone 20 twice daily for 5 days, followed by a 1-week prednisone taper. Daily colchicine (0.6 mg) was initiated after the start of the prednisone taper and continued for 6 months after the flare. Allopurinol (100 mg/day) was begun after the acute gout flare had subsided (Figure Courtesy of Dr. John Stone)

20 mg twice daily for 3–5 days and then taper the glucocorticoids off over the following week. Using parenteral glucocorticoids has no particular advantage over oral administration, unless the subject is NPO or has upper GI symptoms. In these circumstances, one dosing option is triamcinolone acetonide 60 mg IM or its equivalent (Siegel et al. 1994).

Although glucocorticoids are highly effective for the treatment of acute gout, using low-dose oral glucocorticoids for the prevention of gout flares is not evidence based. Glucocorticoids should be withdrawn as quickly as possible after the acute gouty inflammation resolves.

Pearl: "Less is more" when using colchicine in the treatment of acute gout.

Comment: In the past, the typical colchicine regimen for the treatment of acute gout was the administration of one 0.6 mg tablet each hour until the patient improved substantially, developed intolerable side effects (usually nausea and diarrhea), or

J. H. Stone (ed.), *A Clinician's Pearls and Myths in Rheumatology*,
DOI:10.1007/978-1-84800-934-9_36, © Springer Science + Business Media B.V. 2009

reached a predetermined maximum dose (typically 8–12 tablets within 24 h). Nearly all patients' gout attacks benefit from such treatment. Unfortunately, every patient treated in this manner experiences adverse gastrointestinal (GI) effects, yielding a benefit-to-toxicity ratio for colchicine of 1 (Ahern et al. 1987). Moreover, the diarrhea usually begins before relief of the gout flare, with the result that the patient limps off to the bathroom on joints that are still acutely inflamed.

There are better ways than colchicine to treat gout flares in most patients (namely, glucocorticoids or nonsteroidal anti-inflammatory drugs). However, if a patient's comorbidities indicate that colchicine is the preferred therapy, there is a less toxic approach to administering the drug. The European League Against Rheumatism (EULAR) guidelines advocate a regimen of three 0.6 mg colchicine tablets in the first 24 h for treatment of acute gout (Zhang et al. 2006a). Moreover, a recent, large, randomized controlled trial that compared three 0.6 mg colchicine tablets to eight tablets administered within the first 24 h of an acute gout flare demonstrated nearly equal efficacy between the two treatment arms and significantly fewer GI side effects in the lower dose group (Terkeltaub 2008a).

Pearl: Colchicine works best when started in the first day or two of the acute gouty flare.

Comment: If you are going to use colchicine to treat acute gout, then it needs to be started early. The optimal use of colchicine is to instruct the patient to take up to three 0.6 mg tablets orally within 3 h of the first sign of a new gouty flare.

However, it is not prudent to superimpose this therapeutic strategy on a patient already maintained on daily low-dose prophylactic colchicine, as this may enhance colchicine toxicity (Terkeltaub 2003). In short, if the patient has been on colchicine prophylaxis and has been compliant, select another medication for treating an acute gout flare.

Myth: Oral low-dose colchicine for prophylaxis of gout flares is contraindicated in all patients with moderate to severe renal insufficiency.

Reality: Colchicine is eliminated, in part, via renal excretion. Thus, colchicine is contraindicated in patients undergoing dialysis (colchicine is not dialyzable) and in patients with a creatinine clearance less than 10 mL/min. Colchicine neuro-myotoxicity, which can be acute or subacute in onset, is a potentially devastating and slowly reversible consequence of this misstep (Wilbur 2004). Colchicine neuromyotoxicity occurs most frequently in the setting of chronic kidney disease but has also been reported in patients with normal renal function.

Prophylactic low-dose colchicine can be used safely in most patients and even those with chronic kidney disease if there is particular attention to the potential for drug–drug interactions. Medications of particular concern are cyclosporine, some macrolide antibiotics (including erythromycin and

Table 36.1 Dosing guidelines for colchicine in patients with renal dysfunction

Creatinine clearance (mL/min)	Colchicine dose
≥ 50	0.6 mg twice daily
35–49	0.6 mg once daily
10–34	0.6 mg every two 2 or three 3 days
<10, or on hemodialysis, or combined moderate-to-severe renal and hepatobiliary disease	Do not use colchicine

clarithromycin), certain statins, some calcium channel blockers (nifedipine and verapamil), several antineoplastic agents, and HIV protease inhibitors (Niel and Scherrmann 2006; Terkeltaub 2008b). Statins are particularly associated with rhabdomyolysis in the presence of colchicine. The guidelines for the dosing of colchicine in patients with renal dysfunction are shown in Table 36.1.

Patients with combined significant hepatic (and particularly hepatobiliary) disease and renal disease are at particular risk for colchicine toxicity. For patients with severe renal dysfunction, colchicine should not be used more frequently than 0.6 mg every 2 or 3 days. Finally, the impaired colchicine pharmacokinetics in the elderly make it advisable to reduce the daily dosage regimen further by up to 50% in patients above the age of 70.

Only rarely is it necessary for a patient to be treated with prophylactic colchicine for more than 12 months! Colchicine should not be viewed as a chronic medication for gout treatment but rather as a bridge for preventing gout flares until sufficiently low-urate levels are achieved.

Pearl: Keep your eyes on the target level of serum urate.

Comment: Serum urate levels of 6.8 mg/dL (0.41 mmol/L) and higher exceed the saturation limit of urate in solution. Levels above 6.8 mg/dL promote deposition of monosodium urate crystals in connective tissues. To provide some margin for error in treating gout, clinicians should target a serum urate level less than 6.0 mg/dL (0.357 mmol/L). Achieving such a level will eventually lead to fewer gout flares.

Patients with bulky tophi (Fig. 36.2) benefit from having their serum urate levels lowered to the 3.0–4.0 mg/dL to hasten tophus resorption (Perez-Ruiz et al. 2002).

Myth: Serum urate levels do not need to be monitored if the patient is on a standard dose of allopurinol.

Reality: The majority of patients do not achieve target serum urate levels on 300 mg or less of allopurinol daily. The serum urate should be monitored 3–4 weeks after the initiation of urate-lowering therapy and 3–4 weeks after each dose adjustment. Once the serum urate level has been suppressed adequately (<6.0 mg/dL), the urate level should continue to be monitored every 6–12 months.

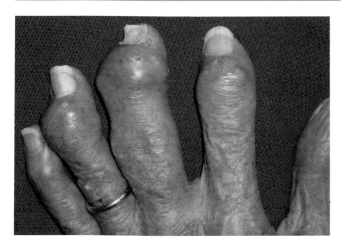

Fig. 36.2 Patients with extensive tophi should have a lower serum urate target level. For most patients with gout, the serum urate target level is 6.0 mg/dL. For those with bulky tophi, resorption will occur more quickly if a serum level of 3.0–4.0 mg/dL can be achieved (Figure Courtesy of Dr. John Stone)

Pearl: Allopurinol is often underdosed.

Comment: Allopurinol is approved by the FDA for the treatment of hyperuricemia in gout at doses up to 800 mg daily. However, more than 98% of all allopurinol prescriptions are written for 300 mg daily or less. This reticence to use higher doses is, in part, due to the fear of precipitating a major allopurinol hypersensitivity syndrome.

The safest clinical practice is the "start low, go slow" approach recommended in the EULAR guidelines (Zhang et al. 2006a). In this model, all patients are started on 100 mg/day, and the serum urate level is monitored 3–4 weeks later. If the target urate level of <6.0 mg/dL has not been achieved by the current dose, the dose is increased by 100 mg every 3–4 weeks until the target serum urate is reached. In subjects with stage 4 or 5 chronic kidney disease, the initial dose may be dropped to 50 mg/day and the subsequent increases made in 50 mg increments every 3–4 weeks.

Remember that while the patient's allopurinol dose is being titrated upwards, the patient should also be on colchicine to prevent disease flares triggered by declining levels of serum urate and associated tophus remodeling.

Myth: Severe allopurinol hypersensitivity syndrome is common.

Reality: Full-blown allopurinol hypersensitivity syndrome is a serious medical illness with a mortality rate of up to 20%. However, it is rare. In contrast, skin rashes develop in approximately 2% of patients who receive allopurinol. Hypersensitivity reactions to allopurinol are hereditary in some patients. Genetic linkage to HLA-B5801 has been described in patients of either European or Han Chinese descent. In other patients, hypersensitivity reactions are dose dependent.

Myth: Allopurinol lowers serum urate and shrinks tophi more effectively than do all uricosuric agents.

Reality: Allopurinol 300 mg daily lowers serum urate by an average of ~33% in subjects with intact renal function (Becker et al. 2005). However, titration of the allopurinol dose is essential to optimize its urate-lowering efficacy. The uricosuric agent benzbromarone (not available in the United States) works at least as well as allopurinol in lowering serum urate levels and shrinking tophi, provided the patient has intact renal function (Perez-Ruiz et al. 2002).

Uricosuric agents are not effective in patients with substantial renal impairment. As an example, probenecid is relatively ineffective in lowering serum urate levels in patients with a creatinine clearance of less than 60 mL/min. In contrast, allopurinol is a reasonable first choice agent for all patients with recurrent gout, regardless of renal function or the patients' status as "overproducers" or "underexcreters" (Terkeltaub 2003).

Pearl: The use of azathioprine and allopurinol together can lead to a severe drug–drug interaction. It is usually better not to use this combination.

Comment: This combination is particularly relevant to the population of patients with organ transplants, many of whom are on azathioprine to prevent graft rejection and many of whom are at risk for gout because of calcineurin inhibitors. Both cyclosporine and tacrolimus alter urate handling, leading to hyperuricemia and gout in a significant number of patients. Xanthine oxidase is involved in the metabolism of azathioprine. As an inhibitor of xanthine oxidase, allopurinol interferes with the metabolism of azathioprine (and its metabolite, 6-mercaptopurine). This can lead to marked elevation of azathioprine levels and the potential for life-threatening bone-marrow toxicity (Duley et al. 2005). Moreover, the inhibition of xanthine oxidase by allopurinol alters azathioprine levels in a variable and unpredictable way. Serious toxicity can occur, despite careful monitoring of hematology and liver function.

The need to consider the combined use of allopurinol and azathioprine is receding because mycophenolate mofetil (MMF) is replacing azathioprine as the immunosuppressive agent of choice. For patients who require both allopurinol and azathioprine and for whom no substitute for either is permitted, the dose of azathioprine should be decreased by 50–75%. Complete blood counts must be followed at frequent intervals until stable doses of the medications and urate levels have been achieved. A second (and lesser) option that is available in patients who do not have extensive tophi is to continue azathioprine but prescribe a uricosuric drug such as probenecid, sulfinpyrazone, or benzbromarone.

Pearl: Renal and heart transplant recipients experience hyperuricemia and gout more frequently than liver transplant patients, but these problems occur in all of these transplant populations.

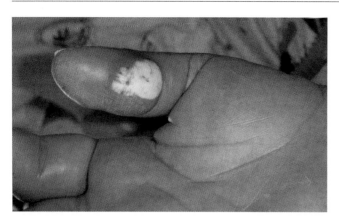

Fig. 36.3 Tophi in patients who develop gout in the setting of organ transplantation often occur over the distal interphalangeal joints (at the site of Heberden's nodes) or as subcutaneous deposits that resemble a local infection (Figure courtesy of Dr. Terence Gibson)

Comment: This is true. However, hyperuricemia and gout certainly occur in liver transplant patients, too. The calcineurin inhibitors cyclosporine and tacrolimus are the principal cause of hyperuricemia in all organ transplant patients. These medications cause hyperuricemia in any clinical situation in which they are used. Cyclosporine and tacrolimus alter urate handling within the kidney and also cause renal dysfunction and hypertension. The hyperuricemic effect is mediated either by a reduction of glomerular filtration or, more likely, by the suppression of uric acid secretion by the proximal tubule (Hansen 1998; Laine 1996).

The renal and heart transplant patients often have additional risk factors for gout. These include the existence of hyperuricemia before renal transplantation (because of end-stage renal disease), the high frequency of renal allograft dysfunction, and a greater likelihood of concomitant diuretic use.

Pearl: Transplant patients are likely to develop tophi without a history of acute gout.

Comment: The accumulation of tophi in the absence of acute arthritis was first emphasized as a manifestation of hyperuricemia in older persons on diuretics (Macfarlane and Dieppe 1985). The tophi in such cases often occur over the distal interphalangeal joints (at the site of Heberden's nodes) or as subcutaneous deposits that resemble a local infection (Fig. 36.3).

Both cyclosporine and diuretics have an intense inhibitory impact on the secretion of urate by the proximal tubule. Both these drugs are often used in transplant patients. As a consequence, hyperuricemia develops and total body urate accumulates very quickly. This rapidity of uric acid accumulation may account for the relative paucity of acute gouty arthritis in transplant patients. The anti-inflammatory effects of immunosuppressive medications used in transplant patients may also contribute.

The development of visible tophi in the absence of typical gout has also been reported in long-term transplant patients who have not been received a calcineurin inhibitor (Braun 1999). These data support for an effect of prednisone and other transplant medications (MMF, azathioprine) on the suppression of clinical gout.

Pearl: Colchicine is best avoided in transplant patients receiving cyclosporine because of the risk of colchicine neuromyotoxicity.

Comment: Most clinicians prudently avoid the use of NSAIDs in renal transplant patients because of their deleterious effect on kidney function. Colchicine might appear to be a safer alternative with regard to potential nephrotoxic effects. However, when colchicine is used for acute gout or in regular low doses as prophylaxis in patients with renal impairment, it carries the risk of proximal myopathy. This adverse effect has been observed most often among transplant recipients who are also on cyclosporine, because cyclosporine interferes with colchicine metabolism (Dupont 2002; Simkin and Gardner 2002).

Colchicine myopathy usually presents as muscle weakness and is associated with an elevated creatine kinase level (Kuncl 1987). Characteristic electromyographic and muscle biopsy abnormalities are present in this condition, and the myopathy can be accompanied by a mild peripheral neuropathy. Symptoms regress over 3–4 weeks after stopping colchicine, but may be permanent. The preferred treatment of acute gout in renal transplant patients is intraarticular or intramuscular injection of a depot preparation of prednisolone, a 7–10 day course of an oral glucocorticoid dose such as prednisone, or an increase in the patient's baseline prednisone dose.

Pearl: Back pain in the transplant patient treated with cyclosporine might be due to gout.

Comment: Back pain due to tophaceous deposits or acute gout can mimic infective diskitis when fever, leukocytosis, and elevated serum inflammatory markers are present (Suk et al. 2007). This is a particularly difficult diagnosis in transplant patients because of their underlying immunosuppression.

Spinal gout is not common, but transplant patients are disproportionately represented among all documented cases (Clive 2000; Hou et al. 2007). Spinal tophi can cause pain, compress emerging nerve roots, and lead to spinal stenosis (Draganescu and Leventhal 2004). The possibility of gout should be considered in patients with a history of hyperuricemia and peripheral articular gout. Spinal infection must be excluded in these cases by image-guided aspiration and biopsy.

Myth: Acute gout is less common than anticipated among hyperuricemic patients in renal failure.

Reality: The clinical impression of less frequent gout in renal failure has been attributed to an antiinflammatory effect of uremia (Hollingsworth 1988; Buchanan et al. 1965). Neither of these assertions is supported by strong clinical evidence. The only comparative study of the frequency of gout among patients with equivalent levels of hyperuricemia but with or without renal failure failed to demonstrate any difference between the two groups in the incidence of acute gout (Youssef et al. 1995).

Myth: A high-protein diet causes hyperuricemia and gout.

Reality: A high-protein meal actually increases uric acid clearance and can reduce serum urate (Matzkies et al. 1980). Low-protein diets have no effect on gout.

Most circulating uric acid derives from the catabolism of endogenous purines that are generated in the liver. Purines that are ingested, in contrast, contribute variably to the total uric-acid pool. The food items that are richest in dietary purines are shellfish, caviar, and organ meats such as liver, kidney, brain, pancreas ("sweetbreads"), and intestines ("chitlins"). Some vegetables, such as legumes, contain more purines than others.

A formula diet that is entirely devoid of purines for several days can reduce the serum urate of a healthy man by 30% (Griebsch and Zollner 1974), but such diets are rarely sustainable over the long term. A general rule of thumb is that lowering the serum urate level by more than 1 mg/dL is not possible by diet alone. Patients with substantial hyperuricemia and frequent symptoms of gout require medication.

Myth: Patients with gout ingest more purines than healthy people.

Reality: There is only one irrefutable dietary association of hyperuricemia and gout, namely, the strong link with alcohol consumption (Rodnan 1980; Choi et al. 2004a, b). There are also broad correlations between measures of obesity and serum uric-acid levels (Acheson and Chan 1969). One dietary study did not find higher levels of total purine consumption among patients with gout compared with controls (Gibson et al. 1983). However, an excess of alcohol was confirmed in the gout population. All forms of alcohol heighten the risk of gout, but beer appears to be a stronger risk factor in this respect than are wine and whiskey (Choi et al. 2004a, b).

Pearl: If a patient's serum urate fails to reach the target level, despite reasonable allopurinol doses, the clinician should be suspicious of noncompliance.

Comment: Hyperuricemia and recurrent gout can be encountered despite a dose of allopurinol that exceeds 600 mg daily. Only 25–50% of patients on allopurinol 300 mg/day achieve a target urate level of <6.0 mg/dL. Lactic acidosis or ketoacidosis can cause hyperuricemia by competitive inhibition of urate secretion in the proximal tubules. All diuretics, with the exception of spironolactone, reduce uric acid excretion by the kidneys, and can interfere with the ability of allopurinol to lower serum urate levels.

Having said that, patient noncompliance is a major issue in the treatment of gout. Noncompliance with allopurinol was reported to be ~50% in one study (Riedel et al. 2004). The question of whether or not a patient is taking his medicine can be settled by the measurement of a serum oxypurinol level. Oxypurinol is the major active metabolite of allopurinol, and its presence in a plasma measurement means the patient is taking at least some of his medication. Therapeutic levels of oxypurinol are between 5 and 15 mg/L.

Allopurinol compliance can also be monitored by the quantification of allopurinol metabolites in the urine. These estimations rely on one or more 24-h urine collections—not always easy to obtain in patients who are inclined to noncompliance.

Myth: There are no therapeutic options for patients who fail or are intolerant to allopurinol.

Reality: Many patients fail to achieve the target suppression of serum urate to <6.0 mg/dL on "standard doses" of allopurinol. A person should not be considered a treatment failure until the dose of allopurinol has been escalated slowly to 800 mg/day. For patients who are intolerant of allopurinol, febuxostat (a daily oral xanthine oxidase inhibitor) and pegloticase (an intravenous pegylated urate oxidase protein given every 2–4 weeks) may both be accessible therapeutic options shortly. Both medications are currently under review by the FDA. Febuxostat use has been approved in Europe (Edwards 2008).

Adjunctive medications that are readily available now include the use of uricosuric agents such as probenecid, losartan, and fenofibrate. Rasburicase is a nonpegylated urate oxidase used primarily for short-term prophylaxis of the tumor lysis syndrome. Its short half-life (~24 h in serum) and high degree of immunogenicity (including anaphylaxis) makes it a poor choice for the treatment of chronic hyperuricemia (Terkeltaub 2007).

Pearl: All forms of intensive urate-lowering therapy actually promote gout flares.

Comment: Any condition that dramatically raises or lowers the serum urate level is likely to induce a flare of gout. Thus, the risk of a gout flare increases when a patient is begun on urate-lowering therapy alone. The increased risk is particularly high within the first 6 months of urate-lowering therapy.

Tophus remodeling is probably responsible for this. The breakup of quiescent, walled-off tophaceous aggregates of urate crystals within the synovium may initially release more inflammatory forms of crystals. These mobilized crystals interact readily with resident synovial cells and initiate the "attack."

As an example, in one study of patients who started allopurinol 300 mg/day, at least a quarter of subjects experienced gout flares following the discontinuation of prophylactic colchicine (Becker et al. 2005). Prophylactic low-dose colchicine therapy should be continued for 6–9 months after the target serum urate is achieved or until the visible subcutaneous tophi have resolved (Borstad et al. 2004).

Myth: Urate-lowering therapy should be halted temporarily during acute gout flares.

Reality: Both rising and falling serum urate levels are associated with increased gouty flares, likely due to changes in the structure of microscopic tophi in the joint space. As a result, urate-lowering therapy should not be initiated during an acute attack, and ongoing urate-lowering therapy should not be halted during acute gout flares.

If the patient is not on urate-lowering therapy at the time of a gout flare, the clinician should wait until at least 1 week after the acute gouty inflammation has resolved before beginning a urate-lowering agent. Daily low-dose colchicine, with doses adjusted for renal dysfunction (see Table 36.1), should begin as the acute flare is resolving. The patient should be on colchicine for at least 1 week before beginning a urate-lowering agent.

Pearl: Show me a gout patient and I'll show you a person in need of a good internist.

Comment: Gout is associated with hypertension, metabolic syndrome, diabetes, hyperlipidemia, chronic kidney disease, diuretic use, and heavy alcohol consumption. Gout and serum urate elevations have been linked with increased coronary artery disease and risk of death due to vascular disease. Several studies have implicated hyperuricemia as an independent risk factor for hypertension, coronary artery disease, and death due to vascular disease (Fang and Alderman 2000). All of these issues require close longitudinal management and patient education. Lifestyle management that includes weight loss should be an early and forceful recommendation for treatment.

Pearl: Losartan and other commonly used drugs can have a beneficial effect on lowering serum urate.

Comment: Thiazide diuretics elevate serum urate levels significantly and can exacerbate gout. In contrast, losartan, an angiotensin II receptor blocker, is uricosuric. In addition, losartan raises the urinary pH and thereby reduces the risk of uric acid urolithiasis promoted by uricosuric therapy (Shahinfar et al. 2000). Changing the drug from hydrochlorothiazide to losartan is a reasonable decision if hypertension is controlled adequately with losartan.

The uricosuric effect of losartan is only moderate, typically leading to only a 10% reduction of serum urate levels. However, the overall effect on urate levels can be substantial if HCTZ is eliminated.

Fenofibrate (micronized fenofibrate 200 mg/day), a medication used for the treatment of hyperlipidemia, is also uricosuric. This drug decreases serum urate levels by up to 27% (Liamis et al 1999). The combination of fenofibrate and losartan can have an even greater impact on urate lowering (Elisaf et al. 1999). Atorvastatin also is uricosuric.

Caution should be exercised, including attention to oral hydration, baseline renal function, and possible uric acid overproducer status, when considering treatment of any hyperuricemic patient with drugs with known substantial uricosuric effects.

Pearl: A baby aspirin is the ideal dose of salicylates in gout patients.

Comment: Low-dose aspirin therapy promotes renal urate reabsorption and hyperuricemia and can therefore exacerbate gout. Decreasing the daily aspirin dose from 325 to 81 mg is advisable in the many gout patients who stand to benefit from low-dose daily aspirin for other reasons.

Myth: Wine intake is beneficial for patients with established gout.

Reality: Incident gout is significantly lower among drinkers of wine than among those who prefer beer or other alcoholic beverages (Choi 2004b). However, this does not mean that wine is good for patients with gout. All forms of alcohol consumption not only elevate serum urate but can also precipitate acute gout flares (Zhang 2006b). Wine and other forms of alcohol should be used at most in moderation in patients with gout.

Myth: The institution of a diet that is low in purines is essential to the effective management of gout.

Reality: Even severely purine-restrictive diets result in a relatively small decrease (1–2 mg/dL) in serum urate levels. Furthermore, such diets are unpalatable to many, and there is no evidence that dietary restriction of vegetables with high purine content protects against incident gout (Choi 2004b). Dietary modifications are in order for patients who consume large amounts of beer, shellfish, and organ meats, because indiscretions with these foodstuffs can exacerbate gout. However, a patient with significant hyperuricemia and frequent gouty episodes, tophi, or uric acid overproduction needs a medication designed to reduce the serum urate level to below the level of urate solubility (target serum in most patients: <6.0 mg/dL).

Weight-reduction diets that stress smaller portion sizes and counteracting insulin resistance appear promising for overweight patients with gout (Dessein et al. 2000).

References

Acheson R, Chan Y. New Haven survey of joint diseases. The prediction of serum uric acid in a general population. J Chronic Dis. 1969; 21:543–5

Ahern MJ, Reid C, Gordon TP, et al Does colchicine work? The results of the first controlled study in acute gout. Aust NZJ Med. 1987; 17:301–4

Becker MA, Schumacher HR Jr, Wortmann RL, et al Febuxostat compared with allopurinol in patients with hyperuricemia and gout. N Engl J Med. 2005;353:2450–61

Borstad GC, Bryant LR, Abel MP, et al Colchicine for prophylaxis of acute flares when initiating allopurinol for chronic gouty arthritis. J Rheumatol. 2004;31:2429–32

Buchanan WW, Klinenberg JR, Seegmiller JE. The inflammatory response to injected microcrystalline monosodium urate in normal, hyperuricaemic, gouty and uremic subjects. Arthritis Rheum. 1965;8:361–7

Choi HK, Atkinson K, Karlson EW, et al Alcohol intake and risk of incident gout in men: a prospective study. Lancet 2004a;363:1277–81

Choi HK, Atkinson K, Karlson EW, et al Purine-rich foods, dairy and protein intake, and the risk of gout in men. N Engl J Med. 2004b;350: 1093–103

Clive D. Renal transplant-associated hyperuricemia and gout. J Am Soc Nephrol. 2000;11:974–9

Dessein PH, Shipton EA, Stanwix AE, et al Beneficial effects of weight loss associated with moderate calorie/carbohydrate restriction, and increased proportional intake of protein and unsaturated fat on serum urate and lipoprotein levels in gout: a pilot study. Ann Rheum Dis. 2000;59:539–43

Draganescu M, Leventhal LJ. Spinal gout: case report and review of the literature. J Clin Rheumatol. 2004;10:74–9

Duley JA, Chocair PR, Florin TH. Observations on the use of allopurinol in combination with azathioprine or mercaptopurine. Aliment Pharmacol Ther. 2005;22:1161–2

Edwards NL. Treatment-failure gout: a moving target. Arthritis Rheum. 2008;58:2587–90

Elisaf M, Tsimilhodimos V, Bairaktari E, et al Effect of micronized fenofibrate and losartan combination on uric acid metabolism in hypertensive patients with hyperuricemia. J Cardiovasc Pharmacol. 1999;34:60–3

Fang J, Alderman MH. Serum uric acid and cardiovascular mortality: The NHANES I epidemiologic follow-up study, 1971–92. JAMA 2000;283:2404–10

Gibson T, Rodgers A, Simmonds H, et al A controlled study of diet in patients with gout. Ann Rheum Dis. 1983a;42:123–7

Griebsch A, Zollner N. Effect of ribomononucleotides given orally on uric acid production in man. Adv Exp Med Biol. 1974;41B:435–42

Hou LC, Hsu AR, Veeravagu A, Boakye M. Spinal gout in a renal transplant patient: a case report and literature review. Surg Neurol. 2007;67:65–73

Janssens HJ, Janssen M, van de Lisdonk EH, et al Use of oral prednisolone or naproxen for the treatment of gout arthritis: a double-blind, randomised equivalence trial. Lancet 2008;371:1854–60

Kuncl RW, Duncan G, Watson D et al Colchicine myopathy and neuropathy. N Engl J Med 1987; 18; 316(25): 1562–8

Liamis G, Bairaktari ET, Eliasf M. Effects of fenofibrate on serumuric acid levels. Am J Kidney Dis. 1999;34:594–8

Macfarlane D, Dieppe PA. Diuretic induced gout in elderly women. Br J Rheumatol. 1985;24:155–7

Matzkies F, Berg G, Madl H. The uricosuric action of protein in man Adv Exp Med Biol. 1980;122A:227–31

Niel E, Scherrmann JM. Colchicine today. Joint Bone Spine. 2006;73:672–8

Perez-Ruiz F, Calabozo M, Pijoan JI, et al Effect of urate-lowering therapy on the velocity of size reduction of tophi in chronic gout. Arthritis Rheum. 2002;47:356–60

Riedel AA, Nelson M, Joseph-Ridge N, et al Compliance with allopurinol therapy among managed care enrollees with gout: a retrospective analysis of administrative claims. J Rheumatol. 2004;31: 1575–81

Rodnan G. The pathogenesis of aldermanic gout: procatarctic role of fluctuations in serum urate concentration in gouty arthritis provoked by feast and alcohol. Arthritis Rheum. 1980;23:737

Shahinfar S, Simpson RL, Carides AD, et al Safety of losartan in hypertensive patients with thiazide-induced hyperuricemia. Kidney Int. 1999;56:1879–85. Published correction appears in 2000; 57:370

Siegel LB, Alloway JA, Nashel DJ. Comparison of adrenocorticotropic hormone and triamcinolone acetonide in the treatment of gouty arthritis. J Rheumatol. 1994;21:1325–27

Simkin P, Gardner G. Colchicine use in cyclosporine treated transplant recipients: how little is too much? J Rheumatol. 2000;27: 1334–7

Suk KS, Kim KT, Lee SH, et al Tophaceous gout of the lumbar spine mimicking pyogenic discitis. Spine J. 2007;7:94–9

Terkeltaub 2008. Semin Arthritis Rheum 2009; 38(6):411–9

Terkeltaub R. Learning how and when to employ uricase as bridge therapy in refractory gout. J Rheumatol. 2007;34:1955–8

Terkeltaub RA. Clinical practice. Gout. N Engl J Med. 2003;349: 1647–55

Wilbur K, Makowsky M. Colchicine myotoxicity: case reports and literature review. Pharmacotherapy 2004;24:1784–92

Youssef P, Brama T, York H, et al Does renal impairment protect from gout? J Rheumatol. 1995;22:494–6

Zhang W, Doherty M, Bardin T, et al EULAR Standing Committee for International Clinical Studies Including Therapeutics. EULAR evidence based recommendations for gout. Part II: Management. Report of a task force of the EULAR Standing Committee for International Clinical Studies Including Therapeutics (ESCISIT). Ann Rheum Dis. 2006a;65:1312–1324

Zhang Y, Woods R, Chaisson CE, et al Alcohol consumption as a trigger of recurrent gout attacks. Am J Med. 2006b;119: 800e13–8

Calcium Pyrophosphate Dihydrate (CPPD) Crystal Deposition Disease

Ann K. Rosenthal and Robert A. Terkeltaub

37.1 Overview of CPPD

> Calcium pyrophosphate dihydrate (CPPD) crystal deposition disease is a clinically heterogeneous disorder that is characterized by the presence of intraarticular CPPD crystals.

> CPPD crystals deposit primarily in cartilage but can traffic within the joint space.

> CPPD crystals form in the normally unmineralized pericellular matrix of articular hyaline and fibrocartilage. The most common sites of involvement are the knee meniscus, the triangular fibrocartilage of the wrist, and the glenohumeral joint. Asymptomatic disease is common in these sites as well as in others (e.g., the symphysis pubis).

> Pathologic cartilage calcification is promoted by changes in inorganic pyrophosphate (PP_i) metabolism, extracellular matrix, and chondrocyte differentiation.

> CPPD deposition disease has a close and complex relationship with osteoarthritis.

> CPPD most commonly afflicts the elderly but can occur in younger patients who have a familial variant of the condition or who are afflicted with any of several metabolic diseases that predispose to CPPD deposition.

> No specific evidence-based therapies for CPPD exist. However, the inflammation promoted by CPPD crystal deposition can be managed successfully in most patients through strategies typically employed for the treatment and prophylaxis of gout.

37.2 Symptoms and Signs

Pearl: CPPD deposition disease can present not only as pseudogout but also as a polyarticular inflammatory arthritis.

Comment: In a small but significant fraction of subjects with CPPD deposition disease, the manifestations of polyarticular CPPD arthropathy overlap substantially with those of rheumatoid arthritis (RA). CPPD deposition disease can mimic RA in its inflammatory signs and symptoms as well as in its ability to involve small and large joints in a symmetric manner (McCarty 1975).

A positive rheumatoid factor (RF) occurs in 10% of patients with CPPD deposition disease (McCarty 1975). This reflects the high frequency of false-positive RF assays in aging. Elevated markers of systemic inflammation are also common in symptomatic CPPD patients, particularly those with polyarticular CPPD deposition disease.

The other side of the coin is this: patients with longstanding RA sometimes develop articular CPPD crystal deposition. This is attributable to the occurrence of secondary osteoarthritis, as well as the effects of aging. In fact, in a study of synovial fluid samples from 93 patients who fulfilled the American College of Rheumatology (ACR) classification criteria for RA, 25% contained CPPD crystals (Gerster et al. 2006).

The response to therapy may not differentiate CPPD crystal deposition disease from RA in all cases. Some studies suggest that patients with refractory, polyarticular CPPD deposition disease also responds to methotrexate, but this finding is not consistent (Chollet-Janin et al. 2007; Doan et al. 2008).

Pearl: CPPD deposition disease can mimic a variety of rheumatic disorders.

Comment: CPPD deposition disease can also present as pseudoseptic arthritis, neuropathic arthritis, polymyalgia rheumatica, masses of the soft tissue and bone, recurrent hemarthrosis, and of course, pseudogout (Terkeltaub 2008).

Pearl: The "crowned dens syndrome" must be excluded in an elderly patient presenting with neurological disturbances and a painful cervical mass.

Comment: Large CPPD crystal deposits can develop in the ligamentum flavum or the transverse ligament at C1, and crystal-induced inflammation can occur at this site (Fig. 37.1). This collection of disease features is termed the "crowned dens syndrome" (Goto et al. 2007). Patients may present with meningismus, cervical canal stenosis, myelopathy, and the

Fig. 37.1 The crowned dens syndrome. Computed tomography scan of the C1 region, showing calcium deposition around the odontoid process of the axis

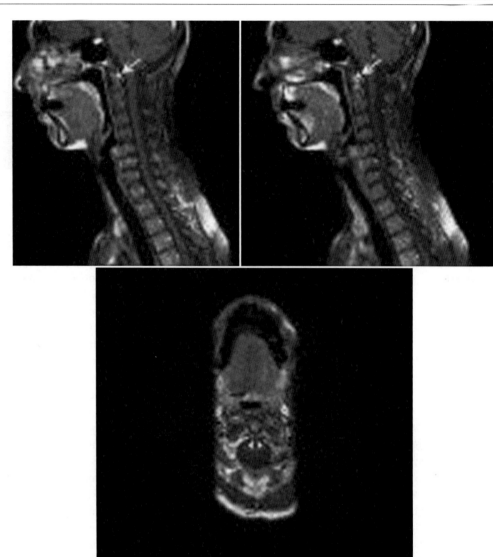

foramen magnum syndrome. Fracture of the odontoid peg precipitated by calcification at C1–C2 has been reported.

Pearl: CPPD deposition disease may be present but unrelated to the cause of the patient's joint pain.

Comment: The prevalence of CPPD deposition disease is remarkably high in the elderly patients. However, CPPD deposition disease is asymptomatic or subclinical in many cases. This disorder is detected often as an incidental finding on radiographs, with calcification of the knee menisci or triangular fibrocartilage of the wrist (Figs. 37.2a, b).

Arthritis in aged patients with preexisting CPPD deposition should not be automatically attributed to CPPD deposition disease. Other disorders must be excluded judiciously, as RA and polymyalgia rheumatica can both coexist with CPPD deposition disease and be mimicked by that condition.

True infectious arthritis is a particular consideration in patients with established CPPD crystal deposition disease. CPPD crystal deposits in the joint, like those of monosodium urate, are detected in some infected joint fluids. This is because CPPD crystals within articular cartilage are "stripmined" by the enzymes associated with joint sepsis.

Pearl: CPPD crystals can be hard to find. Keep looking!

Comment: CPPD crystals vary in size and shape more than do urate crystals. They are generally smaller than urate crystals and typically are rods or rhomboids (Fig. 37.3). CPPD crystals demonstrate weakly positive birefringence or sometimes no birefringence, in contrast to the consistent bright, negative birefringence of monosodium urate crystals.

CPPD crystals, notoriously difficult to detect in some synovial fluids, are missed or misidentified routinely in clinical

Fig. 37.2 Calcium pyrophosphate dehydrate (CPPD) deposition within the meniscal cartilage of the knee (**a**) and the triangular fibrocartilage of the wrist (**b**) (Courtesy of Dr. Richard Chou, Dartmouth-Hitchcock Medical Center)

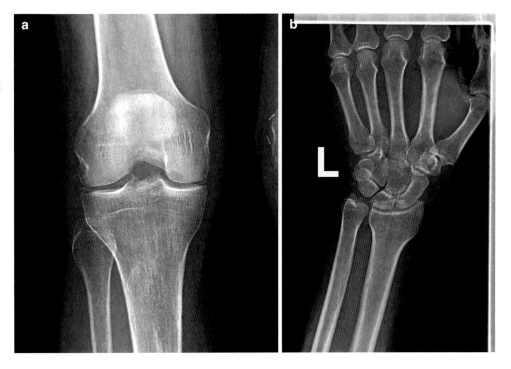

Fig. 37.3 Calcium pyrophosphate dehydrate (CPPD) crystals in synovial fluid. CPPD crystals are often weakly positively birefringent and have a characteristic rectangular shape with blunted ends (Courtesy of Laureen Daft, BS)

specimens (Gordon et al. 1989; Schumacher et al. 1986; Hasselbacher 1987). Several factors and techniques enhance the likelihood of finding such crystals, if present:

- the microscopist's experience and the length of time spent searching for crystals improve the ability to identify them correctly
- phase contrast and high magnification enhance the sensitivity of the procedure
- using the oil objective permits examination for crystals within synovial fluid leukocytes
- second looks can yield the diagnosis.

In one study, two separate examinations of the same synovial fluid 24 h apart significantly increased the number of fluids in which CPPD crystals were detected (Yuan et al. 2003). This phenomenon is probably a function of the time spent searching for crystals (Hearn et al. 1978).

Pearl: Clinical clues help differentiate gout and pseudogout.

Comment: Using the physical examination criteria alone, it is impossible to differentiate among the three major causes of monoarticular arthritis: trauma, infection, and crystal arthritis. Thus, all patients with acute inflammatory monoarticular arthritis should have a joint aspiration. However, certain clinical clues raise the index of suspicion for pseudogout.

- Pseudogout is more likely to present in a large joint (e.g., the knee) or an upper extremity joint than is gout. The classic location for an initial attack of gout of course is the first metatarsophalangeal joint.
- Blood-tinged synovial fluid is more often seen during pseudogout attacks than in acute gout.
- Compared with gout attacks, attacks of pseudogout take longer to peak in intensity, respond more slowly to therapy in general, and often demonstrate less complete treatment responses.
- When gout and CPPD crystals coexist, which is not uncommon, lowering uric-acid levels may not completely ameliorate the arthritis (Fig. 37.4).

Pearl: Pseudogout attacks can be provoked reliably by certain well-defined medical procedures.

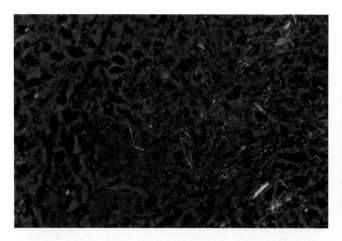

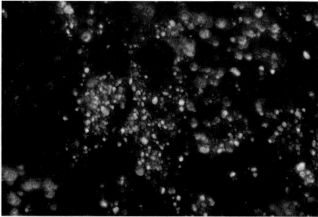

Fig. 37.4 Coexistence of monosodium urate and calcium pyrophosphate dehydrate (CPPD) crystals in a single joint fluid. In this fluid, both monosodium urate and CPPD crystals are seen (Courtesy of Laureen Daft, BS)

Fig. 37.5 Glucocorticoid crystals in synovial fluid. These brightly birefringent crystals are from an intraarticular glucorticoid injection performed several weeks before this joint aspiration (Courtesy of Laureen Daft, BS)

Table 37.1 Medical and surgical procedures known to trigger CPPD flares

Arthroscopy
Intra-articular administration of hyaluronan
Parathyroid surgery for hyperparathyroidism
Parenteral administration of granulocyte colony stimulating factor (G-CSF)
Bisphosphonates

Fig. 37.6 Talc crystals in synovial fluid. These crystals are seen less frequently as less talc is used in the manufacture of gloves. They typically appear as round "beach-ball"-like structures (Courtesy of Laureen Daft, BS)

Comment: Pseudogout can be provoked by minor trauma. In theory, this is the result of a "shaking loose" of CPPD crystals from joint cartilage. However, the precise pathophysiology remains unclear. A variety of medical and surgical procedures can also trigger CPPD flares (Table 37.1).

Pearl: Chronic degenerative arthropathy in CPPD crystal deposition disease commonly affects several joints that are spared in classic cases of primary osteoarthritis.

Comment: The metacarpophalangeal joints, wrists, elbows, and glenohumeral joints are not typical targets for primary osteoarthritis. However, these joints are affected commonly in CPPD crystal deposition disease. If an elderly patient with an inflammatory arthritis of these joints does not have RA, CPPD deposition disease is a good bet.

Pearl: Tumoral deposits of CPPD crystal can present with acute attacks of arthritis and behave as a locally aggressive but benign chondroid tumor.

Comment: Tumoral or pseudotophaceous CPPD crystal deposition has been reported in periarticular structures such as tendons, ligaments, bursae, and also in bones such as the temporal bone, femur, and tibia (close to the joint) (Terkeltaub 2008). The clinical presentation can mimic osteonecrosis. Tumoral CPPD crystal deposition sometimes necessitates surgical removal.

37.3 Diagnosis

Pearl: Beware CPPD mimics in synovial fluid.

Comment: All positively birefringent particulate matter within synovial fluid is not CPPD. Be particularly wary of crystals that are described as very "brightly" birefringent or fluids described as having large quantities of crystals. The most common mimics of CPPD crystals include contaminants such as glucocorticoids crystals (introduced at earlier joint injections (Fig. 37.5) or talc crystals (from gloves (Fig. 37.6)).

Myth: Synovial fluid examinations are worthless unless performed immediately. This is because stored synovial fluid generates artifactual calcium-containing crystals, including CPPD crystals.

Reality: It is a widely held belief that the storage of synovial fluid (e.g., overnight) results in the *de novo* formation of crystals that are of no clinical significance. Several older studies suggested that stored synovial fluids produce brushite, a calcium-containing crystal ($CaHPO_4{\sim}2H_2O$), that is described often as having a star-shaped morphology (Dieppe et al. 1979).

More recent studies do not support the phenomenon of brushite formation. Galvez et al. (2002) showed that, for synovial fluid samples deemed crystal-free on immediate examination, no new crystals appeared following storage in either a refrigerator or freezer. In addition, clinically important crystals were retained, despite refrigeration for at least 72 h, with only minor losses observed with freezing.

These findings support the theory that, based on the known levels of calcium and pyrophosphate in synovial fluids, CPPD crystals are extremely unlikely to form in solution (Hearn et al. 1978).

Myth: Intracellular CPPD crystals are more significant than are extracellular ones.

Reality: Many clinicians believe that, unless CPPD crystals are intracellular, they are clinically irrelevant (Fig. 37.7). Few studies support this belief. On the contrary, in one study, neither the clinical presentation nor the presence or absence of joint inflammation correlated with the location of CPPD crystals (intracellular versus extracellular) (Martinez-Sanchis and Pascual 2005).

Myth: All patients with CPPD deposition disease should undergo an extensive metabolic evaluation.

Reality: The three most common risk factors for articular CPPD deposition are: (1) age; (2) age; and, (3) age. Fifty percent of nonagenarians have articular CPPD crystals (Mitrovic et al. 1988). It is rare for CPPD crystals to be

Table 37.2 The five H club: metabolic causes of CPPD crystal deposition

Hyperparathyroidism
Hemochromatosis
Hypomagnesemia
Hypophosphatasia
(Benign Familial) Hypocalciuric hypercalcemia

Table 37.3 Laboratory evaluation for the younger patient presenting with calcium pyrophosphate dehydrate (CPPD) deposition disease

Calcium
Phosphate
Magnesium
Alkaline phosphatase
Ferritin
Serum iron and total iron binding capacity
Thyroid stimulating hormone
Parathyroid hormone levels (drawn only if the serum calcium level is abnormal)

detected in patients younger than 60 years, unless the disease is familial, caused by trauma to a single joint, or associated with one of a handful of metabolic abnormalities. A 90-year-old patient with chondrocalcinosis on a knee film is unlikely to have an occult metabolic condition.

Young patients should certainly be screened for the metabolic associations of CPPD crystal deposition, of which hyperparathyroidism, hemochromatosis, and hypomagnesemia (Table 37.2) are most common. Gout is also a well-characterized risk factor for CPPD deposition disease. The appropriate laboratory evaluation for these disorders is shown in Table 37.3.

Myth: Findings on plain radiographs correlate reliably with pathological and clinical manifestations in CPPD crystal deposition disease.

Reality: Conventional radiography is most often the initial approach to the evaluation of patients with suspected CPPD deposition disease. However, in one study that employed knee arthroscopy, the correlation between radiographic and pathological findings was only 39% (Fisseler-Eckhoff and Muller 1992). Improved applications to CPPD deposition disease of ultrasonography, advanced imaging, and quantitative physicochemical analyses of joint fluid and tissue crystals are needed to understand better the relationships between the amounts and articular foci of crystal deposition, symptoms, and disease outcome.

37.4 Epidemiology

Myth: CPPD deposition disease is equally prevalent in all ethnic groups.

Fig. 37.7 Intra- and extracellular calcium pyrophosphate dehydrate (CPPD) crystals. Typically, CPPD crystals are seen both intra- and extra-cellularly (Courtesy of Laureen Daft, BS)

Reality: CPPD deposition disease of the wrist and knee is markedly less common among Chinese in Beijing than among whites in Framingham, MA (Zhang et al. 2006). This disparity is evident, despite the higher prevalence of knee osteoarthritis in the Chinese population. Relatively high calcium in drinking water in Beijing, which leads to long-term suppression of parathyroid hormone production, might explain this observation, at least in part.

Myth: Hypothyroidism is a common metabolic cause of secondary CPPD crystal deposition disease.

Reality: In case studies, CPPD crystals have been detected in joint effusions of some patients with severe hypothyroidism, a condition that by itself can cause arthropathy. However, both hypothyroidism and CPPD crystal deposition are highly prevalent among older individuals. This fact alone probably explains the frequent coexistence of these two conditions. Indeed, several cross-sectional studies of patients with radiographically detected CPPD deposition disease have failed to detect a significant association of hypothyroidism with chondrocalcinosis (Visinoni et al. 1993; Job-Deslandre et al. 1993; Komatireddy et al. 1989).

Myth: The clinical presentation of familial CPPD crystal deposition disease is homogeneous.

Reality: Familial CPPD deposition disease is best characterized in Chile and Spain (Zaka et al. 2006; Terkeltaub 2008). Familial CPPD crystal deposition disease usually presents in the third and fourth decades of life, but familial disease can also be detected before the age of 20 or into late middle age.

The ANKH gene, which encodes a transmembrane protein that channels PP_i into and out of the chondrocyte, appears to be important in the pathophysiology of chondrocalcinosis (Zaka 2006; Terkeltaub 2008). Some kindreds with linkages to *ANKH* on chromosome 5p manifest early-onset polyarthritis. The knees and wrists are affected most commonly, but ankylosing intervertebral disease and involvement of the symphysis pubis and sacroiliac joints are also described.

Chondrocalcinosis of late onset has also been reported in some kindreds. In an English kindred with CPPD disease linked to *ANKH* mutation on chromosome 5p, recurrent childhood seizures were associated with development of CPPD deposition disease in later life. Familial CPPD deposition disease can involve more than one joint and manifests a level of clinical intensity comparable with that seen in idiopathic CPPD deposition disease. Premature osteoarthritis is common but not universal.

Pearl: Most elderly patients with chondrocalcinosis of the knee also have radiographic evidence of this disorder in other joints.

Comment: The prevalence of chondrocalcinosis increases progressively with aging. As an example, one study of knee meniscal cartilage calcification detected this abnormality in only 16% of women between the ages of 80 and 89, but in 30% of women older than 89 (Ellman and Levin 1975). Moreover, in a radiographic survey of the hands, wrists, pelvis, and knees, the prevalence of chondrocalcinosis was 44% among individuals older than 84 years, 36% among 75–84-year-olds, and 15% among 65–74-year-olds (Wilkins et al. 1983).

37.5 Pathophysiology

Pearl: The term "pyrophosphate arthropathy" appropriately describes the chronic degenerative changes in cartilage that are associated with CPPD crystal deposition.

Comment: Altered concentrations of calcium, PP_i, and the solubility products of these ions clearly promote CPPD crystal formation. The levels of magnesium in cartilage and the composition of the extracellular matrix also influence the dynamics of CPPD crystal formation. These factors determine the ratio of monoclinic to triclinic CPPD crystals. This ratio is important, because monoclinic CPPD crystals are more inflammatory.

Both calcium and PP_i also exert important effects on gene expression, cell differentiation, and viability in chondrocytes. Excess quantities of PP_i leads to the induction of matrix metalloproteinase-13 and the promotion of apoptosis (Terkeltaub 2008). Hence, "pyrophosphate arthropathy" appropriately describes some of the chronic degenerative changes in cartilage in CPPD crystal deposition disease. These changes are not simply due to the toxic effects on chondrocytes and proinflammatory effects of CPPD crystals.

Pearl: Altered PP_i transport by ANKH is central to the pathogenesis of both idiopathic and familial CPPD crystal deposition disease.

Comment: As noted earlier, ANKH encodes a transmembrane protein that facilitates the transport of PP_i in and out of the chondrocyte (Rosenthal 2006; Zaka et al. 2006; Terkeltaub 2008). "Gain of function" alterations in intrinsic ANKH PP_i channeling activity could lead to chronic, low-grade "PP_i leak" from chondrocytes.

ANKH is increased in osteoarthritic and chondrocalcinotic cartilage chondrocytes. In addition, homozygosity for a single nucleotide substitution (-4 G to A) in the *ANKH* 5'-untranslated region that promotes increased ANKH expression was present in approximately 4% of British subjects with the diagnosis of idiopathic chondrocalcinosis of aging (Zhang et al. 2005). Hence, some patients with late-onset CPPD crystal deposition disease appear to have a familial component.

Two major chromosomal linkages, 8q and 5p, have been identified in studies of familial CPPD deposition disease. Chromosome 5p-linked chondrocalcinosis, which is more widely distributed than 8q-linked disease, is associated with *ANKH* mutations. However, ANKH is not the only modulator of PP_i metabolism that is linked with idiopathic chondrocalcinosis. The disorder also is characterized by excessive NPP1 activity, which leads to the generation of PP_i by chondrocytes (Terkeltaub 2008). Finally, the chondrocyte in idiopathic chondrocalcinosis responds abnormally to growth factors insulin-like growth factor-1 and transforming growth factor, with increased PP_i production (Rosenthal 2006).

37.6 Treatment and Outcomes

Pearl: Systemic glucocorticoids are useful for treatment of acute pseudogout.

Comment: Several studies support use of systemic glucocorticoids for both gout and pseudogout in the short term (Roane et al. 1997; Alloway et al. 1993). Most studies to date have employed either one or two 60 mg intramuscular injections of triamcinolone or oral prednisone for up to 10 days.

On the other hand, prolonged courses or using high doses of prednisone have not been studied thoroughly in acute pseudogout. Such approaches may create more problems than they solve, particularly in the elderly population that is at greatest risk for CPPD deposition disease. Thus, glucocorticoid bursts are helpful in treating acute flares of microcrystalline disease, but "maintenance" prednisone is a bad idea.

Pearl: Intraarticular glucocorticoids are the most effective and often the safest therapy for acute CPPD deposition disease-associated arthritis.

Comment: A variety of therapeutic options for the treatment of acute gout exist. Many of these same therapies are useful for pseudogout, as well, but tend to be less effective in pseudogout. The risks of colchicine and NSAIDs are not trivial in elderly patients. Few controlled trials of any therapy exist, but intraarticular glucocorticoids appear to be more effective than the alternatives and are certainly safer than most systemic therapies (O'Duffy 1976). Glucocorticoids should be used as the treatment of choice unless there is a concurrent infection or, in rare instances, when the involved joint is inaccessible to injection.

Despite using intraarticular glucocorticoids, joint aspiration, and nonsteroidal antiinflammatory drugs (NSAIDs), the average duration of a pseudogout attack in one study was 18 days (Masuda and Ishikawa 1987). Colchicine is useful for prophylaxis against recurrent pseudogout.

Myth: Secondary CPPD crystal deposition in cartilage always worsens the outcome of primary osteoarthritis.

Reality: This appears to be true only in a subset of patients with osteoarthritis. Patients with knee osteoarthritis, with calcium-containing crystals in their joint fluids, have been reported to have more severe radiographic scores and require knee-replacement surgery more often than those with primary osteoarthritis who do not have crystals (Rosenthal 2006). However, this conclusion contrasts with the results of two magnetic-resonance imaging studies of knee osteoarthritis in which the relationship between chondrocalcinosis and the course of osteoarthritis was evaluated longitudinally (Neogi et al. 2006). Knees that demonstrated chondrocalcinosis had a decreased or unchanged risk of cartilage loss, compared with those without chondrocalcinosis (Neogi et al. 2006). When interpreting these studies, it is important to remember that MRI is neither sensitive nor specific for the imaging of CPPD deposition.

Similarly, in a study of 102 consecutive patients sent for total knee replacement, CPPD crystal deposition disease was identified in 53%. No associations were observed between chondrocalcinosis and overall joint function or age at arthroplasty (Viriyavejkul et al. 2006). The dysregulated cartilage matrix repair that generates CPPD crystal deposition may be a biomarker for processes that retard the progression of cartilage tissue loss in some patients with osteoarthritis.

In summary, there is no established direct correlation between extent of cartilage calcification and progression of CPPD deposition arthropathy.

References

Alloway J, Moriarty M, Hoogland Y, et al Comparison of triamcinolone acetonide with indomethacin in the treatment of acute gouty arthritis J Rheumatol. 1993;20:111–3

Chollet-Janin A, Finckh A, Dudler J, et al Methotrexate as an alternative therapy for chronic calcium pyrophosphate deposition disease: an exploratory analysis. Arthritis Rheum. 2007;56:688–92

Dieppe P, Crocker P, Corke C, et al Synovial fluid crystals. Q J Med. 1979;48:533–55

Doan TH, Chevalier X, Leparc JM, et al Premature enthusiasm for the use of methotrexate for refractory chondrocalcinosis: comment on the article by Chollet-Janin et al Arthritis Rheum. 2008;58:2210–1

Ellman MH, Levin B. Chondrocalcinosis in elderly persons. Arthritis Rheum. 1975;18:43–7

Fisseler-Eckhoff A, Muller KM. Arthroscopy and chondrocalcinosis. Arthroscopy 1992;8:98–104

Galvez J, Saiz E, Linares L, et al Delayed examination of synovial fluid by ordinary and polarized light microscopy to detect and identify crystals. Ann Rheum Dis. 2002;61:444–7

Gerster J, Varisco P, Kern J, et al CPPD crystal deposition disease in patients with rheumatoid arthritis. Clin Rheumatol. 2006;25:468–9

Gordon C, Swan A, Dieppe P. Detection of crystals in synovial fluid by light microscopy: sensitivity and reliability. Ann Rheum Dis. 1989;48:737–42

Goto S, Umehara J, Aizawa T, et al Crowned dens syndrome. J Bone Joint Surg Am. 2007;89:2732–6

Hasselbacher P. Variation in synovial fluid analysis by hospital laboratories. Arthritis Rheum. 1987;30:637–42

Hearn P, Russell R, Elliott J, et al Formation products of calcium pyrophosphate crystals in vitro and the effect of iron salts. Clin Sci. 1978;54:29P

Job-Deslandre C, Menkes CJ, Guinot M, et al Does hypothyroidism increase the prevalence of chondrocalcinosis? Br J Rheumatol. 1993;32:177–9

Komatireddy GR, Ellman MH, Brown NL. Lack of association between hypothyroidism and chondrocalcinosis. J Rheumatol. 1989;16:807–8

Martinez-Sanchis A, Pascual E. Intracellular and extracellular CPPD crystals are a regular feature in synovial fluid from uninflamed joints of patients with CPPD related arthropathy. Ann Rheum Dis. 2005; 64:1769–72

Masuda I, Ishikawa K. Clinical features of pseudogout attack: a survey of 50 cases. Clin Orth Rel Res. 1987;229:173–81

McCarty DJ. Diagnostic mimicry in arthritis: patterns of joint involvement associated with calcium pyrophosphate dihydrate crystal deposits. Ann Rheum Dis. 1975;25:804–9

Mitrovic D, Stankovic A, Iriarte-Borda O, et al The prevalence of chondrocalcinosis in the human knee joint. An autopsy survey. J Rheumatol. 1988;15:633–41

Neogi T, Nevitt M, Niu J, et al Lack of association between chondrocalcinosis and increased risk of cartilage loss in knees with osteoarthritis: results of two prospective longitudinal magnetic resonance imaging studies. Arthritis Rheum. 2006;54:1822–8

O'Duffy J. Clinical studies of acute pseudogout attacks. Comments on prevalence, predisposition and treatment. Arthritis Rheum. 1976;19 (Suppl):349–52

Roane D, Harris M, Carpenter M, et al Prospective use of intramuscular triamcinolone in pseudogout. J Rheumatol. 1997;24:1168–70

Rosenthal AK. Calcium crystal deposition and osteoarthritis. Rheum Dis Clin North Am. 2006;32:401–12

Schumacher H, Sieck M, Rothfuss S, et al Reproducibility of synovial fluid analyses. Arthritis Rheum. 1986;29:770–4

Terkeltaub R. Firestein GS, Budd RC, Harris ED, Jr., McInnes IB, Ruddy S, Sergent JS. Diseases associated with articular deposition of calcium pyrophosphate dihydrate and basic calcium phosphate crystals. In: Firestein G et al, editor. Kelley's textbook of rheumatology, 8th ed, WB Saunders, Philadelphia, 2008

Viriyavejkul P, Wilairatana V, Tanavalee A, et al Comparison of characteristics of patients with and without calcium pyrophosphate dihydrate crystal deposition disease who underwent total knee replacement surgery for osteoarthritis. Osteoarthr Cartil 2006;13: 232–5

Visinoni RA, Ferraz MB, Furlanetto RP, et al Hypothyroidism and chondrocalcinosis: new evidence for lack of association between the 2 pathologies. J Rheumatol. 1993;20:1991–2

Wilkins E, Dieppe P, Maddison P, et al Osteoarthritis and articular chondrocalcinosis in the elderly. Ann Rheum Dis. 1983;42: 280–4

Yuan S, Bien C, Wener M, et al Repeat examination of synovial fluid for crystals: Is it useful? Clin Chem. 2003;49:1562–3

Zaka R, Williams CJ. Role of the progressive ankylosis gene in cartilage mineralization. Curr Opin Rheumatol. 2006;18:181–6

Zhang Y, Johnson K, Russell RG, et al Association of sporadic chondrocalcinosis with a -4-basepair G-to-A transition in the 5'-untranslated region of ANKH that promotes enhanced expression of ANKH protein and excess generation of extracellular inorganic pyrophosphate. Arthritis Rheum. 2005;52:1110–7

Zhang Y, Terkeltaub R, Nevitt M, et al Lower prevalence of chondrocalcinosis in Chinese subjects in Beijing than in white subjects in the United States: the Beijing Osteoarthritis Study. Arthritis Rheum. 2006;54:3508–12

Inflammatory Eye Disease

38

James T. Rosenbaum and George N. Papaliodis

38.1 Overview of Inflammatory Eye Disease

> The eye is frequently the target of immune-mediated inflammation, either as the sole organ involved or as part of a multiorgan system disease.

> Systemic inflammatory disorders tend to involve the eye in characteristic manners. As examples, disorders associated with HLA-B27 often cause a highly symptomatic anterior uveitis; Behcet's disease can cause a subclinical but ultimately vision-threatening posterior uveitis; and Wegener's granulomatosis is associated with scleritis, peripheral ulcerative keratitis, and orbital pseudotumor.

> The diagnosis of systemic disease can therefore be inferred from the specific types of ocular involvement.

> The uveal tract is divided into anterior, intermediate, and posterior segments.

> "Anterior uveitis" and "iritis" are synonyms.

Myth: Patients with retinal vasculitis should be evaluated thoroughly for systemic vasculitis.

Reality: "Retinal vasculitis" is a widely misunderstood term. Ophthalmologists use vasulitis in a manner that differs significantly from usage by rheumatologists (Rosenbaum et al. 1991). Rheumatologists generally rely on histopathological confirmation or the finding of a classic angiographic appearance in medium-sized arteries to make the diagnosis of vasculitis. In contrast, ophthalmologists rarely biopsy the retina owing to the morbidity of this procedure. Ophthalmologists diagnose retinal vasculitis either by the appearance of the eye on fundoscopy or by fluorescein angiography. Leakage of fluorescein dye is sufficient evidence for an ophthalmologist to diagnose "vasculitis" (Fig. 38.1).

Endothelial cells are highly diverse. The microvasculature of the retina differs substantially from the blood vessels typically involved in disorders such as polyarteritis nodosa

or Wegener's granulomatosis (WG). In the context of the term used by ophthalmologists, retinal vasculitis can:

- Involve arteries, veins, or both
- Be categorized as either occlusive or nonocclusive
- Be limited to the peripheral retina or a focal area of the retina.

The systemic diseases that are most commonly associated with retinal vasculitis are sarcoidosis, Behcet's disease, and multiple sclerosis (MS).

Pearl: All patients with new diagnoses of scleritis should have a serum assay for antineutrophil cytoplasmic antibodies (ANCA).

Comment: Autoantibodies play a relatively small role in the evaluation of patients with scleritis (Fig. 38.2). A detailed history is by far the most useful tool in establishing a systemic disease as the underlying cause of the eye inflammation (Smith et al. 2007). Antinuclear antibody (ANA) assays seldom yield anything other than "false-positive" results. In a patient with scleritis, a positive ANA assay would not establish the diagnosis of lupus in the absence of other evidence for that disease, because scleritis is not a typical feature of lupus and multiple other conditions can be associated with a positive ANA. Rheumatoid arthritis certainly causes scleritis, but severe ocular inflammation is seldom the initial disease manifestation.

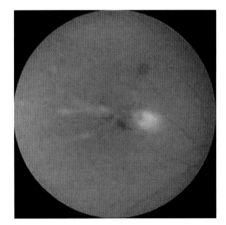

Fig. 38.1 Retinal vasculitis (Courtesy of Dr. James Rosenbaum)

J. H. Stone (ed.), *A Clinician's Pearls and Myths in Rheumatology,*
DOI:10.1007/978-1-84800-934-9_38, © Springer Science + Business Media B.V. 2009

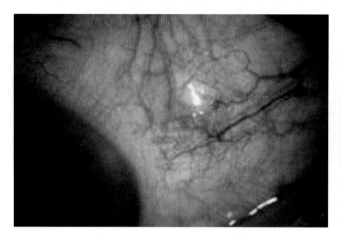

Fig. 38.2 Scleritis (Courtesy of Dr. John Stone)

On the other hand, ANCA assays can be extremely useful in the evaluation of patients with scleritis. Among the "ANCA-associated" vasculitides, WG is by far the most likely to cause scleritis (Hoang et al. 2008). (Microscopic polyangiitis and the Churg–Strauss syndrome rarely cause this ocular condition). In the WG Etanercept Trial, 8 of the 180 patients (5%) had scleritis (Mahr et al. 2008). WG often causes scleritis early in the disease course, when manifestations of "full-blown" disease are absent.

Pearl: The development of peripheral ulcerative keratitis is associated with the presence of an occult systemic disease that may be lethal if not identified and treated aggressively.

Comment: Peripheral ulcerative keratitis (PUK) is a devastating disease in which progressive destruction of the peripheral cornea leads to perforation of the globe and predisposes the patient to ocular infections. The most common disease entities that cause PUK are rheumatoid arthritis and WG.

Pearl: Approximately 50% of patients with WG have ophthalmologic manifestations at some point in their course.

Comment: WG can involve essentially any ocular tissue (orbital inflammatory pseudotumor, conjunctivitis, episcleritis (Fig. 38.3), scleritis, keratitis, and uveitis). However, retinal involvement by vasculitis in WG is relatively uncommon.

Pearl: If an ophthalmologist reports that your patient with WG has retinal vasculitis, the correct diagnosis is probably an infection.

Comment: WG very seldom causes a true retinal vasculitis. The disease has been associated with retinal vasculitis in only a handful of anecdotal reports. On the other hand, patients with WG who are being treated actively with immunosuppression—particularly cyclophosphamide and glucocorticoids—are at substantial risk for an infectious retinitis caused by herpes simplex, herpes zoster, or cytomegalovirus (Fig. 38.4).

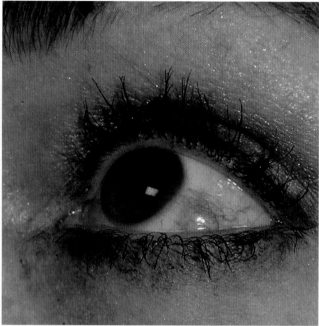

Fig. 38.3 Episcleritis (Courtesy of Dr. John Stone)

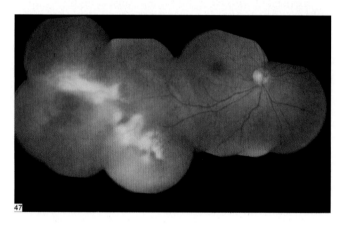

Fig. 38.4 CMV vasculitis (Courtesy of Dr. James Rosenbaum)

Herpes viruses can infect the retina and typically cause both intraretinal hemorrhages and blood vessels that appear abnormal on fluorescein angiography. Thus, these infections are often mislabeled as "retinal vasculitis." Fluorescein angiography usually demonstrates an occlusive vasculopathy in patients with herpes virus infections. Ironically, the treatment for "retinal vasculitis" in a patient with WG is usually to reduce the immunosuppression medications—and treat with an appropriate antimicrobial agent.

Myth: Patients with giant cell arteritis often recover from their visual loss with glucocorticoid therapy.

Reality: In a *New England Journal of Medicine* clinicopathological case conference, the clinician suspected giant-cell arteritis in a patient who had suffered monocular visual loss (Seton et al. 2008). High-dose glucocorticoids were administered and the vision improved. This should have alerted the clinician to the fact that the underlying disease was not giant-cell arteritis (in fact, on autopsy, a disseminated fungal infection was found to be the cause of the patient's temporary monocular blindness).

Patients with giant-cell arteritis frequently experience episodes of amaurosis fugax, which is (by definition) transient visual loss. This symptom may improve without therapy—for a while. Once the visual loss secondary to the ischemia of giant-cell arteritis has been present for 1 day or more, however, the ship has sailed: no intervention will lead consistently to any substantial restoration of vision (Aiello et al. 1993). In fact, marked improvement in acuity following the institution of glucocorticoids therapy should call into question the accuracy of the underlying diagnosis.

Myth: A normal erythrocyte sedimentation rate effectively excludes giant-cell arteritis.

Reality: The great majority of patients with giant-cell arteritis have elevated sedimentation rates (ESRs), but biopsy-proven disease can occur in patients whose ESRs are normal (Salvarani and Hunder 2001). Moreover, at least, one group has found that patients who experience visual loss tend to have lower (but not necessarily normal) ESRs relative to patients with GCA who do not suffer visual loss (Lopez-Diaz et al. 2008). One explanation for this is that clinicians are less likely to suspect GCA in a patient who does not have a strikingly high ESR. Anterior ischemic optic neuropathy and its permanent blindness in the affected eye may be the symptom that announces the presence of GCA.

A normal ESR in the setting of a convincing clinical history for giant-cell arteritis should not dissuade the clinician from obtaining a temporal artery biopsy (and even treating the patient empirically until the biopsy is obtained).

Pearl: Hoarseness is a possible initial manifestation of giant-cell arteritis.

Comment: A rare but established manifestation of giant-cell arteritis is hoarseness. Other less well-appreciated manifestations of GCA include sore throat, nonproductive cough, or an ulceration of the tongue.

Pearl: The aggressive use of topical glucocorticoids early in the course of an iritis exacerbation minimizes the duration of the event and potential for ocular injury.

Comment: Increasing the dosing frequency of a topical glucocorticoid enhances the bioavailability in the anterior chamber. The package insert for prednisolone acetate and prednisolone sodium phosphate suggests BID to QID dosing for ocular inflammation. Most ocular inflammatory disease specialists prescribe the use of topical glucocorticoids every 1 or 2 h at the onset of an acute exacerbation.

Pearl: The most common cause of intraocular inflammation throughout the world is toxoplasmosis.

Comment: Toxoplasma gondii is an obligate intracellular parasite found throughout the world that produces a characteristic retinochoroiditis. This organism is responsible for 30–50% of all cases of posterior uveitis in the United States. The primary site of infection in the eye is the retina or optic nerve, but clinical findings can include vitritis, retinal vasculitis, and iritis.

Myth: Patients who have experienced a single, brief episode of uveitis do not require further evaluation.

Reality: Many ophthalmologists regard a self-limited case of uveitis the way that rheumatologists regard one episode of podagra: generally not worthy of further evaluation or treatment. On the contrary, even a single episode of uveitis that resolves on its own requires a thorough medical evaluation.

The most common systemic disease associated with uveitis in North America and Europe is either ankylosing spondylitis or a related spondyloarthropathy. The uveitis that accompanies this family of systemic conditions is anterior, unilateral, and self-limited; i.e., the eye inflammation resolves completely within several months even without treatment.

Two thirds of the patients with the acute onset of unilateral anterior uveitis in the setting of a spondyloarthropathy are not aware that their chronic low-back pain is caused by sacroiliitis (Rosenbaum 1989). Thus, the first episode of iritis presents an opportunity to recognize a treatable cause of chronic low-back pain. HLA-B27 testing and sacroiliac imaging are appropriate parts of the evaluation of a patient with unilateral anterior uveitis.

Pearl: Intraocular CNS lymphoma is an uncommon malignancy but should be considered in older patients who present with new onset vitritis.

Comment: Documentation of intense intraocular inflammation (in the absence of pain or photophobia), subretinal infiltrates, and lack of a sustained response to glucocorticoid treatment should raise concern about the possibility of intraocular lymphoma. A high index of suspicion is necessary to avoid a delay in diagnosis. The average time between onset of ocular symptoms and definitive diagnosis is approximately 21 months (Whitcup et al. 1993).

Pearl: The treatment of infectious uveitis requires the appropriate antimicrobial agent but often also necessitates the use of systemic glucocorticoids.

Comment: Multiple infectious diseases can involve ocular structures. The cornerstone of therapy for eye infections is the appropriate antimicrobial agent. The host inflammatory response to the infectious agent and the reaction after initiation of antimicrobial treatment can induce significant ocular injury, including cystoid macular edema, vitritis, retinitis, papillitis, and choroiditis. The use of systemic glucocorticoids, although counterintuitive given the etiology of the ocular inflammation, is often required.

Pearl: A normal serum level of angiotensin converting enzyme (ACE) does not exclude sarcoidosis as the cause of uveitis.

Comment: Ocular disease is nearly as common as pulmonary disease as the initial manifestation of sarcoidosis. ACE levels are elevated in approximately 60% of patients with pulmonary sarcoidosis. Early sarcoidosis and disease localized to the eye are associated with a relatively small "burden" of granulomas, the site of ACE production. Thus, serum ACE levels are often normal even when sarcoidosis is the cause of ocular inflammatory disease.

Pearl: A computed tomography (CT) scan of the chest is indicated in the evaluation of patients with uveitis.

Comment: Sarcoidosis is a common cause of uveitis. In fact, ocular disease is nearly as common as pulmonary disease as the initial manifestation of sarcoidosis. Many patients with sarcoid-associated uveitis have no pulmonary symptoms, and chest radiographs often fail to capture hilar or mediastinal lymphadenopathy.

A study from the Cleveland Clinic found that 57% of older women with uveitis who were otherwise asymptomatic had adenopathy detectable on chest CT (Kaiser et al. 2002). Consequently, CT scans of the hilum and mediastinum are considered appropriate for the evaluation of patients with uveitis who do not fit neatly into a specific diagnostic category.

Pearl: Penetrating trauma to one eye can induce ocular inflammation in both eyes.

Comment: Sympathetic ophthalmia is a granulomatous uveitis that occurs after penetrating trauma or after surgical procedures. The disease is uncommon but devastating due to its potentially blinding effects in both the inciting and the sympathizing eye. The presumed mechanism of inducing ocular inflammation is due to exposure of uveal antigens (previously sequestered in immunologically privileged sites in the eye) to the host immune system, with the resultant loss of immune tolerance.

Pearl: Despite advances in diagnostic capabilities, many cases of uveitis remain idiopathic.

Comment: Careful ophthalmologic examination with appropriate serologic and radiologic studies often lead to a definitive diagnosis of a specific disease that is causing intraocular inflammation. However, up to 50% of cases of uveitis remain "idiopathic"; i.e., they cannot be attributed to a particular underlying disease.

Pearl: Certain medications can cause uveitis.

Comment: There are many reports in the literature implicating drugs as causal agents for uveitis. These medications include topical agents, oral medications, intravenous preparations, and vaccinations. The agents most commonly associated with uveitis are the bisphosphonates, rifampin, rifabutin, and cidofovir.

Pearl: Thyroid disease is the most common cause of orbital inflammatory disease.

Comment: Several systemic immune-mediated diseases can cause orbital inflammation (Lutt et al. 2008). Orbital inflammatory disease results in pain, exophthalmos, restricted eye motility, diplopia, and visual loss caused by compression of the optic nerve (Fig. 38.5). The most common cause of orbital inflammation is Graves' disease. The specific diagnosis of thyroid-associated orbital inflammatory disease is sometimes strongly supported by imaging (e.g., MRI) and by testing for thyroid autoantibodies. In some instances, an orbital biopsy is required to establish the diagnosis.

Pearl: Children with uveitis often have asymptomatic disease.

Comment: In adults with uveitis, patients' symptoms include eye pain, eye redness, light sensitivity, and blurry vision. Children with juvenile idiopathic arthritis (JIA) may have significant intraocular inflammation without complaints. Ninety percent of patients who have uveitis associated with JIA have no ocular symptoms (Grassi et al. 2007).

Pearl: Children with a form of uveitis known as pars planitis often present with vitreous hemorrhage.

Comment: The most common form of uveitis in childhood is associated with JIA. The uveitis occurs in the oligoarticular

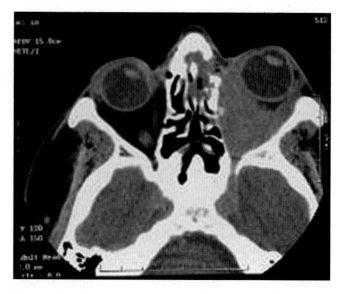

Fig. 38.5 Orbital pseudotumor (Courtesy of Dr. John Stone)

Fig. 38.6 Pars planitis
(Courtesy of
Dr. George Papaliodis)

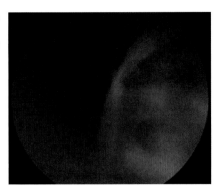

Fig. 38.7 Birdshot
choroidopathy
(Courtesy of
Dr. George Papaliodis)

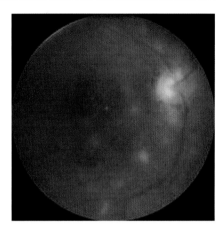

form of JIA and usually affects young girls whose serum tests positively for ANA.

Children can also develop a condition called pars planitis, a form of uveitis associated with inflammatory exudates overlying the peripheral retina which is known as the pars plana. Neovascularization is a common complication of pars planitis, particularly in children. These new vessels are friable and may bleed. This results in a sudden "shower" obscuring vision. A careful evaluation of a child who suffers this type of bleeding known as a vitreous hemorrhage may reveal pars planitis (Lauer et al. 2002). Since the blood usually will not allow an adequate examination of the eye, the first clue to the diagnosis may be a careful examination with indirect ophthalmoscopy of the opposite eye, which is free of hemorrhage (Fig. 38.6).

Pearl: Pars planitis is a risk factor for the development of MS, just as optic neuritis is a risk factor for that diagnosis.

Comment: Uveitis has a rare but well-defined association with MS. Approximately 1% of patients with MS have uveitis, and MS patients comprise about 1.5% of all patients with uveitis in tertiary referral clinics. The uveitis of MS can take several forms, the most common of which is pars planitis.

Patients with MS and pars planitis share common HLA haplotypes. One study found a 20% risk of developing either MS or optic neuritis within 5 years of the diagnosis of pars planitis (Malinowski 1993). This risk may be even higher if the patient is female and has the type of perivascular changes in the retina that are termed peripheral retinal periphlebitis. In experimental autoimmune encephalomyelitis, an animal model of demyelinating disease, the animals often develop uveitis.

Pearl: One of the strongest HLA links to disease susceptibility is the association of HLA-A29 with birdshot retinochoroidopathy.

Comment: Ophthalmologists recognize a variety of "white-dot syndromes" that are caused by inflammation in the retina and the adjacent choroid. These entities, which lead to focal whitening of the retina, include serpiginous choroiditis, the

multiple evanescent white-dot syndrome, punctate inner choroidopathy, multifocal choroiditis, and acute multifocal placoid pigmentary epitheliopathy.

"Birdshot choroidopathy" (Fig. 38.7) another white-dot syndrome, is typically bilateral. The lesions in birdshot choroidopathy are thought to represent focal granulomas. Visual loss with birdshot choroidopathy can be severe, but the process is responsive to immunosuppression. Approximately 95% of patients with birdshot choroidopathy are HLA-A29 positive (LeHoang et al. 1992), making this disorder one of the best examples of a link between an HLA class I antigen and disease susceptibility.

Pearl: HLA-B27 is associated with uveitis secondary to either psoriatic arthritis or inflammatory bowel disease. However, the association is not as strong as that between HLA-B27 and uveitis secondary to ankylosing spondylitis.

Comment: Just as HLA-B27 is associated with the subset of patients with psoriatic arthritis who develop sacroiliitis and the subset of inflammatory bowel disease (IBD) patients who develop sacroiliitis, so HLA-B27 is associated with the subset of either patients with psoriatic arthritis or IBD who develop uveitis (Paiva et al. 2000; Lyons and Rosenabum 1997). Furthermore, just as approximately 50% of patients with sacroiliitis and either psoriasis or IBD are HLA-B27 positive, about 50% of patients with either psoriatic arthritis or IBD who develop uveitis are HLA-B27 positive.

Pearl: Pain is a typical manifestation of scleritis, but pain is not typical of episcleritis.

Comment: The episclera is a superficial layer of tissue that overlies sclera. Patients who have scleritis often have a concomitant component of episcleritis, but the converse is not true; i.e., patients can have episcleritis without scleritis.

Intense, boring pain is nearly universal in patients with scleritis, but absent in episcleritis. Patients with episcleritis often complain of a vague discomfort in the eye, but it does not rise to the level of "pain." Both scleritis and episcleritis cause ocular redness, which may be nodular or elevated and may assume the shape of a wedge (see Fig. 38.3). Thus, distinguishing scleritis from episcleritis on the clinical appearance of the eye redness alone (and without the help of a slit-lamp) can be challenging. The presence or absence of pain is useful in discriminating the two conditions.

Episcleritis and scleritis generally have entirely different implications. Only a small minority of cases of episcleritis are associated with a systemic inflammatory disease, and episcleritis does not pose a risk to vision. In contrast, roughly half of patients with scleritis have an associated systemic disease, the most common of which is rheumatoid arthritis or WG.

Scleritis can cause intraocular complications such as glaucoma, uveitis, or optic neuropathy. It can also cause a "corneal melt," an intensely painful condition that leads to the loss of useful vision in the eye (Fig. 38.8).

Pearl: The syndrome of fever, arthralgias, renal dysfunction, and the sudden onset of bilateral anterior uveitis is often due to tubulointerstitial nephritis with uveitis (TINU), a significantly underappreciated disorder.

Comment: The differential diagnosis for uveitis in association with systemic symptoms includes a broad variety of infections and idiopathic inflammatory conditions. One disease that is arguably the least recognized, but perhaps, the most common explanation of systemic symptoms and uveitis is TINU (Mackensen et al. 2007). This disease usually occurs in patients who are younger than 20 years of age. TINU is the second most common cause of uveitis among children in Japan (Goda et al. 2005).

The uveitis of TINU is sudden in onset and typically involves both anterior chambers simultaneously. However, inflammation may begin in one eye several days before the other is involved clinically. TINU patients experience substantial systemic symptoms, including fever, malaise, and arthralgias. The systemic symptoms may precede the uveitis or begin simultaneously with the eye disease. Rarely, the systemic symptoms follow the eye disease.

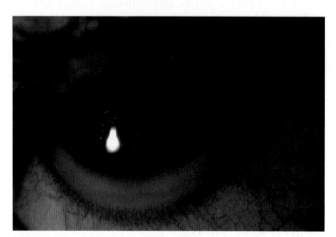

Fig. 38.8 Corneal melt (Courtesy of Dr. George Papaliodis)

Laboratory studies indicate a mild anemia, slightly elevated hepatic transaminases, and a markedly elevated ESR. Serum creatinine elevations are present in many but not all patients. However, a sterile pyuria and elevation of the urinary β-2 microglobulin level are usually detected. The systemic symptoms of TINU usually respond dramatically to modest doses of oral glucocorticoids such as 20 mg of prednisone per day.

Pearl: The differential diagnosis of cotton wool spots includes hypertension, diabetes, lupus, and infection with the human immunodeficiency virus (HIV).

Comment: Cotton wool spots are retinal exudates that indicate local retinal ischemia. In addition to diabetes mellitus and diabetic retinopathy, cotton spots are seen commonly in patients with hypertension, lupus, or HIV. One study of lupus patients followed for as long as 16 years reported that 7% had cotton wool spots at some time (Stafford-Brady et al. 1988). Patients with SLE and cotton wool spots were more likely to have a lupus anticoagulant, central nervous system disease, and a poor prognosis.

Myth: Hydroxychloroquine is a dangerous medication and should be avoided due to ocular toxicity.

Reality: The retinal toxicity of hydroxychloroquine is dependent on dose and duration of treatment. In a prospective cohort study of patients with SLE and RA who were treated with hydroxychloroquine at doses less than or equal to 6.5 mg/kg/day, no retinal toxicity was reported within the first 6 years of treatment (Mavrikakis et al. 2003). Among patients treated with more than 6 years of hydroxychloroquine, 3.4% of Patients with maculopathy caused by the medication, which stabilized when hydroxychloroquine was stopped.

The principal risk factors for hydroxychloroquine toxicity appear to be the use of high doses (i.e., >6.5 mg/kg/day), long durations of treatment, and concomitant renal dysfunction.

Myth: Cataract extraction via phacoemulsification (the most successful surgical technique in modern medicine) is as successful in patients with uveitis as it is in patients without uveitis.

Reality: Advances in cataract surgery and intraocular lens technology have improved the quality of life for patients tremendously. Patients with uveitis pose a special challenge from both a technical and disease-management perspective. Uveitic patients often have small pupillary apertures from episodes of ocular inflammatory disease, unstable zonules and capsular support. Intraocular inflammation, a normal response to surgical trauma, can be significantly exaggerated in uveitis patients. This leads to a higher incidence of macular edema, posterior capsular opacification, or intraocular lens intolerance among patients with histories of uveitis.

In one series of 242 uveitic eyes undergoing cataract surgery, 10.7% had vision loss compared with preoperative visual acuity (Yamane 2007).

Myth: Syphilis rarely involves the eye, and serologic studies to exclude syphilis are unnecessary.

Reality: Syphilis is called the "great imitator" for good reasons. Its ability to involve the eye is no exception. Syphilis can cause episcleritis, scleritis, keratitis, uveitis, retinal vasculitis, papillitis, and iris gummas. In addition, syphilis is enjoying a resurgence. Between 2005 and 2006, the incidence of primary and secondary syphilis increased by nearly 12%. Ocular disease occurs in approximately 10% of syphilis cases.

Pearl: Although included in the differential diagnosis as a cause for uveitis, ocular tuberculosis is extremely rare.

Comment: In the 1940s, tuberculosis was estimated to be responsible for up to 80% of granulomatous uveitis worldwide. Today, ocular tuberculosis is extremely rare, even in regions characterized by a high incidence of tuberculosis. One study of 1,273 patients who presented with uveitis in India found that tuberculosis was the culprit in only five patient (0.4%) (Biswas et al. 1996).

Myth: Roth spots are diagnostic of bacterial endocarditis.

Reality: A Roth spot is an intraretinal hemorrhage with a white center (Fig. 38.9). The white center is a cotton wool spot, which indicates the presence of local ischemia. Septic emboli secondary to subacute bacterial endocarditis are the cause of Roth spots most familiar to medical students. However, lupus can also cause this finding.

Myth: Any tumor necrosis factor (TNF) inhibitor is a good therapeutic choice for a patient with uveitis who has failed other immunosuppressive therapies.

Reality: Systemic disorders associated with uveitis respond differently to TNF inhibitors. Ankylosing spondylitis appears to respond rather uniformly to TNF inhibitors, regardless of which one is used. In contrast, several retrospective studies

have reported that etanercept is not as consistently effective as infliximab for the uveitis associated with Behcet's disease (Galor et al. 2006). The experience with adalimumab is promising but remains limited at the time of this writing.

Although infliximab is often highly effective for uveitis, one prospective study found a surprisingly high morbidity from the medication, including drug-induced lupus and thrombosis (Suhler et al. 2005). One hypothesis is that patients with localized inflammation are more prone to complications from TNF inhibition than are patients with systemic inflammation, who in theory have higher serum levels of TNF. No TNF inhibitor is approved for the treatment of uveitis in the United States, but infliximab has this approval in Japan for patients with Behcet's disease.

References

Aiello P, Trautmann J, McPhee T, et al Visual prognosis in giant cell arterits. Ophthalmology 1993;100:550–5

Biswas J, Narain S, Das D, Ganesh SK. Pattern of uveitis in a referral uveitis clinic in India. Int Ophthalmol. 1996–1997;20(4) 223–8

Galor A, Perez V, Hammel J, et al Differential effectiveness of etanercept and infliximab in the treatment of ocular inflammation. Ophthalmology 2006;113:2137–2323

Goda C, Kotake S, Ichiishi A, et al Clinical features in tubulointerstitial nephritis and uveitis (TINU) syndrome. Am J Ophthalmol. 2005;140:637–41

Grassi A, Corona F, Casellato A, et al Prevalence and outcome of juvenile idiopathic arthritis associated uveitis and relation to articular disease. J Rheumatol. 2007;34(5):1139–45

Hoang L, Lim L, Vaillant B, et al Antineutrophil cytoplasmic antibody-associated active scleritis. Arch Ophthalmol. 2008;126:651–5

Kaiser PK, Lowder CY, Sullivan P, et al Chest computerized tomography in the evaluation of uveitis in elderly women. Am J Ophthalmol. 2002;133:499–505

Lauer AK, Smith JR, Robertson JE, et al Vitreous hemorrhage is a common complication of pediatric pars planitis. Ophthalmology 2002;109:95–8

LeHoang P, Ozdemir N, Benhamou A, et al HLA-A29.2 subtype associated with birdshot retinochoroidopathy. Am J Ophthalmol. 1992;113:33–5

Lopez-Diaz M, Liorca J, Gonzalez-Juanatey C, et al The erythrocyte sedimentation rate is associated with the development of visual complications in biopsy-proven giant cell arteritis. Semin Arthritis Rheum. 2008;38:116–23

Lutt J, Lim L, Phal P et al Orbital inflammatory disease. Semin Arthritis Rheum. 2008;37:207–22

Lyons JL, Rosenbaum JT. Uveitis associated with inflammatory bowel disease compared with uveitis associated with spondyloarthropathy. Arch Ophthalmol. 1997;115:61–4

Mackensen F, Smith J, Rosenbaum JT. Enhanced recognition, treatment, and prognosis of tubulointerstitial nephritis and uveitis syndrome. Ophthalmology 2007;114:995–9

Mahr AD, Neogi T, LaValley MP et al A re-evaluation of item selection and weighting in the Birmingham Vasculitis Activity Score for Wegener's granulomatosis. Arthritis Care Res. 2008;59: 884–91

Malinowski SM, Pulido JS, Folk JC. Long-term visual outcome and complications associated with pars planitis. Ophthalmology 1993;100:818–24

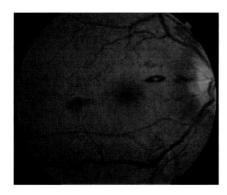

Fig. 38.9 Roth spot (Courtesy of Dr. George Papaliodis)

Mavrikakis I, Sfikakis PP, Mavrikakis E, et al The incidence of irreversible retinal toxicity in patients treated with hydroxychloroquine: a reappraisal. Ophthalmology 2003;110(7):1321–6

McCannel CA, Holland GN, Helm CJ, et al Causes of uveitis in the general practice of ophthalmology. Am J Ophthalmol. 1996: 121:35

Paiva ES, Macaluso DC, Edwards A, et al Characterisation of uveitis in patients with psoriatic arthritis. Ann Rheum Dis. 2000;59: 67–70

Rosenbaum JT. Characterization of uveitis associated with spondyloarthritis. J Rheumatol. 1989;16:792–96

Rosenbaum JT, Robertson JE, Watzke RC. Retinal vasculitis: a primer. West J Med. 1991;154:182–5

Salvarani C, Hunder GG. Giant cell arteritis with low erythrocyte sedimentation rate: frequency of occurrence in a population-based study. Arthritis Rheum. 2001;45:140–5

Seton M, Pless M, Fishman J, et al Case records of the Massachusetts General Hospital. Case 18–2008. A 68 year old man with headache and visual changes after liver transplantation. N Engl J Med. 2008; 358:2619–28

Smith J, Mackensen F, Rosenbaum JT. Therapy insight: scleritis and its relationship to systemic autoimmune disease. Nat Clin Pract 2007; 3:219–26

Stafford-Brady FJ, Urowitz MB, Gladman DD, et al Lupus retinopathy. Patterns, associations, and prognosis. Arthritis Rheum. 1988; 31: 1105–10

Suhler EB, Smith JR, Wertheim MS, et al A prospective trial of infliximab therapy for refractory uveitis: preliminary safety and efficacy outcomes. Arch Ophthalmol. 2005;123:903–12

Whitcup SM, deSmet MD, et al Intraocular lymphoma. Clinical and histopathological diagnosis. Ophthalmology 1993;100:1399–406

Immune-Mediated Inner Ear Disease

39

Yuri Agrawal and Howard W. Francis

39.1 Overview of Immune-Mediated Inner Ear Disease

> Immune-mediated inner ear disease (IMIED) is the preferred term for the syndrome involving cochlear dysfunction, leading to degrees of sensorineural hearing loss and vertigo.

> Although vasculitis has been inferred to be the cause of IMIED in some cases, histopathological proof of vasculitis involving the inner ear in this condition is lacking. The condition does appear to be mediated in some fashion by the immune system; hence, the name IMIED.

> IMIED can occur in association with a recognized autoimmune condition such as Sjögren's syndrome, Wegener's granulomatosis, or giant cell arteritis, or as an isolated entity in which no other organ dysfunction is evident.

> The onset of hearing loss in IMIED is rapid compared with other entities that lead to auditory dysfunction. Hearing loss in IMIED occurs over the course of weeks to months.

> Patients with IMIED-associated hearing loss have problems with both hearing acuity and word discrimination. Following conversations in noisy environments (e.g., in crowded restaurants) may be particularly challenging.

> For patients with IMIED, vestibular problems that result from cochlear damage can be as challenging as the auditory dysfunction, if not more so.

> Up to 70% of patients diagnosed with IMIED demonstrate clinical improvement following glucocorticoid treatment. Prednisone (1 mg/kg/day) is a reasonable starting dose for the treatment of rapidly progressive sensorineural hearing loss secondary to IMIED.

> If the patient regains significant auditory and vestibular function within 2 weeks, tapering of the prednisone dose can begin in a taper designed to discontinue the medication over 2 months.

> For patients with severe or recurrent audiovestibular dysfunction secondary to IMIED, it is not clear whether long-term courses of high-dose glucocorticoids and additional immunosuppressive agents are effective in restoring inner ear function. Such treatment approaches should be used cautiously.

39.2 Definition

Pearl: IMIED is the preferred term for the syndrome of sensorineural hearing loss, tinnitus, and vertigo.

Comment: In 1979, McCabe described a case series of 18 patients with rapidly progressive, bilateral, asymmetric hearing loss (McCabe 1979). These patients' hearing loss was often accompanied by tinnitus and vertigo. In many cases, the patients' symptoms appeared to respond to the combination of glucocorticoids and cyclophosphamide.

McCabe termed this syndrome "autoimmune sensorineural hearing loss," leading to the recognition of this syndrome as a distinct clinical entity. Because hearing loss is often not the sole feature of this disorder and evidence of a true autoimmune basis for this disease is lacking, the term IMIED is a more appropriate designation (Stone and Francis 2000).

Pearl: "Sympathetic otitis" is an antiquated name for IMIED.

Comment: Anticochlear antibodies were hypothesized to contribute to a subset of cases of bilateral sensorineural hearing loss as early as in the 1950s. Further support for immune processes in the inner ear came from the phenomenon of "sympathetic otitis," whereby patients who had sustained an injury in one ear (either traumatic or iatrogenic) later experienced hearing loss in the contralateral ear (Kikuchi 1959). The presumed mechanism of this was the exposure of previously cryptic inner ear antigens as a result of injury, leading to activation of the immune system against these antigens

Fig. 39.1 Anatomy of the temporal bone and audiovestibular apparatus. *AN* auditory nerve; *C* cochlea; *ES* endolymphatic sac; *OC* ossicular chain; *SCC* semicircular canals; *V* vestibule. From (Stone and Francis 2000). Reprinted from Current Opinion in Rheumatology with kind permission from Wolters Kluwer Health

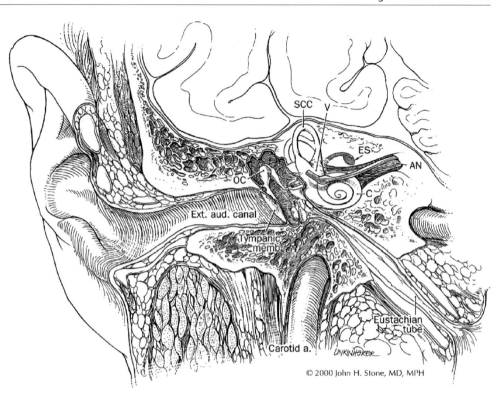

and autoimmune destruction of the remaining healthy inner ear tissue (ten Cate and Bachor 2005; Schindler and Niparko 1998).

Pearl: The main blood supply to the inner ear, the labyrinthine artery, is an end-artery that has minimal collateral anastomoses.

Comment: The inner ear, housed within the temporal bone of the skull, consists of an audiovestibular apparatus collectively referred to as the labyrinth (Fig. 39.1). The principal vascular supply to the inner ear is the labyrinthine artery, which is a branch of the anterior inferior cerebellar artery. The labyrinthine artery, which terminates within the structures of the labyrinth, lacks collateral anastomoses. This renders the inner ear particularly vulnerable to vascular pathologies such as thromboembolism, ischemia, and vasculitis.

Myth: IMIED always occurs in the context of a systemic vasculitis or autoimmune disease.

Reality: IMIED is associated with systemic autoimmune conditions in only about 15–30% of cases (Bovo et al. 2006). Thus, IMIED is more likely than not to be a primary inner ear disease process, without any clear link to an associated systemic disorder.

A large handful of systemic disorders can be associated with sensorineural hearing loss that closely resembles those found in IMIED. Sensorineural hearing loss is an essential feature of Cogan's syndrome (see Chap. 31) and also occurs in patients with systemic lupus erythematosus (SLE), Sjögren's

syndrome, relapsing polychondritis, and sarcoidosis (Stone and Francis 2000). Systemic vasculitides such as Wegener's granulomatosis, polyarteritis nodosa, and Behcet's disease can be associated with sensorineural hearing loss, but the true prevalence of IMIED in these disorders is not known with certainty.

Myth: Wegener's granulomatosis is a common cause of IMIED.

Reality: Ear involvement occurs in a significant percentage of patients with Wegener's granulomatosis. However, the usual focus of ear dysfunction in Wegener's granulomatosis is the middle ear rather than the inner ear (Kornblut et al. 1982a, b). Sinonasal or nasopharyngeal disease in Wegener's granulomatosis can lead to Eustachian tube dysfunction, serous otitis media, and conductive hearing loss (see Chap. 24). Destructive granulation tissue located in the middle ear itself can also lead to chronic otitis media and conductive hearing loss in Wegener's granulomatosis. These complications are much more common in Wegener's granulomatosis than is sensorineural hearing loss.

Myth: The temporal bone histopathologic changes observed in IMIED reflect a form of vasculitis that is localized to the inner ear.

Reality: Very few human temporal bones from patients with IMIED have been examined early in the disease course. This is because it is impossible to obtain tissue from the inner ear at surgery without destroying viable labyrinthine function, thereby defeating the purpose of establishing an early diagnosis.

The few temporal bone specimens from patients with IMIED that have been investigated are generally from patients with longstanding disease treated for lengthy periods with glucocorticoids and other immunosuppressive medications. Features of the original disease process are difficult to discern in these specimens. The available specimens have demonstrated four patterns of temporal bone pathology:

- Endolymphatic hydrops (or fluid-filled distension of the scala media). This is similar to the appearance of the inner ear in Meniere's disease.
- Acute labyrinthitis resulting in atrophy of hair cells and their supporting structures.
- Proliferation of fibrous tissue or bone ("neo-osteogenesis").
- Neuronal atrophy.

Features characteristic of active vasculitis, specifically infiltration of the blood vessel walls with inflammatory cells, leukocytoclasis, and fibrinoid necrosis, have not been observed.

39.3 The Clinical History

Pearl: The time course of symptoms is a key clinical feature of IMIED.

Comment: The onset of hearing loss in IMIED is relatively rapid, occurring over a course of weeks to months. The time course of IMIED distinguishes it from sudden sensorineural hearing loss (e.g., that associated with acute acoustic trauma), which occurs over hours to days. The time course also distinguishes IMIED from slowly progressive hearing loss (e.g., presbycusis), which evolves over years.

Myth: IMIED affects both ears to the same degree.

Reality: The hearing loss in IMIED is typically bilateral, but the magnitude of the hearing loss may be asymmetric. Although one ear can be affected before the other, unilateral disease is followed in most cases by decreased hearing in the contralateral ear within weeks to months. Symptoms may also fluctuate over time.

Pearl: Vestibular symptoms include the illusory sense of motion at rest or with head movements.

Comment: Patients with dysfunction of their peripheral vestibular apparatus typically complain of dizziness. Their symptoms of feeling "dizzy" include vertigo, which is an illusory sense of motion. Vertigo can occur at rest or with movements of the head.

The vestibular apparatus tracks information about the head position. It also contributes to the maintenance of gaze and postural stability via the vestibulo-ocular and vestibulospinal reflexes (Schubert and Minor 2004). The hair cells in

the right and left vestibular organs have a baseline firing rate. If the head is moved towards the right, the hair cells on the right increase their firing rate as those on the left decrease theirs. The opposite changes occur when the head moves to the left. The brain compares the input from right and left vestibular organs in order to gauge the head position.

In patients with vertigo at rest, there is a baseline imbalance in vestibular input between the right and left sides, producing a false perception of motion. This type of vertigo usually results from acute unilateral vestibular hypofunction, which characteristically undergoes central compensation over time.

In motion-induced vertigo, the brain fails to encode changes in head position. This leads to destabilization of gaze and oscillopsia, the sense that stationary objects are moving (Schubert and Minor 2004). Chronic oscillopsia, which typically occurs in the setting of bilateral vestibular hypofunction, has a devastating impact on the patients' quality of life.

Vestibular symptoms in IMIED may fluctuate over time, often in concert with changes in hearing. Imbalance associated with dizziness or vertigo should be distinguished from that resulting from impaired motor coordination due to paresis, decreased proprioception, or cerebellar deficits.

39.4 Physical Findings

Pearl: The vestibular system can be evaluated at the bedside as well as in the otolaryngologist's office.
Comment: The function of the vestibular end-organs cannot be measured directly either at the bedside or in the laboratory. However, routine vestibular tests that evaluate directly observable phenomena such as eye movements are helpful in gauging the degree of vestibular dysfunction.

One of the principal functions of the vestibular system is to maintain gaze stability during head movements. This process is known as the vestibulo-ocular reflex. In order to maintain gaze stability, the vestibular apparatus tracks changes in head position and communicates this information to the oculomotor system, which produces compensatory eye movements in the direction opposite to that of the head movement. The vestibulo-ocular reflex allows the retinal fovea to remain fixed upon on an object, even during head motion. Dysfunction of the vestibular organs leads to unstable gaze fixation and corrective eye movements, which can be observed on physical examination.

The principal part of the bedside vestibular examination is assessment for spontaneous or gaze-evoked nystagmus (Minor and Zee 2003). Nystagmus refers to spontaneous and repetitive eye movements; these can be physiologic in some cases, pathologic in others (Fig. 39.2). Nystagmus consists of both a slow phase and a fast phase. Spontaneous nystagmus, the correlate of spontaneous vertigo (discussed above), is

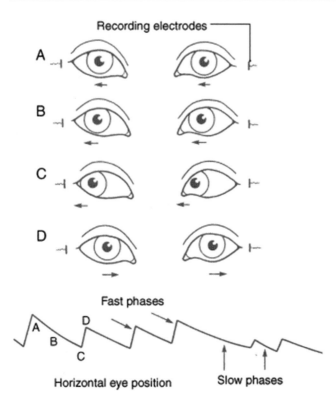

Fast phases

Horizontal eye position   Slow phases

Fig. 39.2 Vestibular nystagmus in the horizontal plane showing slow phase (**a–c**) and fast phase (**d**) eye movements (Figure courtesy of David Dickman, Washington University from http://vestibular.wustl.edu/primer5.html accessed 8/16/2008)

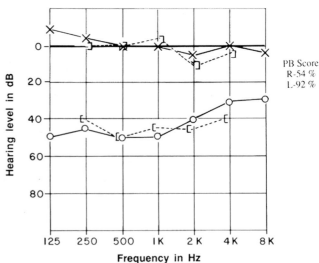

Fig. 39.3 Sample audiogram of a patient with right sensorineural hearing loss. Bone conduction thresholds (R = [, L =]) are measures of auditory function of the cochlea and proximal neural pathway, whereas air conduction thresholds (R = *circle*, L = *X*) measure function of the entire auditory system. *dB* decibel; *PB* Score: percentage correct on speech discrimination test using phonetically-balanced (PB) words

typically pathologic. It is observed usually in acute, unilateral, uncompensated vestibular hypofunction, and suggests asymmetry in the firing rates of the right and left vestibular nerves.

Asymmetric firing of the vestibular nerves leads the brain to think that the head is moving towards the side with the higher discharge rate – away from the side of the lesion. Compensatory eye movements are made in the opposite direction of the presumed head movement towards the side of the lesion (slow phase of nystagmus), followed by rapid refixation of gaze towards the intact side once the brain realizes that the head is not moving (fast phase of nystagmus).

39.5 Auditory and Vestibular Tests

Pearl: The audiogram is a formal test of hearing acuity and speech perception.

Comment: The audiogram is a graphical representation of the lowest volume at which sounds of specific frequencies can be heard by the listener. Audiometry assesses both the speech reception threshold and the discrimination of speech presented at suprathreshold levels. The speech reception threshold is the lowest volume at which the patient can repeat

50% of a list of phonetically-balanced words. The speech reception threshold serves as a valuable crosscheck of pure tone audiometry for the frequencies of normal speech, which range from 500 to 2,000 Hz (Roeser 1996). The speech discrimination test reflects the percentage of words presented above the speech reception threshold that a listener can repeat correctly. An example audiogram is provided in Fig. 39.3.

Changes in pure-tone audiometry over 5 years in a patient with IMIED are presented in Table 39.1. Several features of progressive sensorineural hearing loss are illustrated: the initial involvement of one ear only, the evolution to bilateral disease, and the progression to profound bilateral sensorineural hearing loss.

Myth: The ability to hear soft environmental sounds excludes IMIED as a cause of perceived hearing dysfunction.

Reality: Hearing loss in IMIED can take two forms. First, patients may experience a decline in the ability to perceive sound (hearing acuity). Second, patients may note a decreased ability to identify individual words (word discrimination). A decline in either type of auditory function constitutes a hearing deficit. Assessments of a patient's auditory function must consider both.

Formal audiological assessment uses frequency-specific bone and air conduction thresholds to assess hearing acuity, and speech discrimination testing to assess the clarity of speech perception. An individual whose ability to hear environmental sounds is stable but who experiences a decline in speech clarity has a hearing loss that can be both isolating and disabling. For example, patients with decreased word

Table 39.1 Five-year temporal progression of audiometric thresholds (dB) in a patient with Cogan's syndrome[a]

250 Hz		500 Hz		1,000 Hz		2,000 Hz		4,000 Hz		8,000 Hz	
Right	Left	Right	Left	Right	Left	Right	Left	Right	Left	Right	Left
25	5	35	5	40	5	40	5	50	5	65	5
30	55	35	55	40	50	50	55	70	60	70	65
35	105	35	105	35	105	45	110	65	110	75	95
105	105	105	105	105	105	105	105	105	105	105	105

dB decibels hearing level; *Hz* Hertz
[a]Four audiograms obtained in 5 years

discrimination can have profoundly impaired abilities to follow conversations in settings with significant ambient noise, such as in restaurants.

Pearl: Electronystagmography provides an objective measure of peripheral vestibular function.

Comment: Electronystagmography, an assessment of eye movements in response to a variety of stimuli, is a central part of the assessment of peripheral vestibular dysfunction. In electronystagmography, surface electrodes placed around the orbit are used to detect and record eye movements both at rest and in response to various stimuli of the vestibular system. Standard stimulatory test include caloric stimulation of the ears and changes in head position.

Caloric testing consists of warming and then cooling of the ears. Either air or water irrigation can be applied to the external auditory canals for this purpose. Caloric testing causes a convective movement of endolymph within the horizontal semicircular canals, which are located in proximity to the external auditory canals. The movement of fluid within the horizontal canal alters the firing rate within the vestibular nerve. This elicits, in turn, an eye movement, corresponding to the slow phase of nystagmus (see Fig. 39.2), followed by a rapid corrective saccade that corresponds to the fast phase.

The slow phase eye movement normally is towards the cooled ear and away from the warmed ear. The fast phase is away from the cooled ear and towards the warmed ear (A simple mnemonic: COWS, cold opposite, warm same). Decreased eye movements (<10/s) following caloric stimulation suggest vestibular hypofunction. Unilateral vestibular hypofunction is considered to produce a 20% or greater reduction in eye movement velocity on the affected side when compared with the nonaffected side.

39.6 Differential Diagnosis

Pearl: Several categories of disease must be excluded in the evaluation of a patient with possible IMIED.

Comment: The differential diagnosis of IMIED can be parsed primarily according to the time course of the patient's symptoms (Table 39.2) (Minor et al. 2003). The onset of hearing

loss or vertigo can be sudden (evolving over hours to days); of intermediate duration (evolving over days to several months); or slowly progressive (evolving over several months to years).

The time course of IMIED is typically of intermediate duration, occurring over a period of days to several months. A careful chronology of the inner ear symptoms helps exclude sudden-onset inner ear disease and its associated etiologies (e.g., viral labyrinthitis, acoustic trauma, barotrauma, perilymph fistula) as well as slowly progressive inner ear disease and its associated causes (e.g., presbycusis). Once an intermediate time course of symptoms has been established, the laterality of disease, the relative effects on hearing and balance, and serologic testing serve to distinguish further between the relevant clinical entities.

Major causes of inner ear dysfunction of intermediate onset are acoustic neuromas, spirochetal etiologies, and ototoxic medications. Acoustic neuromas typically are associated with unilateral symptoms. The diagnosis is established by the finding on MRI of an enhancing lesion at the cerebellopontine angle. A diagnosis of syphilis or Lyme disease can be made based on positive FTA-ABS (fluorescent treponemal antibody absorption test) or *Borrelia burgdorferi* serology, respectively (see below for further discussion of otologic manifestations of syphilis).

Ototoxic medications such as gentamicin usually have a preferential effect on the vestibular system as opposed to auditory function. Symptoms of chronic dysequilibrium and signs of bilateral vestibular hypofunction are characteristic of drug-induced ototoxicity.

Pearl: Behcet's disease, Cogan's syndrome, relapsing polychondritis, and sarcoidosis must all be considered in patients with a history of ocular disease and findings consistent with IMIED.

Comment: Ear findings and eye findings often go together. Recognition of characteristic patterns of audiovestibular and ocular inflammatory disease can crack the case. Behcet's disease (Chap. 22), Cogan's syndrome (Chap. 31), relapsing polychondritis (Chap. 32), and sarcoidosis (Chap. 42) must all be considered when ocular inflammation and auditory dysfunction are present. The diagnosis of these and other conditions can be complicated by the fact that ocular findings, audiovestibular symptoms, and disease manifestations in other organ systems do not always occur simultaneously.

Table 39.2 Differential diagnosis of immune-mediated inner ear disease (IMIED)

Time course	Associated disorders	Vestibular symptoms	Distinguishing features
Slowly-progressive (>3 months to years)	Meniere's syndrome	+	Episodic vertigo, unilateral hearing loss, tinnitus, aural fullness
	Presbycusis	−	Symmetrical high frequency hearing loss
	Latent or tertiary syphilis	±	+FTA-ABS, ±RPR
	Acoustic neuroma	±	Unilateral hearing loss, tinnitus; enhancing lesion on MRI
Intermediate (days – 3 months)	IMIED	±	
	Primary		See text
	Secondary (vasculitis, connective tissue disorder)		Signs and symptoms of systemic inflammatory disorders
	Drugs		
	Aminoglycosides	+	Chronic dysequilibrium; signs of bilateral vestibular hypofunction (e.g., oscillopsia)
	Antimalarials		
	Loop diuretics		
	NSAIDs	±	Exposure risk; +*B. burgdorferei* serology
	Lyme disease	±	+FTA-ABS, ±RPR
	Latent or tertiary syphilis	±	Unilateral hearing loss, tinnitus; enhancing lesion on MRI
	Acoustic neuroma		
Sudden (hours to days)	Acoustic trauma	−	Recent intense noise exposure
	Barotrauma	±	Recent deep sea diving, barotrauma
	Perilymph fistula	+	Otolaryngology evaluation
	Viral/bacterial labyrinthitis	+	Acute vertigo and/or hearing loss
	Early or secondary syphilis	+	+FTA-ABS, +RPR
	Acoustic neuroma	±	Unilateral hearing loss, tinnitus; enhancing lesion on MRI

FTA-ABS fluorescent treponemal antibody absorption test; IMIED immune-mediated inner ear disease; MRI magnetic resonance imaging study; NSAIDS nonsteroidal anti-inflammatory drugs; RPR rapid plasma reagin

Myth: The loss of balance accompanied by hearing loss, tinnitus, and ear fullness is Meniere's disease until proven otherwise.

Reality: Vertigo accompanies hearing loss in more than 50% of patients with IMIED (Bovo et al. 2006). In addition, 25–50% of IMIED patients experience tinnitus and aural fullness associated with their hearing loss (Bovo et al. 2006). These features are also characteristic of Meniere's disease. Thus, distinguishing between IMIED and Meniere's disease is challenging in patients who have sensorineural hearing loss, vertigo, tinnitus, and aural fullness.

The principal method for distinguishing between IMIED and Meniere's disease is a consideration of the time course of symptoms. Meniere's disease causes hearing loss over a period of years rather than weeks to months that are characteristic of IMIED. In addition, Meniere's disease is more likely to be unilateral, with progression to the contralateral ear occurring in fewer than 50% of cases (Sajjadi and Paparella 2008).

Distinction between IMIED and Meniere's disease is important because IMIED is more likely to respond to the early initiation of immunosuppressive therapy.

Pearl: Both secondary and tertiary syphilis can mimic IMIED.

Comment: The inner ear complications of syphilis take many forms. The spirochete employs numerous pathologic mechanisms, each of which causes a distinct pattern of injury. Syphilitic infection is divided into three stages, primary, secondary, and tertiary. The second and third stages both have the potential to affect the inner ear (Pletcher and Cheung 2003). In the secondary stage of syphilis, meningeal invasion by the organism can lead to multiple associated cranial neuropathies, including an acute disturbance of the cochleovestibular nerve. The sudden onset of hearing loss and vertigo may evolve over hours to days. The rapid plasma reagin (RPR) assay is invariably positive in the secondary stage of syphilis.

In latent or tertiary syphilis, the spread of gummatous lesions and associated arteritis within the temporal bone is responsible for the subacute to slowly progressive pattern of hearing loss. The time course of hearing loss in the tertiary stage of syphilis can also be similar to the time course of hearing loss in IMIED. Obtaining the FTA-ABS test is critical to distinguish between secondary and tertiary syphilis, because the RPR is negative in many cases of tertiary disease.

Myth: IMIED can be excluded with relative certainty if specialized serologic assays are negative.

Reality: There is no pathognomonic serologic test for IMIED. Nevertheless, numerous candidate molecules have been advanced as being involved in the pathophysiology of IMIED. Most data available are on antibodies that are directed against a 68 kilodalton (kDa) antigen. In a cohort of 72 patients with idiopathic, progressive, bilateral sensorineural hearing loss, higher levels of an antibody to a 68-kDa inner ear protein were observed in patients whose hearing loss responded to glucocorticoid treatment and who had more active disease (Moscicki et al. 1994). This inner ear protein was believed initially to be heat-shock protein 70 (HSP70). Although this hypothesis appeared biologically plausible because of the role of heat shock proteins in inflammation, the findings were not substantiated by subsequent studies (Bloch et al. 1995; Billings et al. 1995; Yeom et al. 2003; Trune et al. 1998).

More recent work has suggested that the antibody to the 68 kDa antigen is the Kresge Hearing Research Institute-3 (KHRI-3) antibody, which binds to an antigen on the supporting cells of the organ of Corti, leading to hair cell depletion and hearing loss (Disher et al. 1997; Nair et al. 1995). Moreover, a protein known as the choline transporter-like-2 (CTL-2) has been identified as the likely 68 kDa antigen (Nair et al. 2004). CTL-2 regulates the function of both choline, a constituent of the neurotransmitter acetylcholine, and phosphatidylcholine, a cell membrane component that is integral to hair cell survival.

Knowledge of a patient's antibody status with regard to the 68 kDa antigen may turn out to be of clinical value. Some data suggest that glucocorticoids are more likely to be effective in patients who are positive for such antibodies (Zeitoun et al. 2005). Commercial assays for antibodies to the 68 kDa protein remain poorly-validated or not widely available (Ruckenstein 2004).

39.7 Treatment

Myth: The symptoms of IMIED are irreversible.

Reality: IMIED is an important diagnosis to make because it is one of the few causes of hearing loss (or vestibulopathy) that is potentially reversible. The natural history of IMIED bears some similarity to that of rapidly progressive glomerulonephritis, in which irreversible renal damage frequently occurs within weeks to several months of onset. As such, IMIED is worth at least one stab at aggressive therapy. Prolonged courses of immunosuppression may not be worthwhile in the absence of a clear treatment response, but few patients are willing to forgo the ability to hear without a trial of immunosuppressive therapy.

Up to 70% of patients diagnosed with IMIED demonstrate clinical improvement following steroid therapy (Harris et al. 2003; Matteson et al. 2001). In the setting of a rapidly progressive sensorineural hearing loss, prednisone of 1 mg/kg/day is a reasonable starting dose. If the patient regains significant auditory and vestibular function within 2 weeks, tapering of the prednisone dose can begin in a taper designed to discontinue the medication over 2 months. Methotrexate is a reasonable steroid-sparing agent to use if patients demonstrate a convincing response to glucocorticoids (Harris et al. 2003).

Pearl: IMIED patients are good candidates for hearing aids or cochlear implants.

Comment: All is not lost for patients with IMIED who fail or cannot tolerate immunosuppressive therapy. Therapeutic options beyond prednisone, cyclophosphamide, and the like are available. Patients who develop moderate unilateral or bilateral hearing loss can derive significant benefit from programmable hearing aids. Those with severe to profound bilateral sensorineural hearing loss and poor word discrimination despite the use of hearing aids are candidates for cochlear implantation.

Hearing aids deliver amplified sound through the ear canal. In contrast, a surgically-placed cochlear prosthesis stimulates the auditory nerve directly, generating electrical representations of speech sounds that patients learn to decode in the auditory portions of their central nervous system. In many patients, cochlear implants provide a return to the land of the hearing.

Myth: Benzodiazepines or meclizine are an effective long-term approach to patients with dizziness.

Reality: The long-term use of vestibular suppressant medications should be limited to short-term management of acute vertigo. Agents such as meclizine impede the development of central vestibular compensation.

A more effective long-term approach to patients with significant peripheral vestibular dysfunction is vestibular rehabilitation. Peripheral vestibular dysfunction can be overcome by compensation of the central nervous system. This process is aided by a program of vestibular rehabilitation, whereby trained physical therapists teach habituation exercises that promote central compensation to peripheral deficits. Physical therapists who focus on vestibular rehabilitation can also provide strategies that minimize fall risk. Patients are challenged to perform the head movements and postural changes that produce vertigo and then coached about compensatory strategies.

References

Billings PB, Keithley EM, Harris JP. Evidence linking the 68 kilodalton antigen identified in progressive sensorineural hearing loss patient sera with heat shock protein 70. Ann Otol Rhinol Laryngol. 1995;104(3):181–8

Bloch DB, San Martin JE, Rauch SD, Moscicki RA, Bloch KJ. Serum antibodies to heat shock protein 70 in sensorineural hearing loss. Arch Otolaryngol Head Neck Surg. 1995;121(10):1167–71

Bovo R, Aimoni C, Martini A. Immune-mediated inner ear disease. Acta Otolaryngol. 2006;126(10):1012–21

Disher MJ, Ramakrishnan A, Nair TS, et al Human autoantibodies and monoclonal antibody KHRI-3 bind to a phylogenetically conserved inner-ear-supporting cell antigen. Ann N Y Acad Sci. 1997;830: 253–65

Harris JP, Weisman MH, Derebery JM, et al Treatment of corticosteroid-responsive autoimmune inner ear disease with methotrexate: a randomized controlled trial. JAMA. 2003;290(14):1875–83

Kikuchi M. On the "sympathetic otitis". Zibi Rinsyo Kyoto. 1959; 52:600

Kornblut AD, Wolff SM, deFries HO, Fauci AS. Wegener's granulomatosis. Otolaryngol Clin N Am. 1982a;15(3):673–83

Kornblut AD, Wolff SM, Fauci AS. Ear disease in patients with Wegener's granulomatosis. Laryngoscope 1982b;92(7 Pt 1): 713–17

Matteson EL, Fabry DA, Facer GW, et al Open trial of methotrexate as treatment for autoimmune hearing loss. Arthritis Rheum. 2001;45(2): 146–50

Mccabe BF Autoimmune sensorineural hearing loss. Ann otol Rhinol Laryngol. Sep-Oct 1979;88 (5pt1):585–589

Minor L, Carey J, Lustig LR. Disorders of balance. In: Lustig LR, Niparko JK, editors. Clinical neurotology: diagnosing and managing disorders of hearing, balance and the facial nerve. New York: Martin Dunitz; 2003. p. 225–44

Minor L, Zee DS. Clinical evaluation of the patient with dizziness. In: Lustig LR, Niparko JK, editors. Clinical neurotology: diagnosing and managing disorders of hearing, balance and the facial nerve. New York: Martin Dunitz; 2003. p. 81–110

Moscicki RA, San Martin JE, Quintero CH, Rauch SD, Nadol JB Jr, Bloch KJ. Serum antibody to inner ear proteins in patients with progressive hearing loss. Correlation with disease activity and response to corticosteroid treatment. JAMA. 1994;272(8):611–16

Nair TS, Kozma KE, Hoefling NL, et al Identification and characterization of choline transporter-like protein 2, an inner ear glycoprotein of 68 and 72 kDa that is the target of antibody-induced hearing loss. J Neurosci. 2004;24(7):1772–9

Nair TS, Raphael Y, Dolan DF, et al Monoclonal antibody induced hearing loss. Hear Res. 1995;83(1–2):101–13

Pletcher SD, Cheung SW. Syphilis and otolaryngology. Otolaryngol Clin N Am. 2003;36(4):595–605, vi

Roeser R. Audiology desk reference: a guide to the practice of audiology. 1 ed. New York: Thieme; 1996

Ruckenstein MJ. Autoimmune inner ear disease. Curr Opin Otolaryngol Head Neck Surg. 2004;12(5):426–30

Sajjadi H, Paparella MM. Meniere's disease. Lancet 2008;372 (9636):406–14

Schindler JS, Niparko JK. Imaging quiz case 1. Transverse temporal bone fractures (left) with subsequent progressive SNHL, consistent with sympathetic cochleolabyrinthitis. Arch Otolaryngol Head Neck Surg. 1998;124(7):814, 816–8

Schubert MC, Minor LB. Vestibulo-ocular physiology underlying vestibular hypofunction. Phys Ther. 2004;84(4):373–85

Stone JH, Francis HW. Immune-mediated inner ear disease. Curr Opin Rheumatol. 2000;12(1):32–40

ten Cate WJ, Bachor E. Autoimmune-mediated sympathetic hearing loss: a case report. Otol Neurotol. 2005;26(2):161–5

Trune DR, Kempton JB, Mitchell CR, Hefeneider SH. Failure of elevated heat shock protein 70 antibodies to alter cochlear function in mice. Hear Res. 1998;116(1–2):65–70

Yeom K, Gray J, Nair TS, et al Antibodies to HSP-70 in normal donors and autoimmune hearing loss patients. Laryngoscope. 2003;113(10): 1770–6

Zeitoun H, Beckman JG, Arts HA, et al Corticosteroid response and supporting cell antibody in autoimmune hearing loss. Arch Otolaryngol Head Neck Surg. 2005;131(8):665–72

Osteoporosis

40

Kenneth G. Saag, Sarah L. Morgan, and Amy H. Warriner

40.1 Overview of Osteoporosis

> Bone continually undergoes a process of renewal called remodeling. In the normal adult skeleton, bone formation and bone resorption are closely coupled: new bone laid down by osteoblasts exactly matches osteoclastic bone resorption.

> The bone mass of an individual in later life is a consequence of the peak bone mass accrued in utero and during childhood and puberty, as well as the subsequent rate of bone loss.

> Genetic factors strongly contribute in determining the peak bone mass. However, hormonal, nutritional, and environmental influences modulate the genetically determined pattern of skeletal growth.

> More than 1.5 million fractures related to osteoporosis occur in the United States every year.

> Ninety percent of all hip and spine fractures are related to osteoporosis.

> Most osteoporotic fractures involve the femoral neck, the vertebral bodies, or the wrist.

> Two types of scores have been used traditionally to quantify bone mineral density (BMD):
>   – The T score is the number of standard deviations of the patient's BMD above or below the young-normal mean BMD.
>   – The Z score is the number of standard deviations of the measurement above or below the age-matched mean BMD.

> The World Health Organization (WHO) defines osteoporosis with a T score ≤ -2.5.

40.2 Osteoporosis Epidemiology

Myth: There is a safe dose of glucocorticoids for bone.

Reality: Glucocorticoids are the most common cause of drug-induced osteoporosis and lead to an increased risk of fractures in a fashion that is dose and time dependent. As many as half of all persons taking glucocorticoids on a long-term basis will experience fracture in their lifetime. Glucocorticoids affect the bone independently of their effects on BMD due to their direct toxicity to osteoblasts and osteocytes (Manolagas, Weinstein 1999; van Staa et al. 2003). The large General Practice Research Database of the United Kingdom has shown that even at doses of glucocorticoid below the physiologic replacement dose (estimated at 7.5 mg/day prednisolone), glucocorticoid use is associated with greater fracture rates at both the hip and spine (van Staa et al. 2000). In normal volunteers, oral glucocorticoids at physiologic doses result in a prompt reduction in osteocalcin as a measure of bone formation (Ton et al. 2005). Similarly, triamcinolone administered intra-articularly also was associated with a reduction in bone formation (Emkey et al. 1996). Finally, inhaled glucocorticoids may also adversely impact bone density and lead to an increased rate of fractures (Israel et al. 2001; Wong et al. 2000).

Pearl: African Americans get osteoporosis, too.

Comment: Although young, healthy African Americans have a 10% greater BMD on an average when compared with Caucasians, osteoporosis and fracture risk are under-appreciated among African. Among older African American women, osteoporosis is a common problem that is less frequently diagnosed and treated than in Caucasian women of similar ages (Looker et al. 1997; Mikuls et al. 2005; Miller et al. 2005; Mudano et al. 2003; Siris et al. 2001). African American women who have already experienced a fracture are 50% less likely to receive subsequent testing or treatment than Caucasian women who have fractured (Mikuls et al. 2005; Miller et al. 2005; Mudano et al. 2003). Furthermore, when African American men and women fracture, they have worse outcomes including longer hospital stays, increased disability, and greater mortality (Furstenberg, Mezey 1987; Jacobsen et al. 1992; Kellie, Brody 1990). Black women older than 65 years of age have a mortality rate from hip fractures that is 1.5 times higher than that of white women. Antiosteoporotic therapies appear to have equal efficacy across races.

Pearl: Men also get osteoporosis.

Comment: Approximately 30% of all fractures in the aging population occur in men. These fractures account for up to 25% of the total osteoporosis costs (Burge et al. 2007; Jones et al. 1994; van Staa et al. 2001), and the risk of recurrent fracture is nearly threefold higher in men than women (Center et al. 2007; Sanders et al. 1999). Fracture-related death rates have been increasing in both men and women, but are noted to be consistently higher in men. The age-related rise in fractures in men tends to occur approximately 5–10 years later, than the increase seen in women (Kudlacek et al. 2000). The use of BMD for fracture-risk prediction also differs between men and women: men develop vertebral fractures at a higher BMD than women (Kudlacek et al. 2000; Orwoll 2000). The difference in body size between men and women partially explains the difference in BMD, but does not fully explain the lower fracture risk that men have when compared to women (Looker et al. 2001; Melton et al. 2005).

Physicians' perception that osteoporosis does not affect men adds a further barrier to successful diagnostic and therapeutic intervention. Similar to women, current guidelines set by the International Society for Clinical Densitometry (ISCD) recommend using a T score of 2.5 standard deviations below the normal male reference levels to diagnose osteoporosis in men over the age of 50 years, unless other secondary causes of low BMD exist (ISCD 2007). However, uncertainty exists on when to start screening for osteoporosis in men. ISCD recommends screening all men over the age of 70, based only on expert opinion (ISCD 2007). In contrast, one analysis suggests that it is only cost-effective to screen and begin treatment in men over the age of 65 with a diagnosis of osteoporosis based on BMD and a history of a fracture, or men over the age of 80 with osteoporosis based on BMD and no history of a fracture (Schousboe et al. 2007). Further investigation into the proper timing for osteoporosis screening and treatment for men is currently ongoing.

Until evidence-based recommendations become available, assessment of clinical risk factors (e.g., prior fracture, use of androgen deprivation therapy for prostate cancer) is important in order to identify men most at risk of a fracture. In terms of treatment options, both bisphosphonates and teriparatide have been shown to reduce fracture risk in men.

Pearl: In young adults with new fractures, hereditary disorders of collagen should be considered.

Comment: Osteogenesis imperfecta and the Ehlers–Danlos syndrome are two of the more common hereditary disorders of collagen synthesis that can lead to fractures in young adults. Severe variants of these conditions are detected by fractures at birth or in childhood, but persons with less severe phenotypes may present with their first of successive fractures in later years. Excessive joint mobility, abnormal wound scarring ("cigarette papering"), blue-tinged sclera, mitral valve prolapse/other cardiac anomalies, short stature, and dental problems are among a number of the historical or physical examination clues that may heighten suspicion for such a condition (See Chap. 47, "Heritable Disorders of Connective Tissue").

Forme frustes or incomplete penetrance of hereditary connective tissue disorders may escape clinical attention for many years and may be concurrently missed by the existing genetic testing evaluating for mutations in COL1A and other related genes affecting collagen productions. In children and adults with osteogenesis imperfecta, bisphosphonate medications have proven effectiveness in lowering fracture rates (Rauch, Glorieux 2004).

Pearl: In older adults, any fracture, regardless of the degree of trauma, may represent osteoporosis.

Comment: Low trauma fractures have historically been linked to osteoporosis due to the subsequent increased risk of a recurrent fracture. In one study, investigators found an increased risk of subsequent fracture following a low-trauma fracture at all fracture sites with only two exceptions: rib fractures in men and ankle fractures in women (Center et al. 2007).

Low trauma falls are the most common cause of fractures in persons over the age of 65 years, and their predominance increases with rising age to nearly 90% in persons over the age of 90 years (Bergstrom et al. 2008). The site of fracture of most of these low trauma falls is the hip or pelvis (Bergstrom et al. 2008). In an earlier study on pelvic fractures, the majority of fractures that occurred as the result of moderate trauma (defined as trauma not usually expected to result in fracture) were in older persons with a mean age of 69 (Melton et al. 1981).

Several studies have shown that the association with osteoporosis is similar for high and low trauma fractures. Regardless of trauma type, individuals with fractures are three times more likely to have osteoporosis at one or more sites (Karlsson et al. 1993; Melton et al. 1993; Sanders et al. 1998). A case-control study found that Australian women older than 50 years of age with high trauma fractures had lower BMD at hip, spine, forearm, and total body sites than population-based samples of older women without fracture (Sanders et al. 1998).

A Swedish study that evaluated hip fractures in men reported that high energy fractures were associated with age-related changes in bone strength (Hedlund, Lindgren 1987). A retrospective cohort study of 1288 individuals of age 35 and older with distal forearm fractures found no difference in the risk of subsequent fracture when stratified based on severity of trauma (i.e., severe vs. low trauma) (Cuddihy et al. 1999). A prospective study of two large osteoporosis cohorts of patients 65 years or older, the Study of Osteoporotic Fractures

(SOF) and Osteoporotic Fractures in Men Study (MrOS), found that each standard deviation reduction in total hip BMD was similarly associated with an increased risk of high trauma fracture and low trauma fracture. The risk of future fracture was 34% higher in women with a history of high trauma fracture and 31% higher in women with an initial low trauma fracture, when compared with women having no history of fracture. Risk of subsequent fracture was not examined for men (Mackey et al. 2007). These findings suggest that any prior fracture, regardless of the degree of trauma, may indicate underlying skeletal fragility and an increased risk of future fracture.

40.3 Osteoporosis Diagnosis: Bone Mass Measurement

Pearl: Both the absolute and relative risks of fractures are important in osteoporosis prevention.

Comment: BMD measurement provides a valid and reliable way to define fracture risk. The "T-score," which represents the number of standard deviations above or below peak bone mass of sex-matched comparisons, has become a standard to characterize the relative risk of fracture and to define the presence or absence of osteoporosis in the absence of fractures. More recently, attention has shifted from the relative risk to absolute risk of fracture, using the WHO FRAX calculator (FRAX 2008; Kanis et al. 2001). FRAX is based on risk-factor modeling of data from numerous international datasets and provides a 10-year absolute fracture risk of the hip and spine.

Absolute fracture risk is a valuable construct that incorporates BMD, but is also derived from other significant risk factors including age, sex, body mass index, previous fracture history, parental history of hip fracture, tobacco smoking, glucocorticoid use, history of rheumatoid arthritis, and other secondary osteoporosis risk factors. Important secondary risk factors include type 1 diabetes mellitus, osteogenesis imperfecta, hyperthyroidism, hypogonadism, premature menopause, chronic malnutrition, malabsorption, and chronic liver disease. The FRAX model can calculate fracture risk in the absence of data related to BMD.

Following development of the FRAX model, the National Osteoporosis Foundation issued new guidelines for osteoporosis treatment that now incorporate FRAX along with revised T-score criteria (NOE 2008). These guidelines were developed based on cost effectiveness considerations. It is recommended that a person with low bone mass by dual-energy X-ray absorptiometry (DXA) (formerly called osteopenia: a T score between −1.0 and −2.5) and a FRAX 10-year absolute probability of fracture of 3% or greater at

the hip or 20% or greater of any major osteoporosis-related fracture be treated with an antiosteoporotic therapy.

Myth: DXA scans from different manufacturers and facilities give comparable results.

Reality: There are numerous manufacturers of machines to measure bone density by DXA. DXA systems and the corresponding data generated from DXA machines by different manufacturers are not interchangeable. Some of the reasons that they are not interchangeable include different methods for dual energy X-ray production (voltage switching vs. K-edge filter), different X-ray detectors, different X-ray acquisition methods (pencil vs. fan beams), different calibration methods (continuous vs. intermittent calibration), different edge detection software, different regions of interest, and different young normal databases.

The ISCD stated that "it is not possible to quantitatively compare BMD or to calculate a least significant change between facilities without a cross-calibration study" (ISCD 2007). Therefore, in order to make quantitative comparisons between successive DXA tests, it is important to scan patients on the *same* DXA system at each study.

Myth: Low bone density in younger women means they have osteoporosis.

Reality: The fracture risk in women before menopause differs from that of postmenopausal women. The criteria set by the WHO to diagnose postmenopausal osteoporosis – namely, a T score of <−2.5 – cannot be applied to premenopausal women. The occurrence of low bone mass in women between the ages of 30 and 40 is unusual: only one such woman at the age of 40 had a T score ≤−2.5 (Khan 2006). In most cases, low BMD in premenopausal women represents low peak bone mass, likely due to genetic factors but with possible environmental contributions as well. Despite their low peak bone mass, the 5- and 10-year fracture risk is very low in these women (Lewiecki 2005).

Estrogen deficiency and glucocorticoid use are the most common identifiable primary and secondary causes of low bone mass in younger women (Moreira Kulak et al. 2000). Estrogen deficiency is generally either due to premature ovarian failure (e.g., because of chemotherapy) or anorexia nervosa. If menstrual irregularities are present, the estrogen status of the patient should be determined. A serum follicle stimulating hormone (FSH) level greater than 20 mIU/L is related to increased bone loss (Khan, Syed 2004). Among premenopausal women with low bone mass, there is also a significant correlation with a family history of osteoporosis (Moreira Kulak et al. 2000), supporting a genetic predisposition.

In addition to consideration of hypogonadism, initial evaluation of low bone mass should include investigation for the underlying causes of bone loss, such as hypovitaminosis

D, medications, thyroid disease, parathyroid disease, dietary causes, and renal or hepatic disease. If fragility fractures have occurred and no secondary causes of bone loss are noted, a bone biopsy should be considered (Khan 2006).

Even if an etiology is identified, the appropriate treatment of premenopausal women found to have low bone mass is unclear. Pharmacologic therapies have not been studied in sufficient detail in this population, and such studies that exist have occurred primarily on patients treated with glucocorticoids (Adachi et al. 2001; Reid et al. 2000; Saag et al. 1998; Wallach et al. 2000). In a case study of bisphosphonate use during pregnancy, no congenital anomalies were noted in the fetuses exposed (Ornoy et al. 2006). However, there continues to be a concern regarding long-term side effects of certain osteoporosis therapies among younger women, especially bisphosphonates, due to the long half-life of these medications. Animal models have shown that bisphosphonates do cross the placenta and skeletal effects have been seen (Patlas et al. 1999). The Federal Drug Administration (FDA) continues to consider bisphosphonates as a class D medication during pregnancy because of these concerns (Novartis 2004).

Information regarding the use of other osteoporosis treatments in premenopausal women is lacking. At the least, younger women with low bone mass should be encouraged to receive adequate calcium, vitamin D, and exercise. Risk factors, such as tobacco use and moderate to heavy ethanol use (i.e., more than one serving of alcohol per day) should be minimized. Such patients should be followed-up around the time of menopause by physicians knowledgeable about osteoporosis.

40.4 Osteoporosis Prevention: Calcium and Sodium Effects

Pearl: Sodium plays a role in bone health.

Comment: A positive relationship exists between dietary sodium intake and calciuria (Heaney 2006a, b). On an average, urinary calcium increases by approximately 1 mmol (40 mg) for each 100 mmol (2300 mg) of sodium ingested. Increased calcium absorptive efficiency is also associated with calciuria (Breslau et al. 1982; Meyer et al. 1976). One of the mechanisms of the relationship between sodium intake and calciuria is the increase in parathyroid hormone (PTH) secretion that occurs in response to a sodium load (50). The amount of calcium consumed in the diet probably have an effect on whether calciuria caused by a sodium load affects calcium balance. Adjustment of a person's daily sodium intake may be beneficial for bone health as well as for hypertension (Teucher et al. 2008).

Mild hyponatremia, a common electrolyte abnormality in the elderly, has been associated with a higher fracture rate (Gankam Kengne et al. 2008). Monitoring selective serotonin reuptake inhibitors and diuretic use is important in preventing hyponatremia.

Myth: If you are elderly or taking a medicine that decreases gastric acid, you must take calcium citrate as a calcium supplement.

Reality: Changes in the gastrointestinal tract have been documented with aging (Bhutto, Morley 2008). It is often suggested that the majority of the elderly have gastric achlorhydria. However, in one study, approximately 90% of elderly subjects had the ability to acidify stomach contents, even in the basal (unstimulated) state (Hurwitz et al. 1997). Among persons with achlorhydria, calcium absorption was superior with calcium citrate when fasting. However, when calcium was administered with a normal breakfast, calcium carbonate absorption was normalized (Recker 1985). The effect of proton pump inhibitors on calcium absorption has been documented to be variable with some studies, suggesting that omeprazole may decrease absorption (O'Connell et al. 2005; Serfaty-Lacrosniere et al. 1995).

Studies of calcium carbonate vs. calcium citrate absorbability from commercial supplements have yielded conflicting results depending upon the methodology used to assess calcium absorbability and whether the calcium salts were taken fasting or with a test meal (Heaney et al. 1999; Heller et al. 2000; Heller et al. 1999). In a randomized, crossover trial that compared commercial calcium carbonate and calcium citrate, there were no significant differences between preparations with regard to urinary calcium or intact PTH levels. A cost-benefit analysis was also completed between the preparations. The authors concluded that calcium carbonate was a good choice based upon bioavailability, cost, and clinical efficacy when given with a meal. The relative bioavailability of calcium from orange juice fortified with calcium citrate malate, skim milk, and a calcium carbonate supplement as a portion of a test meal appeared to be equivalent in a sample of elderly patients (Martini, Wood 2002).

Many other calcium salts besides calcium carbonate and calcium citrate for calcium supplementation are available (Hanzlik et al. 2005). In a four-way crossover study of healthy women treated with 1200 mg of calcium as calcium carbonate, calcium citrate, calcium formate, or placebo, serum calcium rose by 15% with calcium formate and the intact PTH level fell by 70% within 60 min of administration. The authors concluded that calcium formate may be a useful calcium supplement (Hanzlik et al. 2005). When bone markers are followed as an outcome measure, calcium citrate may decrease markers of bone resorption more than calcium carbonate in postmenopausal women (Kenny et al. 2004).

Therefore, in patients with documented achlorydria, if calcium is to be taken while fasting, calcium citrate is an appropriate choice. However, as not all elderly individuals have achlorhydria, calcium citrate is not necessary in all such patients. Calcium carbonate, which is inexpensive and readily available, appears to be absorbed as along with calcium citrate when taken with a meal. Future investigations should center on other calcium salts for supplementation.

Myth: Calcium supplementation as monotherapy is a sufficient therapy following a fracture.

Reality: Randomized controlled trials comparing calcium therapy alone to placebo have shown no benefit in reduction of vertebral and nonvertebral fractures (Grant et al. 2005; Lyons et al. 2007; Prince et al. 2006; Reid et al. 2006). However, these findings may be partially confounded by nonadherence. Patients with adherence of 80% or better did have a reduced risk of fracture in one study (hazard ratio 0.7; 95% CI, 0.4–1.0) (Prince et al. 2006).

Most studies on calcium have evaluated the combination of calcium and vitamin D. Although there is evidence that calcium and vitamin D reduce the risk of fracture, the benefit is not observed in all populations (Chapuy et al. 1992; Dawson-Hughes et al. 1997; Larsen et al. 2004; Bischoff-Ferrari et al. 2005; Heikinheimo et al. 1992; Jackson et al. 2006; Lips et al. 1996; Papadimitropoulos et al. 2002). Both the type and the amount of vitamin D supplementation appear relevant to the reduction of fracture risk (Bischoff-Ferrari et al. 2005). Owing to these multiple confounding issues surrounding the absolute benefit of calcium, it is recommended that all persons take calcium and vitamin D supplements for general bone health. Calcium alone is probably not sufficient to reduce the risk of fracture.

Myth: Taking calcium supplements leads to calcium-containing renal stones.

Reality: Nephroureterolithiasis is a common problem with a rising incidence. Kidney stones arise from a variety of medical conditions and approximately 80% of stones are estimated to contain calcium (Taylor and Curhan 2004). In the Women's Health Initiative (WHI) of 36,282 postmenopausal women who received 1,000 mg of calcium as calcium carbonate and 400 IU of vitamin D3 (cholecalciferol) or placebo each day, the hazard ratio for kidney stones was 1.17 with 95% percent confidence interval of 1.02–1.34 (Jackson et al. 2006). This report raised concern related to nephrolithiasis and calcium consumption. However, the preponderance of the evidence does not support a relationship of higher calcium intake to a greater risk of calcium-containing stones.

The relationship of dietary risk factors and kidney stones was evaluated prospectively in 96,245 females in the Nurses' Health Study II (Curhan et al. 2004). A higher dietary intake of calcium decreased the risk of symptomatic stones, and calcium supplement intake was associated with a "slight and nonsignificant increase in risk" (Curhan et al. 2004).

A randomized trial in men evaluated a "normal" amount of calcium, reduced animal protein (52 g/day), and 50 mmol of salt per day vs. a low-calcium diet in individuals with hypercalciuria and recurrent calcium oxalate stones (Borghi et al. 2002). At 5 years, urinary oxalate excretion increased in the low-calcium diet group and decreased on the normal calcium, low protein, and low sodium diet. The authors concluded that a diet that was restricted in salt and protein and normal in calcium content was more protective than a low calcium diet.

It has been hypothesized that calcium supplementation binds oxalate in the gut, leading to a relative reduction in the proportion of oxalate absorbed in the gut and lowering calcium oxalate stone formation (Williams et al. 2001). Many other nutritional factors, besides calcium, likely contribute to the pathogenesis of calcium-containing stones (Curhan et al. 2004). A prospective cohort study of 45,619 men without a history of kidney stones had self-administered food frequency questionnaires every 4 years (Taylor et al. 2004). After adjusting for age, a higher intake of dietary calcium was associated with a reduced risk of nephrolithiasis. For men older than 60 years of age, no association between dietary calcium and stone formation was observed. Magnesium intake decreased and vitamin C intake increased the risk of symptomatic nephrolithiasis. Dietary phytate intake was associated with a higher risk of kidney stone formation. Higher fluid intake was associated with a lower risk of kidney stones.

The precise recommendations for the prevention of kidney stones depend upon patient's characteristics as well as the composition of the kidney stone (Taylor and Curhan 2006). Therefore, the dictum that all patients who have had renal stones should not consume dietary or supplemental calcium is usually incorrect.

Myth: Taking calcium supplements for osteoporosis increases the risk of cardiovascular disease.

Reality: In a secondary analysis of vascular events from a randomized double-blind, placebo-controlled trial of calcium supplementation ($n = 1,471$), myocardial infarction as well as a composite of myocardial infarction, stroke, and sudden death were more common in the calcium supplement vs. the placebo group. A search of a New Zealand data base for hospital admissions attenuated the calcium effect to borderline significance. The authors concluded that "this potentially detrimental effect should be balanced against the likely benefits of calcium on bone" (Bolland et al. 2008).

Evaluation of data from the WHI of 36,282 postmenopausal women who were randomized to 500 mg calcium and 200 IU of vitamin D twice daily found that women in the calcium and vitamin D arm were not at increased risk for transient ischemic attack, myocardial infarction, stroke, coronary revascularization, angina requiring hospitalization, or transient ischemic attacks (Hsia et al. 2007). In addition, in a cohort of 1,179 women followed for 4 years with a calcium supplement dosage of 1400–1500 mg/day (Lappe and Heaney 2008), the vascular event rate was less than half of the rate seen in an earlier large randomized controlled trial (Bolland et al. 2008).

Thus, the data at this point do not seem to support a detrimental effect of calcium supplementation on vascular events in postmenopausal women. It has been suggested that deteriorating renal function, with vascular calcification related to chronic renal failure, may have contributed to the findings in the study in New Zealand (Lappe and Heaney 2008). Future research is planned to continue to evaluate the hypothesized link between calcium supplementation and vascular disease.

Myth: All calcium-fortified products are good sources of calcium.

Reality: Studies evaluating calcium from calcium-fortified orange juice showed that 48% greater absorption was present with calcium citrate malate fortified juice than tricalcium phosphate/calcium lactate (Heaney et al. 2005). Calcium fortified-soy milk was shown to be absorbed at 75% of the efficiency of cow's milk (Heaney et al. 2000). In addition, it has been shown that in some soy beverages, the added calcium is present as sediment on the bottom of the container (Heaney et al. 2000; Heaney and Rafferty 2006). In the evaluation of eight national brands, the unshaken samples averaged a calcium concentration that was 31% of the labeled calcium content. Shaking the beverages increased the measurable calcium to 59% of the labeled content (Heaney and Rafferty 2006). Therefore, soy beverages are not equivalent to milk in calcium content. High-calcium mineral waters have absorption that is equal to calcium from milk or slightly higher absorption (Heaney 2006a) and can serve as an additional supplement in patients needing calcium supplementation.

In summary, not all calcium-fortified products are good sources of calcium and there is variability in calcium bioavailability. Depending upon the calcium salt selected and interaction of the supplement with the product, calcium absorption can be greatly affected (Rafferty et al. 2007).

40.5 Osteoporosis Prevention: Vitamin D

Pearl: Vitamin D insufficiency is common, but vitamin D level is difficult to measure accurately.

Comment: Vitamin D is important in bone health due to its ability to counter-regulate PTH, a promoter of bone loss, and its stimulation of intestinal and renal calcium absorption. In the presence of inadequate calcium intake or vitamin D deficiency, PTH levels typically rise, resulting in secondary hyperparathyroidism. Despite this knowledge, vitamin D

deficiency is present in up to 90% of the elderly population (Mezquita-Raya et al. 2001), even in southern latitudes (Lips 2001; Visser et al. 2006). Even younger persons have low vitamin D levels with 1/3 of premenopausal women with low levels by the end of winter (Tangpricha et al. 2002). Current recommendations aim to maintain 25(OH) vitamin D at or above 32 ng/mL (80 nmol/dL), the level at which PTH levels plateau.

Obtaining an accurate assessment of vitamin D levels in individuals is also an area of concern. Owing to its extreme hydrophobic characteristics and the presence of two forms of 25(OH) vitamin D {25(OH) D2 and 25(OH) D3}, the precision and accuracy of measuring vitamin D levels has been a historical challenge (Hollis 2008). 25(OH) D3 (cholecalciferol) is formed mainly through ultraviolet radiation of the skin, with only a small amount coming from dietary sources. 25(OH) D2, ergocalciferol, is produced by the irradiation of ergosterol. Some assays provide separate analyses of D2 and D3, but total 25(OH) vitamin D is the level analyzed in most population based studies (Zerwekh 2008).

Currently, great variation can be seen when evaluating 25(OH) vitamin D levels by the assorted analysis methods (Binkley et al. 2004). Concurrent analyses revealed that 15% of tested patients were vitamin D insufficient when tested in one laboratory, whereas 90% were insufficient based on another lab's analysis (Binkley et al. 2004). This variation probably stems from differing methods for evaluating 25(OH) vitamin D status as vitamin D in plasma and serum appears to be very stable (Lissner et al. 1981).

Earlier methods used for evaluating 25(OH) vitamin D levels used a vitamin D binding protein, which not only measured 25(OH)D2 and 25(OH)D3, but also other metabolites, and the process was cumbersome for technicians (Hollis 2008; Haddad, Chyu 1971). In the 1980s, a radioimmunoassay (RIA) technique was developed to simultaneously identify 25(OH) D2 and 25(OH) D3, revealing a total 25(OH) vitamin D level. More recently, direct methods using high performance liquid chromatography (HPLC) and liquid chromatography–mass spectrometry (LC–MS) have largely replaced older methods. HPLC and LC–MS methods evaluate 25(OH)D2 and 25(OH)D3 levels separately (Eisman et al. 1977; Maunsell et al. 2005) and require dedicated technicians and internal standards for the measured compounds (Hollis 2008). HPLC is considered the gold standard by many experts in the field (Hollis 2008). Currently, an updated chemiluminescence RIA method (Diasorin Coorporation) is also available for use and measures the total 25(OH) vitamin D levels (Hollis 2008). LCMS, HPLC, and the more recent RIA methods appear to have improved precision in determining total 25(OH) vitamin D levels, when compared to prior methods, and attempts are being made to ensure continued quality assessment of vitamin D measurements. These variations in vitamin D assays need to be accounted for when evaluating patients in practice and when comparing results from clinical trials.

Myth: Routine exposure to sunshine exposure leads to an adequate 25(OH) vitamin D level.

Reality: Vitamin D forms in the skin after exposure to solar ultraviolet B (UVB) radiation (Holick 2006a). This UVB radiation converts 7-dehydrocholesterol to previtamin D_3 and ultimately vitamin D_3. Excessive exposure to sunlight does not cause vitamin D intoxication because excess vitamin D_3 and previtamin D_3 are also destroyed by sunlight. Many factors decrease the ability to form vitamin D in the skin, including increasing skin melanin, sunscreens, clothing that prevents the sun from reaching the skin, and a reduction in 7-dehydrocholesterol in the skin with aging (Holick 2006a; Holick 2006b; Holick 2007). At some latitudes, in the winter months, the sunlight is not sufficient to produce vitamin D (Holick 2006a). Exposure to 5–10 min of sunlight on the legs between 10 A.M and 3 P.M in the spring, summer, and fall has been shown to be adequate to prevent vitamin D insufficiency (Holick 2006a).

With experimental exposure to UVB light, individuals with a lighter skin tone had greater increases in their 25(OH) vitamin D level than darker skinned individuals (Ton et al. 2005; Armas et al. 2007). Another study in Honolulu, Hawaii, evaluated 25(OH) vitamin D levels in 93 individuals who were under the sun for an average of 28.9 h/week without sunscreen (Binkley et al. 2007). There was a substantial variability of 25(OH) vitamin D levels in the population, with no level exceeding 60 ng/mL. Fifty-one percent of the subjects had a 25(OH) vitamin D level <30 ng/mL. The authors postulated that the individuals with low vitamin D status had inadequate cutaneous production of vitamin D3, enhanced destruction of previtamin D3 or vitamin D3 from sunlight, down-regulation of vitamin D production by sun-induced melanin production, or abnormalities of transport of vitamin D from the skin to the circulation (Binkley et al. 2007). There have been reports of treatment of patients with malabsorption with ultraviolet light to improve vitamin D status (Chandra et al. 2007).

The best gauge of vitamin D status is a 25(OH) vitamin D level (Holick 2008). Owing to many factors detailed earlier, which can affect the production of vitamin D in the skin, sunlight exposure cannot always be counted upon to produce a 25(OH) vitamin D level above 30 ng/mL. However, a combination of supplements and dietary sources and sun exposure can be useful to assure adequate vitamin D status.

40.6 Osteoporosis Treatment: General Considerations

Myth: All prescription osteoporosis medications are equal.

Reality: There is a growing number of prescription therapies available that are approved for the treatment of postmenopausal osteoporosis and other forms of bone loss. Each therapy has been proven to be effective in reducing fractures in some manner. Each treatment option is also associated with unique risks and side effects. Comparisons of efficacy between osteoporosis medications are generally based on nonhead-to-head evaluation of individual clinical trials and the few trials comparing intermediate outcomes. There are currently no studies available that adequately provide a direct head-to-head comparison of fracture risk reduction (Table 40.1).

As a class, bisphosphonates have been found to be effective in reducing the risk of fractures at the spine, hip, and nonvertebral sites with the exception of ibandronate, which is lacking evidence of nonvertebral risk reduction (Black et al. 1996; Chesnut et al. 2004; Delmas et al. 2006; Recker et al. 2004; Stakkestad et al. 2003; Wells et al. 2008a; Wells et al. 2008b). However, newer secondary analysis data on prior ibandronate studies suggest that the currently prescribed doses (in comparison to lower doses used in some clinical trials) do result in a nonvertebral fracture-risk reduction (Cranney et al. 2009). The selective estrogen receptor modulator (SERMs), raloxifene, and calcitonin, reduce the

Table 40.1 Relative risk of a future fracture with use of osteoporosis treatments in a person with a prior fracture; RR (95%CI) (111, 115, 116, 121)

Drug class	Vertebral fracture RR[a]	Nonvertebral fracture (e.g., hip) RR[a]
Bisphosphonates (BPs)	0.39–0.75	0.20–0.41
Alendronate (116)	0.55 (0.43–0.69)	0.77 (0.64–0.92)
Ibandronate	0.62 (0.41–0.75)	Not significant
Risedronate (115)	0.61 (0.50–0.76)	0.80 (0.72–0.90)
Zoledronic acid	0.54 (0.32–0.92)	0.73 (0.55–0.98)
Parathyroid hormone (PTH)	0.65	0.53
Teriparatide		
Selective estrogen-receptor modulators (SERMs)	0.30–0.55%	Not significant
Raloxifene		
Calcitonin	0.23	Not significant

[a]Unless noted, data were obtained from product labeling and are not from head to head studies

risk of vertebral fractures, but also have no significant risk reduction for nonvertebral fractures (Miacalcin® Insert 2003; Evista® Insert 2007). PTH is the only available anabolic agent, whereas the other current therapies are antiresorptive in effect. PTH effectively reduces vertebral and nonvertebral fracture risk (Neer et al. 2001).

Owing to these many considerations, the choice of osteoporosis treatment should be determined for each individual patient, taking into account the risks and benefits of all the therapies. As a result of the strong fracture-risk reduction evidence with bisphosphonate therapy, these medications are currently considered first-line therapy. Gastrointestinal side effects are the most common problems associated with oral bisphosphonates, which can be overcome with the use of intravenous zoledronic acid or ibandronate. There are also reported cases of osteonecrosis of the jaw and atrial fibrillation with the use of bisphosphonates (see other Myths). A full understanding of all putative adverse events is not available. Raloxifene is associated with an increased risk of thromboembolic events. Teriparatide appears safe with rare adverse events, but due to cost and inconvenience of a daily injection, it should be reserved for those with severe osteoporosis or persons who fracture despite bisphosphonate therapy.

40.7 Osteoporosis Treatment: Hormone Replacement Therapy

Myth: Older postmenopausal women should be on long-term hormone replacement for bone health.

Reality: Since the publication of the Women's Health Initiative (WHI) results in 2002, there has been considerable controversy surrounding the risks and benefits of hormone replacement therapy (HRT) (Rossouw et al. 2002). The WHI proved that estrogen is beneficial in preventing bone loss and reducing fracture risk. However, it heightened concerns about the association of HRT on the risk of invasive breast cancer, thromboembolism, and cardiovascular disease.

The WHI evaluated the effect of estrogen only (for women without a uterus) or estrogen plus progesterone (for women with a history of a hysterectomy) in 16,608 women, with primary endpoints of prevention of coronary heart disease (CHD), and secondary effects of other cardiovascular disease prevention and reduction of hip and other fractures (Rossouw et al. 2002). Women treated with combination estrogen plus progesterone were found to have an increased risk of invasive breast cancer (hazard ratio {HR}, 1.2; 95% confidence interval {CI}, 1.0–1.5), as well as stroke, thromboembolism, and pulmonary thromboembolus. The risk of all fractures was reduced in treated women (Hip fracture HR,

0.7; 95% CI 0.7–1.0; other fracture HR, 0.8; 95% CI 0.7–0.8), as was colorectal cancer. The risk of CHD in the treatment group was increased but did not reach statistical significance (HR, 1.2; 95% CI, 1.0–1.5). Estrogen only therapy, on the other hand, was associated with an increased risk of stroke and thromboembolus, a decreased risk of hip and other fractures (Hip fracture HR, 0.6; 95% CI 0.4–0.9; other fracture HR, 0.7; 95% CI 0.6–0.8), and a nonsignificantly reduced risk of CHD and breast cancer. The reduced risk of fracture was seen shortly after the initiation of therapy in both the treatment groups (Rossouw et al. 2002).

There is a debate regarding the applicability of the WHI data to the women seen in practice, since the women participating in the treatment groups were on an average 63 years old and had been postmenopausal for approximately 12–16 years when the therapy was initiated. A meta-analysis found that HRT appeared to be cardioprotective when started in younger women, but no risk reduction was seen when used in older women (Salpeter et al. 2006). Similarly, re-analysis of the WHI data, stratified by the time since menopause, revealed a direct correlation between increasing CHD risk and time since menopause (Rossouw et al. 2007).

Further randomized, controlled trials evaluating the risks and benefits of HRT in younger postmenopausal women are pending. In the interim, the use of HRT should be individualized for each patient, based on age, symptoms, and pertinent risk factors. Although HRT is known to be beneficial in reducing fracture risk and treating menopausal symptoms, there are other treatment options that should be considered if the patient or physician has concerns regarding the use of HRT.

40.8 Osteoporosis Treatment: Bisphosphonates

Pearl: Osteonecrosis of the jaw is uncommon when bisphosphonates are used for osteoporosis.

Comment: Osteonecrosis of the jaw (ONJ), manifested by a nonhealing area of exposed bone in the jaw, has been associated with bisphosphonate therapy (Woo et al. 2006). Most cases reported have occurred in the setting of bisphosphonate use for metastatic breast cancer or myeloma, have followed intravenous bisphosphonate, and have commonly been predated by dental procedures including tooth extraction and dental implants. A large observational experience at the MD Anderson medical center suggests an incidence of 1–2% for patients receiving high dose intravenous bisphosphonates for malignancies (Hoff et al. 2008).

The current incidence of osteonecrosis of the jaw when these bisphosphonates are used for osteoporosis is estimated at just below one per hundred thousand exposed. There have been few controlled studies to adequately address this question. Large clinical trials of intravenous zoledronic acid for treatment of osteoporosis have demonstrated only one potential case in persons exposed to zoledronic acid (and one in those exposed to the control) among over eight thousand persons treated (Lyles et al. 2007; Black et al. 2007). What remains unknown is whether the experience in persons receiving high dose intravenous bisphosphonates (for malignancy) is a precursor to what may become a more common problem as more osteoporosis patients are treated with oral and intravenous bisphosphonates at lower doses but for longer periods of time. With further data pending, the clinician and patient must weigh the risk and benefits with respect to the clear fracture-risk reduction and the putative risk of osteonecrosis of the jaw.

References

Adachi JD, Saag KG, Delmas PD, Liberman UA, Emkey RD, Seeman E, Lane NE, Kaufman JM, Poubelle PE, Hawkins F, Correa-Rotter R, Menkes CJ, Rodriguez-Portales JA, Schnitzer TJ, Block JA, Wing J, McIlwain HH, Westhovens R, Brown J, Melo-Gomes JA, Gruber BL, Yanover MJ, Leite MO, Siminoski KG, Nevitt MC, Sharp JT, Malice MP, Dumortier T, Czachur M, Carofano W, Daifotis A. Two-year effects of alendronate on bone mineral density and vertebral fracture in patients receiving glucocorticoids: a randomized, double-blind, placebo-controlled extension trial. Arthritis Rheum. 2001; 44(1):202–11

Armas LA, Dowell S, Akhter M, Duthuluru S, Huerter C, Hollis BW, Lund R, Heaney RP. Ultraviolet-B radiation increases serum 25-hydroxyvitamin D levels: the effect of UVB dose and skin color. J Am Acad Dermatol. 2007;57(4):588–93

Bergstrom U, Bjornstig U, Stenlund H, Jonsson H, Svensson O. Fracture mechanisms and fracture pattern in men and women aged 50 years and older: a study of a 12-year population-based injury register, Umea, Sweden. Osteoporos Int. 2008;19(9):1267–73

Bhutto A, Morley JE. The clinical significance of gastrointestinal changes with aging. Curr Opin Clin Nutr Metab Care. 2008;11(5): 651–60

Binkley N, Krueger D, Cowgill CS, Plum L, Lake E, Hansen KE, DeLuca HF, Drezner MK. Assay variation confounds the diagnosis of hypovitaminosis D: a call for standardization. J Clin Endocrinol Metab. 2004;89(7):3152–7

Binkley N, Novotny R, Krueger D, Kawahara T, Daida YG, Lensmeyer G, Hollis BW, Drezner MK. Low vitamin D status despite abundant sun exposure. J Clin Endocrinol Metab. 2007;92(6):2130–5

Bischoff-Ferrari HA, Willett WC, Wong JB, Giovannucci E, Dietrich T, Dawson-Hughes B. Fracture prevention with vitamin D supplementation: a meta-analysis of randomized controlled trials. JAMA. 2005;293(18):2257–64

Black DM, Cummings SR, Karpf DB, Cauley JA, Thompson DE, Nevitt MC, Bauer DC, Genant HK, Haskell WL, Marcus R, Ott SM, Torner JC, Quandt SA, Reiss TF, Ensrud KE. Randomised trial of effect of alendronate on risk of fracture in women with existing vertebral fractures. Fracture Intervention Trial Research Group. Lancet 1996;348(9041):1535–41

Black DM, Delmas PD, Eastell R, Reid IR, Boonen S, Cauley JA, Cosman F, Lakatos P, Leung PC, Man Z, Mautalen C, Mesenbrink P,

Hu H, Caminis J, Tong K, Rosario-Jansen T, Krasnow J, Hue TF, Sellmeyer D, Eriksen EF, Cummings SR. Once-yearly zoledronic acid for treatment of postmenopausal osteoporosis. N Engl J Med. 2007;356(18):1809–22

Bolland MJ, Barber PA, Doughty RN, Mason B, Horne A, Ames R, Gamble GD, Grey A, Reid IR. Vascular events in healthy older women receiving calcium supplementation: randomised controlled trial. BMJ. 2008;336(7638):262–6

Borghi L, Schianchi T, Meschi T, Guerra A, Allegri F, Maggiore U, Novarini A. Comparison of two diets for the prevention of recurrent stones in idiopathic hypercalciuria. N Engl J Med. 2002;346(2): 77–84

Breslau NA, McGuire JL, Zerwekh JE, Pak CY. The role of dietary sodium on renal excretion and intestinal absorption of calcium and on vitamin D metabolism. J Clin Endocrinol Metab. 1982;55(2): 369–73

Burge R, Dawson-Hughes B, Solomon DH, Wong JB, King A, Tosteson A. Incidence and economic burden of osteoporosis-related fractures in the United States, 2005–2025. J Bone Miner Res. 2007;22(3): 465–75

Center JR, Bliuc D, Nguyen TV, Eisman JA. Risk of subsequent fracture after low-trauma fracture in men and women. JAMA. 2007;297(4):387–94

Chandra P, Wolfenden LL, Ziegler TR, Tian J, Luo M, Stecenko AA, Chen TC, Holick MF, Tangpricha V. Treatment of vitamin D deficiency with UV light in patients with malabsorption syndromes: a case series. Photodermatol Photoimmunol Photomed. 2007;23(5): 179–85

Chapuy MC, Arlot ME, Duboeuf F, Brun J, Crouzet B, Arnaud S, Delmas PD, Meunier PJ. Vitamin D3 and calcium to prevent hip fractures in the elderly women. N Engl J Med. 1992;327(23): 1637–42

Chesnut IC, Skag A, Christiansen C, Recker R, Stakkestad JA, Hoiseth A, Felsenberg D, Huss H, Gilbride J, Schimmer RC, Delmas PD. Effects of oral ibandronate administered daily or intermittently on fracture risk in postmenopausal osteoporosis. J Bone Miner Res. 2004;19(8):1241–9

Cranney A, Wells GA, Yetisir E, Adami S, Cooper C, Delmas PD, Miller PD, Papapoulos S, Reginster JY, Sambrook PN, Silverman S, Siris E, Adachi JD. Ibandronate for the prevention of nonvertebral fractures: a pooled analysis of individual patient data. Osteoporos Int. 2009;20(2):291–7

Cuddihy MT, Gabriel SE, Crowson CS, O'Fallon WM, Melton LJ III. Forearm fractures as predictors of subsequent osteoporotic fractures. Osteoporos Int. 1999;9(6):469–75

Curhan GC, Willett WC, Knight EL, Stampfer MJ. Dietary factors and the risk of incident kidney stones in younger women: Nurses' Health Study II. Arch Intern Med. 2004;164(8):885–91

Dawson-Hughes B, Harris SS, Krall EA, Dallal GE. Effect of calcium and vitamin D supplementation on bone density in men and women 65 years of age or older. N Engl J Med. 1997;337(10):670–6

Delmas PD, Adami S, Strugala C, Stakkestad JA, Reginster JY, Felsenberg D, Christiansen C, Civitelli R, Drezner MK, Recker RR, Bolognese M, Hughes C, Masanauskaite D, Ward P, Sambrook P, Reid DM. Intravenous ibandronate injections in postmenopausal women with osteoporosis: one-year results from the dosing intravenous administration study. Arthritis Rheum. 2006;54(6): 1838–46

Eisman JA, Shepard RM, DeLuca HF. Determination of 25-hydroxyvitamin D2 and 25-hydroxyvitamin D3 in human plasma using high-pressure liquid chromatography. Anal Biochem. 1977;80(1): 298–305

Emkey RD, Lindsay R, Lyssy J, Weisberg JS, Dempster DW, Shen V. The systemic effect of intraarticular administration of corticosteroid on markers of bone formation and bone resorption in patients with rheumatoid arthritis. Arthritis Rheum. 1996;39(2):277–82

Evista (raloxifene) [package insert]. Indianapolis, IN: Eli Lilly; 2007

FRAX Who Fracture Risk Assessment Tool. http://www.shef.ac.uk/FRAX/ (2008)

Furstenberg AL, Mezey MD. Differences in outcome between black and white elderly hip fracture patients. J Chronic Dis. 1987; 40(10): 931–8

Gankam Kengne F, Andres C, Sattar L, Melot C, Decaux G. Mild hyponatremia and risk of fracture in the ambulatory elderly. QJM. 2008;101(7):583–8

Grant AM, Avenell A, Campbell MK, McDonald AM, MacLennan GS, McPherson GC, Anderson FH, Cooper C, Francis RM, Donaldson C, Gillespie WJ, Robinson CM, Torgerson DJ, Wallace WA. Oral vitamin D3 and calcium for secondary prevention of low-trauma fractures in elderly people (Randomised Evaluation of Calcium or vitamin D, RECORD): a randomised placebo-controlled trial. Lancet 2005;365(9471):1621–8

Haddad JG, Chyu KJ. Competitive protein-binding radioassay for 25-hydroxycholecalciferol. J Clin Endocrinol Metab. 1971;33(6): 992–5

Hanzlik RP, Fowler SC, Fisher DH. Relative bioavailability of calcium from calcium formate, calcium citrate, and calcium carbonate. J Pharmacol Exp Ther. 2005;313(3):1217–22

Heaney RP, Dowell MS, Barger-Lux MJ. Absorption of calcium as the carbonate and citrate salts, with some observations on method. Osteoporos Int. 1999;9(1):19–23

Heaney RP, Dowell MS, Rafferty K, Bierman J. Bioavailability of the calcium in fortified soy imitation milk, with some observations on method. Am J Clin Nutr. 2000;71(5):1166–9

Heaney RP, Rafferty K, Dowell MS, Bierman J. Calcium fortification systems differ in bioavailability. J Am Diet Assoc. 2005;105(5): 807–9

Heaney RP, Rafferty K. The settling problem in calcium-fortified soybean drinks. J Am Diet Assoc. 2006;106(11):1753; author reply 1755

Heaney RP. Absorbability and utility of calcium in mineral waters. Am J Clin Nutr. 2006a;84(2):371–4

Heaney RP. Role of dietary sodium in osteoporosis. J Am Coll Nutr. 2006b;25(3 Suppl):271S6S

Hedlund R, Lindgren U. Trauma type, age, and gender as determinants of hip fracture. J Orthop Res. 1987;5(2):242–6

Heikinheimo RJ, Inkovaara JA, Harju EJ, Haavisto MV, Kaarela RH, Kataja JM, Kokko AM, Kolho LA, Rajala SA. Annual injection of vitamin D and fractures of aged bones. Calcif Tissue Int. 1992;51(2): 105–10

Heller HJ, Greer LG, Haynes SD, Poindexter JR, Pak CY. Pharmacokinetic and pharmacodynamic comparison of two calcium supplements in postmenopausal women. J Clin Pharmacol. 2000; 40(11):1237–44

Heller HJ, Stewart A, Haynes S, Pak CY. Pharmacokinetics of calcium absorption from two commercial calcium supplements. J Clin Pharmacol. 1999;39(11):1151–4

Hoff AO, Toth BB, Altundag K, Johnson MM, Warneke CL, Hu M, Nooka A, Sayegh G, Guarneri V, Desrouleaux K, Cui J, Adamus A, Gagel RF, Hortobagyi GN. Frequency and risk factors associated with osteonecrosis of the jaw in cancer patients treated with intravenous bisphosphonates. J Bone Miner Res. 2008;23(6): 826–36

Holick MF. Deficiency of sunlight and vitamin D. BMJ. 2008;336(7657): 1318–9

Holick MF. High prevalence of vitamin D inadequacy and implications for health. Mayo Clin Proc. 2006a;81(3):353–73

Holick MF. Resurrection of vitamin D deficiency and rickets. J Clin Invest. 2006b;116(8):2062–72

Holick MF. Vitamin D deficiency. N Engl J Med. 2007;357(3):266–81

Hollis BW. Measuring 25-hydroxyvitamin D in a clinical environment: challenges and needs. Am J Clin Nutr. 2008;88(2):507S—10S

Hsia J, Heiss G, Ren H, Allison M, Dolan NC, Greenland P, Heckbert SR, Johnson KC, Manson JE, Sidney S, Trevisan M. Calcium/vitamin D supplementation and cardiovascular events. Circulation 2007; 115(7):846–54

Hurwitz A, Brady DA, Schaal SE, Samloff IM, Dedon J, Ruhl CE. Gastric acidity in older adults. JAMA. 1997;278(8):659–62

ISCD. The International Society for Clinical Densitometry:2007 ISCD Official Positions Brochure. http://www.iscd.org/Visitors/pdfs/ ISCD2007OfficialPositions-Combined-AdultandPediatric.pdf (2007)

Israel E, Banerjee TR, Fitzmaurice GM, Kotlov TV, LaHive K, LeBoff MS. Effects of inhaled glucocorticoids on bone density in premenopausal women. N Engl J Med. 2001;345(13):941–7

Jackson RD, LaCroix AZ, Gass M, Wallace RB, Robbins J, Lewis CE, Bassford T, Beresford SA, Black HR, Blanchette P, Bonds DE, Brunner RL, Brzyski RG, Caan B, Cauley JA, Chlebowski RT, Cummings SR, Granek I, Hays J, Heiss G, Hendrix SL, Howard BV, Hsia J, Hubbell FA, Johnson KC, Judd H, Kotchen JM, Kuller LH, Langer RD, Lasser NL, Limacher MC, Ludlam S, Manson JE, Margolis KL, McGowan J, Ockene JK, O'Sullivan MJ, Phillips L, Prentice RL, Sarto GE, Stefanick ML, Van Horn L, Wactawski-Wende J, Whitlock E, Anderson GL, Assaf AR, Barad D. Calcium plus vitamin D supplementation and the risk of fractures. N Engl J Med. 2006;354(7):669–83

Jacobsen SJ, Goldberg J, Miles TP, Brody JA, Stiers W, Rimm AA. Race and sex differences in mortality following fracture of the hip. Am J Public Health. 1992;82(8):1147–50

Jones G, Nguyen T, Sambrook PN, Kelly PJ, Gilbert C, Eisman JA. Symptomatic fracture incidence in elderly men and women: the Dubbo Osteoporosis Epidemiology Study (DOES). Osteoporos Int. 1994;4(5):277–82

Kanis JA, Johnell O, Oden A, Dawson A, De Laet C, Jonsson B. Ten year probabilities of osteoporotic fractures according to BMD and diagnostic thresholds. Osteoporos Int. 2001;12(12):989–95

Karlsson MK, Hasserius R, Obrant KJ. Individuals who sustain nonosteoporotic fractures continue to also sustain fragility fractures. Calcif Tissue Int. 1993;53(4):229–31

Kellie SE, Brody JA. Sex-specific and race-specific hip fracture rates. Am J Public Health. 1990;80(3):326–8

Kenny AM, Prestwood KM, Biskup B, Robbins B, Zayas E, Kleppinger A, Burleson JA, Raisz LG. Comparison of the effects of calcium loading with calcium citrate or calcium carbonate on bone turnover in postmenopausal women. Osteoporos Int. 2004; 15(4):290–4

Khan A. Premenopausal women and low bone density. Can Fam Physician. 2006;52:743–7

Khan AA, Syed Z. Bone densitometry in premenopausal women: synthesis and review. J Clin Densitom. 2004;7(1):85–92

Kudlacek S, Schneider B, Resch H, Freudenthaler O, Willvonseder R. Gender differences in fracture risk and bone mineral density. Maturitas 2000;36(3):173–80

Lappe JM, Heaney RP. Calcium supplementation: results may not be generalisable. BMJ. 2008;336(7641):403; author reply 404

Larsen ER, Mosekilde L, Foldspang A. Vitamin D and calcium supplementation prevents osteoporotic fractures in elderly community dwelling residents: a pragmatic population-based 3-year intervention study. J Bone Miner Res. 2004;19(3):370–8

Lewiecki EM. Premenopausal bone health assessment. Curr Rheumatol Rep. 2005;7(1):46–52

Lips P, Graafmans WC, Ooms ME, Bezemer PD, Bouter LM Vitamin D. supplementation and fracture incidence in elderly persons. A randomized, placebo-controlled clinical trial. Ann Intern Med. 1996;124(4):400–6

Lips P. Vitamin D deficiency and secondary hyperparathyroidism in the elderly: consequences for bone loss and fractures and therapeutic implications. Endocr Rev. 2001;22(4):477–501

Lissner D, Mason RS, Posen S. Stability of vitamin D metabolites in human blood serum and plasma. Clin Chem. 1981;27(5):773–4

Lyles KW, Colon-Emeric CS, Magaziner JS, Adachi JD, Pieper CF, Mautalen C, Hyldstrup L, Recknor C, Nordsletten L, Moore KA, Lavecchia C, Zhang J, Mesenbrink P, Hodgson PK, Abrams K,

Orloff JJ, Horowitz Z, Eriksen EF, Boonen S. Zoledronic acid and clinical fractures and mortality after hip fracture. N Engl J Med. 2007;357(18):1799–809

Lyons RA, Johansen A, Brophy S, Newcombe RG, Phillips CJ, Lervy B, Evans R, Wareham K, Stone MD. Preventing fractures among older people living in institutional care: a pragmatic randomised double blind placebo controlled trial of vitamin D supplementation. Osteoporos Int. 2007;18(6):811–8

Mackey DC, Lui LY, Cawthon PM, Bauer DC, Nevitt MC, Cauley JA, Hillier TA, Lewis CE, Barrett-Connor E, Cummings SR. High-trauma fractures and low bone mineral density in older women and men. JAMA. 2007;298(20):2381–8

Manolagas SC, Weinstein RS. New developments in the pathogenesis and treatment of steroid-induced osteoporosis. J Bone Miner Res. 1999;14(7):1061–6

Martini L, Wood RJ. Relative bioavailability of calcium-rich dietary sources in the elderly. Am J Clin Nutr. 2002;76(6):1345–50

Maunsell Z, Wright DJ, Rainbow SJ. Routine isotope-dilution liquid chromatography-tandem mass spectrometry assay for simultaneous measurement of the 25-hydroxy metabolites of vitamins D2 and D3. Clin Chem. 2005;51(9):1683–90

Melton LJ III, Atkinson EJ, O'Fallon WM, Wahner HW, Riggs BL. Long-term fracture prediction by bone mineral assessed at different skeletal sites. J Bone Miner Res. 1993;8(10):1227–33

Melton LJ III, Beck TJ, Amin S, Khosla S, Achenbach SJ, Oberg AL, Riggs BL. Contributions of bone density and structure to fracture risk assessment in men and women. Osteoporos Int. 2005;16(5): 460–7

Melton LJ III, Sampson JM, Morrey BF, Ilstrup DM. Epidemiologic features of pelvic fractures. Clin Orthop Relat Res. 1981;155:43–7

Meyer WJ III, Transbol I, Bartter FC, Delea C. Control of calcium absorption: effect of sodium chloride loading and depletion. Metabolism 1976;25(9):989–93

Mezquita-Raya P, Munoz-Torres M, Luna JD, Luna V, Lopez-Rodriguez F, Torres-Vela E, Escobar-Jimenez F. Relation between vitamin D insufficiency, bone density, and bone metabolism in healthy postmenopausal women. J Bone Miner Res. 2001;16(8): 1408–15

Miacalcin® Nasal Spray [Package Insert], East Hanover, NJ: Novartis Pharmaceuticals; 2003

Mikuls TR, Saag KG, George V, Mudano AS, Banerjee S. Racial disparities in the receipt of osteoporosis related healthcare among community-dwelling older women with arthritis and previous fracture. J Rheumatol. 2005;32(5):870–5

Miller RG, Ashar BH, Cohen J, Camp M, Coombs C, Johnson E, Schneyer CR. Disparities in osteoporosis screening between at-risk African-American and white women. J Gen Intern Med. 2005;20(9): 847–51

Moreira Kulak CA, Schussheim DH, McMahon DJ, Kurland E, Silverberg SJ, Siris ES, Bilezikian JP, Shane E. Osteoporosis and low bone mass in premenopausal and perimenopausal women. Endocr Pract. 2000;6(4):296–304

Mudano AS, Casebeer L, Patino F, Allison JJ, Weissman NW, Kiefe CI, Person S, Gilbert D, Saag KG. Racial disparities in osteoporosis prevention in a managed care population. South Med J. 2003;96(5): 445–51

National Osteoporosis Foundation. Physician's guide to prevention and treatment of osteoporosis. Belle Mead, NJ: Excerpta Medica; 2008

Neer RM, Arnaud CD, Zanchetta JR, Prince R, Gaich GA, Reginster JY, Hodsman AB, Eriksen EF, Ish-Shalom S, Genant HK, Wang O, Mitlak BH. Effect of parathyroid hormone (1–34) on fractures and bone mineral density in postmenopausal women with osteoporosis. N Engl J Med. 2001;344(19):1434–41

Novartis API. http://www.fda.gov/cder/foi/label/2005/20036s030lbl. pdf (2004). Accessed 1 Oct 2008

O'Connell MB, Madden DM, Murray AM, Heaney RP, Kerzner LJ. Effects of proton pump inhibitors on calcium carbonate absorption in women: a randomized crossover trial. Am J Med. 2005;118(7): 778–81

Ornoy A, Wajnberg R, Diav-Citrin O. The outcome of pregnancy following pre-pregnancy or early pregnancy alendronate treatment. Reprod Toxicol. 2006;22(4):578–9

Orwoll E. Assessing bone density in men. J Bone Miner Res. 2000;15(10):1867–70

Papadimitropoulos E, Wells G, Shea B, Gillespie W, Weaver B, Zytaruk N, Cranney A, Adachi J, Tugwell P, Josse R, Greenwood C, Guyatt G. Meta-analyses of therapies for postmenopausal osteoporosis. VIII: meta-analysis of the efficacy of vitamin D treatment in preventing osteoporosis in postmenopausal women. Endocr Rev. 2002;23(4):560–9

Patlas N, Golomb G, Yaffe P, Pinto T, Breuer E, Ornoy A. Transplacental effects of bisphosphonates on fetal skeletal ossification and mineralization in rats. Teratology. 1999;60(2):68–73

Prince RL, Devine A, Dhaliwal SS, Dick IM. Effects of calcium supplementation on clinical fracture and bone structure: results of a 5-year, double-blind, placebo-controlled trial in elderly women. Arch Intern Med. 2006;166(8):869–75

Rafferty K, Walters G, Heaney RP. Calcium fortificants: overview and strategies for improving calcium nutriture of the U.S. population. J Food Sci. 2007;72(9):R152–8

Rauch F, Glorieux FH. Osteogenesis imperfecta. Lancet 2004;363(9418): 1377–85

Recker RR, Weinstein RS, Chesnut CH III, Schimmer RC, Mahoney P, Hughes C, Bonvoisin B, Meunier PJ. Histomorphometric evaluation of daily and intermittent oral ibandronate in women with postmenopausal osteoporosis: results from the BONE study. Osteoporos Int. 2004;15(3):231–7

Recker RR. Calcium absorption and achlorhydria. N Engl J Med. 1985;313(2):70–3

Reid DM, Hughes RA, Laan RF, Sacco-Gibson NA, Wenderoth DH, Adami S, Eusebio RA, Devogelaer JP. Efficacy and safety of daily risedronate in the treatment of corticosteroid-induced osteoporosis in men and women: a randomized trial. European Corticosteroid-Induced Osteoporosis Treatment Study. J Bone Miner Res. 2000; 15(6):1006–13

Reid IR, Mason B, Horne A, Ames R, Reid HE, Bava U, Bolland MJ, Gamble GD. Randomized controlled trial of calcium in healthy older women. Am J Med. 2006;119(9):777–85

Rossouw JE, Anderson GL, Prentice RL, LaCroix AZ, Kooperberg C, Stefanick ML, Jackson RD, Beresford SA, Howard BV, Johnson KC, Kotchen JM, Ockene J. Risks and benefits of estrogen plus progestin in healthy postmenopausal women: principal results from the Women's Health Initiative randomized controlled trial. JAMA. 2002;288(3):321–33

Rossouw JE, Prentice RL, Manson JE, Wu L, Barad D, Barnabei VM, Ko M, LaCroix AZ, Margolis KL, Stefanick ML. Postmenopausal hormone therapy and risk of cardiovascular disease by age and years since menopause. JAMA. 2007;297(13):1465–77

Saag KG, Emkey R, Schnitzer TJ, Brown JP, Hawkins F, Goemaere S, Thamsborg G, Liberman UA, Delmas PD, Malice MP, Czachur M, Daifotis AG. Alendronate for the prevention and treatment of glucocorticoid-induced osteoporosis. Glucocorticoid-Induced Osteoporosis Intervention Study Group. N Engl J Med. 1998;339(5): 292–9

Salpeter SR, Walsh JM, Greyber E, Salpeter EE. Brief report: coronary heart disease events associated with hormone therapy in younger and older women. A meta-analysis. J Gen Intern Med. 2006;21(4): 363–6

Sanders KM, Pasco JA, Ugoni AM, Nicholson GC, Seeman E, Martin TJ, Skoric B, Panahi S, Kotowicz MA. The exclusion of high trauma fractures may underestimate the prevalence of bone fragility fractures in the community: the Geelong Osteoporosis Study. J Bone Miner Res. 1998;13(8):1337–42

Sanders KM, Seeman E, Ugoni AM, Pasco JA, Martin TJ, Skoric B, Nicholson GC, Kotowicz MA. Age- and gender-specific rate of fractures in Australia: a population-based study. Osteoporos Int. 1999;10(3):240–7

Schousboe JT, Taylor BC, Fink HA, Kane RL, Cummings SR, Orwoll ES, Melton LJ III, Bauer DC, Ensrud KE. Cost-effectiveness of bone densitometry followed by treatment of osteoporosis in older men. JAMA. 2007;298(6):629–37

Serfaty-Lacrosniere C, Wood RJ, Voytko D, Saltzman JR, Pedrosa M, Sepe TE, Russell RR. Hypochlorhydria from short-term omeprazole treatment does not inhibit intestinal absorption of calcium, phosphorus, magnesium or zinc from food in humans. J Am Coll Nutr. 1995;14(4):364–8

Siris ES, Miller PD, Barrett-Connor E, Faulkner KG, Wehren LE, Abbott TA, Berger ML, Santora AC, Sherwood LM. Identification and fracture outcomes of undiagnosed low bone mineral density in postmenopausal women: results from the National Osteoporosis Risk Assessment. JAMA. 2001;286(22):2815–22

Stakkestad JA, Benevolenskaya LI, Stepan JJ, Skag A, Nordby A, Oefjord E, Burdeska A, Jonkanski I, Mahoney P. Intravenous ibandronate injections given every three months: a new treatment option to prevent bone loss in postmenopausal women. Ann Rheum Dis. 2003;62(10):969–75

Tangpricha V, Pearce EN, Chen TC, Holick MF. Vitamin D insufficiency among free-living healthy young adults. Am J Med. 2002;112(8):659–62

Taylor EN, Curhan GC. Diet and fluid prescription in stone disease. Kidney Int. 2006;70(5):835–9

Taylor EN, Curhan GC. Role of nutrition in the formation of calcium-containing kidney stones. Nephron Physiol. 2004;98(2):p55–63

Taylor EN, Stampfer MJ, Curhan GC. Dietary factors and the risk of incident kidney stones in men: new insights after 14 years of follow-up. J Am Soc Nephrol. 2004;15(12):3225–32

Teucher B, Dainty JR, Spinks CA, Majsak-Newman G, Berry DJ, Hoogewerff JA, Foxall RJ, Jakobsen J, Cashman KD, Flynn A, Fairweather-Tait SJ. Sodium and bone health: impact of moderately high and low salt intakes on calcium metabolism in postmenopausal women. J Bone Miner Res. 2008;23(9):1477–85

Ton FN, Gunawardene SC, Lee H, Neer RM. Effects of low-dose prednisone on bone metabolism. J Bone Miner Res. 2005; 20(3):464–70

van Staa TP, Dennison EM, Leufkens HG, Cooper C. Epidemiology of fractures in England and Wales. Bone. 2001;29(6): 517–22

van Staa TP, Laan RF, Barton IP, Cohen S, Reid DM, Cooper C. Bone density threshold and other predictors of vertebral fracture in patients receiving oral glucocorticoid therapy. Arthritis Rheum. 2003;48(11):3224–9

van Staa TP, Leufkens HG, Abenhaim L, Zhang B, Cooper C. Use of oral corticosteroids and risk of fractures. J Bone Miner Res. 2000;15(6):993–1000

Visser M, Deeg DJ, Puts MT, Seidell JC, Lips P. Low serum concentrations of 25-hydroxyvitamin D in older persons and the risk of nursing home admission. Am J Clin Nutr. 2006;84(3):616–22; quiz 671–2

Wallach S, Cohen S, Reid DM, Hughes RA, Hosking DJ, Laan RF, Doherty SM, Maricic M, Rosen C, Brown J, Barton I, Chines AA. Effects of risedronate treatment on bone density and vertebral fracture in patients on corticosteroid therapy. Calcif Tissue Int. 2000;67(4):277–85

Wells G, Cranney A, Peterson J, Boucher M, Shea B, Robinson V, Coyle D, Tugwell P. Risedronate for the primary and secondary prevention of osteoporotic fractures in postmenopausal women. Cochrane Database Syst Rev. 2008a;(1):CD004523

Wells GA, Cranney A, Peterson J, Boucher M, Shea B, Robinson V, Coyle D, Tugwell P. Alendronate for the primary and secondary prevention of osteoporotic fractures in postmenopausal women. Cochrane Database Syst Rev. 2008b;(1):CD001155

Williams CP, Child DF, Hudson PR, Davies GK, Davies MG, John R, Anandaram PS, De Bolla AR. Why oral calcium supplements may reduce renal stone disease: report of a clinical pilot study. J Clin Pathol. 2001;54(1):54–62

Wong CA, Walsh LJ, Smith CJ, Wisniewski AF, Lewis SA, Hubbard R, Cawte S, Green DJ, Pringle M, Tattersfield AE. Inhaled corticosteroid use and bone-mineral density in patients with asthma. Lancet 2000;355(9213):1399–403

Woo SB, Hellstein JW, Kalmar JR. Narrative [corrected] review: bisphosphonates and osteonecrosis of the jaws. Ann Intern Med. 2006;144(10):753–61

Zerwekh JE. Blood biomarkers of vitamin D status. Am J Clin Nutr. 2008;87(4):1087S–91S

Paget's Disease of Bone

41

Margaret Seton

41.1 Overview of Paget's Disease

> Sir James Paget described the disease as follows: *It begins in middle age or later, is very slow in progress, may continue for many years without influence on the general health, and may give no other trouble than those which are due to the changes of shape, size, and direction of the diseased bones* (Paget 1877).

> Paget's disease is a focal disorder of bone remodeling that occurs in an aging skeleton. Aberrant osteoclast activation is the critical lesion leading to the disease phenotype.

> Paget's disease leads to impaired structural integrity and distortion of bone, the consequences of which include localized bone pain, deformity, fracture, and early arthritis.

> Neurological sequelae such as hearing loss, spinal stenosis, and neuropathies can occur, depending on the sites of affected bones.

> Osteosarcomas arise in pagetic bone in a small number of cases (Seton 2008; Hansen et al. 2006)

> Both familial and sporadic cases of Paget's disease are caused often by a mutation in *SQSTM1*. This mutation results in a C→ T transition mutation (P392L) that in turn results in aberrant osteoclast activation (Laurin et al. 2002). However, not all cases are associated with this disease mutation (Kurihara et al. 2007; Morissette et al. 2006).

> The serum alkaline phosphatase, a marker of *osteoblastic* activity, is a good indicator of skeletal extent and activity of Paget's disease.

> Spot urine assays for *N*-telopeptide levels have replaced 24-h urine collections for hydroxyproline as a measure of antiresorptive activity.

> The goal of treating Paget's disease with antiresorptive agents such as the bisphosphonates and calcitonin is to normalize the serum alkaline phosphatase and urine *N*-telopeptide levels.

> Bisphosphonates are the treatment of choice. However, calcitonin has a role in the elderly patient with renal insufficiency in whom relief of pain rather than remission is a reasonable outcome.

> Resistance to the effects of one bisphosphonate does not predict resistance to another.

Pearl: Most patients with Paget's disease are asymptomatic.

Comment: Despite its remarkable appearance on plain radiographs and bone scintigraphy, most patients with Paget's disease of bone are asymptomatic. The diagnosis typically is made incidentally through findings on radiographs or blood tests ordered for other reasons. Treatment is indicated when pagetic bone affects weight-bearing limbs, approximates a joint, or involves the skull or spine. Treatment is also indicated in patients planning elective total hip or knee replacements that involve pagetic bone, to reduce blood loss from these sites. Treatment rarely restores hearing in patients with Paget's disease of the skull, straighten bowed limbs, or normalize radiographs, but it is expected to ease pain and prevent disease progression. Early treatment is recommended in an effort to avoid complications of long-standing disease.

Pearl: The bones affected by Paget's disease in a given individual remain unchanged over the lifetime of that person.

Comment: Paget's disease tends to present in middle-aged or older individuals. The disorder has a predilection for the skull, axial skeleton, and long bones of the lower extremity. The number of bones involved in Paget's disease tends to be fixed in a given individual, sometimes presenting as monostotic disease and other times as a polyostotic disorder (Fig. 41.1).

The persistence of the disease in certain bones in an individual patient has implications for the initial evaluation of a patient with possible Paget's disease. This is because Paget's disease must be distinguished from cancers metastatic to bone. Paget's disease does not "metastasize" or extend across

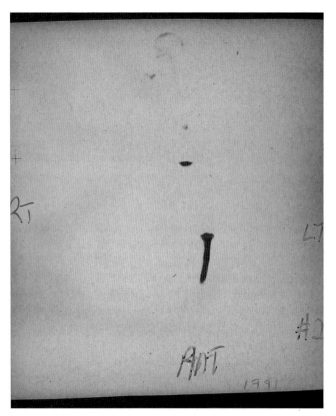

Fig. 41.1 Monostotic Paget's disease, L tibia. Paget's disease can involve one bone only or it can involve multiple bones. However, once its pattern of bone involvement is established in an individual patient, it does not "metastasize" to new bones. Evidence of new bony abnormalities suggests the possibility of metastatic cancer until proven otherwise. (the other site of intense uptake is the bladder)

joints to involve contiguous bone. The involvement of new bones strongly suggests an underlying malignancy.

A bone scan is indicated at diagnosis to identify the distribution of pagetic bone in the skeleton (Fig. 41.2). Bone scintigraphy typically reveals intense uptake beginning at one end of a bone and extending a variable distance through that bone. Radiographs of the affected sites should be obtained to confirm the diagnosis, define the anatomy of the problem, and establish the need for treatment. The subsequent involvement of new bones should be considered metastatic cancer until proven otherwise by biopsy (Cooper et al. 1999; Griffiths 1992; Haddaway et al. 2007).

Myth: Paget's disease occurs in children.

Reality: This is not true. Familial idiopathic hyperphosphatasia, sometimes termed "juvenile Paget's disease," is a separate entity. Familial idiopathic hyperphosphatasia is a rare autosomal-recessive disorder that is ascribed in most cases to a deficiency in osteoprotegerin. The disorder results in ungoverned bone remodeling, deformity, and fractures in children (Whyte et al. 2002).

Pearl: Paget's disease begins in subchondral bone, moving in one direction up or down the affected bone.

Comment: Early Paget's disease is often described as purely lytic. In fact, purely lytic lesions are an uncommon finding on plain radiographs at the time of diagnosis. Patients usually have radiographic evidence of both lysis (osteoclast activity) and thickened bone (osteoblast activity).

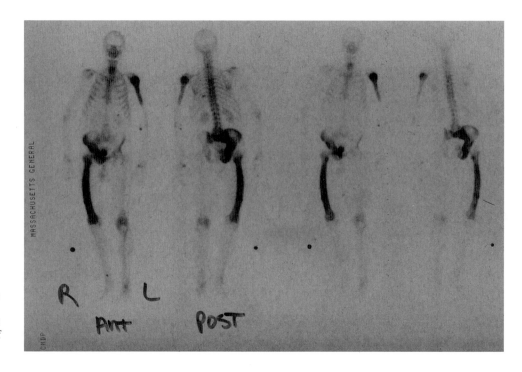

Fig. 41.2 Bone scintigraphy in Paget's disease. Polyostotic Paget's disease evident on bone scan, with the classic bowing of the femur

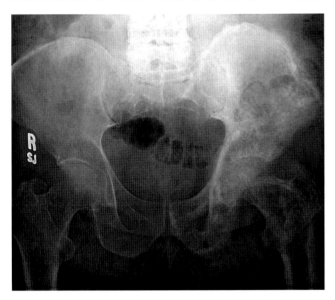

Fig. 41.3 Radiographic findings in late Paget's disease of bone. There is marked bone remodeling. The cortices become thickened. The trabeculae are coarsened, and the bone deformed

Late Paget's disease manifests itself as dense overgrowth of bone. The characteristic radiographic findings in late disease are thickened cortices striped by tunneling osteoclasts, coarsened trabeculae, and marked remodeling of the affected bone (Fig. 41.3). The bone enlarges, softens, and becomes deformed.

Myth: There is no effective treatment for Paget's disease of bone.

Reality: This is one of the most distressing myths of all related to Paget's disease. Bisphosphonates ease pain from pagetic bone effectively, restore bone turnover markers to normal levels, and result in the deposition of normal lamellar bone. Treatment may also result in the radiographic healing of lytic lesions or a reduction in bone scan activity in some patients. No prospective clinical trials have yet been conducted to confirm the clinical suspicion that bisphosphonate therapy prevents long-term complications of Paget's disease.

Alendronate, risedronate, and zoledronic acid all lead to a biochemical remission: i.e., to normalization of serum alkaline phosphatase levels (Reid et al. 1996; Siris et al. 1996; Brown et al. 2000; Miller et al. 1999; Seton and Krane 2007). This is incorrect. Retreatment is often required, prompted by rising serum alkaline phosphatase levels or recurrent bone pain (Hosking et al. 2007; Reid et al. 2005).

Pearl: Etidronate is contraindicated in patients who have lytic lesions in weight-bearing bones.

Comment: Etidronate can worsen bone pain in pagetic limbs and heighten the risk of fracture. This stems from etidronate's narrow therapeutic margin: at the doses required to suppress bone resorption, the drug also causes impaired mineralization (Altman 1985; Eyres et al. 1992; Gibbs et al. 1986).

Myth: Treatment of patients with bisphosphonates invariably eases their pain.

Reality: Paget's disease is a focal disorder of an aging skeleton. Treatment is aimed at preventing the complications of the existing disease, inhibiting disease progression, and easing the symptoms of bone pain at pagetic sites. Treatment will alleviate pain if the pain stems from pagetic bone. However, pain in Paget's patients, many of whom are elderly, can be multifactorial. Symptoms that result from degenerative changes in the spine or hips do not respond well to bisphosphonates or calcitonin. Nonsteroidal antiinflammatory drugs, physical therapy, or surgery may also be required.

Pearl: Teriparatide is contraindicated in patients with Paget's disease.

Comment: Many elderly patients with Paget's disease have osteoporosis, too. There may be some temptation to treat the patient's osteoporosis with teraparatide, a recombinant form of human parathyroid hormone that stimulates bone formation. However, Paget's disease is a contraindication to teriparatide. This is because of the rare but real risk of osteosarcoma arising from pagetic bone. Thus, bisphosphonates and calcitonin are the current mainstays of Paget's disease treatment. Both treat osteoporosis as well as Paget's disease.

References

Altman RD. Long-term follow-up of therapy with intermittent etidronate disodium in Paget's disease of bone. Am J Med. 1985;79(5): 583–90

Brown JP, Chines AA, Myers WR, et al Improvement of pagetic bone lesions with risedronate treatment: a radiologic study. Bone 2000; 26(3):263–7

Cooper C, Dennison E, Schafheutle K, et al Epidemiology of Paget's disease of bone. Bone 1999;24(5 Suppl):3S–5S.

Eyres KS, Marshall P, McCloskey E, et al Spontaneous fractures in a patient treated with low doses of etidronic acid (disodium etidronate). Drug Saf. 1992;7(2):162–5

Gibbs CJ, Aaron JE, Peacock M. Osteomalacia in Paget's disease treated with short term, high dose sodium etidronate. Br Med J (Clin Res Ed). 1986;292(6530):1227–9

Griffiths HJ. Radiology of Paget's disease. Curr Opin Radiol. 1992;4(6):124–8

Haddaway MJ, Davie MW, McCall IW, et al Effect of age and gender on the number and distribution of sites in Paget's disease of bone. Br J Radiol. 2007;80(955):532–6

Hansen MF, Seton M, Merchant A. Osteosarcoma in Paget's disease of bone. J Bone Miner Res. 2006;21(Suppl 2):P58–63

Hosking D, Lyles K, Brown JP, et al Long-term control of bone turnover in Paget's disease with zoledronic acid and risedronate. J Bone Miner Res. 2007;22(1):142–8

Kurihara N, Hiruma Y, Zhou H, et al Mutation of the sequestosome 1 (p62) gene increases osteoclastogenesis but does not induce Paget disease. J Clin Invest. 2007;117(1):133–42

Laurin N, Brown JP, Morissette J, et al Recurrent mutation of the gene encoding sequestosome 1 (SQSTM1/p62) in Paget disease of bone. Am J Hum Genet. 2002;70(6):1582–8

Miller PD, Brown JP, Siris ES, et al A randomized, double-blind comparison of risedronate and etidronate in the treatment of Paget's disease of bone. Paget's Risedronate/Etidronate Study Group. Am J Med. 1999;106(5):513–20

Morissette J, Laurin N, Brown JP. Sequestosome 1: mutation frequencies, haplotypes, and phenotypes in familial Paget's disease of bone. J Bone Miner Res. 2006;21(Suppl 2):P38–44

Paget SJ. On a form of chronic inflammation of bones (osteitis deformans). Med Chir Trans. 1877;LX:29–53

Reid IR, Miller P, Lyles K, et al Comparison of a single infusion of zoledronic acid with risedronate for Paget's disease. N Engl J Med. 2005;353(9):898–908

Reid IR, Nicholson GC, Weinstein RS, et al Biochemical and radiologic improvement in Paget's disease of bone treated with alendronate: a randomized, placebo-controlled trial. Am J Med. 1996;101(4):341–8

Seton M. Paget's disease of bone.. In: Hochberg MC, Silman AJ, Smolen JS, Weinblatt ME, Weisman MH, editors. Rheumatology. 4th ed. Philadelphia: Mosby. 2008

Seton M, Krane SM. Use of zoledronic acid in the treatment of Paget's disease. Ther Clin Risk Manag. 2007;3(5):913–8

Siris E, Weinstein RS, Altman R, et al Comparative study of alendronate versus etidronate for the treatment of Paget's disease of bone. J Clin Endocrinol Metab. 1996;81(3):961–7

Whyte MP, Obrecht SE, Finnegan PM, et al Osteoprotegerin deficiency and juvenile Paget's disease. N Engl J Med. 2002;347(3):175–84

Sarcoidosis

42

Robert P. Baughman and Elyse E. Lower

42.1 Overview of Sarcoidosis

> Sarcoidosis involves systemic inflammatory disorder with noncaseating granulomatous inflammation in affected organs.

> It commonly involves the lungs, eyes, skin, joints, lymph nodes, and upper respiratory tract.

> In the United States, prevalence of sarcoidosis is between 10 and 40 cases/100,000 population. In Sweden, the prevalence is higher, estimated to be between 60 and 80 cases/100,000 population.

> In the United States, the highest incidence of sarcoidosis is observed in young African–American women.

> Löfgren's syndrome, the combination of fever, erythema nodosum, bilateral hilar adenopathy, symmetric polyarthritis, and uveitis, is one mode of acute presentation of sarcoidosis.

> The Heerfordt syndrome, another acute presentation, consists of fever, granulomatous inflammation of the lacrimal and parotid glands, uveitis, bilateral hilar adenopathy, and cranial neuropathies.

> Ninety percent of patients with sarcoidosis have evidence of pulmonary disease on chest radiography. The most common finding is hilar adenopathy.

> Ocular involvement is a common complication of sarcoidosis. The usual ocular manifestations are anterior uveitis and pars planitis. However, posterior uveitis and optic neuritis may also occur.

> Posterior uveitis can remain asymptomatic until it has reached the advanced stages. Thus, screening for ophthalmologic disease is important for sarcoidosis patients.

> The diagnosis of sarcoidosis is established by correlation of the clinical presentation, clinical course, histopathological findings, and response to therapy.

> Glucocorticoids remain the cornerstone of therapy for active sarcoidosis.

Myth: Sarcoidosis occurs only in black patients.

Reality: Sarcoidosis patients in the United States often encounter this Myth: "Hmmm. You're white. I thought only African–Americans got sarcoidosis." On the contrary, sarcoidosis occurs in all ethnic groups. Data shown in Table 42.1 confirm that black Americans have a higher rate of sarcoidosis than white Americans do, but Scandinavians (an overwhelmingly Caucasian population, obviously) have an incidence rate of sarcoidosis that is higher than any group of Americans—black, white, Hispanic, or Asian.

Although the source of this particular myth remains unknown, it probably relates to the diversity of sarcoidosis across various ethnic backgrounds. As an example, in a single clinic in London, West Indian black patients experienced more advanced pulmonary disease and were more likely to develop chronic skin lesions (e.g., lupus pernio) than were patients from other ethnic groups (Honeybourne 1980). In the United States, an epidemiologic study ACCESS (A Case Controlled Etiologic Study of Sarcoidosis) examined more than 700 newly diagnosed sarcoidosis patients. That study found that black patients were more likely than other groups to experience eye, splenic, and bone marrow disease (Baughman et al. 2001). Caucasian patients were more likely to have erythema nodosum, but blacks were more likely to develop other types of cutaneous sarcoidosis. Blacks were also more likely to develop new organ involvement and to experience chronic disease over the 2-year follow-up period (Judson et al. 2003).

Previous epidemiologic studies reported a disease incidence for sarcoidosis that was ten times higher among blacks compared with whites (Gorham et al. 2004; Keller 1971). However, these studies were based on a select group of males in military service. One population-based study reported the risk of sarcoidosis to be only three times higher in blacks compared with whites (Rybicki et al. 1997a, b).

Pearl: A positive family history of sarcoidosis makes the diagnosis more likely.

J. H. Stone (ed.), *A Clinician's Pearls and Myths in Rheumatology,*
DOI:10.1007/978-1-84800-934-9_42, © Springer Science + Business Media B.V. 2009

Table 42.1 Prevalence of sarcoidosis per 100,000

>50	40–50	30–40	20–30	10–20	<10
Denmark	Eire	New York[b]	Cape Town	Canada	Algeria
New York[a]	Germany		Holland	France	Brazil
Sweden			Norway	Japan	China
Uruguay				London	India
				Poland	Spain
				New York[c]	

Based on reports by Hosada (1994) and James (1992)
[a]African–American
[b]Puerto Rican
[c]Caucasian

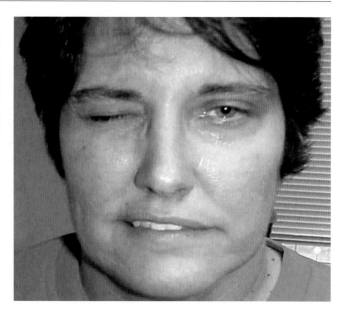

Comment: No single gene mutation causes sarcoidosis, but it is clear that a genetic predisposition exists (Rybicki and Iannuzzi 2007). Five to 10% of Irish–American and African–American patients in the United States report family histories of individuals with the disorder (Rybicki et al. 2001b; Brennan et al. 1984). Thus, when evaluating a patient with possible sarcoidosis, the presence of a positive family history is supportive of the diagnosis.

In an analysis of the first- and second-degree relatives of the 736 newly diagnosed cases of sarcoidosis compared with controls, the siblings of sarcoidosis patients had a relative risk for the disease of 5.8 (Rybicki et al. 2001a, b). Caucasian patients had a markedly higher familial relative risk compared with African–American patients (odds ratio 18.0 vs. 2.8), but this comparison did not reach statistical significance.

Pearl: Bell's palsy sometimes heralds the diagnosis of sarcoidosis.

Comment: The differential diagnosis of seventh cranial nerve palsy is lengthy (Fig. 42.1). Idiopathic occurrences of this problem are termed Bell's palsy (Rahman and Sadiq 2007). Seventh cranial nerve lesions are among the most frequently described abnormalities in neurosarcoidosis (Lower et al. 1997; Zajicek et al. 1999). Glucocorticoids are effective in the treatment of both Bell's palsy and sarcoid-associated seventh nerve lesions (Lower et al. 1997; Zajicek et al. 1999; Stern 2004; Sullivan et al. 2007).

Fig. 42.1 Patient with previously diagnosed sarcoidosis who developed acute onset of left facial weakness. Photograph shows patient closing right eye, with left eye remaining open

In a retrospective study of sarcoidosis patients, the diagnosis of sarcoidosis was not considered in most cases when facial nerve paralysis appeared before other findings (Winget et al. 1994). Moreover, patients often did not link the two problems even after the diagnosis of sarcoidosis. In a patient suspected of having sarcoidosis, a history of facial nerve palsy supports that diagnosis.

For most cases of neurosarcoidosis, treatment with other agents is often needed. These agents include methotrexate, cyclophosphamide, and infliximab (Lower et al. 1997; Sollberger et al. 2004; Doty et al. 2003). Figure 42.2 summarizes the clinical outcome of 71 neurosarcoidosis patients from a group of 542 sarcoidosis patients followed in one sarcoidosis clinic (Lower et al. 1997).

Pearl: The presence of bilateral hilar adenopathy in an asymptomatic individual is likely to be sarcoidosis.

Comment: Sarcoidosis presents as bilateral hilar and right paratracheal adenopathy and clear lung fields in approximately one

Fig. 42.2 The clinical outcome of 71 neurosarcoidosis patients treated at one institution. Of the 23 patients with seventh cranial nerve involvement, all had improvement whether treated with corticosteroids or not. Only one case had a small residual defect, despite corticosteroid therapy. Those with other forms of neurosarcoidosis had a low response to corticosteroids alone. (Adapted from Lower et al. 1997)

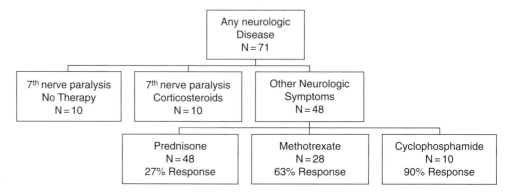

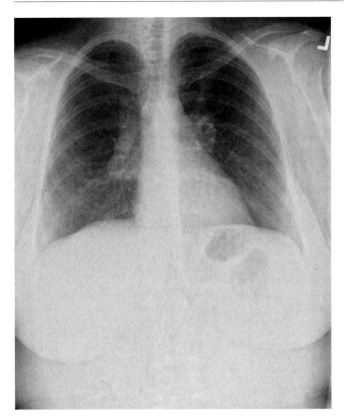

Fig. 42.3 Chest roentgenogram demonstrating bilateral hilar adenopathy due to sarcoidosis

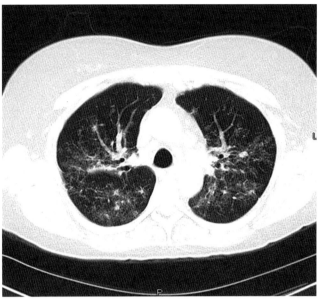

Fig. 42.4 High-resolution CT scan of a sarcoidosis patient. This image demonstrates the fine nodular opacities in a perilymphatic distribution, which is characteristic for sarcoidosis

third of patients (Fig. 42.3) (Baughman et al. 2001; Baughman et al. 2003a). This radiographic pattern is classified as Stage 1 in the scoring system developed by Scadding (1961). Winterbauer et al. (1973) reported that the finding of bilateral adenopathy in an individual who is asymptomatic is highly predictive of sarcoidosis.

Hilar adenopathy can also be associated with lymphoma, metastatic cancer, tuberculosis, and fungal infections. Symmetrical adenopathy is atypical for both tuberculosis and malignancies. Morever, patients with tuberculosis and cancer are usually symptomatic once adenopathy is evident on chest radiography (Sakowitz and Sakowitz 1977). Mediastinal and hilar adenopathy are common among patients infected with HIV but usually less prominent than that associated with sarcoidosis (Pastores et al. 1993).

Pearl: The finding of an increased CD4:CD8 ratio in bronchoalveolar lavage (BAL) fluid strongly supports the diagnosis of sarcoidosis.

Comment: Bronchoscopy with BAL can help confirm the diagnosis of sarcoidosis. An increase in lymphocytes, especially an increased CD4:CD8 ratio, is highly supportive of the diagnosis of sarcoidosis (Drent et al. 2001; Welker et al. 2004; Hunninghake et al. 1999). In addition, transbronchial biopsy reveals noncaseating granulomas in more than 50%

of patients who have only hilar adenopathy on chest radiographs (Koonitz et al. 1976). A transbronchoscopic or ultrasound-guided needle aspirate is also useful in the identification of granulomas in patients with mediastinal adenopathy (Garwood et al. 2007; Wong et al. 2007). However, granulomas can be found also in association with malignancies (Kennedy et al. 2008). Video-assisted mediastinoscopy has become a rapid, safe, outpatient procedure (Karfis et al. 2008).

Myth: Computer tomography is not useful in assessing sarcoidosis.

Reality: The classic radiologic assessment of sarcoidosis remains the routine chest roentgenogram (Hunninghake et al. 1999). However, computed tomography (CT) also has an important role (Vagal et al. 2007). Several radiologic features have been reported in sarcoidosis patients including adenopathy. The hilar lymph nodes in patients with sarcoidosis are usually larger than those of patients with a variety of interstitial lung diseases in whom this finding is encountered. The lymph nodes larger than 2 cm in diameter are most likely caused by sarcoidosis (Niimi et al. 1996). The presence of a fine nodularity with a perilymphatic distribution in the lung parenchyma is a characteristic finding (Fig. 42.4).

Peribronchial thickening is another common CT feature of sarcoidosis (Fig. 42.5). An upper lobe predominance of parenchymal disease is typical of sarcoidosis, but silicosis, hypersensitivity pneumonitis, tuberculosis, and Langerhans cell lung disease also favor the upper lung zones.

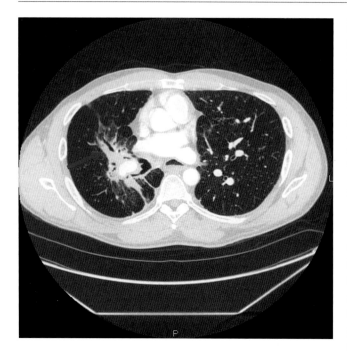

Fig. 42.5 The image demonstrates peribronchial thickening from sarcoidosis (*arrow*)

Fibrotic sarcoidosis often leads to traction bronchiectasis in the upper lobes (Fig. 42.6a). The traction bronchiectasis of sarcoidosis is created by the bronchi themselves rather than the interface between the lung and pleural surface. Hence, these cavities can be quite large and frequently associated with aspergillomas or other mycetomas (Baughman et al. 1991; Tomlinson and Sahn 1987) (Fig. 42.6b).

Myth: If the patient has a normal chest roentgenogram, she cannot have active sarcoidosis.

Reality: This statement was made to the patient in Fig. 42.7, who had active cutaneous sarcoidosis (lupus pernio). The patient had a normal chest radiograph, but she coughed frequently and remained dyspneic due to sarcoidosis in her sinuses. Significant sinus disease is commonly associated with lupus pernio (Baughman et al. 2002).

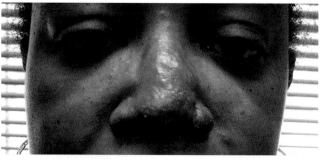

Fig. 42.7 Lupus pernio as a result of sarcoidosis

This case reminds us that sarcoidosis patients may have significant extra-pulmonary disease. Most series suggest that 5–10% of patients with sarcoidosis have no radiographic evidence of lung disease (Baughman et al. 2001; Loddenkemper et al. 1998). Such patients usually have chronic sarcoidosis of the skin, eyes, central nervous system, or heart. In some patients, lung disease present at diagnosis and evident on chest radiography may have resolved over time; yet, significant disease remains in other organs (Judson et al. 2003).

Severe eye disease secondary to sarcoidosis can occur in patients with normal chest roentgenograms. In a study of patients with refractory ocular sarcoidosis, more than half of the patients had normal chest roentgenograms when their eye disease had worsened (Baughman et al. 2005; Bradley et al. 2006). Neurosarcoidosis can exist without any evidence of active pulmonary disease (Bradley et al. 2006). Finally, a retrospective review of 41 patients with cardiac sarcoidosis revealed that only one third had abnormal pulmonary function studies (Chapelon-Abric et al. 2004).

Pearl: Initial disease manifestations can predict chronic sarcoidosis.

Comment: Several sarcoidosis phenotypes are associated with disease resolution, whereas others portend chronic disease (Table 42.2) (Neville et al. 1983; Rizzato et al. 1995). Among the predictive features of chronic disease are lupus pernio (see Fig. 42.7) and fibrotic lung disease (see Fig. 42.6).

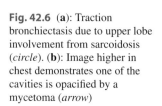

Fig. 42.6 (**a**): Traction bronchiectasis due to upper lobe involvement from sarcoidosis (*circle*). (**b**): Image higher in chest demonstrates one of the cavities is opacified by a mycetoma (*arrow*)

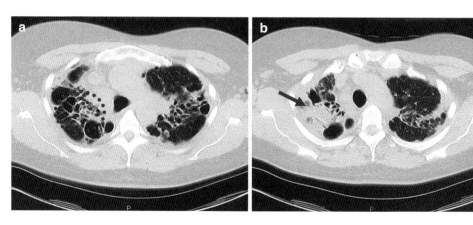

Table 42.2 Features predictive of prognosis in sarcoidosis

Resolution within 2 years	Persistent disease beyond 2 years
Erythema nodosum	Lupus pernio
Hilar adenopathy	Upper lobe traction bronchiectasis
Cranial seventh nerve paralysis	Central nervous system sarcoidosis
Anterior uveitis	Posterior uveitis
	Cardiac disease
	Nephrolithiasis

Lupus pernio tends to be a chronic skin lesion that is unlikely to spontaneously resolve over time (Baughman et al. 2008). Nonfacial skin lesions can also be chronic but seldom comprise a significant cause of morbidity because they can be treated with topical glucocorticoids (Marchell, Judson 2007).

Some data indicate that glucocorticoid treatment is associated with the development of chronic disease (Fig. 42.8) (Gottlieb et al. 1997; Baughman et al. 2006a, c). However, this purported relationship may represent "confounding by indication": the need for systemic therapy may be a surrogate marker for patients who are inherently sicker and therefore more likely to require prolonged treatment.

Myth: Löfgren's syndrome is always associated with a good prognosis.

Reality: Professor Sven Löfgren originally reported that most sarcoidosis patients with erythema nodosum (Fig. 42.9) and hilar adenopathy experience spontaneous remission. This report contained a truly untreated population since his observations preceded the availability of glucocorticoids. Since the original report, the definition of Löfgren's syndrome has been expanded to include periarthritis (Grunewald and Eklund 2007).

Several additional groups have also noted a high rate of disease resolution with erythema nodosum and other signs of sarcoidosis (Neville et al. 1983; Mana and Marcoval 2007). However, 10–20% of patients continue to have active disease at 2 years, and some patients with Löfgren's syndrome develop cardiac and neurologic disease.

A group from Sweden published a 2-year outcomes study of patients who presented with Löfgren's syndrome (Grunewald and Eklund 2007). Disease resolution was experienced within 2 years of diagnosis by 85% of their patients. These investigators confirmed a strong association between Löfgren's syndrome and human leukocyte antigen (HLA) DRB1*0301/DQB1*0201(Sato et al. 2002). In their study, only one of 85 patients with the DRB1*0301/DQB1*0201 allele developed persistent disease. Of the 40 patients negative for DRB1*0301/DQB1*0201 allele, only 22 patients experienced disease resolution within 2 years. Additional investigations are needed to determine whether this Myth can be amended to illustrate a Pearl; namely, that HLA-DRB1*0301/DQB1*0201 is almost always associated with a good prognosis.

Pearl: Fatigue is a common and treatable symptom of sarcoidosis.

Comment: Fatigue is a symptom that frequently afflicts sarcoidosis patients of all ethnic groups and geographic locations (de Vries et al. 2004a, b; Baughman et al. 2007). The etiology of fatigue in sarcoidosis is likely multifactorial, but one potential explanation is the excessive levels of a variety of cytokines released by patients with active disease. These

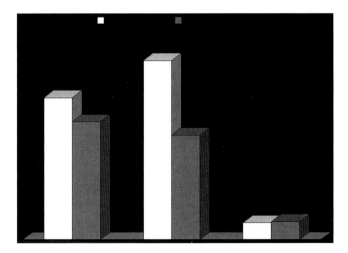

Fig. 42.8 The percentage of patients on systemic therapy for two different studies: one performed in Philadelphia (Gottlieb et al. 1997) and the other a ten-center study done across the United States (ACCESS) (Baughman et al. 2006c). The outcome of patients after at least 2 years is also shown. For those patients given initial therapy, a higher percentage required chronic therapy

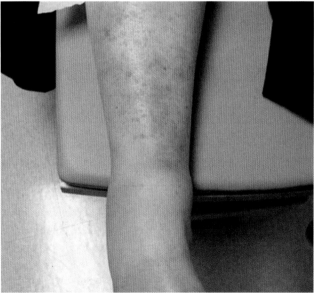

Fig. 42.9 Erythema nodosum on the leg of a sarcoidosis patient

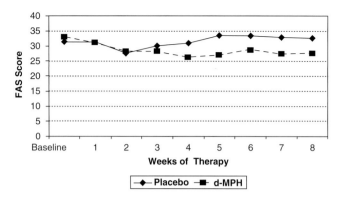

Fig. 42.10 The weekly Fatigue Assessment Score (FAS) during 8 weeks of treatment with either placebo or *d*-methylphenidate of ten patients with sarcoidosis associated fatigue. The higher the FAS, the more the fatigue is. There was a significant improvement in the FAS score during treatment with *d*-MPH ($p < 0.02$). Adapted from (Lower et al. 2008)

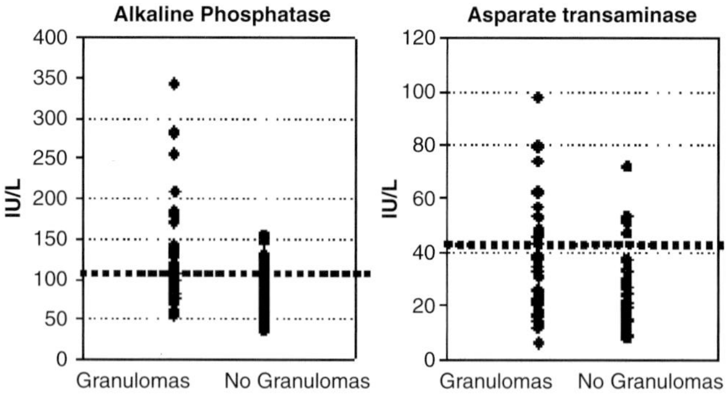

Fig. 42.11 The serum levels of alkaline phophatase and aspirate transaminase before liver biopsy in 84 sarcoidosis patients. The upper limit of normal for each test is indicated by the heavy dashed line. As a group, patients with granulomas in their liver biopsy had higher liver function test results. However, there was significant overlap. (Adapted from Baughman et al. 2003b)

cytokines include tumor necrosis factor (TNF), gamma interferon, and interleukin-2 (Baughman et al. 2003a).

The Fatigue Assessment Scale (FAS) was developed to measure fatigue in sarcoidosis (de Vries et al. 2004a). For this 50-point scale, the higher the number, the more fatigue experienced. Patients with a score of 22 or greater are considered fatigued. Depression contributes to fatigue in some patients (de Vries et al. 2004b). The level of fatigue has also been associated with pulmonary function: more severe fatigue correlates with shorter 6-min walk distance and lower forced vital capacity (Baughman et al. 2007).

Effective treatment of sarcoidosis may relieve fatigue (Fouchier and Moller 2004). However, many patients continue to complain of fatigue, despite using systemic therapy for their sarcoidosis (de Vries et al. 2004b). Methylphenidate may be useful in treating sarcoidosis-related fatigue (Fig. 42.10) (Wagner et al. 2005; Lower et al. 2008).

Pearl: Liver involvement is common but usually asymptomatic in sarcoidosis patients.

Comment: Noncaseating granulomas compatible with sarcoidosis frequently affect the liver (Rose et al. 2008; Warshauer et al. 1994; Klatskin and Yesner 1950). Serum liver function tests are less sensitive than liver biopsy. The results of blood tests do not predict the severity of hepatic disease. Fig. 42.11 demonstrates the levels of alkaline phosphatase and aspirate transaminase from 84 sarcoidosis patients, compared to the findings of their liver biopsies (Baughman et al. 2003b).

Sarcoidosis patients with liver disease can have symptomatic discomfort from hepatomegaly (Fig. 42.12) or splenomegaly and pancytopenia related to splenic sequestration. Most patients with sarcoid-related liver disease have an asymptomatic condition that never requires therapy (Judson 2002). However, a small minority of patients develops cirrhosis and portal hypertension.

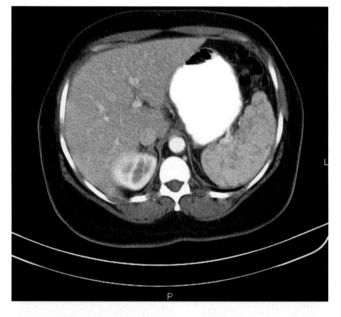

Fig. 42.12 CT scan with contrast of patient with extensive sarcoidosis, including lung, brain, and liver involvement. Massive hepatomegaly led to early satiety and nausea. Hypodense nodules are seen throughout the liver

Myth: Cardiac disease in sarcoidosis is totally unpredictable.

Reality: Cardiac involvement by sarcoidosis is a well-recognized cause of sudden death (Baughman et al. 1997). Congestive heart failure due to cardiomyopathy can be a significant problem, but death is usually due to arrythmias (Chapelon-Abric et al. 2004). Ventricular tachycardia is the most life-threatening arrhythmia in this disorder. Electrocardiography (ECG), 24-h Holter monitoring, and echocardiography are used as screening procedures for cardiac disease (Judson 2005). However, patients with normal baseline ECGs can develop significant arrhythmias (Fig. 42.13).

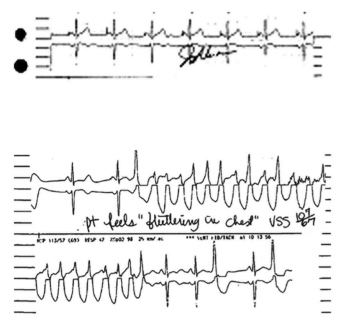

Fig. 42.13 The ECG monitoring a sarcoidosis patient with chest fluttering. The top panel is normal sinus rhythm. The lower two panels demonstrate nonsustained ventricular tachycardia

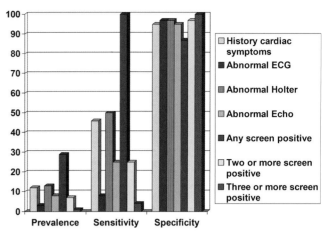

Fig. 42.14 The prevalence of history of cardiac symptoms or abnormal electrocardiography (ECG), 24 Holter monitoring (Holter), or echocardiography (Echo) in 62 sarcoidosis patients. One third of these patients were subsequently determined to the have cardiac sarcoidosis. The sensitivity and specificity of these individual tests are shown. The presence of one or more abnormal test had 100% sensitivity, but only 87% specificity. Presence of three abnormalities was 100% specific but only 4% sensitive. No patient had all four abnormalities. Adapted from (Mehta et al. 2008)

Twenty-four-hour Holter monitoring is more sensitive and specific than other forms of testing (Suzuki et al. 1994). Reports suggest that electrophysiology testing is not as reliable as continuous monitoring in detecting significant cardiac sarcoidosis (Mezaki et al. 2001). Magnetic resonance imaging (MRI) and positive emission tomography (PET) have emerging roles in the evaluation of cardiac sarcoidosis and are used routinely now in the clinical assessment of this disease complication (Skold et al. 2002; Ohira et al. 2008). Findings from MRI and PET may complement each other (Fig. 42.14).

Pearl: Pars planitis and optic neuritis are features shared by both multiple sclerosis and sarcoidosis.

Comment: Ocular disease is a common manifestation of sarcoidosis. Eye findings are often helpful in differentiating sarcoidosis from conditions such as lymphoma or tuberculosis (Ohara et al. 2005). The eye is divided into three chambers—anterior, posterior, and intermediate—based on blood flow (Bradley et al. 2002). Intermediate uveitis occurs in the watershed area between the anterior and posterior circulation. Sarcoidosis and multiple sclerosis are commonly associated with inflammation in this pars planis area (Bradley et al. 2002; Biousse et al. 1999; Prieto et al. 2001).

Multiple sclerosis is frequently associated with ocular disease (Chen and Gordon 2005). In addition to pars planitis, either multiple sclerosis or sarcoidosis can cause optic neuritis. For the patient who presents with both neurologic and ocular diseases, the differentiation between sarcoidosis and

multiple sclerosis can be difficult (Lower and Weiss 2008). Although roentgenographic imaging may be useful, early lesions are nonspecific for both diseases. Disease beyond the central nervous system and eyes does not occur in multiple sclerosis, so the identification of pulmonary, cutaneous, or hepatic disease supports the diagnosis of sarcoidosis.

Myth: A normal angiotensin converting enzyme (ACE) level excludes active sarcoidosis.

Reality: One of the greatest Myths surrounding sarcoidosis is that serum levels of ACE are useful in diagnosing the disease and predicting clinical outcomes (Lieberman et al. 1979; DeRemee and Rohrbach 1980; Buaghman et al. 1983; Gronhagen-Riska et al. 1980). Several factors limit the utility of ACE level in monitoring sarcoidosis.

First, the test is not elevated in all patients with sarcoidosis. Up to 40% of patients with sarcoidosis have normal values at the time of diagnosis (Loddenkemper et al. 1998; Lieberman 1975; Pietinalho et al. 2000). ACE levels are influenced by polymorphisms of the ACE gene. The insertion (I) and deletion (D) polymorphisms lead to three genotypes. The highest ACE levels in normal controls are seen with those with the DD genotype (Tomita et al. 1997).

Second, glucocorticoids suppress ACE levels (Baughman et al. 1983; Gronhagen-Riska et al. 1980). Glucocorticoid withdrawal can lead to the elevation of ACE levels, which does not correlate with a worsening of disease. Figure 42.15 demonstrates the change in ACE levels measured serially in sarcoidosis patients followed in one clinic (Baughman et al. 1983). No relationship was identified between subsequent

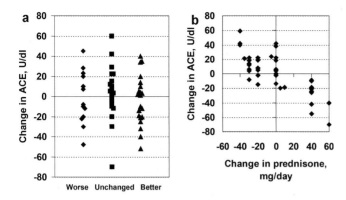

Fig. 42.15 Changes in ACE level over time in sarcoidosis patients followed at one clinic. During the time of observation, prednisone dose was adjusted. There was no relation between the change in ACE level and the change in clinical condition of the patient (a). However, there was a significant negative correlation between the change in prednisone dose and change in ACE level ($R = -0.76$, $p < 0.0001$) (b). Adapted from (Baughman et al. 1983)

clinical course and ACE level. However, a significant inverse correlation existed between change in prednisone dose and ACE level.

Pearl: Hypogammaglobulinemia can cause a granulomatous disease similar to sarcoidosis.

Comment: Sarcoidosis can be associated with a polyclonal hypergammaglobulinemia (Baughman and Hurtubise 1985), but many patients have normal immunoglobulin levels. Glucocorticoids reduce serum levels of immunoglobulin. Therefore, a low immunoglobulin level in a patient with sarcoidosis may be a reflection of treatment.

Approximately 10% of patients with common variable immunodeficiency (CVID) experience a granulomatous disease that mimics sarcoidosis (Mechanic et al. 1997; Park et al. 2005). Bronchiectasis is encountered frequently in CVID patients because of their increased rate of bacterial infections. The radiographic features of CVID include pulmonary nodules and increased reticular markings (Park et al. 2005). In addition, the granulomas that occur in CVID can affect not just the lung but multiple organs. Table 42.3 shows the granulomatous organ involvement documented in 17

Table 42.3 Organ with granulomas identified by biopsy among 17 patients with common variable immunodeficiency syndrome

Organ	Number of patients with documented involvement
Thorax	8
Liver	7
Extra thoracic lymph nodes	6
Spleen	1
Bone marrow	1
Spleen	1

(Adapted from Mechanic et al. 1997). Patients could have more than one organ with documented granulomatous disease.

patients followed at one institution. In that series, serum ACE levels were elevated in seven of the 11 patients (64%) in whom they were measured (Mechanic et al. 1997).

The best treatment for CVID remains unclear. In some patients, the granulomas resolve with immunoglobulin replacement therapy (Pujol et al. 1999). However, many patients do not respond to intravenous immunoglobulin infusions alone (Mechanic et al. 1997). For refractory cases, successful treatment has been reported with agents used to treat sarcoidosis. In our experience, agents such as azathioprine and methotrexate can be beneficial. There have also been reports of successful treatment approaches that employed a targeted inhibitor of TNF (Thatayatikom et al. 2005; Smith, Skelton 2001).

Pearl: "Irreversible" pulmonary sarcoidosis may still be reversible.

Comment: Chronic pulmonary sarcoidosis can lead to pulmonary fibrosis. The finding of pulmonary fibrosis corresponds to Stage 4 of the classification system devised by Scadding (Scadding 1961). The BAL cell population of patients with active pulmonary sarcoidosis in Stages 1–3 usually shows increased numbers of lymphocytes with an increased CD4:CD8 ratio (Baughman and Drent 2001). In contrast, BAL studies from patients with Stage 4 disease demonstrate elevated neutrophil counts and levels of interleukin-8 (Drent et al. 1999; Baughman et al. 1994). These latter findings correlate with pulmonary fibrosis (Baughman and Drent 2001; Lynch et al. 1992).

The finding of fibrosis on chest roentgenogram or CT scan is considered irreversible. However, even lungs explanted at lung transplantation from sarcoidosis patients often still demonstrate some granulomatous inflammation (Padilla et al. 1997), indicative of disease that retains some potential responsiveness to treatment. The insensitivity of our current methods for detecting reversible inflammation within fibrotic areas underscores the importance of considering a course of treatment in any sarcoidosis patient with lung disease, no matter how severe the degree of pulmonary fibrosis.

In a single-center study of nearly 500 sarcoidosis patients, nine patients had at least one vital capacity measurement of less than one liter. The chest roentgenogram findings and low vital capacities in these patients were compatible with "end-stage" lung disease. However, five of those patients (56%) responded substantially to treatment (Baughman et al. 1997). Figure 42.16 reveals the significant improvement experienced by one patient who had been felt to have irreversible pulmonary fibrosis (Baughman et al. 2006b).

Myth: Sarcoidosis patients with interstitial lung disease should always be treated.

Reality: This Myth has led to the treatment of many sarcoidosis patients who have only an abnormal imaging study of

Fig. 42.16 The CT scan of patient with advanced pulmonary sarcoidosis. The image before treatment was felt to show fibrotic changes. The follow-up image was obtained at the same level after 2 months of treatment with infliximab

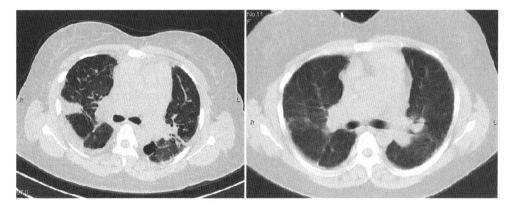

Fig. 42.17 Two levels of the chest of a sarcoidosis patient with no pulmonary symptoms but an abnormal chest roentgenogram. As the prednisone dosage is reduced, the repeat CT scan demonstrates increased nodularity and confluent infiltrates in the parenchyma. However, the patient had no change in pulmonary function or respiratory symptoms. The prednisone was subsequently withdrawn with no deleterious effect to the patient

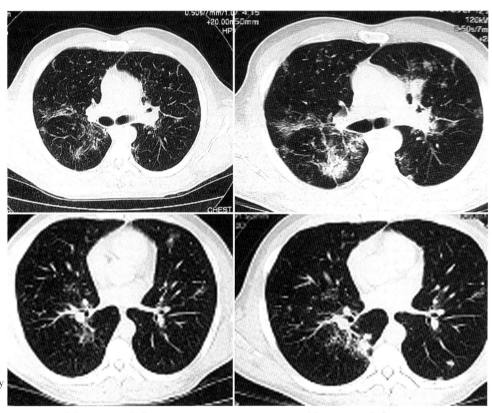

20 mg prednisone   **10 mg prednisone**

the chest. Figure 42.17 demonstrates the CT scans from a sarcoidosis patient who was treated initially with 20 mg/day of prednisone, followed by a reduction to 10 mg/day for 3 months. Because the patient had no pulmonary symptoms, the prednisone therapy was tapered slowly and discontinued over an additional 6 months. The patient has remained off all glucocorticoids for 2 years with no evidence of pulmonary symptoms, despite the persistence of radiologic evidence of interstitial lung disease.

Figure 42.18 demonstrates the clinical outcome of 149 sarcoidosis patients who presented with either stage 2 or 3

disease (Gibson et al. 1996). Only 22% of the patients were symptomatic enough to require therapy in the first 6 months. A high percentage of patients experienced spontaneous remission during the 6 months of observation. However, patients who failed to improve or became symptomatic were randomized subsequently to receive either 18 months of systemic glucocorticoids or observation. Those treated with glucocorticoids experienced a mild but significant improvement in lung function. Twenty percent of the observation group eventually required systemic therapy for their pulmonary symptoms, but the remaining 80% treated with observation

Fig. 42.18 The clinical outcome of 149 sarcoidosis patients who presented with either Stage 2 or 3 disease (Gibson et al. 1996). Only 22% of the patients were symptomatic enough to require therapy in the first 6 months. A high percentage of patients experienced spontaneous remission during the 6 months of observation

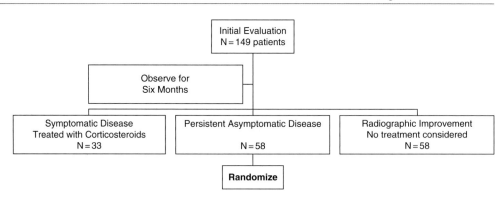

Table 42.4 Incidence of pulmonary hypertension in sarcoidosis patients

First author	Handa et al. (2006)	Bourbonnais and Samavati (2008)	Rizzato et al. (1983)	Sulica et al. (2005)	Baughman et al. (2006a, b, c)	Shorr et al. (2005)
Source of patients	Clinic	Clinic	Clinic	Clinic	Clinic	UNOS
Entry	All patients	All patients	Dyspnea	Dyspnea	Dyspnea	Transplant evaluation
Study to detect pulmonary hypertension	Echo	Echo/Cath	Cath	Echo	Cath	Cath
Number studied	212	162	62	106	53	363
% with pulmonary hypertension	6	15	55	52	60	72

UNOS United Network of Organ Sharing ; *Echo* echocardiography; *Cath* right heart cartherterization

alone never developed pulmonary symptoms. Another study demonstrated that sarcoidosis patients who were asymptomatic at diagnosis had only a 10% chance of developing symptomatic disease during observation (Pietinalho et al. 1999). These studies support the principal of treating only symptomatic patients (Hunninghake et al. 1999).

Pearl: In persistently dyspneic sarcoidosis patient, think of pulmonary hypertension.

Comment: Interstitial lung disease of sarcoidosis often leads to dyspnea, but sarcoidosis also affects the pulmonary vasculature and can cause pulmonary hypertension (Hunninghake et al. 1994). Table 42.4 summarizes several studies of pulmonary hypertension in sarcoidosis. The incidence of pulmonary hypertension in unselected patients appears to be 5–15% (Rizzato et al. 1983; Sulica et al. 2005; Baughman et al. 2006b). However, more than 70% of sarcoidosis patients listed for lung transplant have pulmonary hypertension. Clinical features that suggest pulmonary hypertension are a Stage 4 chest roentgenogram (Rizzato et al. 1983; Sulica et al. 2005), diminished vital capacity (Rizzato et al. 1983; Sulica et al. 2005; Baughman et al. 2006b), reduced 6-min walk distance (Baughman et al. 2007; Bourbonnais and Samavati 2008), and desaturation with exercise (Bourbonnais and Samavati 2008). Pulmonary hypertension in sarcoidosis patients can improve with treatment with a variety of pulmonary vasodilators (Baughman et al. 2006b; Fisher et al. 2006; Milman et al. 2008).

References

Baughman RP, Drent M, Kavuru M, et al Infliximab therapy in patients with chronic sarcoidosis and pulmonary involvement. Am J Respir Crit Care Med. 2006a;174(7):795–802

Baughman RP, Drent M. Role of bronchoalveolar lavage in interstitial lung disease. Clin Chest Med. 2001;22(2):331–41

Baughman RP, du Bois RM, Lower EE. Sarcoidosis. Lancet 2003a; 361:1111–8

Baughman RP, Engel PJ, Meyer CA, et al Pulmonary hypertension in sarcoidosis. Sarcoidosis Vasc Diffuse Lung Dis. 2006b;23:108–16

Baughman RP, Hurtubise PE. Systemic immune response of patients with active pulmonary sarcoidosis. Clin Exp Immunol. 1985; 61:535–41

Baughman RP, Judson MA, Teirstein A, et al Chronic facial sarcoidosis including lupus pernio: clinical description and proposed scoring systems. Am J Clin Dermatol. 2008;9(3):155–61

Baughman RP, Judson MA, Teirstein A, et al Presenting characteristics as predictors of duration of treatment in sarcoidosis. QJM. 2006c;99(5):307–15

Baughman RP, Judson MA, Teirstein AS, et al Thalidomide for chronic sarcoidosis. Chest 2002;122:227–32

Baughman RP, Keeton D, Lower EE. Relationship between interleukin-8 and neutrophils in the BAL fluid of sarcoidosis. Sarcoidosis 1994;11:S217–20S

Baughman RP, Koehler A, Bejarano PA, et al Role of liver function tests in detecting methotrexate-induced liver damage in sarcoidosis. Arch Intern Med. 2003b;163(5):615–20

Baughman RP, Lower EE, Bradley DA, et al Etanercept for refractory ocular sarcoidosis: results of a double-blind randomized trial. Chest 2005;128(2):1062–67

Baughman RP, Ploysongsang Y, Roberts RD, et al Effects of sarcoid and steroids on angiotensin-converting enzyme. Am Rev Respir Dis. 1983;128:631–3

Baughman RP, Shipley RT, Loudon RG, et al Crackles in interstitial lung disease. Comparison of sarcoidosis and fibrosing alveolitis. Chest 1991;100:96–101

Baughman RP, Sparkman BK, Lower EE. Six-minute walk test and health status assessment in sarcoidosis. Chest 2007;132(1):207–13

Baughman RP, Teirstein AS, Judson MA, et al Clinical characteristics of patients in a case control study of sarcoidosis. Am J Respir Crit Care Med. 2001;164:1885–9

Baughman RP, Winget DB, Bowen EH, et al Predicting respiratory failure in sarcoidosis patients. Sarcoidosis 1997;14:154–8

Biousse V, Trichet C, Bloch-Michel E, et al Multiple sclerosis associated with uveitis in two large clinic-based series. Neurology 1999;52(1):179–81

Bourbonnais JM, Samavati L. Clinical predictors of pulmonary hypertension in sarcoidosis. Eur Respir J. 2008;32(2):296–302

Bradley DA, Baughman RP, Raymond L, et al Ocular manifestations of sarcoidosis. Sem Resp Crit Care Med. 2002;23:543–8

Bradley DA, Lower EE, Baughman RP. Diagnosis and management of spinal cord sarcoidosis. Sarcoidosis Vasc Diffuse Lung Dis. 2006; 23(1):58–65

Brennan NJ, Crean P, Long JP, et al High prevalence of familial sarcoidosis in an Irish population. Thorax 1984;39:14–8

Chapelon-Abric C, de ZD, Duhaut P, et al Cardiac sarcoidosis: a retrospective study of 41 cases. Medicine (Baltimore) 2004;83(6):315–34

Chen L, Gordon LK. Ocular manifestations of multiple sclerosis. Curr Opin Ophthalmol. 2005;16(5):315–20

de Vries J, Michielsen H, van Heck GL, et al Measuring fatigue in sarcoidosis: the fatigue assessment scale (FAS). Br J Health Psychol. 2004a;9(Pt 3):279–91

de Vries J, Rothkrantz-Kos S, Dieijen-Visser MP, et al The relationship between fatigue and clinical parameters in pulmonary sarcoidosis. Sarcoidosis Vasc Diffuse Lung Dis. 2004b;21(2):127–36

DeRemee RA, Rohrbach MS. Serum angiotensin-converting enzyme activity in evaluating the clinical course of sarcoidosis. Ann Intern Med. 1980;92(3):361–5

Doty JD, Mazur JE, Judson MA. Treatment of corticosteroid-resistant neurosarcoidosis with a short-course cyclophosphamide regimen. Chest 2003;124(5):2023–6

Drent M, Jacobs JA, Cobben NA, et al Computer program supporting the diagnostic accuracy of cellular BALF analysis: a new release. Respir Med. 2001;95(10):781–6

Drent M, Jacobs JA, de Vries J, et al Does the cellular bronchoalveolar lavage fluid profile reflect the severity of sarcoidosis? Eur Respir J. 1999;13(6):1338–44

Fisher KA, Serlin DM, Wilson KC, et al Sarcoidosis-associated pulmonary hypertension: outcome with long-term epoprostenol treatment. Chest 2006;130(5):1481–8

Fouchier SM, Moller GM, Van Santen-Hoeufft M, et al [Successful treatment with infliximab of a patient with refractory sarcoidosis]. Ned Tijdschr Geneeskd. 2004;148(49):2446–50

Garwood S, Judson MA, Silvestri G, et al Endobronchial ultrasound for the diagnosis of pulmonary sarcoidosis. Chest 2007;132(4):1298–304

Gibson GJ, Prescott RJ, Muers MF, et al British Thoracic Society Sarcoidosis study: effects of long term corticosteroid treatment. Thorax 1996;51(3):238–47

Gorham ED, Garland CF, Garland FC, et al Trends and occupational associations in incidence of hospitalized pulmonary sarcoidosis and other lung diseases in Navy personnel: a 27-year historical prospective study, 1975–2001. Chest 2004;126(5):1431–8

Gottlieb JE, Israel HL, Steiner RM, et al Outcome in sarcoidosis. The relationship of relapse to corticosteroid therapy. Chest 1997;111(3):623–31

Gronhagen-Riska C, Selroos O, Niemisto M. Angiotensin converting enzyme. V. Serum levels as monitors of disease activity in corticosteroid-treated sarcoidosis. Eur J Respir Dis. 1980;61(2):113–22

Grunewald J, Eklund A. Sex-specific manifestations of Löfgren's syndrome. Am J Respir Crit Care Med. 2007;175(1):40–4

Handa T, Nagai S, Miki S, et al Incidence of pulmonary hypertension and its clinical relevance in patients with sarcoidosis. Chest 2006;129(5):1246–52

Honeybourne D. Ethnic differences in the clinical features of sarcoidosis in South-East London. Br J Dis Chest. 1980;74:63–9

Hosada Y. Consensus conference: epidemiology of sarcoidosis. Sarcoidosis 1994;11:17–21

Hunninghake GW, Costabel U, Ando M, et al ATS/ERS/WASOG statement on sarcoidosis. American Thoracic Society/European Respiratory Society/World Association of Sarcoidosis and other Granulomatous Disorders. Sarcoidosis Vasc Diffuse Lung Dis. 1999;16:149–73

Hunninghake GW, Gilbert S, Pueringer R, et al Outcome of the treatment for sarcoidosis. Am J Respir Crit Care Med. 1994;149(4 Pt 1):893–8

James DG. Epidemiology of sarcoidosis. Sarcoidosis 1992;9:79–87

Judson MA, Baughman RP, Thompson BW, et al Two year prognosis of sarcoidosis: the ACCESS experience. Sarcoidosis Vasc Diffuse Lung Dis. 2003;20(3):204–11

Judson MA. Hepatc, splenic, and gastrointestinal involvement with sarcoidosis. Sem Resp Crit Care Med. 2002;23:529–43

Karfis EA, Roustanis E, Beis J, et al Video-assisted cervical mediastinoscopy: our seven-year experience. Interact Cardiovasc Thorac Surg. 2008;7:1015–8

Keller AZ. Hospital, age, racial, occupational, geographical, clinical and survivorship characteristics in the epidemiology of sarcoidosis. Am J Epidemiol. 1971;94:222–30

Kennedy MP, Jimenez CA, Mhatre AD, et al Clinical implications of granulomatous inflammation detected by endobronchial ultrasound transbronchial needle aspiration in patients with suspected cancer recurrence in the mediastinum. J Cardiothorac Surg. 2008;3(8):8

Klatskin G, Yesner R. Hepatic manifestations of sarcoidosis and other granulomatous diseases. Yale J Biol Med. 1950;51:207–48

Koonitz CH, Joyner LR, Nelson RA. Transbronchial lung biopsy via the fiberoptic bronchoscope in sarcoidosis. Ann Intern Med. 1976; 85(1):64–6

Lieberman J, Nosal A, Schlessner A, et al Serum angiotensin-converting enzyme for diagnosis and therapeutic evaluation of sarcoidosis. Am Rev Respir Dis. 1979;120(2):329–35

Lieberman J. Elevation of serum angiotensin converting enzyme (ACE) level in sarcoidosis. Am J Med. 1975;59:365–72

Loddenkemper R, Kloppenborg A, Schoenfeld N, et al Clinical findings in 715 patients with newly detected pulmonary sarcoidosis – results of a cooperative study in former West Germany and Switzerland. WATL Study Group. Wissenschaftliche Arbeitsgemeinschaft fur die Therapie von Lungenkrankheitan. Sarcoidosis Vasc Diffuse Lung Dis. 1998;15(2):178–82

Lower EE, Broderick JP, Brott TG, et al Diagnosis and management of neurologic sarcoidosis. Arch Intern Med. 1997;157:1864–8

Lower EE, Harman S, Baughman RP. Double-blind, randomized trial of dexmethylphenidate hydrochloride for the treatment of sarcoidosis-associated fatigue. Chest 2008;133(5):1189–95

Lower EE, Weiss KL. Neurosarcoidosis. Clin Chest Med. 2008; 29(3):475–92

Lynch JP, Standiford TJ, Rolfe MW, et al Neutrophilic alveolitis in idiopathic pulmonary fibrosis. The role of interleukin-8. Am Rev Respir Dis. 1992;145(6):1433–9

Mana J, Marcoval J. Erythema nodosum. Clin Dermatol. 2007;25(3):288–94

Marchell RM, Judson MA. Chronic cutaneous lesions of sarcoidosis. Clin Dermatol. 2007;25(3):295–302

Mechanic LJ, Dikman S, Cunningham RC. Granulomatous disease in common variable immunodeficiency. Ann Intern Med. 1997;127(8 Pt 1):613–7

Mehta D, Lubitz SA, Frankel Z, et al Cardiac involvement in patients with sarcoidosis: diagnostic and prognostic value of outpatient testing. Chest 2008;133(6):1426–35

Mezaki T, Chinushi M, Washizuka T, et al Discrepancy between inducibility of ventricular tachycardia and activity of cardiac sarcoidosis.

Requirement of defibrillator implantation for the inactive stage of cardiac sarcoidosis. Intern Med. 2001;40(8):731–5

Milman N, Burton CM, Iversen M, et al Pulmonary hypertension in end-stage pulmonary sarcoidosis: therapeutic effect of sildenafil? J Heart Lung Transplant. 2008;27(3):329–34

Neville E, Walker AN, James DG. Prognostic factors predicting the outcome of sarcoidosis: an analysis of 818 patients. Q J Med. 1983; 208:525–33

Niimi H, Kang EY, Kwong JS, et al CT of chronic infiltrative lung disease: prevalence of mediastinal lymphadenopathy. J Comput Assist Tomogr. 1996;20(2):305–8

Ohara K, Judson MA, Baughman RP. Clinical aspects of ocular sarcoidosis. In: Drent M, Costabel U, editors. Sarcoidosis. Wakefiled, UK: The Charlesworth Group; 2005. p.188–209

Ohira H, Tsujino I, Ishimaru S, et al Myocardial imaging with 18F-fluoro-2-deoxyglucose positron emission tomography and magnetic resonance imaging in sarcoidosis. Eur J Nucl Med Mol Imaging. 2008;35(5):933–41

Padilla ML, Schilero GJ, Teirstein AS. Sarcoidosis and transplantation. Sarcoidosis 1997;14:16–22

Park JE, Beal I, Dilworth JP, et al The HRCT appearances of granulomatous pulmonary disease in common variable immune deficiency. Eur J Radiol. 2005;54(3):359–64

Pastores SM, Naidich DP, Aranda CP, et al Intrathoracic adenopathy associated with pulmonary tuberculosis in patients with human immunodeficiency virus infection. Chest 1993;103(5):1433–7

Pietinalho A, Ohmichi M, Lofroos AB, et al The prognosis of sarcoidosis in Finland and Hokkaido, Japan. A comparative five-year study of biopsy-proven cases. Sarcoidosis Vasc Diffuse Lung Dis. 2000; 17:158–66

Pietinalho A, Tukiainen P, Haahtela T, et al Oral prednisolone followed by inhaled budesonide in newly diagnosed pulmonary sarcoidosis: a double-blind, placebo-controlled, multicenter study. Chest 1999; 116:424–31

Prieto JF, Dios E, Gutierrez JM, et al Pars planitis: epidemiology, treatment, and association with multiple sclerosis. Ocul Immunol Inflamm. 2001;9(2):93–102

Pujol RM, Nadal C, Taberner R, et al Cutaneous granulomatous lesions in common variable immunodeficiency: complete resolution after intravenous immunoglobulins. Dermatology 1999;198(2):156–8

Rahman I, Sadiq SA. Ophthalmic management of facial nerve palsy: a review. Surv Ophthalmol. 2007;52(2):121–44

Rizzato G, Fraioli P, Montemurro L. Nephrolithiasis as a presenting feature of chronic sarcoidosis. Thorax 1995;50(5):555–9

Rizzato G, Pezzano A, Sala G, et al Right heart impairment in sarcoidosis: haemodynamic and echocardiographic study. Eur J Respir Dis. 1983;64(2):121–8

Rose AS, Tielker MA, Knox KS. Hepatic, ocular, and cutaneous sarcoidosis. Clin Chest Med. 2008;29(3):509–24

Rybicki BA, Iannuzzi MC, Frederick MM, et al Familial aggregation of sarcoidosis: a case-control etiologic study of sarcoidosis (ACCESS). Am J Respir Crit Care Med. 2001a;164:2085–91

Rybicki BA, Iannuzzi MC. Epidemiology of sarcoidosis: recent advances and future prospects. Semin Respir Crit Care Med. 2007;28(1):22–35

Rybicki BA, Kirkey KL, Major M, et al Familial risk ratio of sarcoidosis in African–American sibs and parents. Am J Epidemiol. 2001b;153(2):188–93

Rybicki BA, Major M, Popovich J Jr, et al Racial differences in sarcoidosis incidence: a five year study in a health maintenance organization. Am J Epid. 1997;145:234–41

Sakowitz AJ, Sakowitz BH. Bilateral hilar lymphadenopathy: an uncommon manifestation of adult tuberculosis. Chest 1977; 71(3):421–3

Sato H, Grutters JC, Pantelidis P, et al HLA-DQB1*0201: a marker for good prognosis in British and Dutch patients with sarcoidosis. Am J Respir Cell Mol Biol. 2002;27(4):406–12

Scadding JG. Prognosis of intrathoracic sarcoidosis in England. Br Med J. 1961;4:1165–72

Shorr AF, Helman DL, Davies DB, et al Pulmonary hypertension in advanced sarcoidosis: epidemiology and clinical characteristics. Eur Respir J. 2005;25(5):783–8

Skold CM, Larsen FF, Rasmussen E, et al Determination of cardiac involvement in sarcoidosis by magnetic resonance imaging and Doppler echocardiography. J Intern Med. 2002;252(5): 465–71

Smith KJ, Skelton H. Common variable immunodeficiency treated with a recombinant human IgG, tumour necrosis factor-alpha receptor fusion protein. Br J Dermatol. 2001;144(3):597–600

Sollberger M, Fluri F, Baumann T, et al Successful treatment of steroid-refractory neurosarcoidosis with infliximab. J Neurol. 2004; 251(6):760–1

Sulica R, Teirstein AS, Kakarla S, et al Distinctive clinical, radiographic, and functional characteristics of patients with sarcoidosis-related pulmonary hypertension. Chest 2005;128(3):1483–9

Sullivan FM, Swan IR, Donnan PT, et al Early treatment with prednisolone or acyclovir in Bell's palsy. N Engl J Med. 2007;357(16): 1598–607

Suzuki T, Kanda T, Kubota S, et al Holter monitoring as a noninvasive indicator of cardiac involvement in sarcoidosis. Chest 1994;106(4): 1021–4

Thatayatikom A, Thatayatikom S, White AJ. Infliximab treatment for severe granulomatous disease in common variable immunodeficiency: a case report and review of the literature. Ann Allergy Asthma Immunol. 2005;95(3):293–300

Tomita H, Ina Y, Sugiura Y, et al Polymorphism in the angiotensin-converting enzyme (ACE) gene and sarcoidosis. Am J Respir Crit Care Med. 1997;156(1):255–9

Tomlinson JR, Sahn SA. Aspergilloma in sarcoid and tuberculosis. Chest 1987;92(3):505–8

Vagal AS, Shipley R, Meyer CA. Radiological manifestations of sarcoidosis. Clin Dermatol. 2007;25(3):312–25

Wagner MT, Marion SD, Judson MA. The effects of fatigue and treatment with methylphenidate on sustained attention in sarcoidosis. Sarcoidosis Vasc Diffuse Lung Dis. 2005;22(3):235

Warshauer DM, Dumbleton SA, Molina PL, et al Abdominal CT findings in sarcoidosis: radiologic and clinical correlation. Radiology 1994;192(1):93–8

Welker L, Jorres RA, Costabel U, et al Predictive value of BAL cell differentials in the diagnosis of interstitial lung diseases. Eur Respir J. 2004;24(6):1000–6

Winget D, O'Brien GM, Lower EE, et al Bell's palsy as an unrecognized presentation for sarcoidosis. Sarcoidosis 1994;11:S368–70

Winterbauer RH, Belic N, Moores KD. A clinical intepretation of bilateral hilar adenopathy. Ann Intern Med. 1973;78:65–71

Wong M, Yasufuku K, Nakajima T, et al Endobronchial ultrasound: new insight for the diagnosis of sarcoidosis. Eur Respir J. 2007; 29(6):1182–6

Zajicek JP, Scolding NJ, Foster O, et al Central nervous system sarcoidosis – diagnosis and management. QJM. 1999;92(2):103–17

Osteoarthritis

43

Nancy E. Lane and Roy D. Altman

43.1 Overview for Osteoarthritis

> Osteoarthritis is a common disease. This chapter will review a number of myths and pearls that will assist clinicians in treating this disease.

Myth: Osteoarthritis (OA) is an unavoidable outcome of aging.

Reality: The prevalence of OA in all joints increases with age. However, more than 30% of people never develop radiographic evidence of OA as they age. In addition, only one third of those who have radiographic evidence of OA develop joint pain. Thus, aging is only one factor in the development of OA (Lawrence et al. 2008).

Myth: The more one uses one's joints, the faster they wear out.

Reality: OA is not a disease of "wear and tear." Regular (but not high impact) joint use is beneficial and necessary for the health of joints lined with synovium. The cartilage needs motion to maintain nutrition. Weight-bearing exercise improves the circulation of blood to the joints because it allows fluid to pass through the synovium. Exercise also facilitates lymphatic drainage, thereby expediting the clearance of oxidative products. In contrast, the lack of joint motion leads to cartilage atrophy, a predecessor to OA (Sutton et al. 2001; Lane et al. 1986; Roos and Dahlberg 2005).

Myth: Inflammation has little role in the pathophysiology of OA.

Reality: The classic findings of joint inflammation are not a cardinal sign of OA. However, as the disease progresses, synovitis develops. This is manifested as the joint warmth that is detected in many patients who have advanced OA of the knee. Synovial effusions are intermittent in OA, but often develop after overuse of the joint in a patient with advanced degenerative changes.

Patients with OA do not always notice or complain of joint swelling, but joint effusions are now recognized with increasing frequency due to the broader use of magnetic resonance imaging and ultrasound. The classic description of inflammation includes heat, redness, pain, swelling, and loss of function. The more modern understanding of inflammation is that it occurs at a cellular and subcellular level. Many of the same mechanisms present in rheumatoid arthritis and other types of arthritis also occur in OA, albeit to a lesser degree (Bonnet and Walsh 2005).

Myth: Recreational running increases the risks of developing lower extremity OA.

Reality: Research on weight-bearing activities that involve both low- and high-impact loading has been reported from retrospective, cross-sectional studies, as well as from longitudinal investigations. One study of middle-aged men and women runners who had jogged approximately 20 miles a week for nine years found no increased risk of radiographic knee OA compared with age-matched controls who did run regularly (Lane et al. 1986).

A follow-up study of that cohort performed ten years later showed no statistical difference between the runners and controls in incident knee OA Lane 1993. However, the runners who did develop radiographic knee OA reported running at a faster pace and were both heavier and older than were runners who did not develop OA. The preponderance of other studies on this question indicate that individuals who run recreationally in the absence of existing injuries are not at increased risks for knee and hip OA. On the other hand, repetitive bending does appear to be a risk factor for knee OA (Schouten et al. 2002; Jensen 2008).

Myth: Cracking one's knuckles leads to hand OA.

Reality: The metacarpophalangeal joint is surrounded by synovial fluid, which contains approximately 15% carbon dioxide in solution. When one cracks one's knuckles, a low-pressure zone (a vacuum) is created within the synovial cavity. The source of the cracking sound is believed to be the drawing in of carbon dioxide and water vapor from the joint fluid. This creates a bubble or a cavity of air that collapses instantly. The influx of fluid from all sides of the bubble generates the noise (Unsworth et al. 1971).

J. H. Stone (ed.), *A Clinician's Pearls and Myths in Rheumatology,*
DOI:10.1007/978-1-84800-934-9_43, © Springer Science + Business Media B.V. 2009

The initial popping of the big bubble leaves small ones that remain for approximately 15 min before the carbon dioxide is totally redissolved. During this time, continued tugging on the finger can cause an expansion of the microbubble into a tiny shock absorber. This probably explains why cracking of the same knuckle in rapid succession is not possible.

There are no data to confirm the old Myth that knuckle-cracking causes OA. The sound of knuckle cracking must be separated from the finding of crepitus that occurs with routine joint activity. Crepitus, caused by uneven joint surfaces, is a symptom of OA (Simkin 1990; Watson et al. 1989; Swezey and Swezey 1975).

Myth: Once joint pain is present with OA, progression of the underlying process is inevitable.

Reality: The joint pain caused by OA is often intermittent and variable. Many patients have prolonged periods of time in which they are free of pain. The cyclical nature of OA relates to one of the etiologies of pain in this condition. OA results from damage to and then loss of articular cartilage. At times, small or even microscopic pieces of cartilage break off and float inside the joint. These fragments cause pain when pressure is exerted on the joint.

The breakdown or removal of these cartilage fragments through natural processes or surgery leads to the recession of joint pain. In addition, overuse of an osteoarthritic joint can create synovitis that resolves spontaneously or with an anti-inflammatory agent (e.g., a glucocorticoid injection).

The progression of OA in most people is quite slow. Intermittent parinful episodes can usually be treated effectively with symptomatic treatment and there is little data to support the notion that NSAIDs accelerate joint degeneration (Haskinson et al. 1992; Rashad et al. 1989)

Myth: Chondrocytes cannot divide in response to injury. Thus, once articular cartilage is damaged, it inevitably "fails."

Reality: The end result of OA is loss of the articular cartilage and changes in the subchondral bone. The structure of cartilage, which is comprised principally of water, is maintained by aggrecan and collagen (Fig. 43.1). The aggrecan is mostly composed of proteoglycans: large, negatively charged groups of molecules that occupy space by imbibing water and electrolytes. This confers elasticity and shear modulus to healthy cartilage. The primary collagen is a special form, collagen type II, which helps contain and bind to the aggrecan, providing tensile strength to the tissue.

When the surface of the cartilage is disrupted, chondrocyte metabolic activity is upregulated with enhanced but defective proteoglycan and collagen production. The chondrocytes proliferate into clones but are eventually lost through apoptosis. It is not clear why the chondrocytes fail. However, it has been postulated that their inability to reform the three-dimensional structure of the cartilage leads to defects, particularly in older individuals. Some data suggest that chondrocytes can repair the articular cartilage if the defects

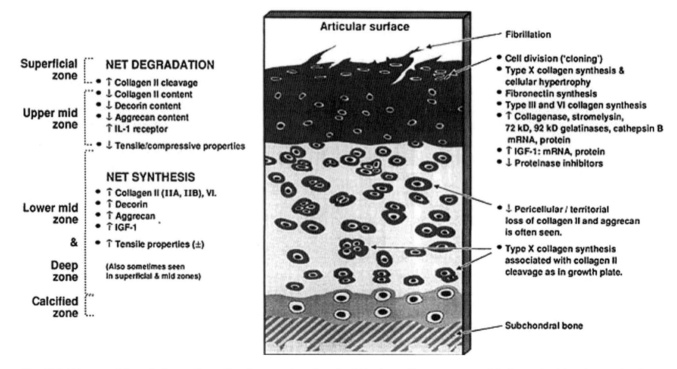

Fig. 43.1 Diagram of the articular cartilage. Chondrocytes, the only cell within the cartilage, are responsible for synthesizing the proteins that make up the articular cartilage and the enzymes that degrade the articular cartilage

occur in a young patient and are small (less than 3 mm) (Goldring and Goldring 2007; Lozado 2005).

Myth: OA is caused by excessive cold.

Reality: Limited clinical data indicate that symptoms of OA worsen with changes in temperature, barometric pressure, or humidity. However, there is no evidence that OA is caused by excesses of either cold or heat in temperature.

Myth: OA is an old person's disease.

Reality: Although OA increases with age, the incidence of this problem begins to rise in the mid-40s (hardly the time of dotage!). Thus, OA is a common cause of joint symptoms and loss of time from work long before someone is considered elderly. OA and back pain (which is often caused by OA; see the Chap. 45) are the largest reasons for loss of time from work (Lawrence et al. 2008).

Myth: Once OA is present, nothing can be done.

Reality: There remains no cure for OA. Current therapy combines physical measures, education, medications, and surgery. With appropriate therapy, most people with OA live normal or near normal lives. Pain from OA is a symptom that is addressable and should be brought to the attention of clinicians (Lozado 2005).

Myth: A highly regulated diet will cure OA.

Reality: The word "diet" translates literally to controlled eating. There are too many proposed diets to summarize. Among them all, only a few have been tested formal studies. None has ever been shown to benefit patients with OA. Numerous dietary supplements are marketed, frequently in health food stores, with unsupported claims of reducing or curing arthritis (Lozado 2005).

The only relevant dietary fact at this time is that a balanced diet that fosters weight reduction can reduce symptoms in patients who are overweight.

Myth: Copper bracelets alleviate the pain of OA.

Reality: There is no deficiency of copper in the body in OA. Indeed, the copper from a bracelet or other amulet does not penetrate the skin. Many patients develop a cutaneous reaction to copper bracelets that results from perspiration and leads to a blue or black discoloration of the skin. Although unseemly in some cases, this skin discoloration is self-limited and has no clinical consequences (Walker and Keats 1976).

Myth: Glucosamine hydrochloride or sulfate and chondroitin sufate compounds slow the progression of knee OA.

Reality: The use of glucosamine and chondroitin compounds has become very popular (Theodosakis 2003). The initial theory to support treatment with these compounds was based on two facts: (1) articular cartilage is composed of proteoglycans, including glucosamine and chondroitins and (2) the

concentration of these compounds is reduced in OA. The theory supporting the use of these medications holds that these compounds are absorbed from the gastrointestinal tract and transported to the joint, where they reinforce articular cartilage and prevent further joint deterioration.

Other investigations suggest that there might be an intracellular regulatory effect associated with the downregulation of inflammatory mediators such as nuclear factor-kappa B (NFκ(kappa)B). Multiple small clinical trials supported by pharmaceutical companies reported that these compounds, either alone or together, were efficacious for pain reduction in OA (McAlindon et al. 2000; MIchel et al.2005; Bellamy 2006b; Towneed et al.2005). Moreover, two other studies (also sponsored by industry) reported reductions in joint space loss and the need for joint arthroplasty at five years among patients treated with crystalline glucosamine sulfate (Reginster et al. 2001; Bruyere et al. 2008). However, a large randomized trial sponsored by the National Institutes of Health showed that neither glucosamine hydrochloride nor chondroitin sulfate improved either pain or function compared to celecoxib (Clegg et al. 2006). A two-year follow-up study found no protection against joint space loss in individuals on glucosamine or chondroitin (Sawitzke et al. 2008).

Myth: Dimethylsulfoxide (DMSO) applied to the joint is an effective treatment for OA.

Reality: DMSO is a topical solvent that penetrates the skin rapidly. The compound is available in many states by prescription. There have been no formal studies of DMSO. No scientific evidence indicates that it has any beneficial effect in OA (Brien et al. 2008).

Myth: Surgery is the only therapy likely to be effective once advanced radiographic changes are evident.

Reality: Only half of all patients with radiographic evidence of OA have symptoms of OA. Although more severe radiographic changes are more likely to be associated with symptoms, such changes per se are not the primary consideration for surgery. The major determinants of the appropriateness of surgery are the severity of the patient's pain and the restriction of function imposed by the OA (Felson 1993).

Myth: Weight-bearing exercise in subjects with knee OA accelerates disease progression.

Reality: On the contrary, numerous studies in subjects with moderately severe knee OA have found that low-impact exercise such as walking and bicycling improves patients' pain and function (Halbert et al. 2001). Aquatic exercise is also helpful for both of these parameters in hip and knee OA (Bartels et al. 2007). Exercise programs for individuals with OA should be monitored by a physician, nurse practitioner, or physical therapist, with the intensity and duration titrated to pain and function. A balanced exercise program is an effective therapeutic modality in OA. In addition, the exercise program assists in weight control.

Pearl: The course of joint degeneration varies substantially among patients with OA.

Comment: Many years can elapse between the time clinical symptoms or radiographic signs begin and the presence of both concurrently. OA probably begins with a change in the articular cartilage or subchondral bone. However, because cartilage has no nerve supply, the inciting event (e.g., an injury) may be asymptomatic. Over time, bone remodeling occurs followed by hypertrophy and changes in the synovium with inflammation. When both articular cartilage and bone changes have occurred, symptomatic pain is more consistent.

The reason for joint pain remains difficult to identify in most individuals with OA. Magnetic resonance imaging studies have revealed that transient bone marrow lesions around the joint affected by OA come and go and are associated with pain when they are present (Figs. 43.2a, b) (Hunter et al. 2006). These bone marrow lesions represent areas of increased vascularity and cellular congestion caused by a lymphatic drainage system that is inadequate to clear the accumulated lymphatic fluid. The increased fluid coming into the lesion increases the pressure.

Approximately 10% of patients with OA have rapid progression of their disease. Bone marrow lesions may be a marker for this disease subset (Hunter et al. 2006; Felson et al. 2007). Additional investigations of such patients are ongoing.

Pearl: Risk factors for OA progression can be modified.

Comment: Individuals with knee OA who lose weight experience a reduction in joint pain and an improvement in joint function. How much weight is a patient required to lose before an impact on the symptoms of OA will be observed? Some studies indicate that a minimum of five kilograms (12 pounds) is necessary (Felson and Chaisson 1997; Felson et al. 2004; Felson et al. 2007; Bierma-Zeinstra and Koes 2007). The optimal place for finishing with weight reduction depends on where one starts. For many patients, the answer is "the more, the merrier."

Pearl: Leg length discrepancy increases the progression of knee and hip OA.

Comment: Some patients have leg length discrepancies from birth. Others develop them as a consequence of arthritis in the knee or hip or after hip arthroplasty. Correction of the leg length discrepancy through the use of orthotic, such as a heel

Fig. 43.2 Magnetic resonance imaging study from a patient with osteoarthritis (OA) of the knee. Note the bone marrow lesions that are adjacent to the joint space. These are known to cause pain in OA patients. (**a**). Right Knee: Normal X-Ray where MRI with degenerative changes (from OAI) Sagittal MRI is Intermediate Weighted Turbo Spin Echo with Fat Suppression (IW TSE FS) through medical compartment showing: Bone Marrow Edema (BME), menscal tear (*black arrow*) and femoral cartilage loss (*white arrow*). (**b**). Left Knee: Large BMEs at baseline (*left*) almost vanished by 24-month follow up (*right*) Sagittal MRI is IW TSE FS through medial compartment showing large femoral BME (*white arrow*) that has become diminished going to tiny BME at 24 month follow up. There is a tibial BME (*white arrow*) at 24 months. This knee also shows full thickness cartilage loss of femur and tibia, a severely damaged meniscus, and osteophytes on femoral condyle

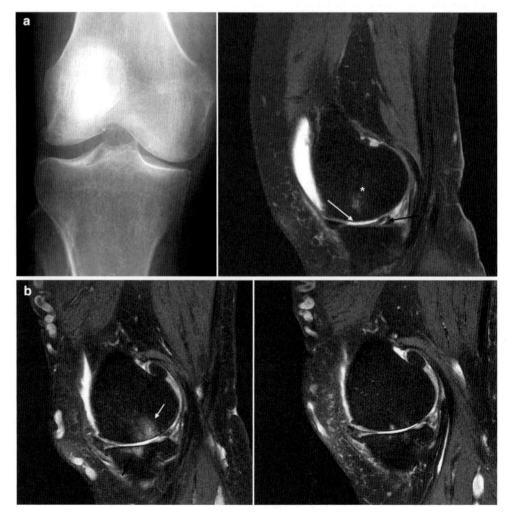

lift, can reduce low back pain and improve joint function (Hofmann et al. 2008; Golightly et al. 2007).

Pearl: Abnormal biomechanical forces across the knee from abnormal heel strike or pes planus can be modified with orthotics. These normalize the biomechanical forces across the joint, slow the pace of cartilage degeneration, and reduce joint pain.

Comment: Pes planus and other biomechanical abnormalities create abnormal mechanical forces across the ankle and knee joints and accelerate the development of OA. Orthotics that provide an external longitudinal arch support across the midfoot mitigate these adverse biomechanical forces and improve exercise tolerance (Lee and Shmerling 2008; Janisse and Janisse 2000).

Pearl: Radiographic findings often correlate poorly with the clinical severity of OA.

Comment: Radiographic evidence of OA usually precedes the onset of clinical symptoms. However, radiographic findings generally lag behind tissue destruction and may underestimate the severity of the disease. In a small number of people with knee OA, the disease may be detected by magnetic resonance imaging before changes on the radiograph.

Magnetic resonance imaging is employed frequently to determine the cause of knee pain and the severity of the underlying lesion. In patients with mild to moderate evidence of OA on plain radiographs, an magnetic resonance imaging study can reveal significant articular cartilage loss, synovitis, and bone marrow lesions, implying disease that is substantially more severe than appreciated on radiographs (Felson 1993). However, in the majority of people, radiography is the only study needed for diagnosis. Magnetic resonance imaging should be reserved for patients whose pain is persistent and unexplained.

Pearl: The method for obtaining knee radiographs is crucial for the determination of OA severity. Each method provides different information about the disease process.

Comment: The standard radiographic method for the assessment of knee OA has the patient standing with approximately 5° of knee hyperextension (Fig. 43.3). This provides information about the presence of osteophytes but often does not assess the severity of joint space narrowing accurately.

If the patient is positioned with 15–20° of knee flexion, the tibial plateau becomes flattened, permitting a reasonable estimate of the width of the tibiofemoral joint space (Fig. 43.4). Narrowing of this joint space is a surrogate measure for status of the articular cartilage. Loss of joint space at the knee correlates highly with articular pain and need for joint replacement (Wolfe et al. 2002). Sunrise views of the knees to evaluate the patellofemoral joint space have a limited clinical role.

Similar radiographic findings are found with hip OA. Pelvic radiographs taken with the patient standing in 15° of toe internal rotation are helpful in assessing the presence and severity of hip OA (Fig. 43.5).

Pearl: Intraarticular injections of glucocorticoids up to four times a year reduce joint pain and improve function.

Comment: Depot glucocorticoid injections are quite effective in the treatment of a knee OA flare. They reduce joint swelling rapidly and lead to improvements in pain and joint function. One randomized, placebo-controlled trial of glucocorticoid injections into the knee joint reported rapid reductions in joint pain (Dieppe et al. 1980 Jones and Doherty 1996). The

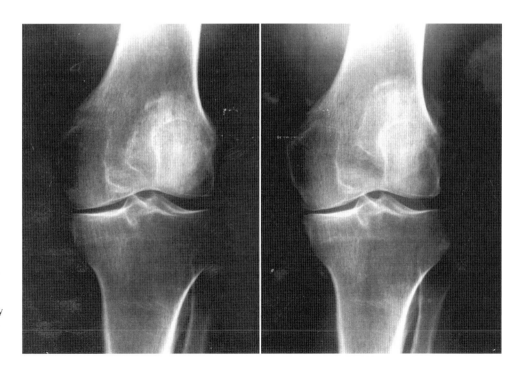

Fig. 43.3 The standard method of assessing knee OA by radiographs. The knee is hyperextended by approximately five degrees. This method is the optimal one for detecting osteophytes

Fig. 43.4 Radiograph of the knee with the patient in 15–20° of flexion. This view flattens the tibial plateau and permits the most accurate assessment of joint space narrowing. (**a**). Normal knee. (**b**). Mild joint space narrowing. (**c**). Moderate joint space narrowing. (**d**). Severe joint space narrowing

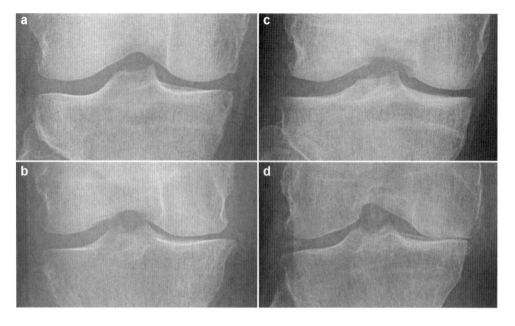

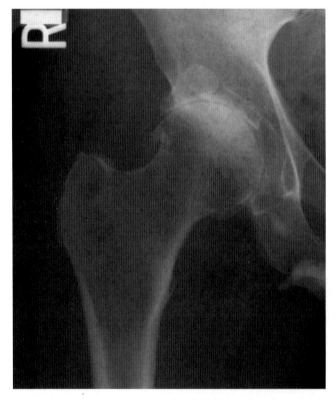

Fig. 43.5 Radiographic view of hip OA. Superolateral joint space narrowing, lateral and medial femoral osteophytes, and subchondral sclerosis of the proximal femur are all present

improvement in overall joint pain persisted through a follow-up period of 14 days. A randomized, controlled trial of intraarticular glucocorticoids for the treatment of hip OA was also effective in reducing joint pain (Lambert et al. 2007).

One Myth about frequent intraarticular glucocorticoid use is that this procedure accelerates the progression of cartilage damage. A two-year study showed no progression of radiographic damage following triamcinolone injections every three months (Raynauld et al. 2003). The American College of Rheumatology recommends intraarticular glucocorticoid injections not more than four times a year (Zhang et al. 2008; Bellamy et al. 2006a).

Pearl: Activities of daily living can be increased with assistive devices.

Comment: The following assistive devices are particularly helpful to some individuals:

- Individuals with hand OA who have poor grip strength can use devices to help open jars.
- Widened spoon, fork, and knife holders can help patients eat.
- Sticks with a pincher at the end can help pick up things from the floor and alleviate bending.
- A cane, held in the hand opposite the knee or hip affected by OA, can help with balance for those with lower extremity OA (Lozado 2005).
- The most common error in the use of a cane is that they are not the proper length. The elbow should be flexed to 12–20° (Lee and Shmerling 2008). Recommendations for choosing and using a case in patients with hip and knee OA are reviewed in Table 43.1.

Pearl: The initial stages of joint degeneration in OA are clinically silent.

Comment: This partially explains the discrepancy between the high prevalence of radiographic disease and lower proportion of patients who eventually develop symptomatic OA. However, even in the later stages of OA, there is a discrepancy between radiographic and clinical symptoms. Articular cartilage has no nerve supply. As a result, once articular cartilage is damaged, there is a delay until the development of symptomatic OA.

Table 43.1 Recommendations for the selection and use of a cane

Consider the functionality of the cane, not only its appearance

Select from the various styles of canes by considering the stability each offers

Choose a cane that is light

To select the proper length for a cane, stand up straight with your shoes on and arms at your sides. The top of the cane should reach the crease on the underside of your wrist

If the cane is a proper fit, your elbow will be flexed 15–20°when you hold the cane while standing

Choose an adjustable cane if you plan to wear different styles of shoes

Make sure you have a good grip of the cane and that the fingers and thumb do not overlap

Shift as much weight to the cane as necessary

Make sure that the tip of the cane is in good condition and that it is replaceable

Hold the cane with the opposite hand of the side that needs extra support

When ascending stairs, step first with the cane and good foot following with the bad side

When descending stairs, step first with the bad foot and follow with the cane and good foot

Carol & Richard Eustice, About.com: Arthritis.

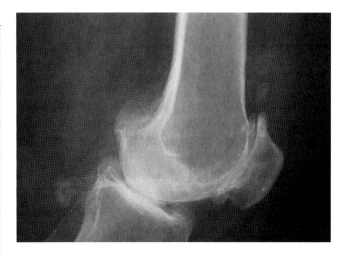

Fig. 43.6 Patellofemoral OA (radiograph)

The time between the initial damage to the cartilage and joint pain depends on a number of factors:

- the age of the patient
- the extent of the injury
- the location of the damaged cartilage within or outside of a weight-bearing area
- the involvement of other joint structures such as the medial menisci or lateral collateral ligaments. Injuries to these structures along with damage to the articular cartilage can render the joint unstable and result in a shorter time to painful disease.

Pearl: Joint pain in OA does not originate from the articular cartilage.

Comment: Articular cartilage has no neural innervation. Thus, joint pain does not arise directly from cartilage injuries. Pain in OA frequently consists of a dull ache and joint stiffness that follows a period of sitting or sleeping. The pain can be aggravated by joint use and can radiate to surrounding joints and other structures. For example, pain that results from hip OA may radiate to the knee or to the lower lumbar spine (Lozado 2005).

Pearl: Pain that originates from the patellofemoral joint is common and often accompanies tibiofemoral joint OA.

Comment: The knee joint is composed of three compartments: the medial and lateral tibiofemoral joints and the patellofemoral compartment. Degeneration of the medial and lateral compartments usually results in a significant amount of knee pain. Disease in either of these compartments is used as a criterion for joint replacement. OA in the patellofemoral compartment can also be a cause of significant pain (Fig. 43.6). Patell-

ofemoral arthritis frequently accompanies the degeneration observed in the other two knee compartments.

Pain arising from the patellofemoral joint degenerative process is exacerbated by walking up and down stairs or inclines. As patients with patellofemoral arthritis ascend stairs or walk on inclines, the patella becomes pushed against the femoral condyle. In the absence of cartilage, this interaction between the patella and femur produces pain. A common complaint with patellofemoral pain is that the symptoms worsen following prolonged sitting in a movie theater (Lozado 2005).

Pearl: There are reversible causes of knee pain in OA.

Comment: Not all knee pain in the patient with OA is caused by OA. The differential diagnosis for pain in the knee includes meniscal and ligament tears, Baker's cysts, anserine bursitis, the patellofemoral syndrome, gout, and calcium pyrophosphate deposition disease. Maintaining a mind that is open to the possibility of other disorders is important for clinicians, because the treatment of many of these other ailments can reduce knee pain and improve function in individuals with OA. These disorders are reviewed in Table 43.2.

Pearl: A major risk factor for hip OA is mild dysplasia of the femoral head and acetabulum.

Comment: Hip dysplasia (Fig. 43.7), a condition with which many are born, results in an abnormal weight-bearing surface and an accelerated pace of hip degeneration with joint use. Other abnormalities from childhood to consider in the adult patient who develops early hip OA are a slipped capital epiphysis and Legg–Calve–Perthes disease (Figs. 43.8 and 43.9) (Reijman et al. 2005b; Lane et al. 2000).

Pearl: Joint pain from hip OA is usually referred to the groin.

Comment: Pain with internal rotation of the hip that is felt in the groin probably represents hip OA. Patients who perceive pain laterally (over the trochanteric region) during internal or

Table 43.2 Common causes of knee pain that are not osteoarthritis

Condition	History	Physical examination	Laboratory findings
Inflammatory arthritis (RA or PSA)	Morning stiffness and joint pain, worse in the A.M.	Evidence of synovitis and warmth on palpation	Can be associated with an elevated ESR of CRP, Inflammatory joint fluid
Crystaline arthritis (gout or pseudogout)	The first MTP or instep of the midfoot may be involved with gout other joints may not be involved with pseudogout	Significant pain on palpation and erythema present during the acute episode	Inflammatory Joint fluid and crystals
Anserine brusitis	Point tenderness with walking	Pain on palpation of the anserine bursa below the knee at the medial side of the tibia	None
Iliotibial band syndrome	Pain that radiates down the lateral thigh to the superior aspect of the tibial/fibular junction. Frequently observed in runners	Pain at the insertion of the iliotibial band	
Meniscal tear	History that the knee may "give out" or buckle	Tenderness on palpation of the tibial femur joint and pain with twisting of the knee with patient lying prone on their abdomen	MRI can identify tears
Chondromalacia patellae	Frequent knee pain in young women, and pain increases going up and down stairs or steps	Pain over patellofemoral joint and with pressing the patella into toward the femur	Usually physical examination or lateral knee radiograph

Adapted from Felson (2006)

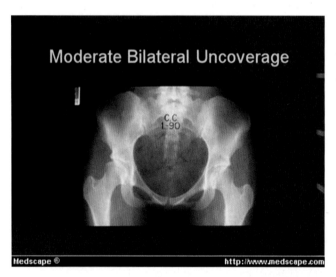

Fig. 43.7 Mild hip dysplasia in a young adult. This condition predisposes the patient to the development of OA of the hip at a young age

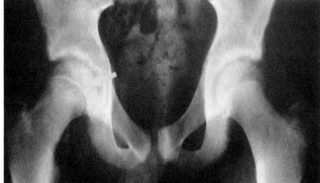

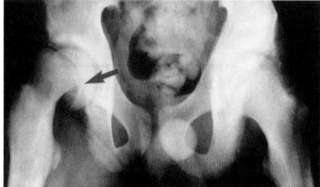

Fig. 43.8 Slipped capital epiphysis (radiograph)

external rotation probably have trochanteric bursitis rather than significant hip OA.

Pain generated by abnormalities of the hip can also be present in the anterior or lateral thigh, the knee, or the lumbar spine. Patients who have symptoms simultaneously lower back and anterior thigh pain are likely to have degenerative disc disease of the lumbar spine.

Pearl: Muscle strength and tone are significantly reduced around a joint affected by OA.

Comment: The muscles around a joint reduce cartilage loading and help protect against joint damage. Maintaining muscle strength and function around an osteoarthritic joint are

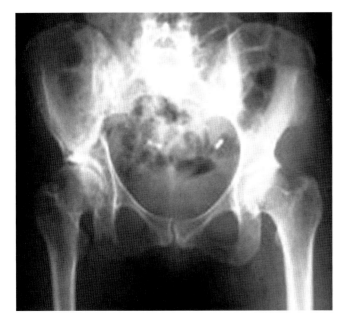

Fig. 43.9 Legg–Calve–Perthes disease (radiograph). Plain radiograph in an adult patient with residual coxa magna and plana deformity with superimposed joint changes

important in reducing joint symptoms. Both muscle strength and range of motion around the OA joints can be improved with a well-defined program of physical therapy that includes isometric and aerobic exercises.

Pearl: Many nonpharmacologic interventions help treat OA joint pain.

Comment: Transcutaneous nerve stimulation, acupuncture, heat, and cold have all been shown to reduce the severity of pain in patients with OA. Although these interventions have only modest effects on the reduction of pain, they provide an alternative to pharmacologic interventions. The use of cushioned footwear such as running or walking shoes can also reduce lower extremity joint pains (Golightly et al. 2007).

Pearl: Prescribed periods of joint rest throughout the day are useful in the management of OA.

Comment: Reduction of joint loading by either rest or use of a cane improves activity levels. Continued or prolonged use of OA joints, especially weight-bearing joints, increases joint pain. Rest time reduces joint pain and prolongs the patient's ability to continue activities.

Pearl: The efficacy of "viscosupplementation" through injections of hyaluronic acid is controversial.

Comment: Hyaluronic acid is a component of synovial fluid and articular cartilage, both of which are reduced in OA. As a result of the decreases in synovial fluid and cartilage, the joint loses much of the lubrication function of hyaluronic acid. Commercial preparations of hyaluronic acid have been developed with the goal of improving joint pain and function.

Injections of hyaluronic acid alter synovial function, reduce the sensitivity of nerve endings, increase the endogenous production of hyaluronate, and have a modest antiinflammatory effect. The FDA has approved a number of hyaluronic acid preparations for patients whose knee pain is not controlled by oral analgesics, NSAIDs, or intraarticular glucocorticoid injections.

All approved hyaluronic acid preparations show that they are significantly more effective than placebo injections in reducing joint pain (Bellamy et al. 2006 b). Studies indicate that approximately two thirds of patients receive benefits from these injections. At the present time, there are no data available to predict patients who are likely to respond to hyaluronic acid injections. Studies are underway to access the efficacy of hyaluronic acid preparations in nonweight-bearing joints, e.g., the shoulder and the elbow (Zhang et al. 2008; Jan et al. 2008; Bellamy et al. 2006 b; Blaine et al. 2008).

Pearl: Joint arthroplasty for OA of the first carpometacarpal joint is not yet ready for prime time.

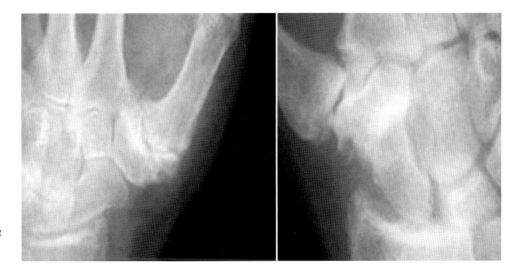

Fig. 43.10 OA of the first carpometacarpal joint. (**a**) Clinical photograph showing squaring of the first carpometacarpal joint at the base of the thumb. (**b**) Radiograph revealing OA of the first carpometacarpal joint

Comment: Degenerative joint disease of the first carpometa-carpal joint is extremely common, particularly among women with hand OA (Fig. 43.10). However, currently there is very little if anything to gain in function with a joint replacement at this site.

References

Bartels EM, Lund H, Hagen KB, et al Aquatic exercise for the treatment of knee and hip osteoarthritis. Cochrane Database Syst Rev. 2007;17(4):CD005523

Bellamy N, Campbell J, Robinson V, et al Intraarticular corticosteroid for treatment of osteoarthritis of the knee. Cochrane Database Syst Rev. 2006a;19:CD005328

Bellamy N, Campbell J, Robinson V, et al Viscosupplementation for the treatment of osteoarthritis of the knee. Cochrane Database Syst Rev. 2006b;19(2):CD005321

Blaine T, Moskowitz R, Udell J, et al Treatment of persistent shoulder pain with sodium hyaluronate: a randomized, controlled trial. J Bone Joint Surg Am. 2008;90:970–9

Bierma-Zeinstra SM, Koes BW. Risk factors and prognostic factors of hip and knee osteoarthritis. Nat Clin Pract Rheumatol. 2007;3(2):78–85

Bonnet CS, Walsh DA. Osteoarthritis, angiogenesis and inflammation. Rheumatology (Oxford) 2005;44:(1):7–16

Brien S, Prescott P, Bashir N, et al Systematic review of the nutritional supplements dimethyl sulfoxide (DMSO) and methylsulfonyl-methane (MSM) in the treatment of osteoarthritis. Osteoarthritis Cartilage. 2008;16(11):1277–88

Bruyere O, Pavelka K, Rovati LC, et al Total joint replacement after glucosamine sulphate treatment in knee osteoarthritis: results of a mean 8-year observation of patients from two previous 3-year, randomised, placebo-controlled trials. Osteoarthritis Cartilage. 2008; 16(2):254–60

Clegg DO, Reda DJ, Harris CL, et al Glucosamine, chondroitin sulfate, and the two in combination for painful knee osteoarthritis. N Engl J Med. 2006;354(8):795–808

Dieppe PA, Sathapatayavongs B, Jones HE, et al Intra-articular steroids in osteoarthritis. Rheumatol Rehabil. 1980;19:212–7

Felson DT, Chaisson CE. Understanding the relationship between body weight and osteoarthritis. Baillieres Clin Rheumatol. 1997;11(4): 671–81

Felson DT, Goggins J, Niu J, et al The effect of body weight on progression of knee osteoarthritis is dependent on alignment. Arthritis Rheum. 2004;50(12):3904–9

Felson DT, Niu J, Guermazi A, et al Correlation of the development of knee pain with enlarging bone marrow lesions on magnetic resonance imaging. Arthritis Rheum. 2007;56(9):2986–92

Felson DT. The course of osteoarthritis and factors that affect it. Rheum Dis Clin North Am. 1993;19(3):607–15

Felson DT. Clinical practice. Osteoarthritis of the knee. N Engl J Med. 2006;354(8):841–8

Goldring MB, Goldring SR. Osteoarthritis. J Cell Physiol. 2007; 213(3):626–34

Golightly YM, Tate JJ, Burns CB, Gross MT. Changes in pain and disability secondary to shoe lift intervention in subjects with limb length inequality and chronic low back pain: a preliminary report. J Orthop Sports Phys Ther. 2007;37:380–8

Halbert J, Crotty M, Weller D, et al Primary care-based physical activity programs: effectiveness in sedentary older patients with osteoarthritis symptoms. Arthritis Rheum. 2001;45(3):228–34

Hofmann AA, Bolognesi M, Lahav A, Kurtin S. Minimizing leg-length inequality in total hip arthroplasty: use of preoperative templating and an intraoperative X-ray. Am J Orthop. 2008;37(1):18–23

Hunter DJ, Zhang Y, Niu J, et al Increase in bone marrow lesions associated with cartilage loss: a longitudinal magnetic resonance imaging study of knee osteoarthritis. Arthritis Rheum. 2006;54: 1529–35

Jan MH, Lin JJ, Liau JJ, et al Investigation of clinical effects of high- and low-resistance training for patients with knee osteoarthritis: a randomized controlled trial. Phys Ther. 2008;88:427–36

Janisse DJ, Janisse E. Shoe modification and the use of orthoses in the treatment of foot and ankle pathology. J Am Acad Orthop Surg. 2000;16(3):152–8

Jensen LK. Hip osteoarthritis: influence of work with heavy lifting, climbing stairs or ladders, or combining kneeling/squatting with heavy lifting. Occup Environ Med. 2008;65:6–19

Jones A, Doherty M. Intra-articular corticosteroids are effective in osteoarthritis but there are no clinical predictors of response. Ann Rheum Dis. 1996;55:829–32

Lambert RG, Hutchings EJ, Grace MG, et al Steroid injection for osteoarthritis of the hip: a randomized, double-blind, placebo-controlled trial. Arthritis Rheum. 2007;56:2278–87

Lane NE, Bloch DA, Jones HH, et al Long-distance running, bone density, and osteoarthritis. JAMA. 1986;7(255):1147–51

Lane NE, Lin P, Christiansen L, et al Association of mild acetabular dysplasia with an increased risk of incident hip osteoarthritis in elderly white women: the study of osteoporotic fractures. Arthritis Rheum. 2000;43(2):400–4

Lawrence RC, Felson DT, Helmick CG, et al Estimates of the prevalence of arthritis and other rheumatic conditions in the United States. Part II. Arthritis Rheum. 2008;58:26–35

Lee YC, Shmerling RH. The benefit of nonpharmacologic therapy to treat symptomatic osteoarthritis. Curr Rheumatol Rep. 2008; 10(1):5–10

Lozado CJ. Management of osteoarthritis. In: Harris ED, Budd RC, Firestein GS, Genovese MC, Seargent JS, Ruddy S, Sledge CB editors Kelley's textboook of rheumatology. 7th edition, Vol II. PA, Elsevier; 2005. p. 1528–40

McAlindon TE, LaValley MP, Gulin JP, Felson DT. Glucosamine and chondroitin for treatment of osteoarthritis: a systematic quality assessment and meta-analysis. JAMA. 2000;283(11):1469–75

Raynauld JP, Buckland-Wright C, Ward R, et al Safety and efficacy of long-term intraarticular steroid injections in osteoarthritis of the knee: a randomized, double-blind, placebo-controlled trial. Arthritis Rheum. 2003;48:370–7

Reginster JY, Deroisy R, Rovati LC, et al Long-term effects of glucosamine sulphate on osteoarthritis progression: a randomised, placebo-controlled clinical trial. Lancet 27;2001;357(9252):251–6

Reijman M, Hazes JM, Pols HA, et al Acetabular dysplasia predicts incident osteoarthritis of the hip: the Rotterdam study. Arthritis Rheum. 2005b;52:787–93

Roos EM, Dahlberg L. Positive effects of moderate exercise on glycosaminoglycan content in knee cartilage: a four-month, randomized, controlled trial in patients at risk of osteoarthritis. Arthritis Rheum. 2005;52:3507–14

Sawitzke AD, Allen D, Shi H, et al The effect of glucosamine and/or chondroitin sulfate on the progression of knee osteoarthritis. Arthritis Rheum. 2008;58(10):3183–91

Schouten JS, de Bie RA, Swaen G. An update on the relationship between occupational factors and osteoarthritis of the hip and knee. Curr Opin Rheumatol. 2002;14:89–92

Simkin PA. Habitual knuckle cracking and hand function. Ann Rheum Dis. 1990;9(11):957

Sutton AJ, Muir KR, Mockett S, Fentem P. A case-control study to investigate the relation between low and moderate levels of physical activity and osteoarthritis of the knee using data collected as part of the Allied Dunbar National Fitness Survey. Ann Rheum Dis. 2001;60:756–64

Swezey RL, Swezey SE. The consequences of habitual knuckle cracking. West J Med. 1975;122(5):377–9

Theodosakis J. The arthritis cure. London: MacMillan Publishers; 2003

Unsworth A Dowson D Wright V. "Cracking joints". A bioengineering study of cavitation in the metacarpophalangeal joint. Ann Rheum. 1971;30:348–58

Walker WR, Keats DM. An investigation of the therapeutic value of the 'copper bracelet'-dermal assimilation of copper in arthritic/rheumatoid conditions. Agents Actions. 1976;6(4): 454–9

Watson P, Hamilton A, Mollan R. Habitual joint cracking and radiological damage. BMJ. 1989;299(6715):1566

Wolfe F, Lane NE, Buckland-Wright C. Radiographic methods in knee osteoarthritis: a further comparison of semiflexed (MTP), schuss-tunnel, and weight-bearing anteroposterior views for joint space narrowing and osteophytes. J Rheumatol. 2002;29: 2597–601

Zhang W, Moskowitz RW, Nuki G, et al OARSI recommendations for the management of hip and knee osteoarthritis, part II: OARSI evidence-based, expert consensus guidelines. Osteoarthritis Cartilage. 2008;16(2):137–62

44.1 Introduction

This chapter is divided into sections based upon the anatomic sites: shoulder, elbow, wrist, hand, coccyx, hip, knee, ankle, and foot. Before focusing on specific musculoskeletal regions, however, we provide one introductory Pearl and then some general comments on the performance of arthrocentesis and joint injection. Some specific pointers on arthrocentesis and the injection of individual joints are found within the appropriate section.

Introductory Pearl: "The number of rheumatologists doing procedures equals the number of different ways of performing them..." (Gardner 2007).

Comment: It is true: there are many ways to skin a cat, and there are also many ways to perform most of the procedures described in this chapter. The preferences of the authors are emphasized herein, but other approaches may also work.

44.2 General Points on Performing Arthrocentesis and Joint Injection

Pearl: The contraindications to performing an intra-articular glucocorticoid injection are different from those for an arthrocentesis.

Comment: No joint should be tapped through an open, weeping, purulent ulcer. Apart from that proviso, there is virtually no absolute contraindication to tapping a joint if the information is needed for the purpose of diagnosis.

Conversely, there are several important contraindications to the injection of glucocorticoids. These are shown in Table 44.1.

Myth: A joint should not be tapped if there is an overlying cellulitis.

Reality: The concern, of course, is the introduction of the cutaneous infection into the joint. However, the price to pay for missing a septic joint is much higher than the chance of introducing infection by tapping into the joint through an overlying cellulitis. In addition, cutaneous erythema overlying a joint may not be secondary to an infection; gout, for example, can also be associated with intense cutaneous erythema. It is critical to distinguish between microcrystalline disease and infection. Never let the skin stand between you and the diagnosis!

Myth: Coagulopathy (INR > 3) and thrombocytopenia are contraindications to arthrocentesis.

Reality: Coagulopathy and thrombocytopenia are only relative contraindications to arthrocentesis. One would prefer not to have to tap a joint under such circumstances, but potential coagulation issues should not stand as impediments to the timely diagnosis of septic arthritis, which is a potentially life-threatening condition. The statement that "No one has ever exsanguinated into a joint" is macho but true.

Arthrocentesis is actually critical to perform in the setting of a suspected hemarthrosis. Bleeding into a joint (e.g., as a complication of hemophilia) can cause chemical synovitis and lead to irreversible joint damage. Evacuation of the blood via a surgical approach may be necessary to preserve joint function. A diagnostic arthrocentesis is therefore essential for management in such cases.

Pearl: When assessing synovial fluid joint counts, the "Rule of Twos" applies.

Comment: The Rule of Twos refers to the number of white blood cells (WBCs) contained within the synovial fluid (Table 44.2):

- Normal synovial fluid contains <200 WBCs/mm^3.
- Noninflammatory fluid contains between 200 and 2000 WBCs/mm^3.
- Inflammatory fluid contains >2,000 (but <50,000) WBCs/mm^3.

Septic arthritis, a condition that does not fit neatly into the Rule of Twos, is generally associated with synovial WBC counts in excess of 75,000/mm^3.

J. H. Stone (ed.), *A Clinician's Pearls and Myths in Rheumatology,*
DOI:10.1007/978-1-84800-934-9_44, © Springer Science + Business Media B.V. 2009

Table 44.1 Contraindications to the injection of glucocorticoids into a joint

Infection: septic joint, periarticular infection/cellulitis, bacteremia
Unstable joint
Intra-articular fracture
Hypersensitivity to the agent or agents to be injected
Joint prosthesis
Poor response to previous injection
Significant coagulopathy

Pearl: Culture of the synovial fluid remains the only way to diagnose septic bursitis.

Comment: The "Rule of Twos" for the synovial fluid of joints does not apply to bursal fluids. Septic bursa fluids can have fewer than 2000 WBCs/mm^3 and a lower percentage of neutrophils when compared to infected joint fluids. Moreover, the systemic symptoms and signs of an infectious process are often absent in patients with septic bursitis. The characteristics of septic and nonseptic bursal fluids are shown in Table 44.3.

Pearl: Glucocorticoid-lidocaine injections should be pain-free procedures, apart from the "bee sting" associated with local anesthesia.

Comment: The immediate pain relief that results from a properly directed injection into a tendon sheath, bursa, enthesis, or nerve area helps to validate the clinician's diagnosis (Petri et al. 1987). The injection, if performed properly, should not cause discomfort to the patient.

Basic principles of intralesional injections include aseptic technique and the use of small needles (25-gauge 5/8", 25-gauge 1½", or a 22-gauge 1½"). (Larger needles may facilitate joint aspiration, when synovial fluid sampling is necessary). A 2% lidocaine solution is preferred over a 1% solution because it is more effective in decreasing discomfort related to the injection. The use of separate syringes for lidocaine and glucocorticoid, hereafter termed the "two-syringe technique," avoids mixing of the substances and permits immediate infiltration of lidocaine, beginning with a small intracutaneous wheal (Kessell 1986).

Large wheals are generally unnecessary and are discouraged because they are more painful than small ones. In addition to the local infiltration of lidocaine, a vapocoolant spray (fluorimethane) can be applied to the injection site to provide topical anesthesia. After the skin is anesthetized, a small amount of lidocaine is injected continuously as the needle is directed to the site of the lesion. When the needle reaches the desired site, additional lidocaine is injected.

The quantity of lidocaine used to anesthetize the lesional area ranges from 0.2 to 1 mL, depending on the problem. The clinician should pause for a few seconds after the lidocaine is injected to ensure a full anesthetic effect. The lidocaine syringe is then changed to the glucocorticoid syringe (leaving the needle in place) and the glucocorticoid solution is injected. A Kelly clamp can facilitate the changing of syringes.

Pearl: No method of sterile skin preparation can eliminate the small risk of joint or soft tissue infection entirely.

Comment: The rate of iatrogenic infection from arthrocentesis is low, but clinicians should not become cavalier when performing this procedure. The lowest estimate – 1 in 10,000 procedures – is derived from the original description of the use of arthrocentesis as a route for the delivery of glucocorticoids (Hollander 1961). The highest, 1 in 2,500, is an unpublished description of anecdotal experience (Roberts WN). A full-time practitioner might be expected to cause three or four joint infections in his or her career.

The best evidence about sterile skin preparation is extrapolated from studies of various surgical preparation techniques. Most such studies rely upon surrogate measures of infection, e.g., colony counts from swabs of skin prepared in a sterile fashion. Trial data indicate that a single chlorhexidine scrub, the most expensive technique, is probably the best (Mimoz et al. 1999). A triple betadine preparation, similar to the technique for obtaining blood cultures, is probably the second most effective. The least effective approach is the use of alcohol swabs alone.

No technique can eliminate the small risk of joint infection entirely (Charalambous et al. 2003). Every procedure, regardless of the details of sterile technique, instills some inoculum of

Table 44.2 Assessing synovial fluid joint counts

	Normal	Noninflammatory	Inflammatory	Septic
Color	Transparent	Transparent	Translucent to opaque	Opaque
Viscosity	Very high	High	Low	Variable
WBC count (#/mm^3)	<200	200–2,000	>2,000 but <50,000	>50,000
Polys (%)	<75	<75	>75	>75
Examples		OA	RA	Bacterial infection
			Gout	
		AVN	CPPD	
		HPOA	Spondyloarthropathy	
			Lupus	
			Serum sickness	

CPPD = calcium pyrophosphate dihydrate deposition; AVN = avascular necrosis; HPOA = hypertrophic osteoarthropathy

Table 44.3 Bursal fluid characteristics (Nonseptic vs. septic)

	Nonseptic	Septic
WBC/cm³	90–11,000	350–395,000
%PMN	0–90	50–100
Gram stain +	0	5–100%

(Zimmermann et al. 1995 and Raddatz et al. 1987)

microorganisms into the joint. The larger cores of skin resulting from the use of larger needles presumably are associated with larger inocula. Diligent attention to preparation of the skin is important, regardless of which cleansing agent is employed.

Pearl: For optimal interpretations, synovial fluid should be evaluated within a couple of hours of arthrocentesis.

Comment: Delay in fluid evaluation can be associated with a fall in the synovial fluid WBC count (Kerolus et al. 1989). The quantity of CPPD and monosodium urate crystals may also fall somewhat with time, but the crystals can still be observed for days after the arthrocentesis, particularly if the fluid is refrigerated.

If synovial fluid is allowed to stand for hours, the fall in the number of CPPD crystals tends to be greater than the decline in monosodium urate crystals. As discussed elsewhere, new crystals do not develop in synovial fluid that has been aspirated and allowed to stand for hours before examination (See Chap. 37).

Pearl: Use of a more water-soluble glucocorticoid preparation decreases the possibility of skin atrophy if some of the injected glucocorticoid remains within the dermis or epidermis.

Comment: If excessive dose of glucocorticoid is injected or if the injection is placed into the subcutaneous tissue or within the skin itself, then skin atrophy, subcutaneous fat atrophy, and skin depigmentation can occur (Gottlieb et al. 1978). Atrophy and depigmentation are observed in particular following injections for lateral epicondylitis and DeQuervain's tenosynovitis.

The use of a water-soluble glucocorticoid preparation diminishes the risk of these complications as well as the risk of glucocorticoid-induced tendon weakness or a postinjection flare of inflammation. Two good options for water-soluble glucocorticoid preparations are betamethasone and triamcinolone (Drendorf et al. 1986).

Pearl: Postglucocorticoid hypopigmentation of the skin can be avoided by the injection of air following the medication.

Comment: Cutaneous hypopigmentation can result from "backleak" of glucocorticoids through the injection track following the injection of a superficial joint or tendon such as the ulnar styloid. After completion of the glucocorticoid injection, the syringe can be unscrewed and replaced with a tuberculin syringe containing 0.3 cc of air. The injection of an "air seal" prevents the leakage of glucocorticoids from the needle track into the dermis, thereby avoiding the potential for skin depigmentation.

Myth: The glucocorticoid preparation and lidocaine solution should be mixed for joint and soft tissue injections.

Reality: Clinical practice on this point varies widely, but the only sound rationale for mixing the two compounds is convenience. The two-syringe technique described earlier has several advantages:

- Less pain with injection
- Lower risk of injecting the glucocorticoid into the soft tissue rather than the joint, which can be associated with skin and subcutaneous atrophy
- Removal of concern about the potential interaction or precipitation of the glucocorticoid and anesthetic.

44.3 Tendinitis: General Points

Myth: Tendinitis is an inflammatory condition.

Reality: The various terms used to refer to tendon injuries or overuse syndromes are confusing. Tendinitis has been the main term for such conditions. However, the histology of this condition reveals degenerative changes and hyaline features in the tendon but few inflammatory cells (Khan et al. 2002). Thus, "tendinosis" may be more appropriate. Nevertheless, the beneficial response to glucocorticoid injections suggests a role for cytokines in the pathophysiology of this disorder.

"Tendinopathy" defers judgment on the contribution of inflammation to the problem. "Tendon insufficiency" refers to a stretching or tearing of the tendon. Finally, "tenosynovitis" and "peritendinitis" refer to an inflammatory response within the tenosynovium or peritenon.

Apart from these musings, we suspect that both the term "tendonitis" and its incorrect spelling (What's a tendin?) are here to stay.

Pearl: When injecting a tendon sheath, the needle should be placed parallel to the tendon fibers, and not into the tendon itself.

Comment: The clinician should not inject glucocorticoids directly into the tendon. This error heightens the risk of tendon rupture. Injection of the glucocorticoids parallel to the tendon sheath generally leads to a good therapeutic effect.

44.4 Shoulder

Pearl: While injecting a joint or a bursa close to a tendon, the use of a small bore needle (25 gauge) can make the difference between injecting glucocorticoids correctly into a joint or a bursa and injecting them in a tendon.

Comment: While injecting the subacromial bursa, the needle tip may enter the top of the rotator cuff. When this occurs, intra-tendinous pressure will not allow the plunger of the syringe to be depressed if a small-bore needle (25-gauge) is used. The small-bore needle thus provides a feedback mechanism. If the clinician encounters excessive resistance, the needle should be pulled back 2–3 mm before injection is attempted again.

Myth: Bursitis is the most common problem of the shoulder.

Reality: The term "bursitis" is often used incorrectly by clinicians and patients to describe the most common cause of shoulder pain. Rotator cuff tendinitis is actually the most common cause of this complaint (Chard et al. 1991). The tendons of the rotator cuff attach at the humeral tuberosities. The subacromial bursa, which lies inferior to the acromion, is contiguous with the subdeltoid bursa that covers the humeral head. Although rotator cuff tendinitis is the primary cause of shoulder pain, secondary involvement of the subacromial bursa occurs in some cases.

Myth: A complete tear of the rotator cuff means that the entire rotator cuff is torn.

Reality: Rotator cuff pathology is another confusing area of nomenclature. A partial or incomplete tear is a nonfull thickness tear. Partial tendon tears can involve the glenohumeral side of the rotator cuff, the bursal side, or the intratendinous portion of the cuff. A complete tear of the rotator cuff, in contrast, refers to a tear that is a "through and through" or full thickness tear that involves both the rotator cuff and the subacromial bursa. Such a rupture creates a direct communication between the glenohumeral joint and the subacromial bursa.

Complete rotator cuff tears vary in size and clinical impact. Some are small and relatively asymptomatic. The patient's ability to abduct the arm to some degree can persist despite small rotator cuff tears. Symptomatic tears, however, result in a range of complaints that extends from severe pain and mild weakness to no pain and marked weakness, or some combination in between. The complete tears are classified as small (1 cm or less), medium (1–3 cm), large (3–5 cm), or massive (>5 cm). Thus, a complete tear of the rotator cuff does not necessarily mean a total avulsion of the rotator off the humeral head.

Pearl: Superior migration of the humeral head detected by plain radiography indicates a significant rotator cuff tear (Fig. 44.1).

Comment: Plain radiography of the shoulder is not the usual method of diagnosing a large tear of the rotator cuff, but such a finding points to a significant rotator cuff lesion.

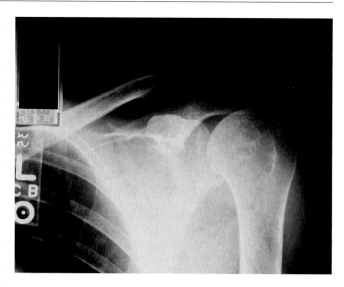

Fig. 44.1 Superior migration of the humeral head in the setting of a complete rotator cuff tear. (Figure courtesy of Dr. Joseph Biundo)

The rotator cuff normally holds the humeral head within the glenoid fossa. When the rotator cuff is torn, the deltoid exerts relatively unopposed upward pull on the humeral head, leading to superior migration. This finding may be noted incidentally on a chest radiograph.

Pearl: Brachial plexopathy is a neurogenic cause of acute, severe shoulder pain.

Comment: Most causes of acute, severe shoulder pain are musculoskeletal in nature. However, severe shoulder pain can also be caused by a neurological lesion. Brachial plexopathy, also known as the Parsonage–Turner syndrome, is such an entity (Misamore and Lehman 1996). Brachial plexopathies can result from trauma, tumor, radiation, vaccinations ("inoculation neuritis"), diabetes, infection, or median sternotomy done for cardiac surgery. They can also be idiopathic.

A brachial plexopathy presents with a deep, sharp shoulder pain that begins rapidly. The pain is exacerbated by abduction and rotation. The severity of the pain is generally quite perplexing at presentation. Its onset is followed by weakness of the shoulder girdle. Muscle atrophy of the deltoid can ensue, and sensory findings can also be present.

The entire brachial plexus or merely individual components can be affected. Plain radiographs and MRI of the shoulder are normal in patients with brachial plexopathy. However, an electromyogram can help confirm the diagnosis by demonstrating positive sharp waves and fibrillations in the involved muscles. Ultrasonography can also be used to evaluate brachial plexus pathology (Graif et al. 2004). The treatment of brachial plexopathy consists mainly of avoiding reinjury or exposure to a metabolic cause of nerve damage. Recovery requires from 1 month to several years, and residual muscle weakness sometimes persists.

Pearl: Microcrystalline disease can cause acute, severe shoulder pain.

Comment: Hydroxyapatite, calcium pyrophosphate, and monosodium urate crystals are all potential causes of acute shoulder dysfunction. In such cases, the rotator cuff and subacromial bursa are apt to become inflamed. Hydroxyapatite crystal deposition leads to a tendinitis that presents with abrupt, excruciating pain. Such cases tend to occur in younger patients and are likely to be associated with calcific deposits within the supraspinatus tendon (Fig. 44.2). A plain radiograph demonstrates these deposits most effectively when the arm is held in external rotation. The deposits appear round or oval and several centimeters in length. A true subacromial bursitis can also result from the rupture of calcific material into the bursa. The hydroxyapatite deposits may resolve spontaneously over a period as short as weeks, but sometimes require longer. The acute episode is best treated with a glucocorticoid injection of the subacromial bursa.

Acute shoulder arthritis due to CPPD deposition also occurs (Hughes et al. 1990). In addition, CPPD deposition may be found in chronic rotator cuff tears. Gout in the shoulder is quite rare, and when present, it is most likely to be part of a polyarticular attack.

Myth: A variety of approaches to injecting the shoulder work equally well.

Reality: This Myth might also be called the "horseshoes and hand-grenades" approach to shoulder injections. There are a couple of reasons why it is not quite true. The fundamental one is that the shoulder is the most complex of joints in terms of the number of compartments and tendon insertions. These compartments communicate poorly or not at all. The shoulder is technically more than one joint, in the sense that the acromio-clavicular joint is entirely separate from both the subdeltoid space and the true glenohumeral joint. The latter two are also separate from one another unless a connection is established in the form of a full-thickness rotator cuff tear.

In a randomized trial conducted at Guys Hospital in London, patients were examined by one orthopedic surgeon. Anatomic diagnoses such as rotator cuff pain, impingement syndrome, biceps tendinitis, and acromion-clavicular osteoarthritis were rendered. The patients were then randomized to have either the anterior glenohumeral approach for injection marked regardless of diagnosis, or to have the approach corresponding to the actual anatomic diagnosis marked. A second blinded surgeon in another room then injected the shoulder according to the approach marked on the skin. Finally, a third blinded surgeon later followed up to evaluate the results of the injection. The group with the injections directed by their anatomically specific diagnosis fared about 15% better in terms of the magnitude and duration of their clinical improvement.

Thus, from the subspecialty point of view, the "horseshoes and hand grenades" dogma of glucocorticoid injection fails. Learning to differentiate among the major causes of shoulder complaints and mastering the individual approaches to shoulder injection are worthwhile.

On the other hand, in general practice, the 15% advantage may not be sufficient to justify abandoning the "one size fits all" approach to shoulder injections. It is impossible to damage the pleura or axillary when approaching the shoulder from the poster-lateral angle with a 1.5 inch needle into the subacromial bursa (Fig. 44.3). For generalists, therefore, it is

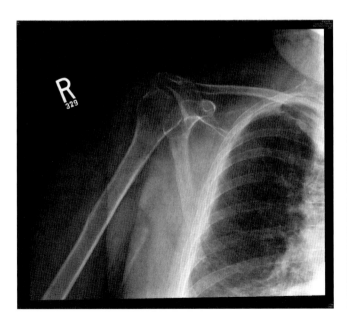

Fig. 44.2 Calcific tendonitis secondary to hydroxyapatite deposition within the supraspinatus tendon. (Figure courtesy of Dr. Richard Chou)

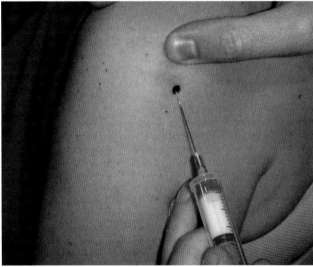

Fig. 44.3 Posterolateral approach to injecting the shoulder. (Figure courtesy of Dr. John Stone)

safer to learn the posterolateral approach to shoulder injections rather than the anterior glenohumeral approach. A remote possibility of pneumothorax or injury to the axillary neurovascular bundle exists with the latter approach.

Pearl: Any palpable effusion in the shoulder should be evaluated carefully.

Comment: Palpable effusions of the shoulder are rare and, when present, should be given careful consideration. The glenohumeral joint lies deep inside many soft tissue structures. Thus, small or even moderate-sized effusions are usually not detected by palpation. Likewise, the presence of warmth or erythema is less frequently detected in this joint, even with acute inflammation or infection.

The anatomy of the normal shoulder capsule includes a dependent, pouch-like projection that extends into the axilla, which remains inaccessible to physical examination. This pouch is apparent only on arthrography or another imaging study. Any effusion of the shoulder fills this pouch first before becoming palpable on the antero-superior aspect of the shoulder.

Palpable swelling of the shoulder might be due to an effusion of only the glenohumeral joint or only of the subacromial bursa, or more likely a combination of the two with a communication via a torn rotator cuff. In fact, shoulder effusions are seen most commonly in association with a torn rotator cuff (Fig. 44.4) (Hollister et al. 1995). These cuff tears are often associated with osteoarthritis. This combination, when severe, is known as "cuff tear arthropathy" (Neer et al. 1983). When associated with hydroxyapatite crystal deposition, it has been termed "Milwaukee shoulder" (Halverson 1981). Shoulder effusions are also found in RA, but less commonly now than before the era of biologic therapies. When shoulder effusions are present, they are frequently associated with torn rotator cuffs (Weiss et al. 1975; Kim et al. 2007).

44.5 Elbow

Pearl: Be alert to the possibility of infection as the cause of olecranon bursitis.

Comment: In septic olecranon bursitis, the major clues are localized erythema and warmth over the bursa, in addition to bursal swelling (Fig. 44.5) (Smith et al. 1989). Some nonseptic inflammatory conditions can also cause erythema over the bursa, but this is atypical in the absence of an active infection. Bursal swelling is also more likely to extend beyond the normal bursal area if an infection is present, and pain is present more frequently when the bursa is infected. However, in contrast to infection within a more confined space (such as a joint), infection of the olecranon bursa does not always cause significant pain.

Additional clues to a septic etiology are the presence of a skin abrasion, puncture, or other superficial trauma to the olecranon as a possible entry site of infection. Bursal fluid should be aspirated, examined for crystals, and submitted for Gram stain and culture. Glucocorticoids should not be administered until an infection has been excluded. WBC counts in bursae do not reach the levels as high as in similar problems of joints (see Table 44.3) (Canoso 1981).

Pearl: One common complication of tapping the olecranon bursa is the creation of a fistula.

Comment: The risk of fistula development can be minimized by taking the "zigzag approach." With this approach to the bursa, the needle is inserted at an angle that will not enter the bursa directly. When the tip of the needle is within the

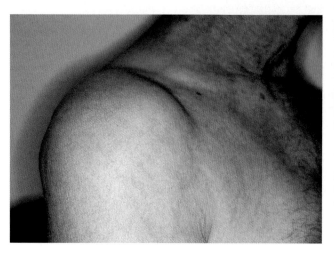

Fig. 44.4 Shoulder effusions are seen most commonly with complete tears of the rotator cuff. (Figure courtesy of Dr. Joseph Biundo)

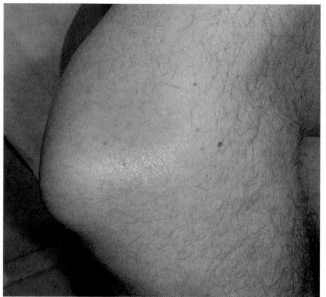

Fig. 44.5 A septic olecranon bursitis. (Figure courtesy of Dr. John Stone)

subcutaneous tissue, it is redirected toward and into the bursa.

Pearl: Swelling of the antecubital area of the elbow is unusual, but may be due to cubital bursitis.

Comment: Swelling of the antecubital area of the elbow is not common. Several known entities may account for the swelling. The first is cubital bursitis, also known as bicipito-radial bursitis. This condition is manifested by swelling in the antecubital fossa and tenderness, with some restriction of pronation. Rheumatoid arthritis or other inflammatory arthritic conditions are the most likely causes of cubital bursitis, but the disorder can also be secondary to trauma or overuse.

Clinicians must also bear in mind the possibility of a partial or complete tear of the distal biceps tendon. An MRI or ultrasound can confirm the diagnosis (Sofka and Adler 2004). Arterial aneurysm from illicit drug injections, accidentally but repeatedly injected arterially instead of intravenously, can also give antecubital swelling.

44.6 Wrist

Myth: Carpal tunnel syndrome (CTS) is caused by overuse among computer and keyboard operators.

Reality: This concept has received much interest in the fields of work-related injuries, occupational medicine, workers' compensation, and disability. However, multiple studies have failed to demonstrate correlations between CTS and the use or overuse of computers and other keyboard devices (Atroshi et al. 2007; Palmer et al. 2007). Work-related CTS, however, has been associated with occupations that require a high force or vibration of the hand. Some nonillness and noninjury factors are also associated with CTS. For example, women are three times more likely than are men to develop CTS.

Wrist shape also appears to be a risk factor for CTS. Persons with "square-shaped" wrists are at greater risk of this condition when compared with patients whose wrists are not "square-shaped." A squared wrist results from an increase in the depth of the wrist in relation to the width. When the depth:width ratio is ≥0.7, the likelihood of CTS increases. Finally, a number of systemic disorders (e.g., amyloidosis) are known to be associated with CTS. The traditional four-part differential diagnosis of simultaneous bilateral CTS is amyloidosis, rheumatoid arthritis, hypothyroidism, and pregnancy. However, nerve conduction studies have shown that idiopathic CTS is often bilateral, even though symptoms may be unilateral.

Pearl: The carpal tunnel can be injected safely, easily, and effectively.

Comment: A glucocorticoid injection can be an effective therapy for CTS if splints worn at night have been ineffective.

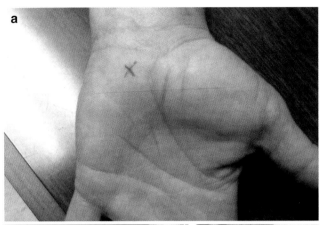
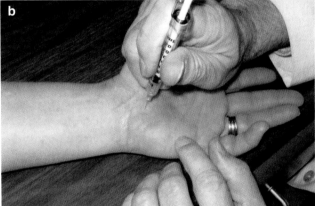

Fig. 44.6 (**a**, **b**) Site, orientation, and angle for a carpal tunnel injection. (Figure courtesy of Dr. Joseph Biundo)

Glucocorticoid injections can also be the treatment of first choice to provide immediate relief for patients with severe neurogenic pain from median nerve compression. In general, milder CTS cases tend to respond more readily to an injection than do chronic cases, in which the patients have already developed substantial prolongation of distal latencies on nerve conduction velocity studies.

The approach to a carpal tunnel injection is via the palmar surface of the hand (Fig. 44.6). The site of injection is about one centimeter distal to the distal wrist crease and about 0.75 cm toward the ulnar side of midline. Caution should be employed not to inject too far to the ulnar side of midline, lest one hit the ulnar artery. The skin should be numbed down to the transverse carpal ligament, using only about 0.2 mL of lidocaine. The clinician can feel the transverse carpal ligament with the needle tip. The 5/8-inch needle should be pushed through the ligament and inserted to the hilt.

Lidocaine that is injected directly next to the median nerve can anesthetize the hand. After reaching the desired area of the flexor tendons beneath the flexor retinaculum, the needle is kept in place, and the syringe with lidocaine is changed to a tuberculin syringe containing 1 mL of 40 mg of methylprednisolone. The median nerve should not be injected directly. If the patient feels tingling when the needle is inserted or when the injection begins, the needle is slightly withdrawn and redirected in a more ulnar orientation.

While injecting the carpal tunnel, ask the patient to flex and extend the fingers. If the needle has lodged within the tendon, then the needle will move along with the finger. If this occurs, simply pull the needle back a millimeter or so and redirect it. Repeat the finger movements to confirm that you are not in the tendon.

Myth: A positive Finkelstein's test is the best maneuver for the diagnosis of deQuervain's tenosynovitis.

Reality: The Finkelstein's test is a venerable maneuver for the diagnosis of deQuervain's tenosynovitis. However, the test has limitations and can lead to false-positive results. For example, osteoarthritis of the first carpal-metacarpal joint often produces local pain on flexion of the thumb and abduction of the wrist, simulating a positive Finkelstein's test. The Intersection Syndrome is another condition that can result in a positive Finkelstein's test (Pantukosit et al. 2001).

The method of performing the Finkelstein's test has often been described erroneously in the literature (Elliott 1992). Finkelstein described the test as follows:"On grasping the patient's thumb and quickly abducting the hand ulnarward, the pain over the styloid tip is excruciating" (Finklelstein 1930). This account does not describe the thumb to be flexed in the palm with a fist being made over the thumb, as often misstated in the literature. In the correct maneuver, the fingers of the involved side are not flexed. The proper performance of this test helps decrease the number of false positives.

44.7 Hand

Pearl: Volar (palmar) flexor tenosynovitis is a common but often overlooked cause of hand pain that can be quite severe.

Comment: Inflammation of the flexor tendon sheaths in the palm is extremely common, but often goes unrecognized. The most common cause of volar flexor tenosynovitis is overuse trauma of the hands. Excessive gripping leads to increased pull on the flexor tendons. However, this tenosynovitis can also be part of inflammatory conditions such as rheumatoid arthritis, psoriatic arthritis, and apatite crystal deposition disease.

Flexor tenosynovitis of the palm is easily overlooked in the setting of PIP or MCP synovitis caused by an underlying arthritic condition, yet the tenosynovitis can be the dominant cause of pain and loss of motion in some patients. Pain in the palm generally occurs upon flexion of the involved digits, but is felt even at rest in severe cases. Patients seldom

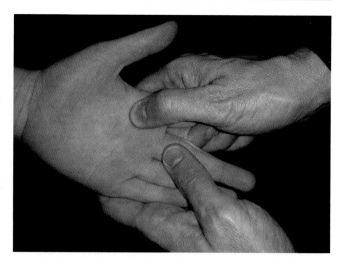

Fig. 44.7 Palpation of the tendon on the palmar surface of the hands, the key to diagnosing tendinitis of the flexor digitorum superficialis and flexor digitorum profundus tendons. Tendinitis of these tendons is a common cause of intense hand pain and is often underdiagnosed, in patients with underlying inflammatory disorders such as rheumatoid arthritis as well as health individuals. (Figure courtesy of Dr. John Stone)

volunteer a clear description of the pain's location. In some cases, the pain is reported as radiating to the PIP and MCP joints on the dorsal side, thus further misleading the examiner.

The only way to identify this condition properly is for the clinician to supinate the hand and palpate the palmar tendons directly (Fig. 44.7). The diagnosis is confirmed by the finding of localized tenderness that reproduces the patient's symptoms and usually swelling of the palmar tendon sheaths. Tenderness is usually present directly over the metacarpal heads or (more likely) just proximal to them. The middle and index fingers are affected most often, but the thumb, ring, and little fingers can also be involved.

Nodules composed of fibrous tissue can often be palpated in the palm just proximal to the MCP joint on the volar side. A nodule can interfere with the normal gliding of the tendon, leading to a triggering or locking (trigger finger). The symptoms of trigger finger are often intermittent and can produce an uncomfortable or even painful sensation. The presenting complaint may be a trigger finger, which can vary from mild triggering to severe. Trigger finger may emerge as a consequence of an earlier or evolving tenosynovitis, but volar flexor tenosynovitis can occur in the absence of triggering.

The technique for injection for volar flexor tenosynovitis is the following. The injection site is determined by careful palpation for tenderness, thickening, and possibly a nodule in one of more of the flexor tendons on the palmar surface. The site is generally about 0.5–2.0 cm proximal to the palmar digital crease. About 0.3 mL of methylprednisolone acetate and 0.3 mL of 2% lidocaine are drawn into two separate 1 mL tuberculin syringes, each of which has a 5/8 inch, 25-gauge needle. The needle with the lidocaine syringe is inserted into the skin at about a 30° angle, going from distal to proximal. About 0.1 mL of lidocaine is injected during the insertion of the needle, with the remainder injected at the lesion site, and then followed by the steroid injection from the separate syringe. The injection is performed parallel to the tendon sheath, avoiding penetration of the tendon itself.

Nodules cannot be injected because of too much back pressure, and the syringe may be knocked off the needle if attempted. A nodule may be bathed with the glucocorticoid in an attempt to decrease the size. When done properly, the procedure is relatively painless. Moreover, an immediate reduction in pain is effected in most cases, validating the diagnosis and the accuracy of the injection.

44.8 Coccyx

Pearl: Coccydynia can be treated successfully by a local injection.

Comment: Many physicians are reluctant to inject this area even in persistent cases of coccydynia, because of the delicate nature of the site involved. Yet the response to a glucocorticoid and lidocaine injection is often dramatic (Ramsey et al. 2003). Tenderness is typically present at the lower part of the coccyx. This bony area is the proper site to inject. The precise injection site is identified by careful palpation.

The patient lies prone and is draped appropriately. The area is cleaned well with alcohol wipes and providone-iodine. Topical and local forms of anesthesia are employed as described elsewhere in this chapter, and the two-syringe technique is used. The injection of 1–2 mL of lidocaine (2%) must be directed down to the coccyx, with the injection needle actually reaching bone. The periosteum of the coccyx is very sensitive and painful when stuck with a needle. Therefore, the approach to the bone is gradual and gentle. The location of the bony target should be maintained during the injection by continued palpation of the site with the index finger of the noninjecting hand. The needle remains at the site as the syringe is changed to one containing 40 mg of methylprednisolone, which is then distributed over the bony area. If the diagnosis of coccydynia is correct and the injection directed properly, lidocaine mediates immediate pain relief.

44.9 Leg Cramps

Pearl: Prophylactic stretching is the most effective treatment for calf cramps.

Comment: Nocturnal calf cramps, a frequent complaint of elderly patients, do not respond well to medications. Quinine-

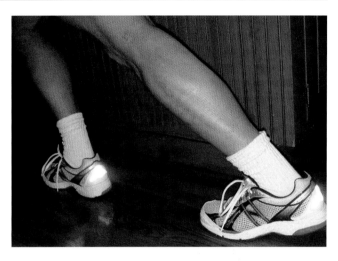

Fig. 44.8 The runner's stretch, for preventing nocturnal leg cramps. (Figure courtesy of Dr. John Stone)

containing compounds and various muscle relaxants are employed by some practitioners as therapy, but the benefits are mixed at best. Calf cramps are often attributed erroneously to hypokalemia, hypocalcemia, or other electrolyte disturbances. Such disturbances are rarely the true cause.

The best therapy for calf cramps is prophylactic stretching of the calf muscles. Many older people have unrecognized tightness of the gastrocnemius and soleus muscles. This muscle tightness can cause vague aching of the lower leg, in addition to being the major predisposing cause of cramps. The tight muscles, which may be acquired over a life time of not stretching, are easily palpable and observed to limit the degree of stretch of the calf.

The proper procedure for stretching the calves is to perform the "runner's stretch": i.e., to stand close to a wall and place one's outstretched hands on the wall. One foot is placed with the toe touching the wall and the other approximately 12–24 inches behind the heel of the front foot. The knee of the front leg is flexed inducing a stretch of the calf of the back leg, which is not flexed at all. Both feet can remain flat on the floor or the heel of the rear foot may be slightly raised (Fig. 44.8). The stretch should be gentle and prolonged, lasting for about 30 sec and repeated for a total of five repetitions on each leg. The stretching should be done nightly before bedtime.

Patients should also be instructed to dorsiflex the foot when a calf cramp occurs. This movement stretches the calf muscles and helps abort the cramp by countering the contraction of the gastrocnemius muscle.

44.10 Hip

Myth: The main pathology in trochanteric bursitis is in the bursa.

Reality: Like many syndromes that are misnamed, trochanteric bursitis is actually a tendinosis of the gluteal medius and/or gluteal minimus tendons. Several bursae are in the area, including the subgluteus medius and the sub-gluteus minimus bursae. These bursae can be involved secondarily, but tendinosis is the main problem. In some chronic cases, a partial or complete tear of these tendons may be present and can be demonstrated by MRI of the hip.

Myth: Trochanteric bursitis is an easy diagnosis to make.

Reality: Trochanteric bursitis is usually considered to be a straightforward diagnosis, characterized by lateral "hip" pain that is exacerbated by walking, lying on the involved side, and moving the proximal leg in various ways. The diagnosis is generally confirmed by the presence of tenderness on palpation over the trochanteric area. However, it is important to remember a few other problems that can cause pain in the trochanteric region.

Pain and point tenderness localized over the trochanteric region is not equivalent to bursitis in all cases. It may be the result of symptoms referred from degenerative arthritis in the lower back, particularly in the L4–5 and L5–S1 facet joints (Traycoff 1991). This type of referred pain is termed somatic, nonradicular referred pain. True radicular pain may be referred to the lateral hip, but is less likely to be localized only to the lateral hip.

An important reason to consider other possible diagnoses is that in 60% of patients with true hip joint pathology, pain emanating from the hip joint radiates not only to the anterior groin region but also to the greater trochanter area. True pain emanating from the hip joint can also be referred to the trochanteric region and can produce referred tenderness, as well.

Other conditions that can mimic the symptoms of trochanteric "bursitis" are fibromyalgia and unrecognized stress fractures, or even the rare impacted hip fracture, which is sometimes poorly seen on plain radiographs. If the diagnosis remains in doubt, the selective use of imaging studies (e.g., MRI or ultrasound) increases the accuracy of the diagnosis in this area, helping to identify tendinitis of the gluteus medius and minimus tendons, tendon tears, and bursal swelling.

None of these caveats and potential alternative diagnoses makes it unreasonable to inject trochanteric tenderness after an appropriate physical examination of the hip region. The injection can serve as both a diagnostic and therapeutic trial. However, not every case of putative trochanteric tenderness responds to the first injection. When it does not, the differential diagnosis must be revisited. In one series of 65 patients diagnosed with trochanteric bursitis, only two-thirds of the cases improved after the first injection (Schapira and Nahir 1986). The remaining one-third took more time and additional glucocorticoid injections.

Pearl: If a trochanteric bursa injection does not help the patient's trochanteric area pain, it may be referred as pain from piriformis syndrome.

Comment: A simple piriformis muscle injection will take care of it. Piriformis muscle is a fan-shaped muscle lying deep to the gluteal muscles. It originates from the lateral border of the sacrum and inserts on the greater trochanter. To inject the piriformis muscle, draw a straight line from the posterior superior iliac spine (the "dimple of Venus") to the greater trochanter. Palpate just lateral to the midpoint of this line. If the patient is very tender on this area, inject it with a 3-inch spinal needle using 3–6 cc of lidocaine.

44.11 Knee

Pearl: The knee is easiest and best joint on which joint injection techniques can be learned.

Comment: The knee joint is large and its surface anatomy landmarks are prominent. The neurovascular bundles, which are located on the lateral aspect of the popliteal fossa, are well removed from potential injection points (If you remember anything about embryology and the rotation of the limbs, then this makes sense; otherwise just accept it as fact).

Three different approaches – anterior, medial, and lateral – are used to inject the knee:

- The anterior approach places the patient in a seated position, with the knee flexed to 90° (Fig. 44.9). This approach is useful when the patient is unable to get onto the examining table easily, because the procedure can be performed with the patient seated in a chair. The anterior approach is also useful if no arthrocentesis is required for diagnostic purposes, but rather only an injection is needed for treatment. This is

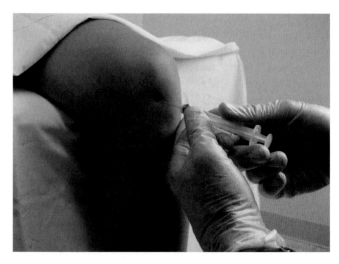

Fig. 44.9 The best way to inject (but not aspirate) a knee. (Figure courtesy of Dr. Ken Fye)

because with the patient positioned for an anterior approach, synovial fluid is forced posteriorly by knee flexion into the popliteal fossa, diminishing the likelihood of a successful joint aspiration. The anterior approach is a poor choice if the diagnosis is unclear and the acquisition of synovial fluid is essential. However, it is the simplest approach to injecting the knee with glucocorticoids or viscosupplementation treatments.

The ease and simplicity of the anterior approach for most knee joint injections cannot be overemphasized. This approach is valuable when there is only a minimal joint effusion (e.g., in osteoarthritis); when the knee is deformed by osteoarthritis, rendering the anatomy difficult; when the patient is morbidly obese and the landmarks around the knee are blunted; and when the patient comes to the clinic in a wheelchair and does not want to get onto the examination table.

Make the patient sit up on the edge of the chair or the examination table with the leg dangling down – foot not resting on ground – so as to open the joint space because of gravitational pull on the leg. Palpate the patellar border and the patellar tendon at the lower end of the patella (this is easily palpable even in morbidly obese patients when they are sitting up). Feel the two "soft spots" on either side of the patellar tendon, half an inch inferior to the lower end of patella. Enter the needle through either of these spots, perpendicular to the skin pointing to the center of the knee.

- The medial approach (Fig. 44.10) has the best landmarks and is easily accessed when the patient is in bed with the hips externally rotated. This approach is preferred when obtaining synovial fluid is essential for the purposes of diagnosis.
- The lateral approach is the essential back-up approach if the medial approach fails to produce fluid.

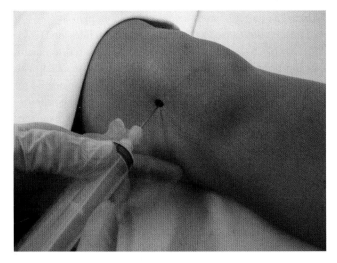

Fig. 44.10 The medial approaches to aspirating the knee. (Figure courtesy of Dr. Ken Fye)

Pearl: A dry tap medially is insufficient to exclude a septic knee.

Comment: If sepsis is suspected, a dry tap through the medial approach is insufficient to exclude infection. Some congenital and acquired variations in anatomy can block aspiration. If no synovial fluid is obtained via the medial approach, then a second attempt via the lateral approach is appropriate. The joint cavity is closer to the skin surface on the lateral side. Thus, any effusion present might be easier to aspirate. A true dry tap virtually rules out septic arthritis.

A study of knee injections and aspirations in patients who did not have a large effusion to guide the operator showed that even experienced operators missed the knee joint 20% of the time (Jackson and Evans 2002). Aspects of chronic synovitis frequently conspire to create "dry tap" situations as shown in the last three images of the figure. The lateral approach for knee aspiration is more successful when one gets an assistant to displace the patella slightly (Anderson 2005).

Pearl: If at first one does not succeed in tapping a knee, think "anatomy."

Comment: When attempting to tap or inject a knee via either the medial or lateral approach, the clinician often strikes bone immediately after entering the joint. In this setting, take a step back and remember the anatomy of the patella. The inferior aspect of this bone is V-shaped (remember its shape on sunrise radiographic view). Thus, the clinician's needle is probably striking the side of the patella, confounding attempts to withdraw fluid. The needle should be partly withdrawn (but not removed entirely) and redirected at a steeper angle in order to attain the retropatellar space.

Myth: In anserine bursitis, the main pathology is bursal inflammation.

Reality: The pes anserinus (Latin for "goose foot") is composed of the conjoined tendons of the sartorius, gracilis, and semitendinosus muscles. The bursa extends between the tendons and the tibial collateral ligament. Although some cases of bursal involvement with swelling have been documented, the pain from this region is more likely to emanate from the entheses in this region, the sites of attachment of the three tendons to the bone.

At the insertion of the pes anserinus on the anterior tibia, the sartorius is the most proximal and anterior tendon (Fig. 44.11). The gracilis lies slightly distal and posterior, and the semitendinosus lies most posterior and distal. One possible mechanism leading to anserine bursitis is the repeated stress on the pes anserinus that occurs in going from a sitting to a standing position. This stress is particularly severe in a person with osteoarthritis of the knees and weakness of the quadriceps. Pain occurs in the pes anserinus region when a patient with poor flexibility of the hips and

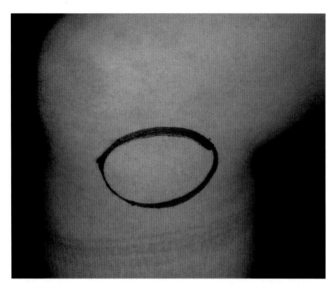

Fig. 44.11 The site of the anserine bursa. Inflammation of this area is often misdiagnosed as "degenerative arthritis" of the knee. (Figure courtesy of Dr. John Stone)

knees climbs stairs. Failure of these joints to flex fully places greater strain on the tendons of the pes anserinus.

A glucocorticoid injection helps anserine bursitis acutely, but the longer term solution lies in physical therapy exercises designed to improve muscle strength and joint flexibility.

Pearl: Anserine bursitis is the major cause of knee pain in some patients with osteoarthritis of the knee.

Comment: Anserine bursitis frequently occurs concomitantly with knee osteoarthritis but is frequently overlooked. Once osteoarthritis of the knee has been diagnosed, it is often blamed for any symptomatology in this region. In many cases, however, anserine bursitis is the principal source of pain. The diagnosis of anserine bursitis is made by eliciting exquisite tenderness to palpation over the pes anserinus.

This area is normally somewhat sensitive to pressure, and care must be exerted to compare the tenderness on one side with that of the opposite leg. The patients are asked the question that is central to all musculoskeletal evaluations: "Is this the same pain as the one that is bothering you?" This diagnosis may be validated by the remission of "knee" pain following the infiltration of approximately 1 mL of lidocaine (2%) into the pes anserinus area. Treatment consists of a glucocorticoid injection, quadriceps strengthening, and stretching of the muscles of the involved tendons.

44.12 Ankle

Pearl: If at first you do not succeed at ankle arthrocentesis, think "anatomy."

Comment: If the needle hits the bone immediately after entering the ankle joint, it is most likely to touch the dome of the talus. Ankle joint is formed by the concave lower end of the tibia and the convex dome of the talus. The commonest mistake that happens is to direct the needle toward the heel, which would touch the talus. Redirecting the needle cephalad (away from the heel, upwards, toward tibia) will enable you to enter the space under the concave inferior surface of the tibia.

Pearl: Heel pain that occurs upon the first step out of bed in the morning is plantar fasciitis.

Comment: Plantar fasciitis is characterized by pain on the plantar surface of the heel. The history is the key to accuracy in diagnosis: clear identification of the specific site of the pain must be extracted from the patient. The pain characteristically occurs in the morning upon arising and is most severe for the first few steps. Thus, it is known as "first step pain." The heel pain then generally lessens after the patient has been on his or her feet for 30 s or so. After this initial improvement, the pain may return later in the day, particularly after prolonged standing or walking.

The symptoms of plantar fasciitis can cause bitter complaints. Physical examination often reveals anteromedial tenderness on the sole of the foot, over the medial calcaneal tubercle at the origin of the plantar fascia (Fig. 44.12).

Pearl: Plantar fasciitis can be treated effectively with a glucocorticoid injection.

Comment: Many clinicians are reluctant to inject plantar fasciitis. This is usually because of uncertainty with regard to the proper approach or concern about causing too much pain. Other clinicians worry about the potential for inducing atrophy of the subcutaneous heel fat pad. The proper site for injection is several millimeters proximal to the distal edge of the calcaneus and several millimeters toward the medial aspect. The target is often tender on deep palpation.

The area is cleansed and anesthetized with lidocaine (2%). A 1.5 inch, 25-gauge needle generally is required to ensure that the periosteal region of the calcaneus is reached. The bony tissue of the calcaneus must be felt with the needle tip to ensure that the injection is performed beneath the subcutaneous tissues. In addition, the fascial fibers involved are those that are attached to the bone itself. The patient can expect immediate relief of pain if the diagnosis is correct and the injection is accurate.

Pearl: A unilateral flat foot may be due to a rupture of the posterior tibialis tendon.

Comment: A progressive flat foot, especially a unilateral one, is often due to the rupture of the posterior tibialis tendon (Churchhill and Sferra 1998). This diagnosis is often overlooked. Trauma or chronic tendon degeneration can cause

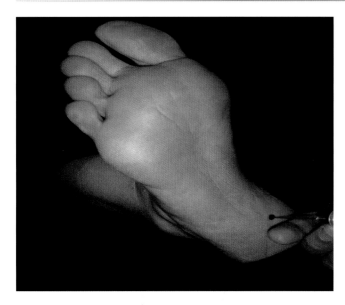

Fig. 44.12 Site of injection of plantar fasciitis. (Figure courtesy of Dr. John Stone)

this tendon to tear. Rheumatoid arthritis is another common culprit.

With rupture of the posterior tibialis tendon, insidious pain and tenderness is noted along the course of the tendon just distal to the medial malleolus. Medial swelling of the hindfoot is also evident. In the setting of a ruptured posterior tibialis tendon, the patient cannot rise onto the ball of the affected foot if the contralateral foot is off the floor (single heel lift test).

Pearl: Aspirating any fluid from the 1st MTP joint in a patient with gout can be difficult. Here are two strategies to increase your success rate of getting a sample out of the MTP joint to look for crystals.

Comment: Use intra-articular anesthetic injection first. This will allow for better positioning, landmark identification, and sometimes one is able to aspirate back the injected anesthetic and identify crystals in that drop of fluid.

Even if no frank fluid is aspirated, the answer may already lie in the needle tip or hub. Tap the contents of the needle, small though they may be, onto a glass slide. This may reveal enough fluid for a diagnostic analysis of crystals.

References

Anderson BC. Guide to arthrocentesis and soft tissue injection. Philadephia: Elsevier Saunders; 2005. p. 132

Atroshi E, Gummesson C, Ornstein E, et al Carpal tunnel syndrome and keyboard use at work: a population study. Arthritis Rheum. 2007;56:3620–5

Canoso JJ. Bursae, tendons and ligaments. Clin Rheum Dis. 1981;7: 189–221

Charalambous CP, Tryfonidis M, Sadiq S, et al Septic arthritis following intra-articular glucocorticoid injection of the knee – a survey of current practice regarding antiseptic technique used during intra-articular glucocorticoid injection of the knee. Clin Rheumatol. 2003;22:386–90

Chard MD, Hazleman R, Hazleman BL, et al Shoulder disorders in the elderly: a community survey. Arthritis Rheum. 1991;34:766–9

Churchhill RS, Sferra JJ. Posterior tibial tendon insufficiency: its diagnosis, management, and treatment. Am J Orthop. 1998;27:339–47

Drendorf H, Mollmann H, Gruner A, et al Pharmacokinetics and pharmacodynamics of glucocorticoid suspensions after intra-articular administration. Clin Pharmacol Ther. 1986;39:313–7

Elliott BG. Finkelstein's test: a descriptive error that can produce a false positive. J Hand Surg Eur Vol. 1992;17:481–2

Finklelstein H. Stenosing tenovaginitis at the radial styloid process. J Bone Joint Surg. 1930;12:509–40

Gardner GC. Teaching arthrocentesis and injection techniques: what is the best way to get our point across? J Rheumatol. 2007;34:1448–50

Gottleib NL, Penneys NS, Brown HEJR. Periarticular perilymphatic skin atrophy after intra-articular corticosteroid injections. JAMA. 1978;240:559–60

Graif M, Martinoli C, Rochkind S, et al Sonographic evaluation of brachial plexus pathology. Eur. Radiol. 2004;14:193–200

Halverson PB, Cheung HS, McCarty DJ et al "Milwaukee shoulder": Association of microspheroids containing hydroxyapatite crystals, active collagenase, and neutral protease with rotator cuff defects. II. Synovial fluid studies. Arthritis Rheum 1981;24:474–83

Hollander JL. Intrasynovial corticosteroid therapy: a decade of use. Bull Rheum Dis. 1961;11:239–40

Hollister MS, Mack LA, Patten RM, et al Association of sonographjcally detected subacromial/subdeltoid bursal effusion and intraarticular fluid with rotator cuff tear. Am J. Roent. 1995;165:605–8

Hughes GM, Biundo JJ, Scheib JS, et al Pseudogout and Pseudosepsis of the shoulder. Orthopedics 1990;13:1169–72

Jackson DW, Evans NA. Thomas: accuracy of needle placement into the intra-articular space of the knee. J Bone Joint Surg Am. 2002; 84A:1522–7

Kerolus G, Clayburne G, Schumacher HR. Is it mandatory to examine synovial fluids promptly after arthrocentesis? Arthritis Rheum. 1989;32:271–8

Kessell L. A colour atlas of rupture of the rotator cuff. Netherlands: Wolfe Medical; 1986. p.22

Khan KM, Cook JL, Kannus P, et al Time to abandon the tendinitis "myth" (Editorial). BMJ. 2002;324:626–7

Kim HA, Kim SH, Seo Y. Ultrasonographic findings of the shoulder in patients with rheumatoid arthritis and comparison with physical examination. J Korean Med Sci. 2007;22:660–6

Mimoz O, Karim A, Mercat A, Cosseron M, Falissard B, Parker F, Richard C, Samii K, Nordmann P. Chlorhexidine compared with povidone-iodine as skin preparation before blood culture. A randomized, controlled trial. Ann Intern Med. 1999 ;131(11):834–7

Misamore GW, Lehman DE. Parsonage–Turner syndrome (acute brachial neuritis). J Bone Joint Surg. 1996;78-A:1405–8

Neer CS, Craig EV, Fukuda H. Cuff-tear arthropathy. J Bone Joint Surg. 1983;65:1232–44

Palmer KT, Harris EC, Coggon D. Carpal tunnel syndrome and its relation to occupation: a systematic literature review. Occup Med. 2007;57:57–66

Pantukosit S, Petchkrua W, Stiens SA. Intersection syndrome in Buriram hospital: a 4-yr. prospective study. Am J Phys Med Rehabil. 2001; 80:656–61

Petri M, Dombrow R, Brower R, et al Randomized double-blind placebo controlled study of the treatment of the painful shoulder. Arthritis Rheum. 1987;30:1040–5

Raddatz DA Hoffman GS, Franck WA. Septic bursitis: presentation, treatment and prognosis. J Rheumatol. 1987;14:1160–3

Ramsey ML, Toohey JS, Neidre A, et al Coccygodynia: treatment. Orthopedics 2003;26:403–5

Smith DL, McAfee JH, Lucas LM, et al Septic and Nonseptic olecranon bursitis: utility of the surface temperature probe in the early differentiation of septic and nonseptic cases. Arch Intern Med. 1989;149:1581–5

Schapira D, Nahir M, Scharf Y. Trochanteric bursitis: a common clinical problem. Arch Phys Med Rehabil. 1986;67(11):815–7

Sofka CM, Adler RS. Sonography of cubital bursitis. AJR. 2004;183: 51–3

Traycoff RB. Pseudotrochanteric bursitis. The differential diagnosis of lateral hip pain. J Rheumatol. 1991;18:1810–2

Weiss JJ, Thompson GR, Doust V, et al Rotator Cuff Tears in Rheumatoid Arthritis. Arch Intern Med. 1975;135:521–525

Zimmermann B, Mikolich DJ, Ho G Jr. Septic bursitis. Semin Arthritis Rheum. 1995;24:391–10

Low Back and Neck Pain

45

Rajiv K. Dixit and Joseph H. Schwab

45.1 Overview

> Low back pain is the most common musculoskeletal complaint. An estimated 80% of the population will experience low back pain over the course of their lifetime.

> The surgical treatment of common lumbar disorders accounts for over $20 billion as hospital fees each year in the United States.

> The rate of procedures directed at the lumbar spine is increasing faster than the aging of the population. Yet, the indications for and the efficacy of surgical interventions for common lumbar disorders have been a source of controversy.

> Low back pain affects the area between the lower rib cage and gluteal folds, and frequently radiates into the thighs.

> Neck pain is also a common complaint, affecting approximately 70% of the population at some time in their lives. Neck pain typically affects the posterior aspect of the neck and frequently radiates into the shoulder blades and deltoid muscles, even in the absence of nerve root or spinal cord involvement.

> An understanding of the basic anatomy of the spine is essential for the diagnosis and management of lower back and neck conditions (Fig. 45.1).

> Randomized trials have evaluated the surgical management of lumbar herniated discs, lumbar spinal stenosis, and lumbar spondylolisthesis with stenosis. These trials have improved our ability to advise patients regarding the expectations of nonoperative vs. operative management.

> Spinal stenosis is caused by encroachment upon the spinal nerves by bulging intervertebral discs, hypertrophied facet capsules, osteophytes, and bulging ligamentum flavum.

> Some individuals are predisposed to spinal stenosis by virtue of congenitally narrowed spinal canals.

45.2 General Considerations

Myth: Patients with low back pain never get better.

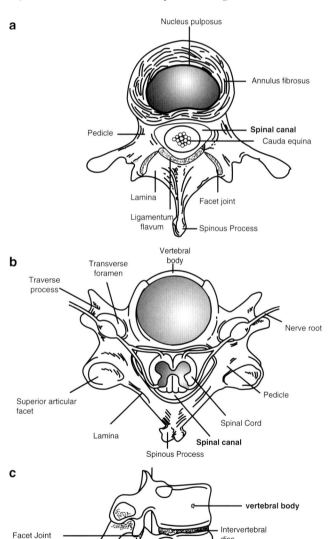

Fig. 45.1 Schematic representation of the superior aspect of a lumbar vertebra (**a**), mid-cervical vertebra (**b**), and a lateral view of the spine (**c**)

J. H. Stone (ed.), *A Clinician's Pearls and Myths in Rheumatology,*
DOI:10.1007/978-1-84800-934-9_45, © Springer Science + Business Media B.V. 2009

Reality: Approximately 90% of patients with acute low back pain improve spontaneously within 4 weeks. The problem is the 5–7% of patients who develop a chronic low back pain syndrome.

Myth: Surgery is the final common pathway in the management of low back pain.

Reality: The vast majority (>85%) of patients with low back pain have transient symptoms. In fact, most will not seek medical attention at all. Those patients who do seek medical attention often respond to activity modification, over-the-counter pain medications, and time.

The surgical treatment of low back pain without neurologic symptoms is controversial. Two prospective, randomized clinical trials have evaluated the efficacy of lumbar fusion surgery for low back pain (Fritzell et al. 2001; Brox et al. 2003). The first study included 294 patients from 19 medical centers in Sweden, enrolled over a 6-year period (Fritzell et al. 2001). The patients enrolled had low back pain without evidence of nerve root compression. All had tried conservative management before trial entry. Patients were randomized into one of four groups, including three groups that received spinal fusion by different methods and one nonoperative group. At 2 years, an independent observer found that the surgical group had "excellent or good" results in 46% of cases, compared with 18% for the nonoperative group. The surgical group was statistically superior to the nonoperative group with regard to pain, disability, and return to work status.

The major criticism of this study was the method by which the conservative group was treated. The patients in that group had already failed conservative treatment yet were randomized to receive additional conservative therapy. This flaw biases the trial results in favor of surgery. However, proponents of surgery cite the trial as evidence that fusion surgery is a viable option for patients whose clinical features fit that of patients enrolled in this study: low back pain without evidence of nerve root compression.

A second prospective, randomized trial compared lumbar fusion followed by postoperative physical therapy with a "modern" rehabilitation program that featured intensive exercise sessions guided by principles of cognitive/behavioral therapy (Brox et al. 2003). This trial revealed no differences between the two treatment modalities with regard to pain, disability, or return to work.

At this point, broad conclusions based on the current literature are not possible. A well-designed trial is needed to shed more light on the optimal management of this common clinical problem.

Myth: Low back pain that radiates into the lower extremities probably represents sciatica.

Reality: In the vast majority of patients who have low back pain that radiates into the lower extremities, the pain arises from pathology within the disc, facet joints, or paraspinal muscles and ligaments (Dixit and Dickson 2008). This pain is said to be "sclerotomal," and it is not neurogenic in nature.

In contrast to the pain caused by sciatica, sclerotomal pain is nondermatomal in distribution and dull in quality. It does not radiate below the knee and is not associated with paraesthesias. Sciatica results from nerve root compression and is generally caused by a herniated disc. This produces lancinating pain that has a dermatomal distribution. Sciatica typically radiates below the knee and may be accompanied by sensory and motor deficits.

Pearl: The vast majority of patients with low back pain have a mechanical cause.

Comment: More than 95% of low back pain is mechanical (Deyo and Weinstein 2001). Degenerative changes, sometimes termed as lumbar spondylosis, occur in both the intervertebral disc and facet joint. These are the most important causes of mechanical low back pain.

Systemic disorders, which include malignancies, infections, and the seronegative spondyloarthropathies, account for only 1% of patients with low back pain. Nonsystemic visceral disease accounts for only 2%. A patient with normal blood cell counts, erythrocyte sedimentation rate, and radiographs of the lumbar spine is unlikely to have an underlying systemic disease as the cause of low back pain.

Myth: A careful evaluation yields a definitive pathoanatomic diagnosis in most patients with low back pain.

Reality: Eighty percent of patients who present with low back pain defy a clear-cut pathoanatomic diagnosis. This is largely because of the weak association between symptoms and the findings on imaging studies. Imaging abnormalities, often the result of age-related degenerative changes, are frequently present even in healthy individuals who are entirely asymptomatic. Conversely, some patients with severe low back pain have minimal findings on imaging studies. Furthermore, even when one is certain that the cause of low back pain is lumbar spondylosis, identification of the "pain generator" is challenging. The precise disc or discs or facet joint or joints responsible for the patient's pain is difficult to localize.

Myth: Strain and sprain are common, well-defined causes of low back pain.

Reality: The diagnostic uncertainty with regard to low back pain has resulted in the use of nonspecific terms such as "strain," "sprain," and "lumbago." These terms have never been characterized anatomically or histologically. Therefore, idiopathic low back pain is perhaps a more accurate label for these patients who have a mostly self-limited syndrome of back pain.

45.3 History and Physical Examination

Pearl: Careful history taking helps differentiate mechanical causes of low back pain from inflammatory etiologies.

Comment: Mechanical low back pain is due to an anatomic or functional abnormality that is not associated with inflammatory or neoplastic disease. Mechanical low back pain typically increases with physical activity and upright posture, and is relieved by rest and recumbency. Nonmechanical low back pain, especially when accompanied by nocturnal pain, suggests the possibility of an underlying infection or neoplasm.

Inflammatory causes of low back pain such as ankylosing spondylitis are associated with marked morning stiffness that lasts for more than 30 min. The pain frequently improves with exercise but not with rest. Pain is often worse during the second half of the night. Some patients complain of alternating buttock pain (Rudwaleit et al. 2006).

Pearl: Physical examination can often differentiate structural from functional scoliosis.

Comment: Scoliosis is associated with structural changes of the vertebral column and sometimes the rib cage, as well. In adults, structural scoliosis is usually secondary to degenerative changes, although some individuals have a history of adolescent idiopathic scoliosis. With forward flexion, structural scoliosis persists. In contrast, in functional scoliosis, which usually results from a paravertebral muscle spasm or leg length discrepancy, usually disappears.

Pearl: Neurologic evaluation of the lower extremities in a patient with sciatica can identify the specific nerve root involved.

Comment: The nucleus pulposus in a degenerated disc may prolapse and push out the weakened annulus. This usually occurs in a posterolateral direction. Evidence of disc herniation is commonly observed in many asymptomatic adults, but sometimes, this herniation leads to nerve root impingement (Fig. 45.2). In general, the more caudal nerve root is impinged by the herniated disc; that is, the L5 nerve root is impinged by an L4–5 herniation, and the S1 nerve root by an L5–S1 herniation. Neurologic evaluation of the lower extremities including motor testing, reflex testing, and tests for dermatomal sensory loss help to identify the specific nerve root involved (Fig. 45.3).

Pearl: Organs that share segmental innervation with the spine may refer pain to the spine.

Comment: Pelvic diseases can refer pain to the sacral area; lower abdominal diseases to the lumbar area; and upper abdominal diseases to the lower thoracic spine. However, in such cases, local signs of disease such as tenderness to palpation, paravertebral muscle spasm, and increased pain on spinal motion are absent.

Pearl: The focus of the initial evaluation is to identify the few patients with systemic disease or significant neurologic involvement.

Comment: Patients with underlying systemic disorders or incipient neurological involvement may require specific interventions on an urgent basis; e.g., antibiotics for

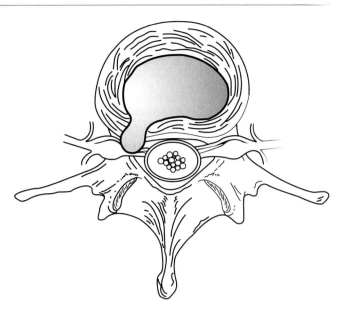

Fig. 45.2 Posterolateral disc herniation resulting in nerve root impingement

Lower Extremity Dermatomes	Disc	Nerve Root	Motor Loss	Sensory Loss	Reflex Loss
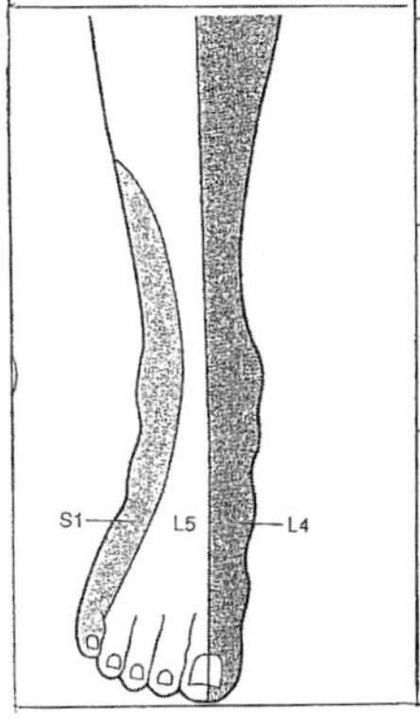	L3-4	L4	Foot Dorsiflexion	Medial Foot	Knee
	L4-5	L5	Great-toe Dorsiflexion	Dorsal Foot	None
	L5-S1	S1	Foot Plantarflexion	Lateral Foot	Ankle

Fig. 45.3 Neurologic evaluation of the lower extremities including motor testing, reflex testing, and tests for dermatomal sensory loss help to identify the specific nerve root involved

vertebral osteomyelitis or surgical decompression for the cauda equina syndrome.

In the rest of the patients with low back pain (>95% of all comers with low back pain), the precise pathoanatomic cause cannot be determined or when it is determined, no specific treatment is available. These patients are managed conservatively along similar lines, at least initially.

Pearl: Pseudoclaudication can be distinguished from claudication by elements of the history.

Comment: "Pseudoclaudication" refers to the nonvascular origin of pain that occurs in the legs during walking but not at rest. Pseudoclaudication is also known as neurogenic claudication. This condition is caused by spinal stenosis. Lumbar MRI studies can reveal spinal stenosis clearly, and arterial Doppler studies are a reliable way of documenting peripheral arterial insufficiency or confirming adequate blood flow. Nevertheless, astute clinical judgment is required to interpret the results of such studies in light of the patient's symptoms. Radiologic abnormalities often translate into findings of trivial clinical importance.

The pain from neurogenic claudication is usually located in the buttocks and hamstrings. Vascular claudication, in contrast, is more likely to be reported as calf symptoms and may be relieved by a 5 min period of rest that restores the tissue oxygen balance. This makes the time course more similar to that of coronary angina than to neurogenic claudication. Neurogenic claudication is also relieved by rest and diminished by forward flexion, but complete relief may take longer (10–20 min) because the symptoms are allegedly related to physical compression of small vessels on the surface of the cord. The classic patient report in neurogenic claudication is of improvement that accompanies bending over to push a grocery cart.

The presence of hair on the toes, which indicates good local blood supply, makes a vascular etiology of the patient's complaint less likely. However, the simplest physical examination maneuver to distinguish between neurogenic and vascular claudication is to feel the dorsalis pedis pulse. If the pulse is present, then vascular claudication is unlikely. Unfortunately, expensive imaging studies are ordered even before the peripheral pulses are palpated.

45.4 Imaging

Pearl: Diagnostic testing is rarely indicated in patients with low back pain unless symptoms persist beyond 6 weeks.

Comment: Early imaging studies are required in the small proportion of patients who have evidence of a significant or progressive neurologic deficit and those in whom an underlying systemic disease is suspected as the cause of low back pain (Chou et al. 2007). Table 45.1 lists the features ("red flags") that suggest the underlying systemic disease or serious neurological involvement.

However, the great majority of patients with low back pain do not need early imaging. Ninety percent of patients with low back pain recover spontaneously within 4 weeks and will do so irrespective of whether or not they have had lumbosacral radiographs or an MRI. The careful selection of patients for imaging studies avoids unnecessary testing and the cascade of follow-up studies that can result from the finding of "incidentalomas." It is worth noting that radiation exposure to the female gonads from standard views of the

lumbar spine is equivalent to that of a daily chest radiograph for several years (Jarvik and Deyo 2002).

Myth: Imaging evaluation usually helps to identify the precise cause of low back pain.

Reality: A major problem with all imaging modalities is that many of the anatomic abnormalities identified are common in asymptomatic individuals. These abnormalities, usually the result of age-related degenerative changes, may have no relationship whatsoever to the patient's chief complaint.

Degenerative changes in the spine are among the earliest degenerative changes observed in the body. They frequently begin appearing in early adult life. Abnormalities such as single disc degeneration, facet joint degeneration, Schmorl's nodes, spondylolysis, mild spondylolisthesis, transitional vertebrae (the "lumbarization" of S1 or "sacralization" of L5), spina bifida occulta, and mild scoliosis are equally prevalent in persons without low back pain as they are in patients who have low back symptoms. Thus, the exercise of making causal inferences based on imaging abnormalities in the absence of corresponding clinical findings is hazardous, and leads to unnecessary and costly interventions.

Myth: An MRI study is appropriate for all patients with significant acute back pain.

Reality: An MRI is not indicated in the evaluation of acute low back pain. Several reasons justify restraint in the ordering of these studies. First of all, the vast majority of patients with this complaint have self-limiting episodes that require no intervention. Moreover, an MRI is likely to detect multiple "abnormalities" that have no relationship to the patient's complaints. Knowledge of these "findings" is not helpful in managing the patient and indeed can be counterproductive

Table 45.1 Red flags

Symptom or condition	Potential diagnosis
Severe morning stiffness	Spondyloarthropathy
Pain improves with exercise, not rest	
Pain during second half of night	
Alternating buttock pain	
Urinary incontinence	Cauda equina syndrome
Overflow incontinence	
Fecal incontinence	
Bilateral or progressive motor deficit	
Saddle anesthesia	
Age > 50 years	Cancer or infection
History of cancer	
Unexplained weight loss	
Immunosuppression	
Injection drug use	
Nocturnal pain	
Elderly	Fracture
Prolonged glucocorticoid use	
Recent trauma	

for a variety of reasons, not the least of which is that some patients fixate on such "abnormalities."

If a patient's symptoms and signs suggest the possibility of a systemic disease, then plain radiographs and simple laboratory tests are more helpful as first steps in defining the etiology (Jarvik and Deyo 2002).

Pearl: Imaging is warranted in a patient with low back pain without radiculopathy when the patient's clinical profile is worrisome for an inflammatory, infectious, or malignant process.

Comment: Patients older than 50 years of age who have low back pain that persists for more than 6 weeks should have plain radiographs performed (Jarvik and Deyo 2002). In that setting, infections and malignancies must be excluded as causes of the patient's symptoms. A radiograph should be the first study, as it provides a significant amount of information at relatively low cost (Chou et al. 2007). By viewing a plain radiograph first, an experienced clinician can gain a sense of the patient's bone stock, evaluate the spinal alignment, detect gross bony destruction, and assess for spinal instability. Additional imaging may be appropriate based on the findings on plain radiography.

Pearl: Imaging is warranted in the case of low back pain with radiculopathy when the symptoms have persisted for more than 6 weeks and the patient is a candidate for an intervention such as an injection or surgery.

Comment: Low back pain with radiculopathy is caused commonly by herniated lumbar intervertebral discs. If a patient's symptoms persist and the patient is a candidate for an epidural glucocorticoid injection, then an MRI should be performed. The clinician must carefully correlate any imaging findings with the patient's history and physical examination before recommending an intervention.

Pearl: Cross-sectional imaging studies of the spine are vastly overused.

Comment: MRI and computed tomographic (CT) studies of the spine should be reserved for patients in whom there is a clinical suspicion of underlying infection or cancer, and for patients who are surgical candidates on clinical grounds (e.g., the presence of a significant or progressive neurologic deficit). MRI is generally the preferred modality for low back imaging because it is more sensitive for infections and metastatic cancer. When bony anatomy is critical, CT is preferable.

Pearl: Disc bulges and herniations are commonly identified by CT and MRI studies, even in asymptomatic adults.

Comment: Disc abnormalities, such as bulges or herniations, protrusions or extrusions, often have little to no relationship with the patient's symptoms. One should interpret these "abnormalities" cautiously.

A bulge is a symmetrical, circumferential extension of the disc material beyond the interspace. A herniation is a focal or asymmetric extension of the disc bulge. Herniations are classified according to whether they are protrusions or extrusions. Protrusions are broad-based. In contrast, extrusions have a "neck," so that the base is narrower than the extruded material. Bulges (52%) and protrusions (27%) are common in asymptomatic adults but extrusions (1%) are rare (Jarvik and Deyo 2002).

45.5 Disc Herniation

Pearl: A negative straight leg raise (SLR) test makes a clinically significant lumbar disc herniation unlikely.

Comment: SLR places tension on the sciatic nerve roots (L4, L5, S1, S2, S3). If any of these nerve roots is irritated such as by impingement from a herniated disc (see Fig. 45.2), further tension on the nerve root by SLR will result in radicular pain that extends below the knee.

The great majority of clinically significant disc herniations occur at L4–5 or L5–S1. The SLR test is very sensitive (95%) but not specific (40%) for clinically significant disc herniations. False-negative tests can be observed at herniations above the L4–5 level. The crossed SLR test, with sciatica reproduced when the opposite leg is raised, is insensitive (25%) but highly specific (90%) for disc herniation (Dixit 2007). The SLR is usually negative in patients with spinal stenosis.

Pearl: Bladder incontinence in a patient with sciatica makes the exclusion of a cauda equina syndrome imperative.

Comment: Cauda equina syndrome usually occurs from a centrally herniated disc (usually L4–5) that compresses the cauda equina. It can also develop secondary to compression by neoplasia, abscess, or hematoma. Cauda equina syndrome is a true surgical emergency because the neurological results are affected by the time to decompression. Patients usually present with unilateral or bilateral sciatica and motor deficits. Sensory loss in the perineum (saddle anesthesia) is common. Urinary retention with overflow incontinence is usually present.

Myth: If a patient has clinical and radiographic evidence of radiculopathy from herniated disk, surgery should be performed to relieve the pain.

Reality: Several prospective, randomized trials have compared surgery with nonoperative management for the treatment of herniated lumbar discs (Weinstein et al. 2006a; Weinstein et al. 2006b; Peul et al. 2007). These trials have shown that surgery improves leg pain and function more quickly than does nonoperative management. However, over time, the differences between the two treatment approaches disappear.

These data have been taken by some to mean that surgery is never indicated for disc herniation leading to radiculopathy. Such a conclusion, however, is not correct in all cases. The value of more rapid improvement in pain and function must be balanced against the risks of surgery. For some patients, depending on a variety of individual circumstances, the decision to undergo surgery is justified. For others, nonoperative management is more appropriate.

Myth: There is never an indication for acute surgical management of a herniated lumbar disc.

Comment: Compression of sacral nerve roots by a herniated disc can cause a cauda equina syndrome. The most sensitive symptom of cauda equina syndrome is urinary retention, which is often followed by overflow urinary incontinence. Bowel dysfunction and saddle anesthesia are also hallmarks of cauda equina syndrome. A cauda equina syndrome is a surgical emergency.

A relative indication for surgical decompression is a significant loss of motor function in the distribution of the compressed nerve. For instance, if a patient is unable to dorsiflex the foot against gravity, surgery may be considered more acutely. The word "considered" is important in that last sentence, because no good studies have examined the effect of surgery in patients with significant motor dysfunction. Such patients have been excluded deliberately from clinical trials because of ethical concerns.

45.6 Spinal Stenosis

Myth: Radicular symptoms indicate a herniated disc.

Reality: Patients with spinal stenosis can also have radicular leg pain. Severe neurological deficits are rarely seen in spinal stenosis, and the physical examination is usually unimpressive. Unsteadiness of gait is a frequent complaint in patients with spinal stenosis. The lumbar component of pain is frequently mild. Lumbar range of motion may be normal.

Making the diagnosis is all about taking a good history: listening to the patient and asking the right questions. The diagnosis is confirmed most easily by MRI.

Myth: Lumbar spinal stenosis is rare.

Reality: Lumbar spinal stenosis is defined as a narrowing of the spinal canal, its lateral recesses, and neural foramina that may result in compression of neural structures.

As many as 20% of asymptomatic adults aged 60 years or older have imaging evidence of spinal stenosis (Jarvik and

Table 45.2 Acquired and congenital causes of lumbar spinal stenosis

Acquired causes
Degenerative
Hypertrophy of the facet joints
Hypertrophy of the ligamentum flavum
Disc herniation
Spondylolisthesis
Iatrogenic
Postlaminectomy
Postsurgical fusion
Miscellaneous
Paget's disease
Diffuse idiopathic skeletal hyperostosis
Fluorosis
Congenital causes
Achondroplastic
Idiopathic

Deyo 2002). However, the prevalence of symptomatic stenosis is unknown.

Pearl: Degenerative changes in the spine are the cause of lumbar spinal stenosis in the vast majority of cases (Table 45.2).

Comment: Any herniation of a degenerated disc will narrow the anterior part of the spinal canal and a hypertrophied degenerated facet joint may result in a narrowing of the lateral recess or intervertebral foramen. Intervertebral discs lose vertical height as they degenerate. This can result in a buckling of the now redundant, and often hypertrophied, ligamentum flavum resulting in a narrowing of the posterior aspect of the spinal canal. Thus, a series of degenerative changes in the spinal column lead to spinal stenosis.

Pearl: The hallmark of spinal stenosis is pseudoclaudication (neurogenic claudication).

Comment: Patients with pseudoclaudication often have bilateral symptoms of pain, weakness, and sometimes paresthesias in the buttocks, thighs, and legs. These symptoms are induced by standing or walking, but relieved by sitting or flexing forward. Forward flexion increases the canal diameter and may lead to the adoption of a simian stance. Factors that favor a diagnosis of pseudoclaudication over vascular claudication include the preservation of pedal pulses, provocation of symptoms by standing just as readily as by walking, and localization of the maximal discomfort to the thighs rather than to the calves.

Myth: Spinal stenosis is purely a radiographic diagnosis.

Reality: Clinical spinal stenosis is manifested as neurogenic claudication. Pain radiates into the buttocks and often down into the lower leg. Pain is worsened by spinal extension and relieved by flexion. The so-called "shopping cart sign" is a useful means by which to assess for neurogenic claudication: many people with spinal stenosis find that they can walk much further while leaning forward, as when pushing a shopping cart.

The reason for this improvement is not entirely clear. One theory is that the spinal canal dimensions are increased when the spine is flexed forward. Another theory is that venous congestion along the spinal nerves is relieved by bending forward and worsened by extending the spine, leading to pain. Pain caused by neurogenic claudication is sometimes but not always accompanied by paresthesia or weakness (Katz and Harris 2008).

The clinical components of spinal stenosis as described earlier are generally accompanied by radiologic evidence of this condition. However, the converse is not true: radiologic evidence of spinal stenosis may be largely or entirely asymptomatic. For example, one study reported an incidence of asymptomatic spinal stenosis in 20% in individuals over the age of 60 years (Boden et al. 1990) Distinguishing the clinical components of spinal stenosis from radiologic evidence of this condition that is asymptomatic is critical in astute management of these patients.

Pearl: Surgical management for lumbar stenosis is a reasonable option for those patients who have failed conservative management.

Comment: Two randomized trials have compared nonoperative management with lumbar laminectomy for the treatment of symptomatic lumbar stenosis (Malmivaara et al. 2007; Weinstein et al. 2008). The first trial showed clinical and statistical improvement at 1 year with regard to back and leg pain among patients randomized to receive surgery (Malmivaara et al. 2007). The difference began to narrow after 2 years. The second trial also demonstrated statistically significant improvement among patients in the surgical arm with regard to leg pain, function, and disability scores. This study was limited by significant crossover, with the result that the as-treated analysis probably biased the study in favor of surgery. However, the results of an observational cohort study performed in parallel with the clinical trial support the trial's conclusions (Weinstein et al. 2008).

45.7 Spondylolisthesis

Myth: Degenerative spondylolisthesis occurs equally in all ethnic groups and genders.

Reality: Degenerative spondylolisthesis occurs more commonly in women than in men. In fact, this condition is approximately four times more common in women. Degenerative spondylolisthesis nearly always between L4 and L5 is diagnosed most easily by a standing lateral radiograph of the lumbar spine. The forward slippage of L4 on L5 narrows the spinal canal and can cause spinal stenosis (Fig. 45.4).

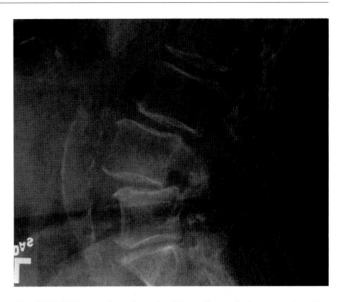

Fig. 45.4 This standing, lateral, plain radiograph demonstrates slippage of L4 onto L5. This is the most common location for degenerative spondylolisthesis to occur. This particular patient has had a lumbar laminectomy which provided short-term relief of her leg pain. After several months, her symptoms of neurologic claudication returned

Pearl: Degenerative spondylolisthesis may be missed if standing lumbar radiographs are not obtained.

Comment: An unstable spinal segment may be missed if one relies upon supine plain radiographs when evaluating a patient with neurogenic claudication (Fig. 45.5a, b). Films obtained while the patient is standing are essential. Similarly, if one relies upon an MRI or CT study, both of which obtained while the patient is supine, then the dynamic nature of their condition can be overlooked. Neurogenic claudication caused by spinal stenosis and that caused by spondylolisthesis cannot be distinguished by details of the history and physical examination. Weight-bearing images are essential to identify spondylolisthesis as the cause of neurogenic claudication in a patient with spinal stenosis.

Pearl: Surgical decompression and fusion for patients with lumbar degenerative spondylolisthesis who present with neurogenic claudication secondary to spinal stenosis is a reasonable alternative to nonoperative management.

Comment: A prospective, randomized trial compared nonoperative management with decompression and fusion for patients with lumbar degenerative spondylolisthesis who presented with neurogenic claudication secondary to spinal stenosis (Weinstein et al. 2007). The authors performed three separate analyses. The intention-to-treat analysis failed to show any benefit from surgery. However, because of significant crossover that occurred between the two treatment arms – with many patients in the nonoperative arm eventually opting for surgery – the authors also performed an "as treated" analysis that demonstrated significant improvement in pain,

Fig. 45.5 (**a**). This supine MRI demonstrates slippage of L4 onto L5. The degree of slippage is just over 5 mm. When one compares the supine MRI with the standing image in (**b**), one can appreciate the dynamic quality of this problem. The L4 vertebra has slipped to over 9 mm. The patient subsequently underwent decompression and posterolateral spinal fusion with complete relief of her symptoms

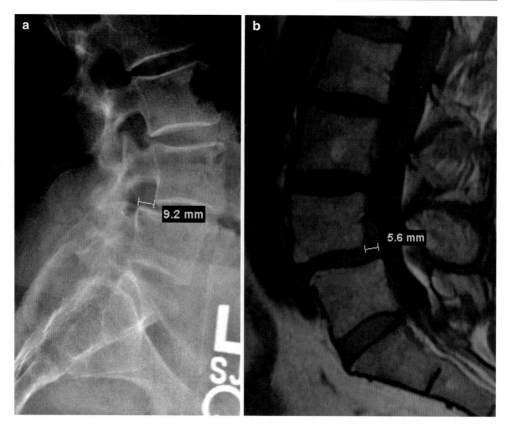

function, and disability for the patients treated surgically. A third analysis, performed in an observational cohort, also showed significant benefits from surgical management in pain, function, and disability. This trial is the best study to date in evaluating the role of surgery in the management of this problem. One can conclude that surgery remains a viable alternative to continued nonoperative management in patients who have neurogenic claudication as a result of spondylolisthesis.

45.8 Miscellaneous but Important Causes of Low Back Pain

Pearl: Severe, acute mechanical low back pain in a postmenopausal woman should trigger suspicion of an osteoporotic vertebral compression fracture.

Comment: This is particularly true if there are additional risk factors for osteoporotic fractures such as a history of a previous fracture, a family history of osteoporosis, or frailty. The pain associated with osteoporotic fractures is generally self-limited, with resolution over a few weeks. Kyphoplasty and vertebroplasty, two technically demanding procedures with the potential for complications, are rarely needed for the treatment of osteoporotic compression fractures.

Pearl: The thoracic spine is the most common site of involvement in diffuse idiopathic skeletal hyperostosis (DISH).

Comment: DISH is characterized by florid hyperostosis of the spine. Marginal bony proliferation leads to the formation of osseous ridges that fuse, giving the appearance of flowing wax. Lesions are most prominent anteriorly and along the right lateral aspect of the spine. Involvement of the left lateral aspect in patients with situs inversus has lead to speculation that the descending thoracic aorta plays a role in the location of calcification.

The thoracic spine is invariably involved in DISH, but the cervical and lumbar regions can be involved, as well. Intervertebral disc spaces are preserved and the facet joints appear normal unless there is co-existing lumbar spondylosis. The absence of sacroiliac joint involvement helps to differentiate DISH from spondyloarthropathies.

45.9 Other Approaches to Evaluation and Treatment

Myth: Provocative discography is a reliable test for identifying "pain generators" in the low back prior to the correction of such problems through surgery or other means.

Reality: Provocative discography involves the injection of dye into an intervertebral disc and then assessing the character of the induced pain. The assumption is that if the injection reproduces a patient's usual low back pain, then that disc must be the cause of the problem. These patients are given a diagnosis of "internal disc disruption" or labeled as having "discogenic low back pain."

The validity of this technique is controversial. The injection of dye into a disc can simulate the quality and location of pain known not to originate from that disc. Furthermore, disc injections are painful 30–80% of the time for patients who do not have symptomatic disc disease but who have had previous disc surgery or who have psychological distress, remote chronic pain, or disputed compensation claims (Carragee 2005). The interpretation of provocative discography procedures should be viewed with caution.

Pearl: Laboratory studies play a limited role in the investigation of low back pain.

Comment: Laboratory studies are used primarily to identify patients with systemic causes of low back pain. For patients whose findings suggest systemic disease or who have back pain that has not improved after 6 weeks of conservative care, a normal complete blood cell count, erythrocyte sedimentation rate, and lumbar spine radiographs exclude systemic disease with a high degree of likelihood (Jarvik and Deyo 2002).

Myth: In patients with acute low back pain, bed rest is an important part of the treatment program.

Reality: Bed rest should be discouraged. Continuing ordinary activities within the limits permitted by pain leads to more rapid recovery than bed rest (Malmivaara et al. 1995).

Myth: A large number of therapies, including physical therapy modalities, injection techniques, and invasive procedures, are effective in the treatment of low back pain.

Reality: Multiple modalities are now employed for the management of low back pain. Most have not been tested rigorously. Uncontrolled studies can produce a misleading impression of efficacy in a condition with fluctuating symptoms and a favorable natural history. A list of therapies that are unproven, controversial, or downright ineffective (but still commonly employed) is shown in Table 45.3.

Myth: Lumbar epidural glucocorticoid injections are helpful for a broad spectrum of patients with low back pain.

Reality: The use of epidural glucocorticoid injections is increasing remarkably rapidly despite the lack of consistent evidence regarding the efficacy of this procedure. Epidural glucocorticoid injections may offer temporary symptomatic relief in some patients with radicular pain, but appear to offer no significant functional benefit and do not reduce the need for surgery.

Table 45.3 Unproven, controversial, or downright ineffective therapies for low back pain

Trigger point injections
Sacroiliac joint injections
Facet joint injections
Ultrasound
Shortwave diathermy
Transcutaneous electrical nerve stimulation (TENS)
Lumbar braces
Traction
Acupuncture
Biofeedback
Prolotherapy
Radiofrequency denervation of nerves to the facet joints
Spinal cord stimulation
Intraspinal drug infusion systems for intrathecal delivery of morphine
Intradiscal electrothermal annuloplasty (IDET)

Limited data suggest that epidural injections in patients with lumbar spinal stenosis temporarily relieve leg pain. They do not, however, influence functional status or subsequent need for surgery (Katz and Harris 2008). There is no evidence that lumbar epidural injections are effective for acute or chronic low back pain in the absence of radicular symptoms.

For a problem in which effective interventions are few, many patients are willing to consider a broad range of treatment options. In some cases, the potential for the temporary relief of pain may justify an epidural glucocorticoid injection. Expectations about the long-term benefit of the procedure, however, should be realistic.

Pearl: The goals for the treatment of patients with chronic low back pain are relief of the pain and restoration of function.

Comment: The majority of patients with chronic low back pain continue working. However, the results of treatment are often unsatisfactory, and complete relief of pain is an unrealistic goal for most.

Many patients respond to a program that includes analgesic agents, education, back exercises, aerobic conditioning, and the loss of excess weight. Low-dose tricyclic antidepressants (e.g., amitriptyline 10–75 mg at bedtime) may help some patients, but anticholinergic side effects are common. Some data support intensive rehabilitation programs that emphasize cognitive behavioral therapy.

45.10 Surgery

Myth: Patients with chronic low back pain who fail conservative care are good candidates for surgery.

Table 45.4 Indications for surgery in spinal stenosis, spondylolisthesis, and disc herniation

Spinal stenosis
Severe or progressive neurologic deficit
Disabling pseudoclaudication or sciatica (elective)
Spondylolisthesis
Severe or progressive neurologic deficit
Disabling pseudoclaudication or sciatica (elective)
Disc herniation
Cauda equina syndrome (emergency)
Severe or progressive neurologic deficit
Greater than 6 weeks of sciatica (elective)

Reality: The pathophysiology of pain in degenerative disease of the lumbar spine remains elusive, and a definitive patho-anatomic cause of back pain cannot be identified in most patients. Thus, it is not surprising that surgical procedures such as spinal fusion or the insertion of artificial discs, aimed at relieving isolated back pain, often yield disappointing results. Spinal fusion surgery is effective for some conditions in some patients, but its efficacy for the most common conditions (e.g., isolated low back pain secondary to degenerative disc disease) remains unclear and controversial (Carragee 2005; Deyo et al. 2004).

Pearl: The major indications for surgery in patients with low back pain are the presence of a severe neurological deficit or a progressive neurological deficit (Table 45.4).

Comment: Nerve root compression syndromes usually result from acute disc herniation, and less often from spinal stenosis or spondylolisthesis. The natural history of acute disc herniation is favorable. Sequential MRI testing reveals that the herniation tends to regress with time and radicular pain resolves. In the absence of a severe or progressive neurologic deficit, patients with disc herniations should be managed conservatively. Fewer than 10% of these patients require surgical decompression. When necessary, decompression is usually accomplished by a laminotomy with limited discectomy. Elective surgery is often performed in patients who have sciatica that does not resolve within 6 weeks (Peul et al. 2007).

The symptoms of spinal stenosis remain stable for years in many patients. In the absence of a severe or progressive neurological deficit, patients are treated conservatively with a program that includes analgesia, loss of excess weight, physical conditioning, and back exercises designed to reduce lumbar lordosis. Epidural glucocorticoids may provide temporary symptomatic relief. Patients with disabling pseudo-claudication or radicular pain may benefit from decompressive surgery. The goal of the surgery is to relieve pressure on neural elements by increasing the area of the spinal canal and neural foramen. The most common surgical procedure for spinal stenosis is a decompressive laminectomy, sometimes accompanied by fusion. This procedure involves removing various parts of the vertebra including the lamina, ligamentum flavum, enlarged facets, osteophytes, and bulging disc material.

45.11 Neck Pain

Pearl: There are a remarkable number of similarities in the clinical features and management of patients with neck pain and low back pain.

Comment: These include the following statements regarding neck pain:

- The natural history of neck pain is favorable in the majority of patients.
- In most patients with radiant neck pain (to the back of the head, shoulder, scapula, or arm), the cause is nonneurogenic, sclerotomal pain. This usually arises from pathology within the disc, facet joint, or paraspinal muscles and ligaments. It is not radicular pain secondary to nerve root compression.
- Degenerative changes in the cervical spine (sometimes termed as cervical spondylosis) are the most commonly identified cause of neck pain. The pain is usually exacerbated by movement and relieved by rest.
- A definitive pathoanatomic diagnosis cannot be made in most patients with neck pain.
- Early diagnostic testing is rarely indicated unless there is a significant or progressive neurologic deficit or some indication that an infection or malignancy might be causing the pain. The major focus of the initial evaluation is the identification of these few patients, as they need urgent, specific interventions.
- Imaging abnormalities identified in patients with neck pain are common in asymptomatic individuals. These abnormalities are often the result of age-related degenerative changes.
- Laboratory tests are useful only in the small minority of patients with a systemic disorder causing neck pain.
- Most patients with neck pain respond to a conservative treatment program that may include NSAIDS, analgesics, muscle relaxants, and range-of-motion and strengthening exercises.
- The major surgical indication in patients with neck pain is the presence of a significant or progressive neurologic deficit.

Pearl: Most neck pain is mechanical in nature.

Comment: Degenerative change in the spine is the most important contributor to mechanical neck pain. The prevalence of neck pain and degenerative change increases with age.

Myth: Electrodiagnostic testing should be prescribed for most patients with neck pain and neurologic symptoms in the upper extremities.

Reality: Electrodiagnostic testing (electromyography and nerve conduction studies) is overused. In most patients with neck pain (or low back pain) who have neurological symptoms, the diagnosis is clear to the astute clinician following a careful history and physical examination. These patients do not require electrodiagnostic testing.

Electrodiagnostic testing can be helpful when the relationship between symptoms, physical findings, and imaging results is unclear. For example, a number of diagnoses could explain the patient with neck pain, paresthesias of the fifth digit, and wasting of the intrinsic muscles of the hand. Among these are a spinal cord lesion, a C8 radiculopathy, a lower trunk brachial plexopathy, and an ulnar neuropathy. Electrophysiologic findings in this scenario might be essential in guiding the clinician to the correct diagnosis.

Electromyographic abnormalities depend upon the development of muscle denervation following nerve injury. This can require 4–6 weeks in the distal musculature.

Pearl: Acute nonspecific neck pain is a common, benign, and self-limited condition.

Comment: The etiology of pain and spasm in acute cervical strains, also termed as "myofascial pain," is unknown. There is usually no history of significant trauma. Pain is often predominantly on one side of the neck and may radiate to the top of shoulder along the superior portion of the trapezius, as well as inferiorly to the periscapular region. Paracervical muscle spasm with secondary loss of cervical lordosis is common. Tender points and trigger points may be present.

Most episodes of acute cervical strain resolve spontaneously within 2 weeks, but may recur. No investigation other than a careful history and physical examination is required. Treatment involves reassurance, analgesics, NSAIDS, gentle mobilization with the help of local heat, and time.

Myth: A whiplash injury has the same excellent prognosis as cervical strain.

Reality: A whiplash is a rapid flexion/hyperextension (acceleration/deceleration) injury to the neck. Whiplash usually results from a rear or side-impact car accident. The paracervical muscles, ligaments, and facet joint capsules become stretched and may sustain injury. In severe cases, the patient develops vertebral fractures or damage to the intervertebral discs. Radiographic evaluation should always be obtained.

Neck pain and stiffness develops within a few hours but may be delayed until the next day. Patients may also complain of headaches, dizziness, anxiety, paresthesias, and insomnia. Physical examination usually reveals paracervical spasm and a decreased range of motion of the cervical spine.

Most patients with whiplash injuries improve within 4 weeks of treatment with a combination of analgesics, NSAIDS, and gentle neck mobilization exercises. However, in some patients – as many as 30% in some estimates – the pain persists for many months or years. The reason for this is unclear, particularly because the response to treatment is often unrelated to the severity of the whiplash injury. Patients with persistent pain may benefit from a noninvasive multi-disciplinary pain management program. In some patients, the persistence of neck pain is associated with depression, the pursuit of disability compensation, or litigation.

Pearl: An older patient with chronic mechanical neck pain almost invariably has evidence of cervical spondylosis on neck imaging.

Comment: On the other hand, many older patients without chronic mechanical neck pain also have evidence of cervical spondylosis on neck imaging! Chronic mechanical neck pain is common in older people. The prevalence of cervical spondylosis, i.e., degenerative changes in the disco-vertebral, facet, and uncovertebral joints, increases with age. Although the neck pain in such patients is often attributed to cervical spondylosis, no consistent relationship exists between radiographic changes – either their presence or their degree – and the complaint of neck pain, the response to treatment for neck pain, or the prognosis of neck pain.

Patients with neck pain secondary to cervical spondylosis often present with a background of chronic discomfort with intermittent acute attacks that last a few days. The neck pain often radiates along the superior portion of the trapezius to the shoulder, to the scapular region, and to suboccipital areas. Neck movement is restricted during most such exacerbations of neck pain. Conservative treatment, which includes reassurance and education, analgesics, NSAIDS, and neck exercises, is usually effective.

Although a small number of patients with cervical spondylosis develop cervical radiculopathy caused by disc herniation or cervical myelopathy secondary to spinal stenosis, most causes of acute neck pain are caused by mechanisms that remain obscure but have self-limited courses.

Pearl: In a patient with radicular symptoms in the upper extremity, a careful neurologic evaluation helps identify the specific nerve root involved.

Comment: Cervical root irritation generally results from either posterolateral disc herniation or osteophyte pressure. The C5–C6 level is the most common site of disc herniation, and results in a C6 radiculopathy (As with low back pain, the more caudal nerve root is impinged). A C7 radiculopathy caused by a C6–C7 disc herniation is the second most common such lesion in the neck.

Radiculopathy symptoms can be exacerbated by Valsalva maneuvers, which lead to increased intrathecal pressure. The

Fig. 45.6 Neurological evaluation of the upper extremities including motor testing, reflex testing, and tests for dermatomal sensory loss help to identify the specific nerve root involved

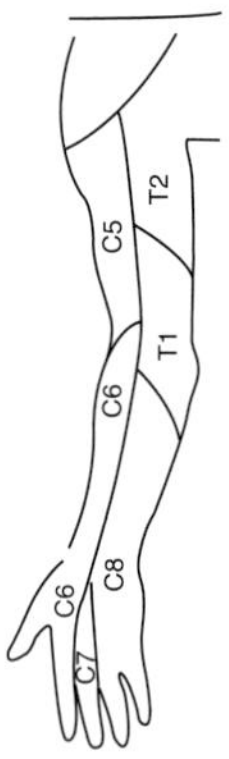

Upper Extremity Dermatomes	Disc	Nerve Root	Motor Loss	Sensory Loss	Reflex Loss
	C4–5	C5	Deltoid	Lateral deltoid	Biceps
	C5–6	C6	Biceps	Index finger and thumb	Supinator, Biceps
	C6–7	C7	Triceps	Middle finger (sometimes index)	Triceps
	C7–T1	C8	Hand*	Ring and little finger	None

*Intrinsic muscles of the hand – the lumbricals and the interossei. Weakness of finger flexion, abduction, and adduction. There may be weakness of grip strength.

Spurling test, a combination of lateral flexion and rotation of the neck to the affected side, also exacerbates symptoms of cervical radiculopathy.

MRI is the most effective technique for localizing the site of disc herniation and nerve root impingement. Most patients respond to conservative care. Surgery is indicated only in patients with a significant or progressive neurologic deficit (Fig. 45.6).

Myth: Cervical myelopathy causes severe neck pain.

Reality: Cervical myelopathy in and of itself is a painless condition. Only one-third of patients with cervical myelopathy complain of neck pain (Borenstein 2007). However, patients with cervical myelopathy can have neck pain or radicular symptoms caused by coexistent cervical spondylosis or cervical nerve root compression.

Myelopathy is a potentially devastating sequela of cervical canal stenosis. This condition usually results from cervical spondylosis. Osteophytes from the discovertebral and facet joints encroach on the spinal canal. The canal is narrowed further by disc herniation and hypertrophy and buckling of the ligamentum flavum.

Cervical canal stenosis leads to compression of the spinal cord or nerve roots. Individual patients present with symptoms that can be predominantly myelopathic, predominantly radicular, or both. Patients with cervical myelopathy complain of symptoms such as paresthesias in all extremities. Symptoms of cervical myelopathy are shown in Table 45.5. The diagnosis of cervical myelopathy should be considered in a patient with progressive spastic paraparesis, paresthesias of hands and feet, or wasting of the intrinsic hand muscles. The most efficient means of confirming the diagnosis is through an MRI.

Table 45.5 Symptoms and signs of cervical myelopathy

Slowly progressive spastic paraparesis
Brisk deep tendon reflexes in the lower extremities
Extensor plantar responses
Diminution of vibratory sense in the legs
Gait difficulty
Urinary incontinence
Radicular arm pain and other neurologic features of cervical radiculopathy

The natural history of spondylitic cervical myelopathy is one of gradual progression. Mild cases of myelopathy that involve only mild arm and hand symptoms may improve with conservative care. However, progressive myelopathy requires surgical decompression before severe neurologic deficits appear.

References

Boden SD, Davis DO, et al Abnormal magnetic-resonance scans of the lumbar spine in asymptomatic subjects. A prospective investigation. J Bone Joint Surg Am. 1990;72(3):403–8

Borenstein D. Approach to the patient with neck pain. In: Imboden J, Hellman D, Stone J editors. Current rheumatology diagnosis and treatment. 2nd ed. NY: McGraw Hill; 2007

Brox JI, Sorensen R, et al Randomized clinical trial of lumbar instrumented fusion and cognitive intervention and exercises in patients with chronic low back pain and disc degeneration. Spine 2003;28(17):1913–21

Carragee EJ. Persistent low back pain. N Engl J Med. 2005;352:1891–8

Chou R, Qaseem A, et al Diagnosis and treatment of low back pain: a joint clinical practice guideline from the American College of

Physicians and the American Pain Society. Ann Intern Med. 2007;147:478–514

Deyo RA, Nachemson A, et al Spinal fusion surgery – the case for restraint. N Engl J Med. 2004;350:722–6

Deyo RA, Weinstein JN. Low back pain. N Engl J Med. 2001;344: 363–70

Dixit RK, Dickson J. Low back pain. In: Adebajo AO, editor. ABC of rheumatology. 4th ed. London: Blackwell Publishing; 2008

Dixit RK. Approach to the patient with low back pain. In: Imboden J, Hellmann D, Stone J, editors. Current rheumatology diagnosis and treatment. 2nd ed. NY: McGraw Hill; 2007

Fritzell P, Hagg O, et al 2001 Volvo Award Winner in Clinical Studies: lumbar fusion versus nonsurgical treatment for chronic low back pain: a multicenter randomized controlled trial from the Swedish Lumbar Spine Study Group. Spine 2001;26(23):2521–32; discussion 2532–4

Jarvik JG, Deyo RA. Diagnostic evaluation of low back pain with emphasis on imaging. Ann Intern Med. 2002;137:586–97

Katz JN, Harris MB. Lumbar spinal stenosis. N Engl J Med. 2008;358: 818–23

Malmivaara A, Hakkinen U, et al The treatment of acute low back pain – bed rest, exercises, or ordinary activity? N Engl J Med. 1995; 332: 351–5

Malmivaara A, Slatis P, et al Surgical or nonoperative treatment for lumbar spinal stenosis? A randomized controlled trial. Spine 2007; 32(1):1–8

Peul WC, et al Surgery versus prolonged conservative treatment for sciatica. N Engl J Med. 2007;356:2245–56

Rudwaleit M, Metter A, et al Inflammatory back pain in ankylosing spondylitis: a reassessment of the clinical history for application as classification and diagnostic criteria. Arthritis Rheum. 2006;54: 569–78

Weinstein JN, Lurie JD, et al Surgical versus nonsurgical treatment for lumbar degenerative spondylolisthesis. N Engl J Med. 2007;356(22): 2257–70

Weinstein JN, Lurie JD, et al Surgical vs nonoperative treatment for lumbar disk herniation: the Spine Patient Outcomes Research Trial (SPORT) observational cohort. JAMA. 2006a;296(20): 2451–9

Weinstein JN, Tosteson TD, et al Surgical versus nonsurgical therapy for lumbar spinal stenosis. N Engl J Med. 2008;358(8): 794–810

Weinstein JN, Tosteson TD, et al Surgical vs nonoperative treatment for lumbar disk herniation: the Spine Patient Outcomes Research Trial (SPORT): a randomized trial. JAMA. 2006b;296(20): 2441–50

Amyloidosis

George H. Sack Jr

46

46.1 Overview of Amyloidosis

> The diagnosis of amyloidosis depends on finding deposits with congo red birefringence in affected tissue.These deposits comprise fibrils of highly ordered proteins or protein fragments that generally contain prominent β-pleated sheet domains.

> Many proteins have regions that can aggregate into amyloid fibrils.Often only a small fragment of a larger molecule is compatible with fibril geometry and thus fibril formation occurs after cleaving the parent protein.

> Amyloid deposits can be found in any tissue.However, some depostis have no pathologic consequence while others can cause serious organ dysfunction by interrupting individual cellular physiology, cell-cell interactions and/or tissue integrity.

> When specific organ dysfunction has been identified, biopsy of that tissue often is the simplest diagnostic method(*e.g.*heart,kidney,liver). An alternative diagnostic approach for systermic amyloidosis is to examine tissue derived by aspiration of the abdominal fat pad.

> Both prognosis and treatment are based on identifying the protein in the fibril.Often, this protein can be identified by immunofluorescence.

> Amyloid proteins vary widely and include immunoglobulins,inflammatory molecules, hormone precursors and inherited variants of normal serum proteins.

> Inherited forms of amyloidosis are uncommon but well-recognized. They often involve specific organs– *e.g.* heart,peripheral nerves,or blood vessels. Most have autosomal dominant inheritance.

> In America, the most common form of amyloidosis (called "Primary" amyloidosis) is derived from immunoglobulin light chains. This is usually due to overproduction from a plasma cell clone. The light chain often can be detected by protein electrophoresis of serum or urine; λ light chains are more frequently involved than κ.

> In tropical regions, "Secondary" amyloidosis can be associated with chronic or episodic inflammatory or infectious diseases. In such cases, the parent protein is the acute phase reactant serum amyloid A (SAA).

> Amyloid deposits in the brain in Alzheimer disease comprise a small fragment (Called Aβ) derived by cleavage of a much larger precursor molecule called the β-protein.

> Successful treatment of any form of amyloidosis depends on eliminating or reducing the available parent protein. For "primary" disease this generally involves chemotherapy; for "secondary" disease the underlying infection or inflammatory process must be controlled.

> Amyloid deposits are relatively inert chemically and intrinsically stable. Thus, successful treatment often must be given for an extended time to permit gradual elimination of the fibrils and restoration of organ function.

Myth: Amyloid tissue is largely composed of carbohydrate.

Reality: The term "amyloid," introduced by Virchow in 1858, is etymologically incorrect. Amyloid is derived from the Latin word for starch, but there is virtually *no* carbohydrate in amyloid deposits, which are composed of protein. Nevertheless, the term has persisted.

Myth: Amyloidosis is rare.

Reality: Amyloid deposits are encountered frequently. Autopsy studies reveal a frequency as high as 25%. However, all deposits of amyloid are not necessarily associated with clinical manifestations.

Myth: Amyloid is amorphous.

Reality: Although light microscopy is generally unrevealing, electron microscopy reveals that all amyloids are composed of masses of highly ordered microfibrillar protein assemblies. β-pleated sheet protein domains are prominent in amyloid

J. H. Stone (ed.), *A Clinician's Pearls and Myths in Rheumatology,*
DOI:10.1007/978-1-84800-934-9_46, © Springer Science + Business Media B.V. 2009

fibrils. Amyloidosis is a disorder of protein folding. However, different types of amyloid fibrils differ in their detailed three-dimensional folding patterns (Dobson 2003).

Myth: Amyloid is a disease of the liver and kidneys.

Reality: Amyloid deposits can be found in any organ or system. The disease can be both widespread throughout multiple organs or involve individual organs in a localized fashion (Biewend et al. 2006; Rocken and Sletten 2003).

Myth: Amyloid reflects similar pathophysiology wherever it is found.

Reality: Many different molecular types of amyloid are known (Table 46.1). These include products of neoplasia (Kyle et al. 2002), inflammatory molecules (Cunnane and Whitehead 1999), genetic protein variants (Connors et al. 2003), and local deposits. In the U.S., about 90% of the cases of amyloidosis are due to fragments of immunoglobulin light chains (AL amyloid: the "L" stands for light chain). AL amyloid is generally secondary to a monoclonal gammopathy. In parts of the world where chronic infections and poorly treated inflammatory diseases are common, much of the amyloid is "secondary" to an underlying process. In such cases, amyloidosis is caused by the deposition of fragments of the serum amyloid A (SAA) protein, the levels of which are elevated as part of an inflammatory response (Sack et al. 1989).

Pearl: The diagnosis of amyloid requires tissue study with specific staining.

Comment: The *definition* of amyloid is that it shows apple-green birefringence when stained with Congo red dye and viewed under cross-polarized light (Fig. 46.1). This is the case of *all* types of amyloid, regardless of etiology.

Pearl: The most important diagnostic and prognostic feature of amyloid is the type of protein present in the fibrils. This is the basis for classifying amyloid disease.

Comment: Identification of the type of protein within amyloid fibrils shows the nature of the underlying condition. Moreover, this identification is essential for determining the patient's prognosis and for recommending treatment. The type of protein present within amyloid fibrils can often be identified by immunofluorescence, but sequence analysis of the protein or gene is required in some cases to distinguish among inherited forms. Table 46.1 presents the main categories and their associated nomenclature.

Table 46.1 Amyloid disease nomenclature

Constituent amyloid protein	Protein precursor	Variant(s)	Clinical
AA	Serum amyloid A (SAA)		Secondary (reactive)
			Familial Mediterranean fever (FMF)
			Muckle–Wells syndrome
AL	κ, λ light chains		Idiopathic (primary), MGUS
			Myeloma-associated
			Macroglobulin-associated
AH	IgG 1 (γ1) heavy chain	Aγ1	Idiopathic (primary)
			Myeloma-associated
ATTR	Transthyretin	>80 mutants	Familial amyloid polyneuropathy
			Familial amyloid cardiomyopathy
			Tenosynovial deposition
AApoA1	apoA1	Arg 26	Familial amyloid polyneuropathy
			Aortic deposition
AGel	Gelsolin	Asn 187	Familial amyloidosis (Finnish)
Aβ	β protein precursor	Gln 618	Alzheimer dementia
			Down syndrome
			Hereditary cerebral hemorrhage
			Aging
Aβ_2M	β_2-microglobulin		Complication of chronic dialysis
APrP	PrP – cellular prion	PrP^{Sc}, PrP^{CJD}	Spongiform encephalopathies
ACal	(Pro)calcitonin	(Pro)calcitonin	Medullary thyroid carcinoma
AANF	Atrial natriuretic factor		Isolated atrial amyloid
AIAPP	Islet amyloid polypeptide		Type II diabetes, insulinoma
APro	Prolactin		Aging pituitary
			Prolactinomas
ALys	Lysozyme		Familial
ACys	Cystatin C		Familial
AFib	Fibrinogen α-chain		Familial

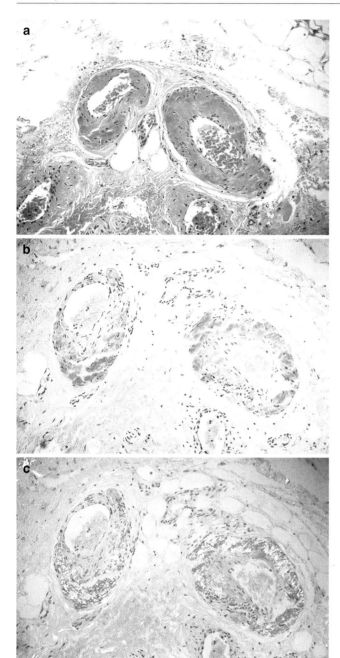

nerves, and heart, all involved commonly, may be appropriate sites for biopsy.

Pearl: Aspiration of the abdominal fat pad offers a minimally invasive source of tissue for analysis in the absence of a flagrantly involved organ.

Comment: Fat pad aspiration, a simple and safe procedure, is often the first approach to the diagnosis of amyloid disease (Duston et al. 1989; Olsen et al. 1999). Proper interpretation of the aspirated material requires an experienced pathologist, because the tissue planes can become distorted as an artifact of the procedure. Figure 46.2 shows material from such a study.

Pearl: Several otherwise unusual clinical features make the diagnosis of amyloidosis more likely.

Comment: Macroglossia may be prominent, leading to stiffening of the tongue and indentation by the teeth (Fig. 46.3). This may interfere with eating and cause hoarseness.

Easy bruising with capillary fragility may be prominent. Purpura in the periorbital tissues is virtually diagnostic of AL amyloidosis (Fig. 46.4).

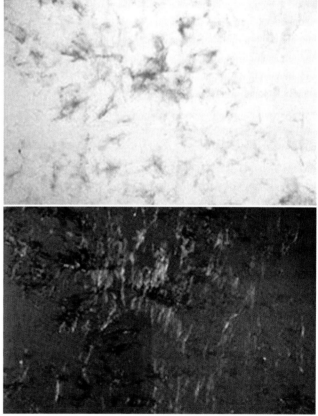

Fig. 46.1 (**a–c**) Serial tissue sections showing deposition of amyloid in the wall of a blood vessel. (**a**). conventional hematoxylin and eosin staining. Note the amorphous quality of the depositions with effacement of normal tissue details. (**b**). Congo red staining with regular illumination. The amyloid appears pink without distinct features. (**c**). Viewing tissue stained with congo red using polarized light shows the diagnostic "apple-green" birefringence. This is the basis for the diagnosis of all amyloid deposits

Pearl: Tissue from the affected organ offers an ideal source for amyloid diagnosis.

Comment: Clinically evident abnormalities generally guide the selection of biopsy site. The liver, kidney, peripheral

Fig. 46.2 Tissue from abdominal fat pad aspiration stained with hematoxylin and eosin (*above*) and congo red (*below*). Note the prominent birefringence on the lower image despite the poorly-defined anatomy characteristic of adipose tissue.

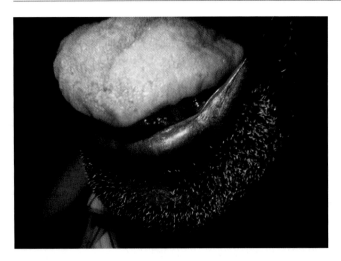

Fig. 46.3 Macroglossia is a relatively common finding in AL amyloidosis. Chewing, swallowing, breathing, and speech all can be affected by this change

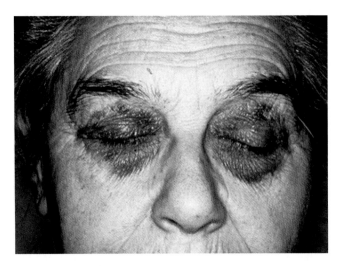

Fig. 46.4 Periorbital purpura is virtually diagnostic of amyloid infiltration. In this case, the changes developed following a colonoscopy: "postproctocopic purpura"

Pearl: Several clinical clues betray cardiac involvement in amyloid disease.

Comment: The heart is involved in up to 50% of patients with AL amyloidosis (Falk 2005). Weight loss, dyspnea, and edema are frequent presentations. Electrocardiographic changes include:

1. Low QRS voltage (limb leads < 5 mm in height).
2. Otherwise nonspecific ST- and T-wave changes including a so-called "pseudoinfarction pattern."
3. Conduction disturbances (various forms of block).

Echocardiography can also help, by revealing:

1. An increased estimated left ventricular mass with wall thickening.

2. A restrictive left ventricular filling pattern with progressive diastolic dysfunction.
3. Prominent valves, consistent with amyloid infiltration.

Myth: The echocardiogram in patients with cardiac amyloidosis has a "sparkling" or "ground-glass" appearance.

Reality: Although often described with earlier technology, improved image processing has made the "ground-glass" appearance of the myocardium is less prominent on the new generation of echocardiography technology. However, increased echogenicity of both valves and myocardium is notable as amyloid deposition progresses.

Pearl: In AL amyloidosis, the protein constituent of the amyloid fibril is unique for each patient.

Comment: At least 90% of the cases of amyloidosis diagnosed in the U.S. result from light chain deposition. Lambda light chains are twice as common as kappa light chains in cases of amyloidosis, and there is a predominance of the λ_{VI} subgroup. The tight fibril packing characteristic of amyloidosis imposes constraints on the light chains; usually, only a short portion of the light chain can fit within the β-pleated sheet. The polypeptide incorporated into the β-pleated sheet generally includes at least part of the variable region of the light chain. As a result, only a *small* fraction of light chains contribute to the formation of amyloid fibrils. Because the *variable* region is commonly involved, the protein constituent of the fibril is likely *unique for each patient.* Hence, the clinical distribution and consequences of AL amyloid are unpredictable.

In effect, at the molecular level, each individual has a novel disease. The long lists of "complications" described conventionally in AL amyloid are unlikely to be encountered in every patient. The clinician must be prepared for surprises.

Pearl: Overproduction of the light chain in AL disease may be due to aggressive plasma cell growth, such as in myeloma. Alternatively, it may arise from a single plasma cell clone that proliferates without causing the other known complications of myeloma.

Comment: The common feature in each case is overproduction of a *specific* light chain that can be cleaved to yield a fragment capable of meeting the stringent constraints of fibril formation. This fragment usually includes at least part of the variable region.

Pearl: The overproduced immunoglobulin in AL amyloidosis is generally detectable through immunoelectrophoresis of serum or urine (i.e., an SPEP or UPEP).

Comment: Because the overproduction of immunoglobulins in amyloidosis usually leads to light chain excess, the light chains pass into the urine where they become detectable by electrophoresis. About 80% of AL patients have proteinuria. Some of the light chains have the solubility characteristics of Bence–Jones proteins. Consequently, any patient suspected of having amyloidosis should be evaluated for the presence of Bence–Jones proteinuria.

Pearl: Monoclonal gammopathies are often detected in asymptomatic individuals.

Comment: This phenomenon is termed monoclonal gammopathy of unknown significance, or "MGUS." Individuals with MGUS represent one end of a broad spectrum of plasma cell proliferation. At the other end of the spectrum is multiple myeloma (Kyle et al. 2002). A small fraction of people on this spectrum produce an immunoglobulin that can cause amyloid fibril formation. The ability of these immunoglobulins to cause amyloidosis is unrelated to the aggressiveness of the plasma cell biology; neither myeloma nor high quantities of aberrant immunoglobulins is required for amyloidosis to develop. The "amyloidogenicity" is related entirely (it seems) to the structural features of the individual patient's protein.

Long-term follow-up of individuals with MGUS indicates that progression from a clinical curiosity to more aggressive changes occurs at a rate of ~1% per year. Such progression may or may not be associated with amyloid deposition.

Pearl: "Secondary" amyloid (AA) can accompany a wide variety of chronic conditions: rheumatologic, inflammatory, infectious, and inherited.

Comment: The distribution of AA amyloid varies across different regions of the world. Still's disease is a very rare cause of AA amyloid in the U.S., but apparently more common in England and Europe. AA amyloid secondary to tuberculosis, leishmaniasis, and other chronic infections is more frequent in Africa and Southeast Asia. Familial Mediterranean fever (FMF), an autosomal recessive disorder, is encountered primarily in individuals from the eastern Mediterranean, from Turkey to Egypt.

The feature common to all of these conditions is overproduction of the small serum protein, SAA (Sack et al. 1989). The production of this protein is caused by high levels of interleukin-6 and tumor necrosis factor. These cytokines are the proximal inducers of SAA synthesis in the liver and other cells.

Pearl: Colchicine prevents the development of amyloidosis in FMF.

Comment: FMF is notable for recurrent episodes of pyrexia, serositis, and serum changes characteristic of the acute phase response. The disorder is caused by mutations in the gene for pyrin, an inflammatory protein expressed in granulocytes. Untreated homozygous individuals are at risk for renal failure secondary to cumulative renal insults with deposition of AA amyloid. Fortunately, long-term treatment of patients predisposed to FMF with colchicine minimizes the frequency and severity of attacks, thereby reducing the likelihood of renal amyloidosis. The usual dose of colchicine in the treatment of FMF is 0.6 mg taken three times daily.

Pearl: Treating individuals with amyloid disease generally requires eliminating the source of the aberrant (or excess) protein.

Comment: Amyloid deposits themselves are largely inert and resolve very slowly. Thus, the goals of therapy are to minimize the expansion or appearance of these deposits elsewhere and to attenuate the local consequences of tissue deposition (Cohen and Kelly 2003). Specific treatments vary according to the responsible protein. The approaches to therapy for the major types of amyloidosis are shown in Table 46.2.

Pearl: Transthyretin (TTR), a small serum protein of 127 amino acids, has more than 80 known mutations, most of which cause the amyloid disease termed ATTR.

Comment: Some TTR mutations (e.g., Val30Met) cause a progressive, debilitating neuropathy. Others (e.g., Thr60Ala) lead to cardiac failure (Connors et al. 2003). Small molecules may stabilize the native TTR tetramer to minimize fibril formation. Identifying the mutation in individuals at risk can be accomplished by tracing the autosomal dominant transmission in the patient's kindred and sequencing the responsible protein or gene.

Most TTR, including the aberrant forms, is produced by the liver. Complications of TTR neuropathies have been mitigated by performing orthotopic liver transplantation before the patient becomes symptomatic. Cells of the transplanted liver do not have the TTR mutation, and therefore produce normal TTR protein.

Pearl: The other major site of TTR production is the choroid plexus.

Comment: Despite the presence of TTR mutations in choroid plexus cells, symptoms referable to central nervous system involvement are rare. Several isolated kindreds with the

Table 46.2 Treatment approaches to major variants of amyloidosis

Variant	Treatment approach
AL	Diminish the production of light chains by plasma cells
AA	Reduce source of chronic inflammation by treating the underlying infection or rheumatologic disorder
Inherited forms	Orthotopic liver transplantation when the liver is the source of the mutant protein (e.g., liver in ATTR)
	Inhibit synthesis of mutant allele (RNAi)
	Colchicine treatment for FMF
Organ-limited	Local excision but removal may not be necessary if there is no dysfunction

so-called "oculoleptomeningeal amyloidosis" have been described.

Pearl: Without a change in the production of the amyloid constituent protein, clinical progression is likely.

Comment: Once fibril formation has begun, the physiologic conditions and supplies of monomers are adequate to cause sustained tissue deposition. It can be assumed under those circumstances that fibril formation will be unimpeded. In vitro studies show that existing fibrils hasten formation of additional fibrils. This means that clinical signs and symptoms, including any evident organ dysfunction, will progress.

Pearl: Alzheimer's dementia is associated with two characteristic changes in brain tissue: neurofibrillary tangles and amyloid plaques.

Comment: The amyloid plaques are formed from fibrils that comprise a small fragment of the so-called "amyloid β protein." Hence, this type of amyloid is called Aβ (Selkoe 1989). The small fragment that gets deposited within the brain, which is usually a polypeptide 40–42 amino acids long, is derived from a much larger protein by specific cleavages. There are three forms of the precursor molecule, each of which is about 700 amino acids long.

Mutations in the Aβ protein itself as well as in the enzymes responsible for the cleavages can be associated with familial forms of Alzheimer's dementia, but such mutations are rare. Histopathologic changes consistent with Alzheimer's disease are also common among individuals with Down's syndrome. This is consistent with the fact that the gene for the Aβ protein is located on chromosome 21; patients with Down's syndrome have three copies of this chromosome (trisomy 21).

Pearl: Prion disorders involve the formation of amyloid-like fibrillar arrays.

Comment: The prion diseases (e.g., Creutzfeldt–Jakob disease) are categorized frequently as "transmissible spongiform encephalopathies." These conditions reflect alternative folding patterns for normal cellular proteins. The transmission of such alternative structures can lead to fibril propagation within neighboring cells. However, some of these disorders develop in the presence of specific mutations that enhance the transition to monomer structures compatible with fibril formation (Caughey and Baron 2006).

References

Biewend ML, Menke DM, Calamia KT. The spectrum of localized amyloidosis: a case series of 20 patients and review of the literature. Amyloid 2006;13:135–42

Caughey B, Baron GS. Prions and their partners in crime. Nature 2006;443:803–10

Cohen FE, Kelly JW. Therapeutic approaches to protein-misfolding diseases. Nature 2003;426:905–9

Connors LH, Lim A, Prokaeva T, Roskens VA, Costello CE. Tabulation of human transthyretin (TTR) variants, 2003. Amyloid 2003;10:160–84

Cunnane G, Whitehead AS. Amyloid precursors and amyloidosis in rheumatoid arthritis. Baill Clin Rheumatol. 1999;13(4):615–28

Dobson CM. Protein folding and misfolding. Nature 2003;426:884–90

Duston MA, Skinner M, Meenan RF, Cohen AS. Sensitivity, specificity, and predictive value of abdominal fat aspiration for the diagnosis of amyloidosis. Arthritis Rheum. 1989;32:82–5

Falk HR. Diagnosis and management of the cardiac amyloidoses. Circulation 2005;112:2047–60

Kyle RA, Therneau TM, Rajkumar V, et al A long-term study of prognosis in monoclonal gammopathy of undetermined significance. N Engl J Med. 2002;346:564–9

Olsen KE, Sletten K, Westermark P. The use of subcutaneous fat tissue for amyloid typing by enzyme-linked immunosorbent assay. Am J Clin Pathol. 1999;111:355–62

Rocken C, Sletten K. Amyloid in surgical pathology. Virchows Archiv. 2003;443:3–16

Sack GH Jr, Talbot CC Jr, Seuanez H, O'Brien SJ. Molecular analysis of the human serum amyloid A (SAA) gene family. Scand J Immunol. 1989;29:113–9

Selkoe DJ. Aging, amyloid, and Alzheimer's disease. N Engl J Med. 1989;320(22):1484–7

The Ehlers–Danlos Syndrome

47

Fransiska Malfait and Anne De Paepe

47.1 Overview of the Ehlers–Danlos Syndrome

> The Ehlers–Danlos syndrome (EDS) comprises a clinically heterogeneous group of connective tissue diseases, the principal features of which result from generalized but variable tissue fragility.
> EDS is a congenital disorder, but the age of onset of symptoms varies from birth to the fifth or even sixth decade of life.
> The major characteristics of EDS are, to a varying degree, present in all EDS subtypes. These include skin hyperextensibility (see Fig. 47.1), poor wound healing causing wide, thin, atrophic scars ("cigarette paper scars") (see Fig. 47.2), easy bruising, joint hypermobility (see Fig. 47.3) with recurrent dislocations, and generalized tissue fragility.
> During childhood, patients may present to the pediatrician with complaints as diverse as hypotonia or delayed neuromotor development, easy bruising, or abnormal wound healing.
> Later in life, patients may present to the hematologist due to unexplained bleeding diathesis; to the rheumatologist with complaints of joint hyperlaxity and arthralgias; to the orthopedic surgeon due to recurrent dislocations; or to the (vascular) surgeon with arterial or bowel rupture.

Pearl: EDS is a disease with many faces.

Comment: The severity of EDS and the impact of this disorder on the patient's quality of life differ substantially according to the different disease subtypes. Inter and intrafamilial variability in severity of disease expression is encountered in many of the EDS subtypes. Moreover, each subtype displays specific additional clinical manifestations that help to determine the EDS subtype.

The EDS is extremely heterogeneous, not only at the clinical level but also at the molecular basis of disease. Mutations in at least ten different genes have been identified to date: *COL1A1, COL1A2, COL3A1, COL5A1, COL5A2, PLOD1, ADAMTS2, TNX-B, β4-Gal-T7,* and *SLC39A13*. Almost every family affected by EDS harbors a unique mutation in one of these genes. In addition, there remain many unclassified EDS variants, the molecular defects of which are unknown.

The upshot of this variation is that EDS is even more heterogeneous than the current classification system indicates. The 1997 Villefranche Nosology recognizes only six subtypes, a substantial under-representation of the variability of this condition (Beighton et al. 1998) (Table 47.1).

Pearl: EDS is more than a collagenopathy.

Comment: The recognition of ultrastructural abnormalities of collagen fibrils in EDS patients led to the concept that EDS is a disorder of fibrillar collagen metabolism. A number of EDS subtypes display abnormalities in the expression or structure of the fibrillar collagen types I, III, and V. Others result from enzymatic abnormalities in the posttranslational modification and processing of these collagens (such as lysyl hydroxylases I and procollagen aminoproteinase or ADAMTS2) (see Table 47.1) (Beighton et al. 1998).

The molecular basis of the common hypermobile variant of EDS is unresolved, as is the basis for some other EDS phenotypes. Following the identification in EDS of mutations in a noncollagenous protein, tenascin-X (TNX), it became clear that the search for EDS candidate genes should extend beyond collagens and their modifying enzymes (Burch et al. 1997; Zweers et al. 2003). TNX is regarded widely as a regulator of in vivo collagen deposition (Mao et al. 2002; Bristow et al. 2005). Other noncollagenous extracellular matrix proteins have been suggested as candidate molecules for EDS by transgenic mice studies, especially the group of small, leucine-rich proteoglycans (SLRPs) such as decorin, fibromodulin, and lumican (Ameye and Young 2002). These SLRPs are involved in regulation of collagen fibril diameter and fibril–fibril interactions. SLRP-deficient mice show clinical and ultrastructural characteristics reminiscent of EDS, but no defects in these SLRPs have been associated with human EDS to date.

Mutations in *SLC39A13*, a gene that encodes a membrane-bound zinc transporter, were identified in a new EDS subtype,

J. H. Stone (ed.), *A Clinician's Pearls and Myths in Rheumatology,*
DOI:10.1007/978-1-84800-934-9_47, © Springer Science + Business Media B.V. 2009

Table 47.1. Proposal for updated EDS-nosology

Clinical subtype	Clinical manifestations		IP	Gene
	Cardinal features	Additional features		
Classic	Skin hyperextensibility	Easy bruising	AD	*COL5A1*
	Widened atrophic scarring	Molluscoid pseudotumors		*COL5A2* (~50%)
	Smooth and velvety skin	Subcutaneous spheroids		(Malfait et al. 2005)
	Joint hypermobility	Muscular hypotonia		Unknown (~50%)
		Complications of joint hypermobility		
		Surgical complications		
		Positive family history		
"Classic –like"	Skin hyperextensibility	Smooth and velvety skin	AR	*TNX-B* (Burch et al. 1997)
	Easy bruising	Complications of joint hypermobility		
	Joint hypermobility			
Hypermobility	Generalized joint hypermobility	Recurring joint dislocations	AD	*TNX-B* (Zweers et al. 2003)
	Mild skin involvement (mild skin hyperextensibility, mild atrophic scarring, soft skin)	Chronic joint pain		*COL5A1* (Malfait et al. 2006a)
		Positive family history		Unknown (majority)
Vascular	Excessive bruising	Acrogeria	AD	*COL3A1*
	Thin, translucent skin	Early-onset varicose veins		
	Arterial/intestinal/	Hypermobility of small joints		
	Uterine fragility or rupture	Tendon and muscle rupture		
	Characteristic facial appearance	Arteriovenous or		
		Carotid-cavernous sinus fistula		
		Pneumo (hemo)thorax		
		Positive family history, sudden death in close relative(s)		
"Vascular-like"	Skin hyperextensibility	Thin, translucent skin	AD	*COL1A1* (Malfait et al. 2007)
	Atrophic scarring	Joint hypermobility		
	Easy bruising	Complications of joint hypermobility		
	Arterial rupture	Positive family history		
"Cardiac-Valvular"	Severe cardiac valvular disease	Atrophic scarring	AR	*COL1A2* (Malfait et al. 2006b)
	Skin hyperextensibility	Easy bruising		
	Joint hypermobility	Bluish sclerae		
		Increased bone fragility		
Kyphoscoliotic	Severe muscular hypotonia at birth	Tissue fragility, including atrophic scars	AR	*PLOD1*
	Generalized joint laxity	Easy bruising		Unknown
	Kyphoscoliosis at birth	Arterial rupture		
	Scleral fragility and rupture of the globe	Marfanoid habitus		
		Microcornea		
		Bluish sclerae		
		Osteopenia		
EDS/OI overlap syndrome	Joint hypermobility	Easy bruising	AD	*COL1A1*
	Mild skin involvement	Recurring joint dislocations		*COL1A2* (Cabral et al. 2005)
	Blue sclera	Kyphoscoliosis		
	Increased bone fragility	Chronic joint pain		
		Arterial rupture		
		Positive family history		
Arthrochalasis	Severe generalized joint hypermobility with recurrent subluxations	Easy bruising	AD	*COL1A1*
		Muscular hypotonia		*COL1A2*
	Congenital bilateral hip dislocation	Kyphoscoliosis		
	Skin hyperextensibility	Mild osteopenia		
	Widened, atrophic scars			
Dermatosparaxis	Severe skin fragility	Soft, doughy skin texture	AR	*ADAMTS-2*
	Sagging, redundant skin	Premature rupture of membranes		
	Excessive bruising	Progressive		
	Characteristic facies	Paperscar-formation		
	Postnatal growth deficiency, short hands and feet	Progressive generalized joint hypermobility		
	Umbilical hernia	Delayed gross motor development		
	Delayed closure of fontanels	Palmar wrinkling		
		Bladder rupture		
		Rupture of diaphragm		

Table 47.1. (Continued)

Clinical subtype	Clinical manifestations		IP	Gene
	Cardinal features	Additional features		
Progeroid	Mental retardation	Variable skin involvement	AR	*β4Gal-T7*
	Wrinkled, loose skin on the face	Easy bruising		
	Curly fine hair	Joint hypermobility		
	Scanty eyebrows and eyelashes			
Periodontotic	Severe early-onset periodontal disease	Variable skin involvement	AD	Unknown
	Discrete, chronically inflamed pretibial plaques	Easy bruising		
		Joint hypermobility		
Spondylo-cheiro dysplastic form	Postnatal growth retardation	Tissue fragility, including atrophic scars	AR	*SLC39A13* (Giunta et al. 2008)
	Hypermobility of small joints, later contractures	Bluish sclerae		
	Slender, tapering fingers, palmar wrinkling, (hypo)thenar atrophy	Osteopenia		
	Platyspondyly			
	Widened metaphyses			

The presence of more than 1 cardinal feature is highly suggestive for the diagnosis of a specific subtype of EDS, while the additional features contribute to the diagnosis of the specific subtype
IP inheritance pattern; *AD* autosomal dominant; *AR* autosomal recessive

characterized by EDS-like features and a mild skeletal dysplasia (Giunta et al. 2008). This shows that genes other than the fibrillar collagens and their known modifying enzymes participate in the complex process of collagen fibrillogenesis and the organization of extracellular matrix architecture. Given that many EDS subtypes are still unexplained, still other undiscovered noncollagen genes probably account for the clinical manifestations in some EDS patients.

Myth: EDS is a rare disorder.

Reality: The prevalence of EDS is not known with any precision. Beighton (1970) estimated a prevalence of 1 in 156,000 in southern England. Others, however, have only claimed that EDS is the most common heritable disorder of connective tissue. The perceived incidence is likely to increase as awareness of the phenotypic variability increases among clinicians.

Some of the severe subtypes, such as the arthrochalasis, kyphoscoliosis, and dermatosparaxis subtype, are indeed rare. The prevalence of "classic" EDS has been estimated at 1:20,000 (Byers 2001). However, some individuals with mild disease manifestations do not come to medical attention and therefore remain subclinical (or at least undiagnosed). The minimum prevalence of vascular EDS is on the order of 1 in 250,000 (Pepin and Byers 2008). However, because many families with the vascular type of EDS are identified only after a severe complication or death, proportion of individuals or families with a milder phenotype who do not come to medical attention is probably considerably higher.

The prevalence of the hypermobility syndrome is unknown. Estimates range from 1:5,000–1:20,000 (Levy 2008), but this is likely to be an underestimate because of the substantial clinical variability of this disorder.

Pearl: The skin is the window to the diagnosis of EDS.

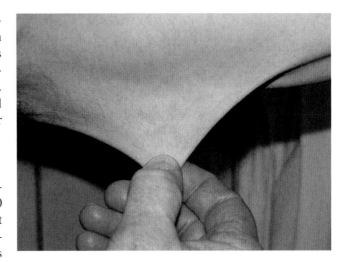

Fig. 47.1 Skin hyperextensibility in the Ehlers–Danlos syndrome

Comment: Not every double-jointed individual has EDS. The cutaneous features of a patient's disease are often the key to the diagnosis. A careful physical examination with particular attention to the skin is critical to making the correct diagnosis. Patients with EDS usually have soft, smooth skin that has a velvety, doughy feel. Some degree of skin hyperextensibility is typical (Fig. 47.1). Cutaneous scars in EDS have an atrophic appearance.

In the vascular subtype of EDS, the skin is not hyperextensible but rather thin and transparent. A venous pattern is evident over the chest, abdomen, and extremities. Other classic physical examination features of the vascular EDS subtype are widespread ecchymoses and varicose veins.

Myth: Ultrastructural abnormalities of the skin are characteristic for a specific EDS subtype.

Reality: A common Myth surrounding EDS is that the ultra-structural findings within the dermis can confirm or exclude a diagnosis of specific EDS subtypes. Ultrastructural examination of the skin, performed by electron microscopy, usually reveals abnormalities of collagen fibrillogenesis. These include irregular, disrupted collagen fibrils ("collagen-flowers") and variability within the diameter of the individual collagen fibrils. However, these abnormalities are found in several EDS variants and are usually insufficient to discriminate between individual EDS subtypes.

There is one exception to this rule. In the dermatosparaxis subtype of EDS, a pathognomonic ultrastructural aspect of the collagen fibril architecture is observed. The finding of this architecture confirms the clinical diagnosis. Collagen fibrils in the dermatosparaxis subtype lose their normal cross-sectional circular aspect and have instead an irregular, branched, "hieroglyphic" appearance (Pierard and Lapiere 1976; Malfait et al. 2004). Clinical diagnosis remains the primary means of identifying all EDS subtypes.

Myth: EDS and cutis laxa are related disorders.

Reality: EDS and the cutis laxa syndromes are different disorders clinically and genetically. From the clinical point of view, the "hyperextensible" skin in EDS must be distinguished from that of "cutis laxa" syndromes. Hyperextensibility, a characteristic of EDS, refers to skin that extends easily and snaps back after release. This should be tested at a "neutral site"; i.e., one not subjected to mechanical forces or scarring. The volar surface of the forearm is one such neutral site.

Hyperextensibility is quantified by pulling the skin until resistance is felt (Fig. 47.2). Cutaneous hyperextensibility is observed to a varying degree in all subtypes of EDS with the exception of the vascular subtype. (In the vascular subtype, the skin is thin and transparent.) In the cutis laxa syndromes, the skin is redundant: it hangs in loose folds and returns very slowly to its former position. The skin in cutis laxa is not fragile, and wound healing is normal.

The EDS subtypes are caused by defects in within the fibrillar collagens (types I, III, or V) or in other proteins involved in collagen fibrillogenesis. In contrast, the cutis laxa syndromes result from the loss or fragmentation of the elastic fiber network. This is caused by mutations in the elastin gene or other genes that encode proteins related to elastic fiber development or homeostasis (e.g., the fibulins).

Pearl: EDS should be considered in the differential diagnosis of child abuse.

Comment: In children with EDS, excessive bruising following minor trauma is often the presenting complaint to the pediatrician. If pronounced, it sometimes raises suspicion of child abuse. Careful evaluation of medical and family history and rigorous clinical examination with special attention to subtle skin features that are characteristic for EDS is

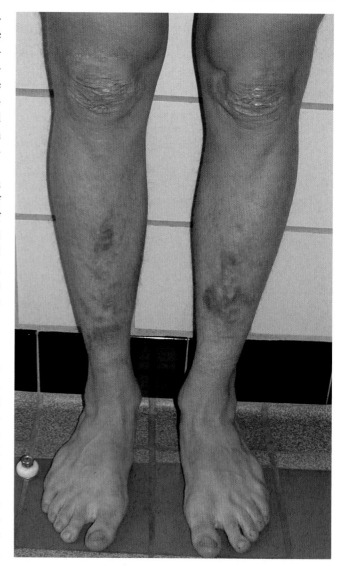

Fig. 47.2 "Cigarette paper" scarring and hemosiderin deposition as a result of repetitive trauma on knees and shins of a patient with the classic Ehlers-Danlos syndrome

necessary to distinguish this disorder from other causes of bruising. Laboratory investigation of clotting factors, platelet aggregation, and bleeding time is usually normal in patients with an EDS or related connective tissue disorders (De Paepe and Malfait et al. 2004).

Myth: Patients with EDS can be recognized by their blue sclerae.

Reality: Most patients with EDS, especially with the more common subtypes, such as the hypermobile, classic, or vascular variants of EDS, do not present blue sclerae. Blue sclerae are commonly present in osteogenesis imperfecta, caused by genetic defects in type I collagen. However, blue–grey sclerae are observed in some of the rare EDS subtypes that are associated with defects in the structure or the processing of type I collagen. As examples, the dermatosparaxis and arthrochalasis subtypes have much phenotypic overlap with osteogenesis imperfecta, and patients with those EDS subtypes can have blue–grey sclerae.

Pearl: Collagen studies allow confirmation of the diagnosis of certain EDS subtypes.

Comment: In certain EDS subtypes, biochemical and molecular analysis can be very helpful to confirm the diagnosis. To this purpose, a skin biopsy is required to obtain cultured skin fibroblasts. Biochemical study of the collagen types I, III, and V includes SDS-polyacrylamide gel electrophoresis of radiolabeled collagens, extracted from the cultured fibroblasts. In the vascular subtype of EDS, biochemical analysis of type III procollagen identifies more than 95% of all patients. Molecular screening of the *COL3A1* gene identifies virtually all mutations.

Characterization of a type III collagen defect enables asymptomatic, but affected family members to be aware of their condition, to learn about appropriate treatments for possible complications of the disorder, to restriction high-impact sports, and to undergo elective surgery, arteriograms, and other possibly risky procedures in an informed manner.

Biochemical analysis can also be helpful in the diagnosis of the arthrochalasis, kyphoscoliosis, dermatosparaxis, and some other rare subtypes of EDS, where distinct abnormal migration patterns of type I (pro)-collagen chains are observed. These findings guide further molecular analysis of the correct genes. When a disease-causing mutation is identified, prenatal and preimplantation genetic diagnosis becomes possible.

Pearl: Genetic counseling is an essential part of EDS management.

Comment: Provision of genetic counseling is an important issue in the management of patients with EDS. The different subtypes of EDS are associated with differences in modes of inheritance, subtype-specific risks, and variable long-term prognoses. Unnecessary or unrealistic fear for certain risks in patients with specific EDS subtypes, misunderstandings and wrong perceptions, are sometimes the result of wrong information, or the wrong interpretation of it, as supplied by various Internet sites or by the media.

Families should be provided with detailed information regarding the inheritance pattern, risk of recurrence, and identification of at-risk family members. Screening of other individuals in the family for subtle signs and symptoms of the condition should be offered, regardless of whether signs or symptoms are suggested by the family history. The prognosis and natural history of the particular EDS type, as well as the possibility of prenatal of preimplantation genetic diagnosis, should be discussed with the family. Another key element in the genetic counseling process includes triage toward appropriate medical services and provision of information about national patient support groups.

Pearl: It is unknown whether hypermobile EDS and (benign) joint hypermobility syndrome represent the same entity.

Comment: The hypermobility type of EDS is characterized by generalized joint hypermobility and joint instability. This causes recurrent subluxations and dislocations, and chronic musculoskeletal pain. Skin abnormalities are usually mild (see Table 47.1). Considerable clinical overlap exists between the EDS hypermobility subtype and two related disorders, the (benign) joint hypermobility syndrome, and familial articular hypermobility syndrome.

The familial articular hypermobility syndrome, formerly known as EDS type XI, is an autosomal dominant connective tissue disorder characterized by severe joint hypermobility and occasional congenital hip dislocation, but no skin involvement (Beighton et al. 1988). The joint hypermobility syndrome is also an autosomal dominant connective tissue disorder, which was first recognized as a distinct condition in 1967 (Kirk et al. 1967). In the original description of the disorder, the joint hypermobility syndrome was defined as "the occurrence of musculoskeletal problems in hypermobile but otherwise healthy persons."

A variety of nonarticular symptoms and signs, including fragility of the skin and other connective tissues, can be associated with the joint hypermobility syndrome. In 1998, Grahame and coworkers presented a set of major and minor diagnostic criteria for this disorder known as the Brighton criteria (Grahame et al. 2000) (Table 47.2). With the recognition of the presence of mild fragility of connective tissues other than the joints, it was suggested that JHS is itself an

Table 47.2 1998 Revised Brighton criteria for benign joint hypermobility syndrome (BJHS)

Major Criteria
Beighton score of ≥ 4/9 (either historically or currently)
arthralgia for > 3 months in 4 or more joints
Minor criteria
Beighton score of 1–3 (0–3 if aged ≥ 50+)
Arthralgia (>3 months) in 1–3 joints or back pain (>3 months), spondylosis, or spondylolysis/spondylolisthesis
Dislocation/subluxation in more than one joint, or in one joint on more than one occasion
Three or more soft tissue lesions (e.g., epicondylitis, bursitis, tenosynovitis)
Marfanoid habitus (tall, slim, span/height ratio > 1.03, upper/lower segment ratio < 0.89, arachnodactyly)
Skin striae, hyperextensibility, thin skin or abnormal scarring
Eye signs: drooping eyelids, myopia, or antimongoloid slant
Varicose veins, hernia uterine or uterine/rectal prolapsed

BJHS is diagnosed in the presence of two major criteria, or one major and two minor criteria, or four minor criteria. Two minor criteria will suffice where there is an unequivocally affected first-degree relative. BJHS is excluded in the presence of Marfan syndrome or EDS other than hypermobility type. From Grahame et al. (2000). Reprinted with permission from The Journal of Rheumatology

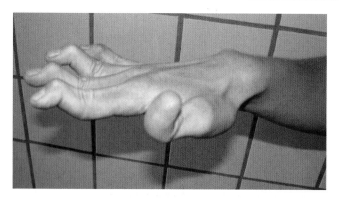

Fig. 47.3 Joint hypermobility in the EDS

under-recognized heritable disorder of connective tissue. Some authorities consider the joint hypermobility syndrome and hypermobile EDS to be essentially indistinguishable if not identical disorders (Grahame 1999).

Pearl: The hypermobility subtype of EDS is more than a circus act.

Comment: Because the hypermobility subtype of EDS is not associated with major skin manifestations or vascular fragility, it is generally considered the least severe of all EDS subtypes. Joint hypermobility is common in the general population, but in the majority of individuals it does not cause major complaints. Joint hypermobility is often considered a curiosity rather than a medical problem, by clinicians as well as the general public (Fig. 47.3).

Joint hypermobility continues to be under-recognized, poorly understood, and managed inadequately. However, significant complications of this disorder can occur. Subluxations and dislocations are common and can be very painful. The predominant presenting complaint is pain. This is often widespread and chronic, leading to major physical and psychosocial distress (Sacheti et al. 1997). It is variable in age of onset, number of sites, duration, quality, severity, and response to therapy. There is often a discrepancy between the extent of pain and the paucity of objective signs on physical or radiological examination. In addition to the pain, there are many other joint symptoms such as stiffness, clicking and popping of the joints, the feeling of joint instability or weakness, and many individuals describe the condition as being imprisoned in an "old" or "dysfunctional" body.

Pearl: Hypermobile EDS: it is not all about the joints!

Comment: In addition to the articular problems, patients with EDS hypermobility type may suffer from a wide variety of extraarticular manifestations. Complications of soft connective tissue fragility are shown in Tables 47.1 and 47.2. Other problems include proprioception difficulties (Hall et al. 1995; Ferrell et al. 2004); poor responses to local anesthetics, e.g., during dental care (Arendt-Nielsen et al. 1991);

fatigue and sleep disturbance; autonomic dysfunction, causing symptoms such as atypical chest pain, palpitations (at rest and/or upon exercise), dizziness, faintness, syncope or presyncope, postural orthostatic tachycardia syndrome, orthostatic hypotension, and gastrointestinal disturbance (Gazit et al. 2003; Hakim and Grahame 2004).

This apparent autonomic dysfunction has several potential explanations, such as exaggerated blood pooling in the lower extremities due to weakened vascular tissue elasticity; impaired peripheral vasoregulation due to neuronal or adrenoreceptor abnormalities; impaired central sympathetic control; or deconditioning due to muscle disuse through pain or fear of pain (Rowe et al. 1999; Gazit et al. 2003; Hakim and Grahame 2004).

Autonomic dysfunction is also frequently encountered in fibromyalgia and chronic fatigue syndrome, two conditions that show many overlapping symptoms with EDS hypermobility type and JHS. Many patients with EDS hypermobility have been diagnosed with fibromyalgia or chronic fatigue syndrome (or both) prior to the recognition of their joint hypermobility. It remains currently unclear whether presence of chronic pain, autonomic dysfunction, and other overlapping symptoms in these populations are the result of a common pathway, or merely reflects the co-occurrence of these three relatively common syndromes.

The impact of this wide spectrum of symptoms can have a devastating impact on sleep, work, physical activities, and social and sexual relationships of affected patients. This leads to the patients being misunderstood or misdiagnosed as having psychosocial problems, hypochondriasis, or depression. Hypermobility is also associated with anxiety and panic attack (Bulbena et al. 1993; Martin-Santos et al. 1998; Hakim and Grahame 2003).

Myth: Mitral valve prolapse is encountered frequently in EDS.

Reality: Mitral valve prolapse was considered at one time to be a manifestation common to all subtypes of EDS. However, this has not been confirmed in rigorous studies (Dolan et al. 1997). Mitral valve prolapse (and, less frequently, tricuspid valve prolapse) appears to be limited to the more severe forms of classic EDS (McDonnell et al. 2006).

Pearl: Patients with vascular EDS require a special approach.

Comment: Some prophylactic measures are critical for patients with the vascular subtype of EDS. The vascular subtype is dominated by generalized vascular fragility that affects large vessels on both sides of the circulatory system, as well as small arteries, veins, and capillaries.

Vascular fragility and bleeding may occur at any site in the body and can present in various ways: acute abdominal pain, stroke, hemoptysis, hematemesis, renal colic and hematuria, retroperitoneal bleeding, muscular swelling, shock, and sudden death. The most common locations of life-threatening arterial bleeding are in the abdominal cavity, where they involve medium-sized arteries such as the renal or splenic arteries. The aorta itself is seldom involved. In some individuals, there is evidence of aneurysmal degeneration and dissection or of arteriovenous fistulae, but in other patients ruptures occur at locations that appear completely normal by angiography (Steinmann et al. 2002). The necessity for periodic arterial screening is therefore uncertain and controversial. Some authors advice not to pursue any additional investigation or surveillance, because a conservative approach will be used irrespective of the findings. Others recommend noninvasive surveillance by means of echocardiogram, carotid ultrasound, and noninvasive imaging of chest and abdomen, because knowledge of incidental lesions may favorably affect survival (Oderich et al. 2005).

Invasive vascular procedures such as arteriography and catheterization in these patients should be avoided because of the risk of vascular ruptures (Cikrit et al. 1987; Freeman et al. 1996). Whenever possible, invasive vascular procedures should be replaced by ultrasonography, computed tomography, or magnetic resonance angiography.

Surgical interventions are discouraged in the vascular subtype of EDS. If surgery is unavoidable, the surgeon should be aware of the diagnosis. Manipulation of vascular and other tissues should be done with extreme care. Finally, patients with vascular EDS should refrain from anticoagulation therapy and from drugs that interfere with platelet function (Steinmann et al. 2002).

Myth: Patients with vascular EDS should not get pregnant.

Reality: Pregnancy for women with the vascular type of EDS is a high-risk venture. The risk of maternal death is as high as 12% from uterine rupture or peripartum arterial rupture (Pepin et al. 2000). On the other hand, some women with vascular EDS have had one or several successful pregnancies prior to the recognition of their underlying condition. It is not known whether elective cesarean sections are preferred to vaginal deliveries.

Myth: There is no treatment for EDS.

Reality: No treatment for the underlying defect is available presently for EDS. However, a series of "preventive" guidelines are applicable to all subtypes of this disorder. These are listed below in a series of Pearls related to skin care, bruising, joint protection, and emotional support.

47.2 Skin Care

- Patients with EDS should be instructed to avoid undue trauma to the skin and other organ systems. Children with pronounced skin fragility should wear protective pads or bandages over the forehead, knees, and shins from an early age.

- Dermal wounds should be closed without tension, preferably in two layers. Deep stitches should be applied generously.
- Cutaneous stitches should be left in place twice as long as usual.
- Fixation of skin adjacent to stitches with adhesive tape can help prevent stretching of the scar.

47.3 Bruising

- Patients with pronounced bruising should avoid contact sports and heavy exercise (Pepin and Byers 2008).
- Protective pads and bandages are also useful in the prevention of bruises and hematomas.
- Supplementation of ascorbic acid, a cofactor for cross-linking of collagen fibrils, ameliorates the tendency toward bruising in some patients (Steinmann et al. 2002).
- DDAVP (desamino-D-arginin-vasopressin) may be useful in EDS patients with chronic bruising or epistaxis, or perioperatively (e.g., for tooth extraction), in whom bleeding time is normalized by DDAVP (Stine and Becton 1997).

47.4 Joint Protection

- In children with hypotonia and delayed motor development, a physiotherapeutic program is important. Nonweight-bearing muscular exercise, such as swimming, is useful to promote muscular development, strength, and coordination.
- Patients should avoid excessive or repetitive heavy lifting and other movements that produce undue strain on the already hypermobile joints.
- They should not "show off" by demonstrating their joint laxity to others. Excessive stretching of the joints further exacerbates the underlying disorder.

47.5 Emotional Support

- Emotional support and behavioral and psychological therapy may be indicated in all subtypes of EDS to accept and cope with the handicap. Patient support groups are available and can be very beneficial.

Pearl: Some but not all patients with EDS should have an annual echocardiogram.

Comment: A baseline echocardiogram should be performed in all patients with EDS to evaluate aortic root diameter, as adjusted for age and body surface area, and to evaluate cardiac valvular abnormalities. Because longitudinal data on progression of aortic dilation are not available, specific recommendations for follow up in individuals with a normal aortic diameter do not exist. However, if no abnormalities are found on echocardiogram in an adult, a follow-up echocardiogram is probably not necessary. For children and adolescents, it is reasonable to repeat the echocardiogram, approximately every 3 years until adulthood. Annual echocardiograms are warranted only if an abnormality such as aortic dilatation or mitral valve prolapse is present.

Pearl: Patients with EDS require a multidisciplinary approach.

Comment: As EDS affects many systems in the body, a number of specialists may need to be involved, depending on the severity of the symptoms of an individual. Each patient will have an individual set of clinical problems, requiring a treatment plan that is tailored to his or her particular needs. One doctor should have a coordinating role ensuring that all areas of the syndrome are covered, preferably the clinical geneticist, who will also provide genetic counseling. The key aspects of management include cardiovascular work-up, physiotherapy, pain management, and psychological follow up.

Besides prescription of physiotherapy, the rheumatologist and/or physical therapist may also provide assisting devices such as braces, ring splints, soft collar necks, while the occupational therapist may provide tools that make the living and working environment more user-friendly for the patient. Many patients will have undergone one or more orthopedic procedures prior to the diagnosis of EDS, such as arthroplasty and capsulorraphy. The degree of joint stabilization, pain reduction, and duration of improvement are usually far less in patients with EDS than in those without this disorder. It is often appropriate to delay surgery in EDS patients in favor of physical therapy and bracing.

Pain management is also very important. Pain medication should be tailored to the individual's subjective symptoms. Cognitive behavioral therapy can be beneficial in patients with hypermobility and chronic pain. Finally, psychological follow up designed to explore coping strategies and to recognize and treat depression is of utmost importance.

References

Ameye L, Young MF. Mice deficient in small leucine-rich proteoglycans: novel in vivo models for osteoporosis, osteoarthritis, Ehlers–Danlos syndrome, muscular dystrophy, and corneal diseases. Glycobiology 2002;12:107R–16R

Arendt-Nielsen L, Kaalund S, Hogsaa B, et al The response to local anaesthetics (EMLA-cream) as a clinical test to diagnose between hypermobility and Ehlers Danlos type III syndrome. Scand J Rheumatol. 1991;20:190–5

Beighton P. The Ehlers–Danlos syndrome. London: William Heinemann Medical Books; 1970

Beighton P, De Paepe A, Danks D, et al International nosology of heritable disorders of connective tissue, Berlin, 1986. Am J Med Genet. 1988;29:581–94

Beighton P, De Paepe A, Steinmann B, et al Ehlers–Danlos syndromes: revised nosology, Villefranche, 1997. Ehlers–Danlos National Foundation (USA) and Ehlers–Danlos Support Group (UK). Am J Med Genet. 1998;77:31–7

Bristow J, Carey W, Egging D, et al Tenascin-X, collagen, elastin, and the Ehlers–Danlos syndrome. Am J Med Genet C Semin Med Genet. 2005;139:24–30

Bulbena A, Duro JC, Porta M, et al Anxiety disorders in the joint hypermobility syndrome. Psychiatry Res. 1993;46:59–68

Burch GH, Gong Y, Liu W, et al Tenascin-X deficiency is associated with Ehlers–Danlos syndrome. Nat Genet. 1997;17:104–8

Byers P. Disorders of collagen biosynthesis and structure. In: Scriver CR, Beaudet AR, Sly WS and Valle D, editors. The metabolic and molecular bases of inherited disease. 2nd ed. Edinbugrh: Churchill Livingstone; 2001. p. 1065–81

Cabral WA, Makareeva E, Colige A, et al Mutations near amino end of alpha 1(I) collagen cause combined OI/EDS by interference with N-propeptide processing. J Biol Chem. 2005;280:19259–69

Cikrit DF, Miles JH, Silver D. Spontaneous arterial perforation: the Ehlers–Danlos specter. J Vasc Surg. 1987;5:248–55

De Paepe A, Malfait F. Bleeding and bruising in patients with Ehlers–Danlos syndrome and other collagen vascular disorders. Br J Haematol. 2004;127:491–500

Dolan AL, Mishra MB, Chambers JB, et al Clinical and echocardiographic survey of the Ehlers–Danlos syndrome. Br J Rheumatol. 1997;36:459–62

Ferrell WR, Tennant N, Sturrock RD, et al Amelioration of symptoms by enhancement of proprioception in patients with joint hypermobility syndrome. Arthritis Rheum. 2004;50:3323–8

Freeman RK, Swegle J, Sise MJ. The surgical complications of Ehlers–Danlos syndrome. Am Surg. 1996;62:869–73

Gazit Y, Nahir AM, Grahame R, et al Dysautonomia in the joint hypermobility syndrome. Am J Med. 2003;115:33–40

Giunta C, Elcioglu NH, Albrecht B, et al Spondylocheiro dysplastic form of the Ehlers–Danlos syndrome – an autosomal-recessive entity caused by mutations in the zinc transporter gene SLC39A13. Am J Hum Genet. 2008;82:1290–305

Grahame R. Joint hypermobility and genetic collagen disorders: are they related? Arch Dis Child. 1999;80:188–91

Grahame R, Bird HA, Child A. The revised (Brighton 1998) criteria for the diagnosis of benign joint hypermobility syndrome (BJHS). J Rheumatol. 2000;27:1777–9

Hakim A, Grahame R. Joint hypermobility. Best Pract Res Clin Rheumatol. 2003;17:989–1004

Hakim AJ, Grahame R. Non-musculoskeletal symptoms in joint hypermobility syndrome. Indirect evidence for autonomic dysfunction. Rheumatology (Oxford) 2004;43:1194–5

Hall MG, Ferrell WR, Sturrock RD, et al The effect of the hypermobility syndrome on knee joint proprioception. Br J Rheumatol. 1995;34:121–5

Kirk JA, Ansell BM, Bywaters EG. The hypermobility syndrome. Musculoskeletal complaints associated with generalized joint hypermobility. Ann Rheum Dis. 1967;26:419–25

Levy HP. Ehlers–Danlos syndrome, hypermobility type. http://www.genetests.org. Accessed September 16, 2008

Malfait F, Coucke P, Symoens S, et al The molecular basis of classic Ehlers–Danlos syndrome: a comprehensive study of biochemical and molecular findings in 48 unrelated patients. Hum Mutat. 2005;25:28–37

Malfait F, De Coster P, Hausser I, et al The natural history, including orofacial features of three patients with Ehlers–Danlos syndrome, dermatosparaxis type (EDS type VIIC). Am J Med Genet A. 2004;131:18–28

Malfait F, Hakim AJ, A De Paepe A, et al The genetic basis of the joint hypermobility syndromes. Rheumatology (Oxford). 2006a;45: 502–7

Malfait F, Symoens S, Coucke P, et al Total absence of the alpha2(I) chain of collagen type I causes a rare form of Ehlers–Danlos syndrome with hypermobility and propensity to cardiac valvular problems. J Med Genet. 2006b;43:e36

Malfait F, Symoens S, De Backer J, et al Three arginine to cysteine substitutions in the pro-alpha (I)-collagen chain cause Ehlers–Danlos syndrome with a propensity to arterial rupture in early adulthood. Hum Mutat. 2007;28:396–405

Mao JR, Taylor G, Dean WB, et al Tenascin-X deficiency mimics Ehlers–Danlos syndrome in mice through alteration of collagen deposition. Nat Genet. 2002;30:421–5

Martin-Santos R, Bulbena A, Porta M, et al Association between joint hypermobility syndrome and panic disorder. Am J Psychiatry. 1998;155:1578–83

McDonnell NB, Gorman BL, Mandel KW, et al Echocardiographic findings in classical and hypermobile Ehlers–Danlos syndromes. Am J Med Genet A. 2006;140:129–36

McKusick VA In: McKusick VA, editor. Heritable disorders of connective tissue. 1st ed. Saint Louis: Mosby; 1972. p. 292–371

Oderich GS, Panneton JM, Bower TC, et al The spectrum, management and clinical outcome of Ehlers–Danlos syndrome type IV: a 30-year experience. J Vasc Surg. 2005;42:98–106

Pepin M, Byers PH. Ehlers–Danlos syndrome, vascular type. . http://www.genetests.org. Accessed September 16, 2008

Pepin M, Schwarze U, Superti-Furga A, et al Clinical and genetic features of Ehlers–Danlos syndrome type IV, the vascular type. N Engl J Med. 2000;342:673–80

Pierard GE, Lapiere M. Skin in dermatosparaxis. Dermal microarchitecture and biomechanical properties. J Invest Dermatol. 1976;66: 2–7

Rowe PC, Barron DF, Calkins H, et al Orthostatic intolerance and chronic fatigue syndrome associated with Ehlers–Danlos syndrome. J Pediatr. 1999;135:494–9

Sacheti A, Szemere J, Bernstein B, et al Chronic pain is a manifestation of the Ehlers–Danlos syndrome. J Pain Symptom Manage. 1997;14: 88–93

Steinmann B, Royce P, Superti-Furga A. The Ehlers–Danlos syndrome. In: Royce P and Steinmann B, editors. Connective tissue and its heritable disorders. 2nd ed. New York: Wiley-Liss; 2002. p. 431–523

Stine KC, Becton DL. DDAVP therapy controls bleeding in Ehlers–Danlos syndrome. J Pediatr Hematol Oncol. 1997;19:156–8

Zweers MC, Bristow J, Steijlen PM, et al Haploinsufficiency of TNXB is associated with hypermobility type of Ehlers–Danlos syndrome. Am J Hum Genet. 2003;73:214–7

Osteonecrosis

Michael G. Zywiel, Mike S. McGrath, and Michael A. Mont

48.1 Overview of Osteonecrosis

> Osteonecrosis, literally "bone death," is the loss of viable bone tissue

> Up to 10% of all hip replacement procedures in the U.S. are performed for osteonecrosis.

> Major risk factors for osteonecrosis include glucocorticoid use, alcohol, cigarette smoking, systemic lupus erythematosus (SLE), scuba diving, and major hip trauma, leading to disruption of the vascular supply to the femoral head.

> Patients who have identifiable risk factors for osteonecrosis are said to have secondary osteonecrosis.

> Idiopathic osteonecrosis occurs in some individuals without overt risk factors for the disorder.

> Clinical outcomes are better in patients who are treated at early stages of the disease.

> Patients who have large osteonecrotic lesions or femoral head collapse at the time of presentation will typically progress to end-stage degenerative disease requiring joint arthroplasty.

> Magnetic resonance imaging (MRI) is the study of choice for patients in whom there is a high index of suspicion of osteonecrosis.

> Core decompression is a relatively noninvasive joint preservation technique that may be effective if applied to patients with early disease.

> Hip resurfacing is a joint arthroplasty technique that requires less resection of native bone compared with traditional joint arthroplasty procedures.

Pearl: A patient treated with high-dose glucocorticoids who develops pain in the area of a single major joint should undergo screening of the affected area for osteonecrosis.

Comment: Glucocorticoid use is implicated in almost 70% of advanced cases of secondary osteonecrosis (Zywiel et al. 2009). Some data are also consistent with a correlation between cumulative glucocorticoid use and the development of osteonecrosis. Thus, osteonecrosis is in the differential diagnosis for any patient who has a substantial history of glucocorticoid use and the new onset of joint pain.

Plain radiographs do not detect osteonecrosis at an early stage, the time at which treatment is most effective. Thus, if a significant question of osteonecrosis exists, MRI should be performed to exclude or diagnose the condition definitively (Fig. 48.1).

Pearl: Smoking tobacco rivals alcohol consumption as a risk factor for secondary osteonecrosis.

Comment: Glucocorticoid use, excessive alcohol consumption, and SLE are cited most frequently as the top risk factors for secondary osteonecrosis. However, cigarette smoking is also a significant risk factor, and a history of smoking increases suspicion for the diagnosis of secondary osteonecrosis in patients with a compatible clinical presentation.

Myth: Osteonecrosis can develop after minor trauma to the hip.

Reality: Minor trauma can lead to subchondral fracture and spontaneous focal bone necrosis in patients who have markedly compromised bone strength, but it is not a causative factor for true osteonecrosis. On the other hand, the femoral head is susceptible to circulatory disruption after major trauma because its blood flow originates in the relatively narrow neck of the femur. Dislocation of the hip can compromise the medial femoral circumflex artery, which traverses the posterior superior aspect of the femoral neck. Disruption of the medial femoral circumflex artery reduces or eliminates perfusion to the femoral head and leads to osteonecrosis. Subcapital femoral fractures, particularly when displaced, also carry a high risk of disruption of the blood supply to the femoral head and the development of osteonecrosis (Fig. 48.2).

Pearl: Minor trauma actually helps some patients by highlighting the presence of early, preexisting osteonecrosis.

Comment: Early stages of osteonecrosis are marked often by the gradual, insidious onset of pain in the affected joint. Because it increases slowly and often seems more irritating than worrying, patients frequently delay seeking medical care. Minor trauma sometimes brings patients fortuitously to

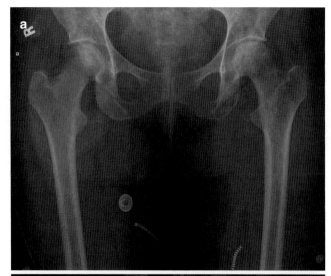

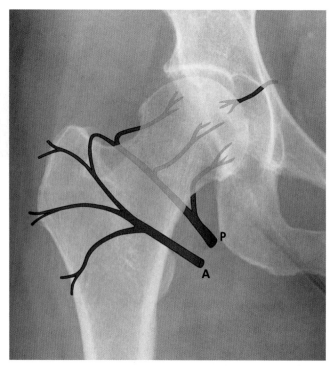

Fig. 48.2 Blood is primarily supplied to the femoral head in retrograde flow from the posterior (*P*) and anterior (*A*) femoral circumflex arteries. Subcapital fractures and/or dislocations of the femoral head can easily disrupt this supply

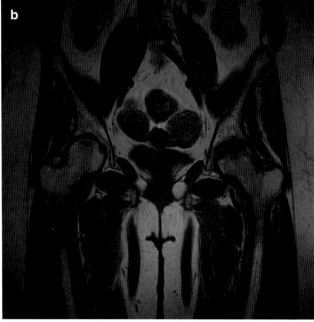

Fig. 48.1 Comparison of the appearance of a stage I osteonecrotic lesion on plain radiograph (**a**) and T1-weighted MRI (**b**)

medical attention and provides an opportunity to make the diagnosis of osteonecrosis at an early stage. Thus, rather than cause osteonecrosis, minor trauma can actually lead to an earlier diagnosis of the condition.

Myth: Patients with osteonecrosis of large joints should be screened for osteonecrosis of the jaw.

Reality: Osteonecrosis of the jaw was described as early as the mid-19th century. "Phossy jaw" – necrosis of the mandible induced by phosphorus exposure in match-factory workers – is a memorable historic example (Anonymous 1867). A tremendous resurgence of interest in jaw osteonecrosis has accompanied reports of this disorder in association with bisphosphonate treatment (Marx 2003). Although osteonecrosis of the jaw and

osteonecrosis of large joints share common pathologic feature of dead necrotic bone, they are otherwise unrelated. There is no need to screen for jaw lesions in patients with osteonecrosis of large joints.

Myth: Patients who have secondary osteonecrosis should undergo bone scintigraphy to detect occult disease foci in other joints.

Reality: Bone scintigraphy has poor sensitivity for osteonecrotic lesions and is therefore of limited value. One study of bone scintigraphy reported that this modality identified only 50% of symptomatic foci (Mont et al. 2008). Bone scans also not effective for detecting lesions at an early stage, rendering them particularly unsuitable for use as a screening tool.

A screening strategy that is more effective than the performance of bone scintigraphy is to remain vigilant for any new onset of pain or ache in the large joints of patients at risk for osteonecrosis. Such patients should be screened with MRI of the symptomatic joint upon the first appearance of symptoms.

Pearl: All patients who present with secondary osteonecrosis should be referred for MRI scans of the hips.

Comment: Up to 90% of patients who present with symptomatic osteonecrosis of one or more joints other than the hip have osteonecrotic lesions of the femoral head. Thus, MRI studies of the hips should be ordered for any patient who has secondary osteonecrosis in a nonhip joint (e.g., the knee or shoulder) (Mitchell et al. 1986).

Myth: All patients with secondary osteonecrosis should be followed with serial MRIs.

Reality: Once a patient is diagnosed with secondary osteonecrosis, MRI adds little to the management of the condition. Two primary treatment concerns exist in osteonecrosis. First, the patient's clinical symptoms of pain and any associated functional limitations must be managed. Second, progression of the disease to subchondral collapse must be delayed or prevented whenever possible. Radiographs or computed tomography scans are both excellent modalities for the monitoring of bony collapse and progressive joint degeneration. They are also substantially cheaper than MRI.

Pearl: Insufficiency fractures of the knee can mimic the clinical and radiographic signs of secondary osteonecrosis.

Comment: Subchondral stress fractures of a femoral condyle sometimes present with pain and a lesion that suggests bone necrosis on plain films or MRI. Although the initial presentation can be similar to secondary osteonecrosis, this is a condition with a different etiology marked by the absence of true bone necrosis and a relatively benign course. Symptoms resolve in the majority of patients who are treated nonoperatively with protected weight bearing. Known as spontaneous osteonecrosis of the knee (SPONK), this condition is characterized by the sudden onset of pain in older individuals who do not have classic risk factors for secondary osteonecrosis (Zywiel et al. 2009). Radiographic imaging shows a single epiphyseal lesion in most cases.

Similar clinical scenarios have been reported in the femoral head (Legroux Gerot et al. 2004). Stress fractures of the femoral head have also been reported in younger patients who have experienced sudden, dramatic increases in physical activity levels (e.g., military conscripts) (Lee et al. 2009).

Pearl: The bone marrow edema syndrome is not true osteonecrosis and has a more benign course generally than osteonecrosis.

Comment: The bone marrow edema syndrome is a disorder distinct from secondary osteonecrosis. Intra-osseous edema occurs in both syndromes, but the elevated intra-osseous pressure in the bone marrow edema syndrome does not lead to bone death. Mild analgesia and protective weight bearing as required for pain is generally sufficient treatment, with edema and pain typically resolving within a few months of the onset of symptoms.

Pearl: Early, appropriate therapy is the key to achieving optimal clinical outcomes in osteonecrosis.

Comment: Treating osteonecrosis in early stages of the disease, before subchondral collapse, can result in good clinical outcomes. Nonoperative treatment does not prevent disease progression in most cases. One study demonstrated, for example, that nearly 80% of patients developed femoral head collapse within 4 years of their osteonecrosis diagnosis (Mont et al. 1996). A proposed treatment algorithm is shown in Fig. 48.3.

Core decompression is an excellent treatment option for osteonecrosis in which the femoral head has not collapsed. The contemporary percutaneous approach employs a small-diameter drilling technique through the skin (Figs. 48.4a–c).

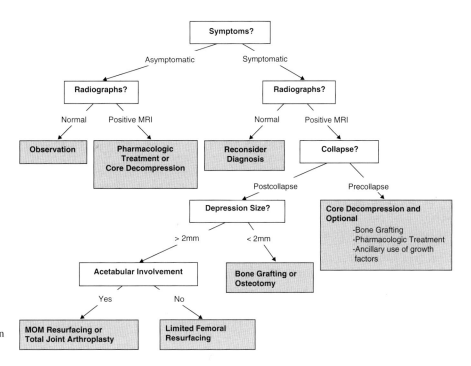

Fig. 48.3 Proposed treatment algorithm for secondary osteonecrosis (from Seyler et al. 2008). Reprinted with kind permission from Springer Science + Business Media

Fig. 48.4 Core decompression of the femoral head using modern percutaneous techniques (**a**) under fluoroscopic control (**b**) is a quick and relatively simple procedure than can be performed on an outpatient basis. The resulting skin wound (**c**); indicated by arrowhead can be closed with an adhesive bandage

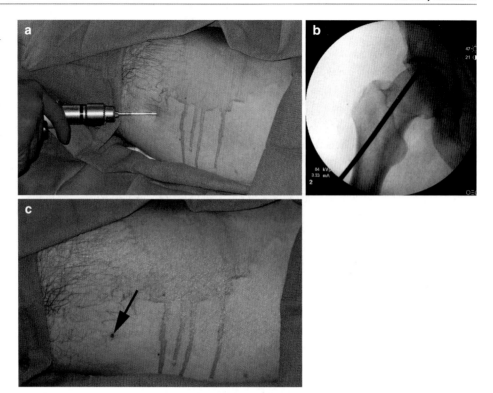

One study reported good clinical outcomes in three-fourths of patient who had a mean follow-up of 11 years (Mont et al. 1997). In contrast, patients who present with collapse of the femoral head invariably progress to total joint replacement.

Pearl: Core decompression is a minimally invasive procedure that can be performed on an outpatient basis.

Comment: Core decompression for osteonecrosis is not a completely risk-free procedure. It does carry the hazards of surgical anesthesia and the remote possibility of inducing joint damage. The early iterations of this technique involved significant surgical disruption of the bony architecture with a large-diameter trephine (Fig. 48.5). In contrast, modern core decompression is performed percutaneously using a small-diameter drill bit (usually 3.2 mm). The procedure requires only minutes to complete and is usually conducted in the outpatient setting. The wound is closed with a self-adhesive bandage, and patients can bear weight and ambulate as tolerated as soon as they have recuperated from the effects of the surgical anesthesia. Many patients report almost immediate pain reduction.

Myth: Core decompression should be attempted in all patients who have osteonecrosis.

Reality: Once osteonecrosis has progressed to the point of femoral head collapse, core decompression will not halt further disease progression. In addition, patients with very large lesions are at extremely high risk of subchondral collapse, regardless of therapy. The risks associated with core

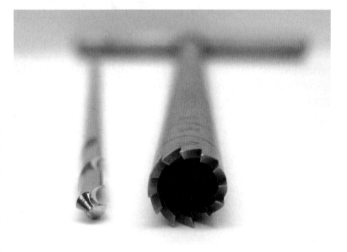

Fig. 48.5 Traditional core decompression used a 6–10-mm trephine (8 mm shown, *right*), removing more of the patient's bone than modern percutaneous techniques, which are often performed using a 3.2-mm drill bit (*left*)

decompression are small, but the absence of any potential benefit makes core decompression an inappropriate treatment choice for patients who have already suffered femoral head collapse or those with large lesions.

Myth: The cessation of glucocorticoid use is a necessary prerequisite for successful treatment of secondary osteonecrosis.

Reality: Glucocorticoid use is the strongest risk factor for osteonecrosis, but is neither a prerequisite for the condition

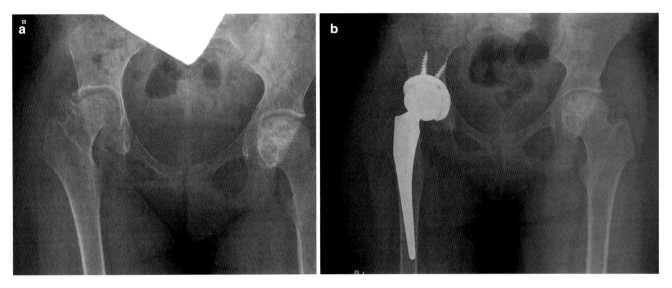

Fig. 48.6 Antero-posterior radiograph of stage IV osteonecrosis (**a**), with collapse of the femoral head, and degenerative changes of the acetabulum. This patient was treated with total hip arthroplasty (**b**)

nor an absolute impediment to the successful treatment of the problem. Tapering and even discontinuation of glucocorticoids are worthy goals (under most circumstances), but effective control of some disorders may require their continued use. Core decompression promotes healing of the necrotic lesion regardless of the patient's glucocorticoid dose.

Pearl: Patients with hip osteonecrosis who have degenerative changes in the acetabulum have only one treatment option: arthroplasty.

Comment: Degenerative changes in the acetabular surface in a patient who has osteonecrosis lead to joint destruction. They are therefore the acetabular equivalent of femoral head collapse. The only option for restoring the patient's joint function and mobility in this setting is total joint arthroplasty (Figs. 48.6a, b).

Pearl: Hip resurfacing is an effective intervention for treating femoral head collapse.

Comment: Secondary osteonecrosis tends to affect younger patients compared to spontaneous disease. Thus, joint arthroplasty for those who require it is usually performed at a relatively young age (e.g., 45 years of age (Johansson, Zywiel, Marker et al. unpublished data)). Many patients eventually require revision surgery – a more challenging procedure than the initial arthroplasty.

Hip resurfacing, a femoral bone-preserving hip arthroplasty technique, is particularly desirable in this setting. Hip resurfacing replaces only the affected portion of the femoral head and acetabulum, retaining as much of the patient's native bone stock as possible. The efficacy of hip resurfacing appears

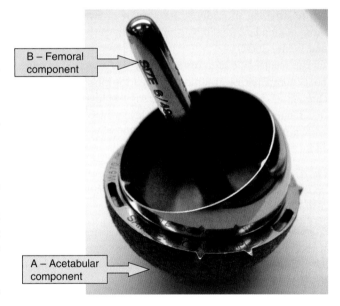

Fig. 48.7 Modern hip resurfacing implant, showing the metal-on-metal articulation of the acetabular (**a**) and femoral (**b**) components

comparable to that of total hip arthroplasty for both osteonecrosis and osteoarthritis (Mont et al. 2006; Revell et al. 2006)

Myth: Hip resurfacing is associated with high rates of implant failure.

Reality: Modern hip resurfacing implants combine a thin-shelled, cementless metal acetabular component that articulates directly with a large-diameter, stemmed, cemented metal bearing (Fig. 48.7). This technology is fundamentally

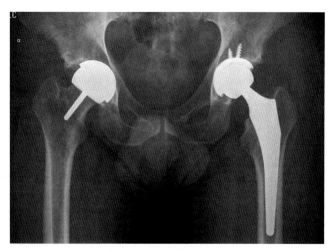

Fig. 48.8 Antero-posterior radiograph of a patient with total hip arthroplasty of the left side, which necessitated removal of significantly more of the patient's bone as compared to the total hip resurfacing of the right side

different from the older metal-on-polyethylene implants that were associated with high failure rates. Joint survival rates in hip resurfacing procedures are similar or even superior to those of standard total hip arthroplasty over 10 years (Buergi and Walter 2007).

Hip resurfacing requires markedly less resection of native bone compared to traditional hip arthroplasty procedures (Fig. 48.8). In addition, some data suggest higher postoperative range-of-motion and activity levels in patients treated with hip resurfacing (Pollard et al. 2006; Vail et al. 2006; Mont et al. 2009; Zywiel et al. 2009).

Pearl: Small, precollapse lesions have a good clinical prognosis. Large, postcollapse lesions are likely to require arthroplasty.

Comment: Several different staging and lesions sizing systems have been reported for describing osteonecrotic lesions. The clinically relevant radiographic factors are: (1) whether the lesions are pre or postcollapse and (2) their size. Regardless of what system is used, small precollapse lesions are amenable to nonoperative or joint-preserving surgical treatment and generally have good outcomes. In contrast, large postcollapse lesions almost always require one joint arthroplasty technique or another.

Myth: Secondary osteonecrosis is a predictor of poor outcomes in total hip arthroplasty.

Reality: Arthroplasty techniques for osteonecrosis have been associated historically with less favorable results compared to patients who underwent the procedure for osteoarthritis. More recent data indicate that the outcomes for these two groups are similar if modern implant designs and second-generation cementing techniques are employed.

Greater differences are observed among patients with different risk factors for osteonecrosis. Patients with sickle cell disease or end-stage renal disease appear to have higher rates of failure and revision compared to those without such risk factors (Johansson, Zywiel, Marker et al. Unpublished Data).

Pearl: Patients with multi-focal osteonecrosis that involves six or more joints are less likely to progress to articular surface collapse than are those with less widespread disease.

Comment: Secondary osteonecrosis presents with a wide range of clinical and functional severity. Some patients present with a single joint lesions that cause only mild discomfort and never experience another symptomatic disease recurrence. Others develop painful lesions that limit function profoundly in several large joints at once. Patients in the latter group undoubtedly experience more profound effects on their daily lives as a result of the disease, in the authors' experience such patients progress to joint collapse less frequently than patients who have less disseminated disease.

Pearl: Patients who have osteonecrosis can have a normal life.

Comment: For some patients, the diagnosis of secondary osteonecrosis represents the start of profound life changes, marking the beginning of a relentless process that progresses to pain and decreased function of large joints and requiring multiple primary and revision arthroplasties. However, the large majority of patients who have secondary osteonecrosis lead very normal lives. Modern joint-preserving surgical treatments such as core decompression have good long-term

Table 48.1 Spontaneous vs. secondary osteonecrosis

Characteristic	Spontaneous osteonecrosis	Secondary osteonecrosis
Age	55 and greater	Below 45
Gender	3:1 ♀:♂	♀:♂ with SLE as associated factor; ♂:♀ with alcohol as associated factor
Onset of pain	Sudden	Gradual
Bilaterality	<5%	>80%
Number of lesions	One	Multiple
Location on bone	Epiphysis	Epiphysis, metaphysis, and diaphysis
Number of joints involved	Single hip or knee joint	Can simultaneouly affect multiple knees, shoulders, ankles
Associated factors	None	Corticosteroids, alcohol, tobacco, other
Associated diseases	None	SLE, sickle cell, caisson disease, Gaucher's disease, thrombophilia, hypofibrinolysis
Pathology	Fibrotic bone, healing fracture	Necrotic bone

outcomes when used during early disease stages. Even patients who have late-stage disease of the hips or knees can expect excellent results with modern total joint arthroplasty techniques (Table 48.1).

References

Anonymous. Necrosis of the lower jaw in makers of Lucifer matches. Am J Dent Sci. 1867;1(series 3):96–7

Buergi ML, Walter WL. Hip resurfacing arthroplasty: the Australian experience. J Arthroplasty 2007;22(7 Suppl 3):61–5

Lee YK, Yoo JJ, Koo KH, et al Collapsed subchondral fatigue fracture of the femoral head. Orthop Clin N Am 2009;40:259–65

Legroux Gerot I, Demondion X, Louville AB, et al Subchondral fractures of the femoral head: a review of seven cases. Joint Bone Spine 2004;2(71):131–5

Seyler TM, Marker D, Mont MA. Osteonecrosis. In: Klippel JH, Stone JH, Crofford LJ, White PH, eds. Primer on the rheumatic diseases. 13th ed. New York: Springer Science+Business Media; 2008:565–572

Seyler TM, Marker D, Mont MA. Osteonecrosis. In: Primer on the Rheumatic Diseases. Klippel JH, Stone JH, Crofford LJ, White PH. Springer 2008

Marx RE. Pamidronate (Aredia) and zoledronate (Zometa) induced avascular necrosis of the jaws: a growing epidemic. J Oral Maxillofac Surg. 2003;9(61):1115–7

Mitchell MD, Kundel HL, Steinberg ME, et al Avascular necrosis of the hip: comparison of MR, CT, and scintigraphy. AJR Am J Roentgenol. 1986;1(147):67–71

Mont MA, Carbone JJ, Fairbank AC. Core decompression versus nonoperative management for osteonecrosis of the hip. Clin Orthop Relat Res. 1996;324:169–78

Mont MA, Marker DR, Smith JM, et al Resurfacing is comparable to total hip arthroplasty at short-term follow-up. Clin Orthop Relat Res. 2009;467:66–71

Mont MA, Seyler TM, Marker DR, et al Use of metal-on-metal total hip resurfacing for the treatment of osteonecrosis of the femoral head. J Bone Joint Surg Am. 2006;88(Suppl 3):90–7

Mont MA, Tomek IM, Hungerford DS. Core decompression for avascular necrosis of the distal femur: long term followup. Clin Orthop Relat Res. 1997;334:124–30

Mont MA, Ulrich SD, Seyler TM, et al Bone scanning of limited value for diagnosis of symptomatic oligofocal and multifocal osteonecrosis. J Rheumatol. 2008;8(35):1629–34

Pollard TC, Baker RP, Eastaugh-Waring SJ, Bannister GC. Treatment of the young active patient with osteoarthritis of the hip. A five- to seven-year comparison of hybrid total hip arthroplasty and metal-on-metal resurfacing. J Bone Joint Surg Br. 2006;5(88): 592–600

Revell MP, McBryde CW, Bhatnagar S, et al Metal-on-metal hip resurfacing in osteonecrosis of the femoral head. J Bone Joint Surg Am. 2006;88(Suppl 3):98–103

Vail TP, Mina CA, Yergler JD, Pietrobon R. Metal-on-metal hip resurfacing compares favorably with THA at 2 years followup. Clin Orthop Relat Res. 2006;453:123–31

Zywiel MG, McGrath MS, Seyler TM, et al Osteonecrosis of the knee: a review of three disorders. Orthop Clin North Am. 2009;40: 193–211

Zywiel MG, Marker DR, McGrath MS, Delanois RE, Mont MA. Resurfacing matched to standard total hip arthroplasty by preoperative activity levels - a comparison of postoperative outcomes. Bull NYU Hosp Jt Dis 2009;67(2):116–9

Index